Nuclear Medicine   THE REQUISITES

SERIES EDITOR **James H. Thrall,** MD
Radiologist-in-Chief,
Department of Radiology,
Massachusetts General Hospital,
Boston, Massachusetts

Nuclear Medicine

THE REQUISITES

JAMES H. THRALL, MD

Professor of Radiology,
Harvard Medical School;
Radiologist-in-Chief,
Department of Radiology,
Massachusetts General Hospital,
Boston, Massachusetts

HARVEY A. ZIESSMAN, MD

Professor of Radiology,
Director, Division of Nuclear Medicine,
Georgetown University Hospital,
Washington, D.C.

with 574 illustrations

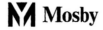 Mosby

St. Louis Baltimore Boston Chicago London Madrid Philadelphia Sydney Toronto

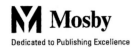
Mosby
Dedicated to Publishing Excellence

Publisher: George S. Stamathis
Editor: Susan Gay
Developmental Editor: Lynne Gery
Project Manager: Carol Sullivan Weis
Production Editor: Christine Carroll
Designer: Betty Schulz

Printed in the United States of America

Mosby-Year Book, Inc.
11830 Westline Industrial Drive
St. Louis, Missouri 63146

Editorial Production by V&M Graphics
Illustration Preparation by Color Associates, Inc.
Printing/Binding by Maple-Vail Book Manufacturing Group

Library of Congress Cataloging in Publication Data

Thrall, James H.
    Nuclear medicine : the requisites / James H. Thrall, Harvey A. Ziessman.
        p.   cm. — (Requisites series)
    Includes bibliographical references.
    ISBN 0-8016-6674-0
    1. Nuclear medicine.   I. Ziessman, Harvey A.   II. Title.   III. Series.
    [DNLM: 1. Radionuclide Imaging.   2. Diagnosis, Radioisotope.
    3. Nuclear Medicine.   WN 445 T529n 1994]
    R895. T498   1994
    616.07'575—dc20
    DNLM/DLC   94-27986
    for Library of Congress   CIP

        96   /   9   8   7   6   5   4   3

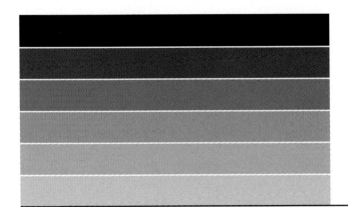

Preface

Nuclear Medicine: The Requisites is the fourth book in a series designed to provide core material in major subspecialty areas of radiology for use by residents during their initial training and for the practicing radiologist seeking a concise review.

The specialty of nuclear medicine is so dynamic that it is impossible to "capture" the entire subject in a textbook. Rather, in our book we have sought to provide a scope or span of information that can serve as an introductory knowledge base for the field.

In the basic science chapters, we have sought to present concepts of physics, instrumentation, and radiopharmacy in the context of clinical nuclear medicine. Where appropriate, we have illustrated or reinforced basic concepts with examples from the practice of nuclear medicine that the resident or practicing radiologist will actually encounter. We hope that this linkage will help "demystify" some of the basic science aspects of nuclear medicine.

The unifying theme in the clinically oriented chapters is the establishment of a logical progression from basic principles to clinical applications. We have tried to stress tracer mechanisms in detail, aiming to provide deductive tools for the analysis of images rather than simply presenting representative illustrations. Scintigraphic patterns represent the convolution of disease pathophysiology with tracer pharmacokinetics. Because no textbook or atlas can present every possible scintigraphic pattern, an understanding of these fundamental principles that underlie the creation of scintigraphic images permits diagnostic inference and the ability to tackle previously unencountered problems.

Another feature of this book is the inclusion of image acquisition protocols for the major procedures. We recognize that each nuclear medicine laboratory must develop its own protocols based on available equipment and other individual considerations. There is probably no single, "correct" way to perform any nuclear medicine procedure. This is particularly true for single photon emission tomography in which observer preference varies widely among physicians and the potential variation in study parameters for different acquisition sequences and processing algorithms are infinite. The included protocols have all been successfully used in our practices and can be taken as "points of departure" for thinking about study acquisition and postprocessing.

One of the novel features of this book is our chapter entitled "Pearls, Pitfalls and Frequently Asked Questions." Textbooks can be very dry, and readers may not recognize the importance of a particular point in a traditional didactic presentation. This chapter is designed to have a little fun for the purpose of reemphasizing and highlighting some of the material presented in previous chapters. We hope you enjoy the chapter.

In keeping with the philosophy of the *Requisites in Radiology* series, we hope that residents will find our book useful in rapidly acquiring a working knowledge of nuclear medicine that will make their initial clinical experiences more meaningful and from which they can continue to build throughout their careers.

James H. Thrall
Harvey A. Ziessman

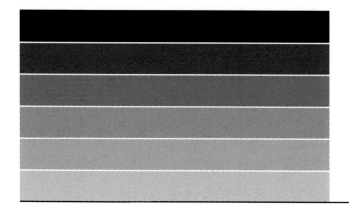

Acknowledgments

We would like to acknowledge the help and support that we have received in preparing *Nuclear Medicine: The Requisites* from colleagues across the country.

Original illustrations and artwork were beautifully done by David M. Klemm and computer graphics by John R. Vaillant, both in Educational Media at Georgetown University Medical Center. Computer graphics and drawings were also done by Nancy Speroni, Director of the Radiology Photography Laboratory at the Massachusetts General Hospital. Illustrations were contributed by many colleagues, including Patrice K. Rehm, M.D., Vijay Varma, M.D., Patrick J. Peller, M.D., Ernest Campanovo, M.D., Douglas F. Eggli, M.D., Kenneth Levin, M.D., Eric Geslein, M.D., David Parker, M.D., Manuel L. Brown, M.D., Kenneth McKusick, M.D., William Strauss, M.D., Tsunehiro Yasuda, M.D., and Merrill Johnson, M.D. Help with special illustrations was also provided by John Hergenrother, Frank Maltais, Avis Loring, and Donna Scannell. Doreen Flynn did an excellent job preparing manuscripts, and she was very patient despite innumerable changes.

Appreciation goes to Frank Atkins, Ph.D., Scott Williams, M.D., Patrice K. Rehm, M.D., Loren Niklason, Ph.D., Ron Callahan, Ph.D., and Steve Dragotakes, M.S., who were kind enough to review chapters and give valuable constructive criticism.

Thanks must also go to all our past residents and students; they were also our teachers and the inspiration for this book.

J.H.T. and H.A.Z.

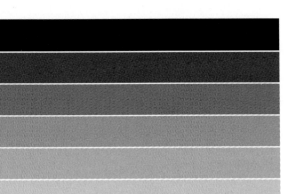

Contents

BASIC PRINCIPLES

Basic Physics for Nuclear Medicine

Medical imaging is based on the interaction of energy with biological tissues. The kind of diagnostic information available in each modality is determined by the nature of these interactions. In conventional x-ray imaging, the differential absorption of x-rays in air, water, fat, and bone allows the distinction of these tissues in the image. In ultrasonography, the differing reflective properties of tissues are the basis for creating images. In magnetic resonance imaging the differences in hydrogen content and in the chemical and physical environments of hydrogen nuclei provide the basis for distinguishing tissues.

In nuclear medicine, the body is imaged "from the inside out." Radiotracers, often in the form of complex radiopharmaceuticals, are administered internally. Diagnostic inference is gained by recording the distribution of the radioactive material in both time and space. Tracer pharmacokinetics and selective tissue uptake form the basis of diagnostic utility. To understand nuclear imaging procedures, it is necessary to understand a sequence of concepts, beginning with the physics of radioactivity and continuing through the process of detecting radiation, the selection of appropriate radiopharmaceuticals, and then the understanding of the uptake and distribution of those pharmaceuticals in health and disease.

ATOMS AND THE STRUCTURE OF MATTER

Atoms are the building blocks of molecules and are the smallest structures that represent the physical and chemical properties of the elements. Each atom consists of a nucleus surrounded by orbiting electrons (Figure 1-1). The nuclei are composed of protons and neutrons collectively referred to as *nucleons*. *Proton*s are positively charged particles, weighing approximately 1.67×10^{-24} grams. Their positive charge is equal in magnitude and opposite to the charge of an electron (Box 1-1). The element the atom belongs to is determined by the number of protons in the nucleus. Neutrons are slightly heavier than protons and are electrically neutral, as the name implies.

By convention, a shorthand notation has been developed to uniquely describe or define specific atoms. The notation is as follows:

$$^A_Z X_N$$

[handwritten annotation: nucleon = proton or neutron]

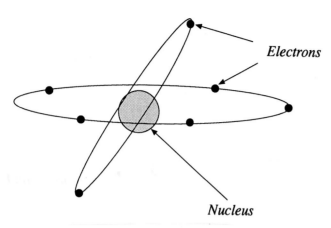

Electrons

Nucleus

Fig. 1-1   Schematic of the Bohr model of the atom. The nucleus contains protons and neutrons and has a radius of 10^{-14} m. The protons in the nucleus carry a positive charge. The orbital electrons carry a negative charge.

Z = atomic # = # protons

Box 1-1   Summary of Physical Constants

Speed of light in a vacuum (c)	3.0×10^8 m/sec
Elementary charge (e)	4.803×10^{-10} esu
	1.602×10^{-19} coulomb
Rest mass of electron	9.11×10^{-28} g
Rest mass of proton	1.67×10^{-24} g
Planck's constant (*h*)	6.63×10^{-27} erg sec
Avogadro's number	$6.02 \times 10^{23} \dfrac{\text{molecules}}{\text{gram mole}}$
1 electron volt (eV)	$1,602 \times 10^{-12}$ erg
1 calorie (cal)	4.18×10^7 erg
1 angstrom (Å)	10^{-10} m
Euler's number (*e*)	2.718

where X is the symbol for the element, Z is the number of protons, N is the number of neutrons, and A is the total number of neutrons and protons. Z is also referred to as the *atomic number* and A as the *mass number* or *atomic mass number*. A *nuclide* is an atom with a given number of neutrons and protons. A *radionuclide* is simply an unstable nuclide or nuclear species that undergoes radioactive decay.

Several terms help define special relationships between different nuclides. The term *isotope* is used to denote nuclides with the same number of protons (Z), that is, the same element but different numbers of neutrons (N). For example, there are more than 20 isotopes of the element iodine. All except one (I-127) are radioisotopes or radionuclides, and several are of medical interest, including I-123, I-125, and I-131, which have the following notation:

$$^{123}_{53}\text{I}_{70} \qquad ^{125}_{53}\text{I}_{72} \qquad ^{131}_{53}\text{I}_{78}$$

Other special terms that are used are *isobar* to indicate the same A but different N and Z, *isotone* to indicate the same number of N but different Z and A, and *isomer* to indicate different *energy states* in nuclides with identical A, Z, and N. The most important isomers in nuclear medicine are technetium-99 and technetium-99m, where the *m* denotes a *metastable* or prolonged intermediate state in the decay of molybdenum-99 to technetium-99.

Bohr Model of the Atom

In the classic Bohr model of the atom, electrons are arranged in well-defined orbits around the nucleus (Figure 1-1). The number of orbital electrons in each atom equals the atomic number, Z (the number of pro-

tons in the nucleus). The closest orbit is referred to as the K shell, followed by the L, M, and N shells, and so forth. The maximum number of electrons in the K shell is 2, in the L shell it is 8, in the M shell it is 18, and in the N shell it is 32, except no more than 8 electrons can be in the outermost shell of an atom. Figure 1-2 illustrates a simplified schematic of the Bohr model for potassium. The term *valence electron* is used to designate electrons in the outermost shell (Box 1-2). These electrons are important in defining the chemical properties of elements. For example, atoms with the outermost shell maximally filled are chemically unreactive. These are the inert gases, helium, neon, argon, krypton, xenon, and radon.

Electrons have a negative charge equal to 1.6×10^{-19} coulomb; as previously noted, protons have a positive charge of equal magnitude. Electrons are bound in their orbits by the electrical force between their negative charge and the positive charge of the nucleus. The highest binding energy is in the electrons in the shell closest to the nucleus (the K shell), with progressively lower binding energies in the more distant shells. To remove an electron from its shell, the binding energy must be overcome. Interactions involving orbital electrons and ionizing electromagnetic radiation (x-rays and gamma rays) are central to the way medical images are made and to the quality of the images

It has long been recognized that the Bohr Model of the atom is too simplistic to accurately portray many atomic phenomena. Very sophisticated wave-mechanical or quantum mechanical models have been developed by nuclear physicists. In these models, probability density functions are used to describe spatial and temporal properties of electrons. However, the Bohr model can still be used to describe the basic interactions of interest in nuclear medicine.

Box 1-2 Terms Used to Describe Electrons

TERM	DEFINITION
Electron	Basic elementary particle
Orbital electron	Electron in one of the shells or orbits of an atom
Valence electron	Electron in the outermost shell of an atom; responsible for chemical characteristics and reactivity
Auger electron	Electron ejected from an atomic orbit by energy released during an electron transition
Photoelectron	Electron ejected from an atomic orbit as a consequence of an interaction with a photon (photoelectric interaction) and complete absorption of the photon's energy
Conversion electron	Electron ejected from an atomic orbit because of *internal conversion* phenomenon as energy is given off by an unstable nucleus

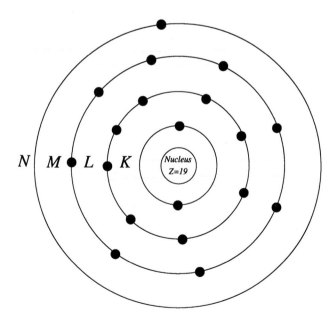

Fig. 1-2 Schematic diagram of the potassium atom. Potassium has an anatomic number of 19, with 19 protons in the nucleus and 19 orbital electrons.

Characteristic Radiation

When an orbital electron is removed from its shell, there is a vacancy that is rapidly filled by an electron from a shell farther from the nucleus. In this process the "cascading" electron gives up energy as it fills the vacancy and becomes more tightly bound. Most often the energy is emitted in the form of electromagnetic radiation, also referred to as a *photon.* The unit of energy used to describe these radiations is the *electron volt* (one electron volt is defined as the kinetic energy of an electron accelerated through a potential difference of 1.0 volt. One electron volt = 1.6×10^{-19} joule or 1.6×10^{-12} erg.)

Photons with energy greater than 100 eV are classified as x-rays. Lower energy photons may be in the range of ultraviolet or visible light. The electromagnetic radiations that arise in the process of filling a vacancy are called *characteristic radiations* or *characteristic x-rays* where applicable because their energy is uniquely defined by the difference in the binding energy of the donor shell and the shell where the vacancy is being filled (that is, the x-ray energy is "characteristic" of the respective transition). In some applications of radionuclides, detection of characteristic x-rays is the primary means of forming the image or measuring the amount of radioactivity.

An alternative process to the emission of characteristic radiation is the ejection of another electron by the energy released in filling a vacancy. An electron ejected in this way is termed an *Auger electron* (Box 1-2).

RELATIONSHIP OF MASS AND ENERGY

In 1905, Albert Einstein published his famous equation, $E = mc^2$, where E is energy in ergs, m is mass in grams, and c is the velocity of light in a vacuum (3×10^{10} cm/sec). From this equation it is possible to calculate the energy equivalent of the various subatomic particles. By definition the unified or universal *atomic mass unit* (U) is equal to $\frac{1}{12}$th the mass of a carbon-12 atom. One U = 1.66×10^{-24} gram. Using this value for mass in Einstein's equation yields the following result:

$$E = (1.66 \times 10^{-24} \text{g/U}) \times (3.0 \times 10^{10} \text{cm/sec})^2$$
$$E = 1.5 \times 10^{-3} \text{erg/U}$$
$$(1 \text{ erg} = 1 \text{gcm}^2/\text{sec}^2)$$

Inserting the conversion factor between ergs and electron volts (Box 1-1) yields the relationship, 1 U = 931.5 MeV. Table 1-1 provides the mass and energy relationships for the basic subatomic particles. The most important of these relationships in clinical nuclear medicine is the energy equivalence of an electron, which is 511 keV.

Table 1-1 Mass-Energy Equivalence for Atomic Particles

Particle	Mass (U)	Energy (MeV)
Electron	5.486×10^{-4}	0.511
Proton	1.0073	938.20
Neutron	1.0087	939.5

[handwritten annotations: "= 1 b/c C_{12}", "= 6p + 6n", "= 12 Amu (u)", "$U = \frac{1}{12}$ mass of C_{12}"]

The relationships between mass and energy are of fundamental importance in nuclear physics. By carefully determining the weight of atomic nuclei, physicists have shown that the theoretical sum of the component nucleons is always greater than the actual observed mass of the respective atomic nuclei. The difference is known as the *mass deficit*. The *nuclear binding energy* is defined as the energy equivalent of the mass deficit.

Energy equal to the difference in nuclear binding energy of the pre- and post-transformation nuclei is released in atomic fusion and atomic fission. The energy of hydrogen and atomic bombs comes from energy released when trillions of new atomic nuclei are formed. This implies that the aggregate mass deficit with the post-transformation nuclei after a fusion or fission reaction is greater than that of the original nuclei.

The concept of mass deficit is also fundamental to the use of radionuclides in medical imaging. As a more stable atomic configuration is formed in the radioactive decay process, the mass deficit always increases. In many radio nuclide decay schemes, part of the mass deficit is given off in the form of energetic electromagnetic radiation (photons) that can be detected and used to form medical images.

RADIONUCLIDES AND THEIR RADIATIONS

Because of their physical properties, certain nuclides are unstable and undergo radioactive decay. For each radionuclide the type of radiation emitted, the energy of the radiation(s), and the half-life of the decay process are physical constants. These parameters are important in determining the suitability of a given radionuclide for medical use. The daughter product in radioactive decay is always at a lower energy state than the parent. The energy difference between parent and daughter is equal to the energy embodied in the radiations given off. The types of radiation important in nuclear medicine are gamma rays, characteristic x-rays, negatrons (beta$^-$ particles), positrons (beta$^+$ particles), and alpha particles. (By definition the term *gamma ray* is used for photons originating in the nucleus and *x-ray* for photons originating outside the nucleus.)

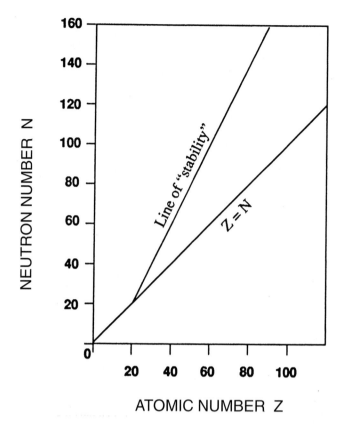

Fig. 1-3 Graphical representation of the ratio of neutrons to protons. For low atomic number elements the two are roughly equal (Z = N). As the atomic number increases the relative number of neutrons increases. Stable nuclear species tend to occur along the line of "stability."

Among the lighter atomic elements the number of protons and neutrons in the nucleus are roughly equal. As the atomic number (Z) increases, the ratio of neutrons to protons in stable nuclei increases. A plot of this ratio versus atomic number defines an empirical "line of stability" (Figure 1-3). That is, the "N/P" ratio is greater than 1 for stable nuclei in the middle and upper atomic numbers. This observation is important in predicting the mode of radioactive decay of unstable nuclides. In general, the decay process tends to return the daughter nucleus closer to the "line of stability." That is, if an unstable nucleus contains more neutrons than do stable isotopes of the same element, the mode of decay will reduce the N/P ratio, and vice versa for nuclei with fewer neutrons than predicted by the line of stability.

Alpha Decay

Alpha particles are essentially helium nuclei with a +2 charge and an atomic mass number of 4. Alpha decay is common in the higher atomic number range of the periodic table of elements. For example, radium-226 decays

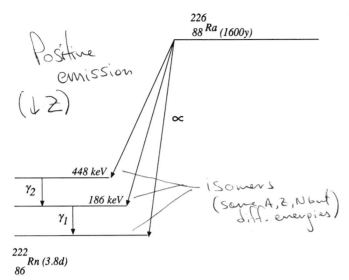

Positive emission (↓Z)

isomers (same A, Z, N but diff. energies)

Fig. 1-4   Simplified decay scheme for radium-226. Decay is by alpha particle emission to the daughter product, radon-222. The emission of an alpha particle results in a decrease in atomic number of 2 and a decrease in atomic mass of 4.

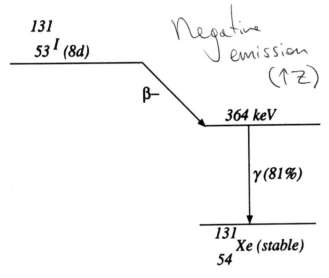

Negative emission (↑Z)

Fig. 1-5   Simplified decay scheme for iodine-131. Decay is by negatron emission. In negatron or beta minus decay the atomic mass does not change (isobaric transition). The atomic mass number increases by 1. The daughter, xenon-131, has one more proton in the nucleus.

to radon-222 by emitting an alpha particle (Figure 1-4).

A system of schematic diagrams has been developed to graphically illustrate radioactive decay schemes. Positive emissions (alpha particles and positrons) and electron capture result in the daughter nucleus having a lower atomic number. This is indicated by an arrow pointing down and to the left (Figure 1-4). Following negative emissions (beta⁻, negatron), the daughter nucleus has a higher atomic number, which is indicated

by an arrow pointing down and to the right (Figure 1-5).

Complete decay schemes can be very complex, with multiple pathways from parent to daughter. For practical purposes the decay schemes in this book are simplified to illustrate important general principles and specific aspects relevant to clinical nuclear medicine.

In the simplified scheme shown for Ra-226, three different alpha particles are shown (see Figure 1-4). One reaches the ground state of Rn-222 directly. The other two result in an excited state of Rn-222 with subsequent gamma ray emission to reach the ground state. (In the complete decay scheme for Ra-226 there are additional alpha particles, but they occur in low abundance.)

In all radioactive decay processes there is conservation of mass and energy. The *transition energy* is the total energy released during the decay process. For alpha decay, this energy is in the form of the kinetic energy of the alpha particle and energy released in the form of gamma radiation.

Alpha particles are undesirable in diagnostic applications because they result in high radiation to the patient. No currently used diagnostic radiopharmaceuticals include alpha-emitting radionuclides. On the other hand, a number of therapeutic agents have been designed to incorporate alpha particle emitters.

Negatron Decay   *n → p + e⁻ + antineutrino*

The negatron decay process involves the conversion of a neutron into a proton, an electron, and an antineutrino. The electron is ejected from the atomic nucleus, thereby giving the decay process its name. The term *negatron* is used to distinguish negative electrons from positive electrons, or *positrons*. Negatron decay is also called *beta decay* or *beta⁻ decay*.

The N/P ratio decreases as a result of negatron decay, and one would predict that this mode of decay occurs in neutron-rich nuclei. That is, it occurs in nuclei with more neutrons than stable species in the respective part of the atomic chart. For example, stable iodine has a mass number of 127 (53 protons, 74 neutrons). By comparison, I-131 has 78 neutrons. This is a higher number than stable iodine, and I-131 undergoes beta⁻ decay (see Figure 1-5).

The transition energy in negatron decay is given off in the form of kinetic energy of the beta particle, the energy in the antineutrino, and the energy in any associated gamma radiation. The maximum kinetic energy (E_{max}) that a beta particle can have is a physical constant of the decay process. Beta particles are emitted with a continuous spectrum of energies lower than the maximum. The mean kinetic energy of beta particles is approximately one-third of the maximum. For beta particles with less than the maximum kinetic energy, the energy is shared between the beta particle and the antineutrino.

Energy of $E_{max} = \beta^- +$ antineutrino energies

It must be stressed again that a decay scheme can have more than one pathway from the parent to the daughter. For many radionuclides decaying by negatron decay, beta particles with different maximum kinetic energies are given off. Because the total transition energy must be the same for each pathway, the energy of associated gamma radiation is also correspondingly different. For example, the decay scheme for I-131 presented in Figure 1-5 illustrates only one pathway from parent to daughter, the one of most interest and importance in clinical practice. In reality, there are beta particles given off with six different energies and there are 19 different gamma rays. However, the most abundant gamma ray occurs in 81% of transitions and has an energy of 364 keV.

A number of beta-emitting radionuclides have been used in clinical nuclear medicine. Iodine-131, the first radionuclide of importance in medicine, is still used in current practice. The disadvantage of beta emitters is the high radiation dose received by the patient from the beta particles. For radioiodine-131 this disadvantage becomes an advantage when the radionuclide is used in the therapy of thyroid cancer and hyperthyroidism.

Positron Decay and Electron Capture

As the name implies, in *positron decay* a positive electron or positively charged beta particle is ejected from the nucleus. This results in a decrease in the atomic number between the parent and the daughter nuclei and an increase in the N/P ratio. Positron decay occurs in nuclides that are neutron poor, with N/P ratios lower than those occurring on the line of stability. Positron decay is illustrated in Figure 1-6 for fluorine-18. The transition energy is embodied in the kinetic energy of the positrons and any associated gamma rays. For positrons given off with less than maximum kinetic energy, the energy difference is embodied in neutrinos. In both negatron and positron decay the neutrinos (or antineutrinos) carry away a substantial portion of the transition energy. The likelihood of neutrinos reacting in soft tissue is small, and the energy in neutrinos is not important in calculating radiation dosimetry for clinical applications.

The minimum transition energy required for positron decay is 1.02 MeV, which is the energy equivalent of the mass of two electrons. In unstable nuclei where the maximum available transition energy is less than 1.02 MeV, decay of neutron-poor radionuclides is by electron capture (Figure 1-7). In *electron capture* an electron from one of the orbital shells (typically close to the nucleus) is incorporated into the nucleus, converting a proton into a neutron. The captured electron is usually from the K shell. The resulting vacancy is filled by transition of an electron from a shell farther from the nucleus. The energy released from this electron transition appears either as characteristic x-radia-

$$\beta \rightarrow n + \beta^+ + neutrino$$

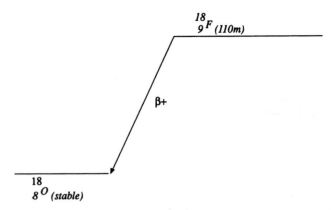

Fig. 1-6 Simplified schematic of the decay of fluorine-18 by positron emission. The daughter product, oxygen-18, has one less proton in the nucleus. Positron decay is another example of an isobaric transition without change in atomic mass number between parent and daughter.

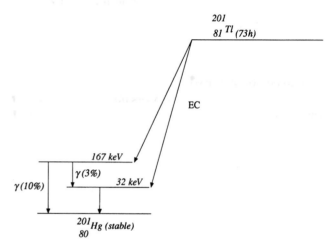

Fig. 1-7 Schematic of thallium-201 decay by electron capture to mercury-201. The daughter nucleus has one less proton than the parent.

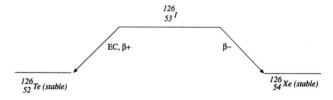

Fig. 1-8 Iodine-126 undergoes decay through multiple processes. The diagram indicates decay by electron capture and by the emission of both positrons and negatrons.

tion or as the kinetic energy of an Auger electron.

Some radionuclides decay by multiple modes, including electron capture, positron decay, and negatron decay (Figure 1-8). The likelihood of electron capture increases as the available transition energy decreases. The probability of electron capture also increases with increasing atomic number.

Isomeric Transition and Internal Conversion

No radionuclide undergoes true radioactive decay just by the emission of gamma radiation. However, in some decay schemes there are intermediate species with measurable half-lives that exist in a *metastable* state. The concept of metastability is arbitrary. Most gamma rays are emitted almost immediately ($<10^{-12}$ seconds) after the primary decay process, whether it be alpha decay, negatron decay, positron decay, or electron capture. When the intermediate excited state lasts longer than 10^{-9} seconds, the term *metastable* is used and an *m* is placed after the mass number to indicate the phenomenon. The transition from the metastable state to the ground state is *isomeric* because there is no change in atomic number.

The most important example of a metastable state in nuclear medicine practice is technetium-99m, which occurs in the decay of molybdenum-99 to technetium-99 (Figures 1-9, 1-10). The metastable state for Tc-99m has a half-life of 6 hours; this allows time for the separation of the metastable species from the parent radionuclide. Tc-99m is very attractive from a radiation safety or health physics standpoint because it is essentially a pure gamma emitter not associated with primary particulate radia-

tions. Its use as a radiolabel is associated with favorably low radiation dosimetry.

The energy released in isomeric transitions may be used to dislodge an orbital electron instead of being emit-

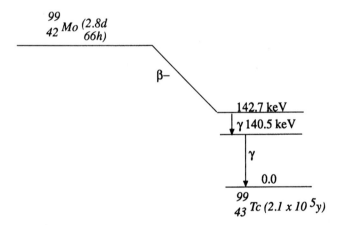

Fig. 1-9   Simplified schematic of the decay of molybdenum-99 by negatron emission to technetium-99.

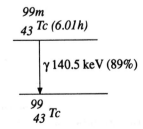

Fig. 1-10   Diagram illustrating the isomeric transition of technetium-99m to technetium-99.

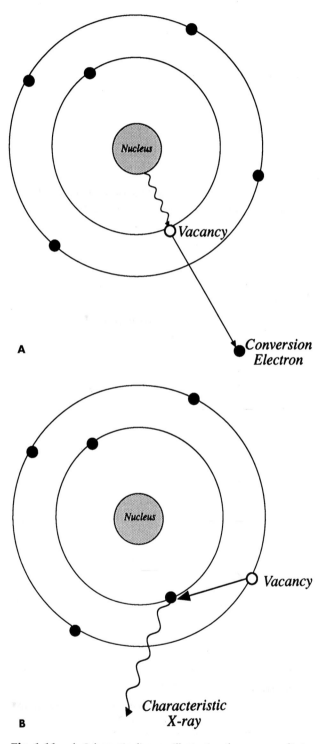

Fig. 1-11   **A,** Schematic diagram illustrating the process of internal conversion. Instead of the emission of a gamma ray, an orbital electron is ejected from its shell. **B,** A characteristic x-ray is then given off as a consequence of the electron vacancy being filled.

ted as a gamma ray. This process is called *internal conversion* (Figure 1-11). The kinetic energy of the electron (conversion electron) is equal to the difference between the gamma ray energy and the binding energy of the electron. The internal conversion process reduces the number of usable, detectable gamma photons for imaging. It also results in a higher radiation dose to the patient because the conversion electron is absorbed in tissue close to its site of origin. In the "decay" of Tc-99m a 140 keV gamma ray is given off 89% of the time, and internal conversion accounts for most of the remaining transitions.

Gamma Ray Emission

As discussed above, many radioactive decay processes result in the release of gamma rays or gamma photons. These are ionizing electromagnetic radiations that originate in the excited, unstable atomic nucleus. They have discrete energies defined by the decay scheme for the respective radionuclide. Gamma rays occur over a wide range of energies. Those most useful in conventional nuclear medicine have energies between approximately 80 keV and 400 keV. Modern nuclear medicine imaging equipment has been optimized for this energy range. Photons with energies below 80 keV present difficulties because of their relatively high attenuation in tissue and their scattering properties. Also, they are less reliably localized by standard imaging devices because of the smaller amount of total energy available in the detection process. Gamma rays with energies significantly higher than 400 keV are progressively more difficult to image. The detection efficiency in widely used detector systems is less at higher energies. Spatial resolution is also lost through difficulty in collimating high-energy photons.

Mathematics of electromagnetic radiation The relationship between the energy of gamma rays (or other electromagnetic radiations) and their frequencies is given by the following equation:

$$E = h\nu,$$

where ν is the frequency and h is Planck's constant (Box 1-1).

Electromagnetic radiation travels with the speed of light (c). The relationship between frequency and wavelength is given by:

$$c = \nu\lambda,$$

where λ is the wavelength. Rearranging this equation to solve for ν and substituting it into the previous equation yields:

$$E = \frac{hc}{\lambda}$$

Taking wavelength in angstroms (Å) and energy in keV, this becomes:

$$E(\text{keV}) = \frac{12.4}{\lambda(\text{Å})}$$

TERMINOLOGY, UNITS, AND MATHEMATICS OF RADIOACTIVE DECAY

Units of Radioactivity

Two systems for expressing decay or disintegration rates are in widespread use and are potentially confusing. The more widely used system historically was based on the *curie*. This unit was based on the disintegration rate of 1 gram of radium and was defined as 3.7×10^{10} disintegrations per second (dps). It is now known that the disintegration rate of 1 gram of radium is slightly different than 1 curie, but the quantitative definition has been widely used throughout the world. Most medical diagnostic applications involve amounts of radioactivity in the microcurie (3.7×10^4 dps) or millicurie (3.7×10^7 dps) range.

An alternative to the curie in the international system of units is the becquerel (Bq), which is equal to 1 disintegration per second. The relationship between the curie and the becquerel is straightforward if somewhat confusing to those used to the older term. One millicurie equals 37,000,000 Bq, or 37 MBq. Both terminology systems are used widely in the literature both in the United States and internationally (Table 1-2).

Half-life and Decay Constant

The mathematics of radioactive decay follow from direct physical measurements. The fundamental empirical observation determined early in the history of work with radionuclides is that the number of atoms undergoing decay during any finite period of time is proportional

Table 1-2   Conversion from CGS to SI Units

	CGS Unit	SI Unit	Conversion Factor
Work	erg	joule (J)	10^7
Radioactivity	curie (Ci)	becquerel (Bq)	3.7×10^{10}
Radiation absorbed dose	rad	gray (Gy)	100
Radiation exposure	roentgen (R)	coulomb/kg	2.58×10^{-4}
Dose equivalent man	rem	sievert (Sv)	100

to the number of radioactive atoms in the sample. This can be written as

$$\frac{-dN_t}{dt} \, \alpha N_t \, ,$$

where N_t is the number of radioactive atoms in the sample at time t. The term dN_t/dt is mathematical notation expressing the change in the number of radioactive atoms over a short interval of time. The negative sign in the equation denotes that the number of radioactive atoms decreases over time.

For any given radioactive species the equation may be rewritten as:

$$\frac{-dN_t}{dt} = \lambda N_t \, .$$

The term λ is the constant of proportionality and is a mathematical constant for each radionuclide. It is also called the *decay constant* and has units of 1/time.

The last equation can be rearranged and integrated and provides the classic equation:

$$N_t = N_0 e^{-\lambda t}.$$

The term N_0 represents the number of radioactive atoms at time $t = 0$, and e is Euler's number (Box 1-1). The equation says in words that the number of radioactive atoms at any later point in time is equal to the product of the original number times an exponential factor that takes into account the rate of decay and the length of time after the initial measurement. Because the activity of the sample is proportional to the number of atoms in that sample, the equation can be rewritten as:

$$A_t = A_0 e^{-\lambda t},$$

where A indicates activity in either curies or becquerels. The decay curve plotted on standard coordinates with time on the x-axis and activity on the y-axis for a radioactive sample shows an exponentially decreasing function that approaches but never reaches zero. On semilog graph paper the function is a straight line.

From these fundamental equations it is possible to derive the concept of physical half-life, which turns out to be a more intuitive and useful way of describing radioactive decay than using the decay constant. The *half-life* is simply defined as the time required for the number of radioactive atoms in a sample to decrease by exactly one half or 50%. Mathematically the value of the half-life can be derived from the above equations by substituting $\frac{N_0}{2}$ and $T_{1/2}$ on the two sides respectively as follows:

$$\frac{N_0}{2} = N_0 e^{-\lambda T_{1/2}}$$

$$\frac{1}{2} = e^{-\lambda T_{1/2}}$$

Because $e^{-0.693} = \frac{1}{2}$, this equation can be simplified to yield:

$$\lambda T_{1/2} = 0.693$$

$$T_{1/2} = \frac{0.693}{\lambda}$$

From these equations it is apparent that the decay constant and the physical half-life have reciprocal units of time. The half-life can be expressed in seconds, minutes, hours, days, or years. Radionuclides with long physical half-lives have smaller values for the decay constant. That is, a lower fraction of the radioactive atoms undergo disintegration in any given unit of time the longer the physical half-life. From a practical standpoint, most radionuclides used in clinical nuclear medicine must have half-lives of hours or days. This permits shipping from the manufacturing site to the hospital, preparation of the radiopharmaceutical, and imaging. Use of shorter-lived agents is feasible in institutions with radionuclide production facilities such as cyclotrons or special accelerators.

In certain cases radionuclides are obtained from "generator" systems, and the practical limitation is then the half-life of the parent compound. For example, the half-life of Tc-99m is 6 hours. The half-life of its parent, molybdenum-99, is 2.7 days (Figures 1-9, 1-10). The Mo-99/Tc-99m generator system provides the dual advantage of a longer-lived parent, which permits commercial distribution and prolonged on-site availability, while the short half-life of the Tc-99m daughter reduces radiation exposure to the patient compared to longer-lived agents.

Mean Life

The concept of the mean life of a radionuclide is useful in thinking about radiation dosimetry. The mean life is given as:

$$\bar{t} = \frac{1}{\lambda}$$

or,

$$\bar{t} = 1.44 T_{1/2}$$

The concept of mean life is more difficult to understand intuitively than the concept of physical half-life but may be thought of as the average length of time of the radioactive atoms in a sample before they undergo disintegration. Another way of thinking about it is to imagine extrapolating the decay curve to infinity. The mean life is the point on the time axis where half the area under the curve is on each side.

Biological Half-life and Effective Half-life

An important concept in determining radiation exposure to patients is the *biological half-life* and the corollary concept, *effective half-life*. The term *biological half-life* is used to describe the biological clearance of the radionuclide from a particular tissue or organ system. Thus, the actual half-life or *effective half-life* of a radiopharmaceutical in a biological system is dependent on both the physical half-life and the biological clearance. Because physical decay and biological clearance occur simultaneously in parallel, the relationship between them and the effective half-life is given by:

$$\frac{1}{T_{1/2eff}} = \frac{1}{T_{1/2p}} + \frac{1}{T_{1/2b}}$$

Rearranging terms, this becomes:

$$T_{1/2eff} = \frac{T_{1/2b} \times T_{1/2p}}{T_{1/2b} + T_{1/2p}}$$

The concept of biological half-life is not as mathematically clear-cut as the physical half-life. It can vary between subjects and does not necessarily follow a regular exponential process. For example, the biological half-time of radioactivity in the bladder is determined by the time at which a patient chooses to void. The half-time of xenon-133 in the lung during pulmonary ventilation studies is determined by the rate and depth of respiration, as well as by the presence of pulmonary disease. Nonetheless, the term biological half-life is useful in thinking about the amount of exposure the patient actually receives during a nuclear medicine procedure.

INTERACTIONS OF RADIATION WITH MATTER

Negatrons (Beta Particles)

Negatrons or beta particles cause ionization in tissues by electrostatic interactions with orbital electrons. They give up energy through a series of such interactions along a tortuous path. As a rule of thumb, the maximum penetration of beta particles in soft tissue in centimeters is equal to the maximum kinetic energy of the negatron in MeV divided by 2. Thus, the radiation dose delivered by negatrons in soft tissue is relatively close to their source. For example, the maximum kinetic energy of the most abundant beta particle in the decay of I-131 is .606 MeV. The majority of the radiation dose delivered in I-131 therapy is within 0.3 cm of the location of the nucleus undergoing decay.

Positrons

Positrons also give up their kinetic energy through electrostatic ionizations. As the positron approaches thermal energy it undergoes *annihilation* by combining with a negatively charged electron (Figure 1-12). Two gamma photons are given off, 180° apart. Each has an

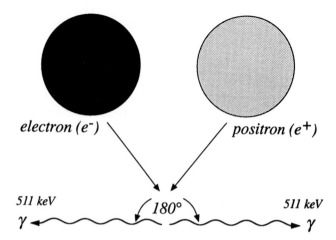

Fig. 1-12   In positron annihilation the mass of a positron and an electron are converted to energy in the form of two photons. The photons each have an energy of 0.511 MeV and are given off 180° apart.

energy of 0.511 MeV, the energy equivalent of positron-electron mass. This unique phenomenon of annihilation radiation 180° apart is the basis for positron emission tomography, or PET.

Gamma Rays and X-Rays

There are three processes through which gamma rays and x-rays are attenuated in tissues. Photons can be completely absorbed by the *photoelectric effect* or in *pair production*. They can also undergo scattering or deflection from their original path by the *Compton effect* or *Compton scattering* phenomenon, in which photons give up part of their original energy.

Pair production   Pair production requires a photon with a minimum energy of 1.02 MeV. The photon energy is converted into one negative and one positive electron. Because the energy required is greater than the photon energies used in medical imaging, this form of attenuation is not important in nuclear medicine.

Photoelectric absorption   Photoelectric absorption occurs when the total energy of an x-ray or gamma ray photon is transferred to an orbital electron (Figure 1-13A). The photon must possess energy greater than the binding energy of the electron. The electron is displaced from its orbit or shell and is either lifted to a higher shell or ejected from the atom (Figure 1-13B). Ejected electrons are termed *photoelectrons*.

As a consequence of the photoelectric interaction, there is an electron cascade to fill the vacancy, with the subsequent emission of characteristic x-rays or Auger electrons (Figure 1-13C). Photoelectric absorption is most likely to occur when the photon energy is just above the electron binding energy. The kinetic energy of the photoelectron is equal to the difference between the energy of the incident photon and the electron binding energy.

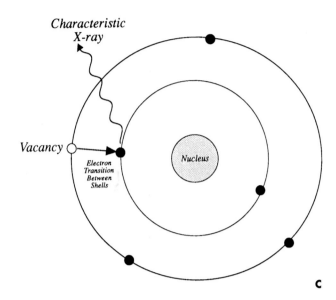

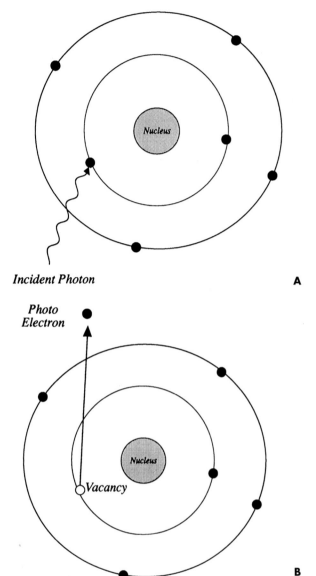

Fig. 1-13 **A**, In the photoelectric absorption process an incident photon interacts with an orbital electron. **B**, The electron is ejected from its shell creating a vacancy. The electron is either ejected from the atom or moved to a shell farther from the nucleus. **C**, The orbital vacancy is filled by the transition of an electron from a more distant shell. A characteristic x-ray is given off as a consequence of this transition.

As photon energy increases the likelihood of a photoelectric event decreases. The photoelectric interaction is important in soft tissues up to an energy of approximately 50 keV. Radionuclides with associated photon energies lower than 50 keV are less desirable for clinical applications because of the high absorption of these photons in soft tissue due to photoelectric interaction. Although photoelectric absorption is undesirable in body tissues, it is fundamental to the detection of ionizing radiation. In both nuclear medicine and roentgenography the creation of images depends on energy absorption in a detecting medium through the photoelectric interaction.

Compton scattering or Compton effect In Compton scattering a photon interacts with a weakly bound outer shell electron. Instead of being completely absorbed as in the photoelectric interaction, in the Compton process the photon is deflected from its original direction and continues to exist but at lower energy (Figure 1-14).

The energy difference is transferred to the recoil electron as kinetic energy. Compton scattering is the dominant mode of gamma ray and x-ray interaction in soft tissues between 30 keV and 30 MeV.

Because the Compton scattered photon gives up energy in the interaction, its wavelength increases. The formula for this is:

$$\Delta\lambda = 0.0243(1 - \cos\phi),$$

where $\Delta\lambda$ is the change in wavelength and the angle ϕ is the angle through which the photon is scattered.

The significance of Compton scattering in nuclear imaging is that scattered photons reaching the imaging detector must be discriminated against and not allowed to form part of the image. Because Compton-scattered photons give up part of their energy, one way to discriminate against them is through setting an "energy window" for acceptance of events in the detector. However, photons

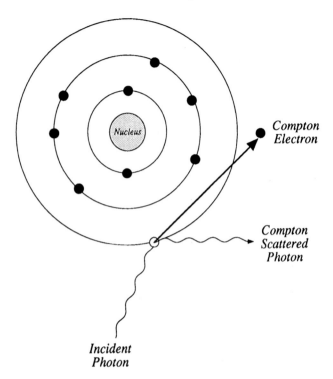

Fig. 1-14   In the Compton scattering process an incident photon interacts with an outer or loosely bound electron. The photon gives up a portion of its energy to the electron and undergoes a change in direction at a lower energy.

scattered through a relatively narrow angle lose only small amounts of energy and may not be effectively excluded by pulse height analysis and the setting of an energy window. Thus, Compton-scattered photons contribute to the loss of spatial resolution in nuclear medicine images. The problem is progressively worse for lower energies because the change in energy for a given scattering angle is less, the lower the original photon energy.

STATISTICS OF RADIOACTIVE DECAY

The time of decay of any single unstable radioactive nucleus is unpredictable and is not influenced by the decay of other nuclei or the physical or chemical environment of the nucleus. Because radioactive decay is random in nature, the actual observed number of nuclei undergoing decay in any given finite period of time is subject to statistical uncertainty; this is a practical problem in clinical nuclear medicine. In any setting where a quantitative measurement is required such as determining the amount of radioactivity in a radiopharmaceutical to be given to the patient, the amount of radioactivity in a blood sample used in calculating a physiologic parameter, or in the quality control of nuclear instrumentation, estimates of statistical certainty are necessary.

Radioactive decay follows *Poisson statistics* or the Poisson probability law. The Poisson probability density function is similar but not identical to the gaussian or normal probability density function. Curves expressing the Poisson and gaussian probability density functions are more closely matched as the number of observed events is increased.

For data obeying the Poisson probability distribution, the standard deviation (SD) is given by:

$$SD = \sqrt{r}$$

where *r* is the true mean. Because the true mean is usually estimated from an average of a number of individual measurements, the estimated standard deviation is:

$$SD(est) = \sqrt{r}\,(est)$$

It is often useful to express standard deviation as a fraction or a percent. The *fractional standard deviation* is simply $1/\sqrt{r}$. The *percent fractional standard deviation* (% SD) is the fractional standard deviation $\times 100$. For example, if 2,500 counts are recorded in a picture element or "pixel" in an image, the fractional standard deviation of the measurement is $1/\sqrt{2,500} = 0.02$. The percent fractional standard deviation is 2%. This can also be expressed in the equation:

$$\%SD = \frac{100}{\sqrt{n}},$$

where *n* is the number of counts observed.

This kind of calculation is useful in determining the number of counts to obtain in the measurement of a radioactive sample or in a scintigraphic image for statistical certainty. The larger the number of counts, the lower the percent fractional or relative standard deviation and the greater the ability to distinguish a true difference in the amount of radioactivity in two different samples. Likewise, in imaging, the greater the number of counts per pixel, the more likely it is that observed differences in the image actually represent true differences in the amount of activity between two locations in the image.

SUGGESTED READINGS

Hendee WR: *Medical radiation physics*, ed 3, St. Louis, 1992, Mosby-Yearbook.

Johns HE and Cunningham JR: *The physics of radiology*, ed 4, Chicago, 1983, Thomas Books.

Rollo FD: *Nuclear medicine physics, instrumentation and agents*, St. Louis, 1977, CV Mosby Co.

Sorenson JA and Phelps ME: *Physics in nuclear medicine*, ed 2, Philadelphia, 1987, WB Saunders Co.

Weber DA, Eckerman KF, Dillman LT and Ryman JC: MIRD: *Radionuclide data and decay schemes*, New York, 1989, Society of Nuclear Medicine.

Radiation Detection and Instrumentation

Detection of radioactivity is fundamental to the practice of nuclear medicine. The amount and type of radioactivity being administered to patients must be measured and documented, and the areas in which people work must be monitored to ensure safety to both health care personnel and patients. Radioactivity emanating from the patient must be detected to allow the temporal and spatial localization necessary to create scintigraphic images. The <u>common denominator</u> in all of the devices used in contemporary nuclear medicine practice for calibration of administered dosages, area monitoring, and imaging is the <u>conversion of energy in the form of ionizing radiation into electrical energy</u>. In modern imaging equipment these electronic signals are often recorded and processed by dedicated nuclear medicine computer systems. Nuclear medicine imaging devices, including the <u>gamma scintillation camera</u>, can be thought of as specialized radiation detection devices, highly modified and adapted to record the <u>temporal and spatial localization of radioactivity in the patient</u>.

RADIATION DETECTION

Ionization Chambers, Proportional Counters, and Geiger-Müller Counters

One important approach to radiation detection is the use of an <u>ionization chamber.</u> The generic design concept is a gas-filled chamber with positive and negative electrodes, at opposite sides of the chamber. A potential difference is created between the two electrodes, but no current flows in the absence of exposure of the chamber to radiation. The interaction of ionizing radiation with the gas in the chamber creates positive and negative ions, which move to the electrodes, creating an electrical current.

The basic concept of the ionization chamber is extremely versatile; specialized devices have been designed for a wide variety of applications. For example, the problem of detecting alpha and beta radiation is quite different from that of detecting gamma radiation because of differences in both their power of penetrating different materials and their likelihood of interaction with matter. Also, the problem of surveying a wide area to determine the presence or absence of radiation is quite different from the problem of accurately calibrating the millicuries of activity to be administered to a patient. Three of the important subtypes of ionization chamber with nuclear medicine applications are the basic ionization chamber, the proportional counter, and the Geiger-Müller counter.

Basic ionization chambers   The voltage difference between the electrodes in the basic ionization chamber is calibrated to be just high enough to "harvest" all of the ions from the sensitive volume of the chamber, but not high enough that the ions in the chamber are accelerated to the point of creating additional secondary ionizations. The effect of this voltage calibration strategy is that the current resulting from any single event is very small and not measurable with any accuracy. Rather, the ionization chamber is used to measure the total current resulting from multiple events over a certain integration time in a given radiation detection setting.

A number of devices routinely used in nuclear medicine clinics operate on the principle of the ionization chamber. Radiation survey meters including the cutie-pie, some pocket dosimeters, and radionuclide dose calibrators are all examples of specialized ionization chambers. The survey meters are typically calibrated to provide units of exposure such as milliroentgens per hour. Dose calibrators are set up to provide readings in the units of radioactivity used in clinical practice. Some laboratories express these units in becquerels; other laboratories have retained the Ci, mCi, and μCi convention. The amount of energy converted to electrical current per unit of radioactivity is different and unique for each radionuclide, and radionuclide dose calibrators must be calibrated for each desired radionuclide to be measured.

Proportional counters   The main difference in a proportional counter compared with the basic ionization chamber is greater applied voltage between the electrodes. The higher voltage results in secondary ionizations in the sensitive volume of the chamber. The term *gas amplification* describes this phenomenon. It can result in increased ionization by a factor of 10^3 to 10^6. The resulting current pulse is large enough to be

measured individually and is proportional to the energy originally deposited in the gas chamber. The name of the device follows from this proportionality of total ionization to the total energy of the ionizing radiation. Proportional chambers do not have wide applicability in clinical nuclear medicine.

Geiger-Müller counter   In the Geiger-Müller counter the voltage is increased even higher than in the proportional chamber application. The voltage is high enough that the initial ionization results in an "avalanche" of secondary ionizations such that the gas is essentially completely ionized. This mode of operation of an ionization chamber allows individual events to be detected, but not their energy (i.e., pulse counting). Another important characteristic of the Geiger-Müller counter is detector dead time. Because the gas in the chamber is completely ionized, it takes a significant amount of time to become ready for the next event. The net effect of the dead time problem is that Geiger-Müller counters are not useful in the presence of large amounts of radioactivity. Rather, they are widely used as area survey meters and have special value in detecting radiation contamination.

Scintillation Detectors: Thallium-Activated Sodium Iodide Crystals

Gas-filled ionization chambers of the kinds described above are very insensitive to x-rays and gamma rays because of the low likelihood of ionizing interactions. The "stopping power" of gas is low. In current practice, thallium-activated sodium iodide crystals, NaI (Tl), are used as the detector medium for single photon imaging systems. These crystals are optically transparent and have sufficient stopping power for sensitive detection of gamma rays (Table 2-1).

As noted earlier an important common denominator of many types of radiation detectors is the conversion of the energy in ionizing radiation to electrical energy. For scintillation detector systems the conversion process is rather interesting. Valence electrons take on energy during photoelectric or Compton interactions from x-rays

Table 2-1 Half-Value Layers of Selected Radionuclides				
		Half-Value Layer (cm)		
Radionuclide	**Energy (keV)**	**Lead**	**Water***	**NaI**
Tc-99m	140	0.028	4.50	0.265
Tl-201	70 } Pb-x-rays	0.0005	3.85	0.048
	81		4.08	0.069
I-131	364	0.220	6.35	1.50

*Soft tissue.

or gamma rays entering the sodium iodide crystal. The imparted energy raises the electrons into the conduction band of the crystal lattice. The energy difference between the valence band and the conduction band is on the order of a few electron volts. As the electrons give up energy in the transition back from the conduction band to the valence band, photons of light are given off. The light photons have a spectrum of energies, but for sodium iodide crystals the spectrum peaks at a wavelength of 4,150 Å, or approximately 3 eV. The energy conversion efficiency in the NaI (Tl) crystal is approximately 13%. The remainder is dissipated in the crystal in the form of molecular motion or heat. The scintillation decay time or length of time for the scintillation event is approximately 1.0 microsecond (10^{-6} seconds).

The next step in the detection process is the interaction of the light photons arising in the crystal with the photocathode of a photomultiplier tube (Figure 2-1). In the typical sodium iodide detector system, whether it is a simple probe or a gamma scintillation camera, the crystal is optically coupled to the photocathode by a light guide or light pipe to ensure the efficiency of light collection. The light photons dislodge electrons from the photocathode. These electrons are then accelerated by a series of electrodes (dynodes) in the photomultiplier tube. With each acceleration the number of electrons is increased. The electrons are collected at the anode or collector of the photomultiplier tube. The multiplication factor is on the order of 3 to 6 per dynode stage and up to several million overall. The resulting voltage pulse from the photomultiplier tube is then available for further processing. This processing may take the form of amplification followed by pulse analysis to determine either the energy deposited in the crystal (pulse height analysis) or the spatial location of the event (position analysis) in the case of gamma scintillation cameras.

A key point to understand in the scintillation detection process is that proportionality is maintained at each step. That is, the number of light photons given off in the NaI (Tl) crystal is proportional to the energy deposited in the crystal from the x-ray or gamma ray. The number of electrons dislodged from the photocathode is proportional to the number of light photons, and the electrical output of the photomultiplier tube is proportional to the number of electrons dislodged from the photocathode. Thus the height of the electrical pulse coming from the photomultiplier tube is proportional to the energy of the radiation absorbed in the crystal. This allows different radionuclides with different energies to be distinguished from one another by *pulse height analysis*. It also permits the distinction of primary photons versus photons that have undergone Compton scattering events before detection. Compton-scattered photons are less energetic than the primary photons and have lower pulse heights. This is very critical in imaging applications of scintillation detec-

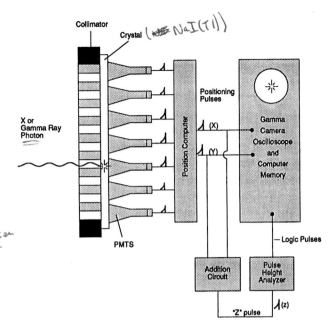

Fig. 2-1   Simplified schematic of gamma scintillation camera. The diagram shows a photon reaching the crystal through the collimator and undergoing photoelectric absorption. The photomultiplier tubes (PMTs) are optically coupled to the NaI (Tl) crystal. The electrical outputs from the respective photomultiplier tubes are further processed through positioning circuitry to calculate x, y coordinates and through addition circuitry to calculate the Z pulse. The Z pulse passes through the pulse height analyzer. If the event is accepted, it is recorded spatially in the location determined by the x, y positioning pulses.

tion because only primary photons are desired to create the image.

Thallium-activated sodium iodide crystals have become the pervasive scintillation detector in nuclear medicine applications for a number of reasons. The crystals are relatively inexpensive and afford great flexibility in size and shape. The stopping power of the sodium iodide crystals is good for the energy range employed in clinical nuclear medicine for single photon applications (i.e., 70 to 365 keV) (Table 2-1). The thallium impurities in the sodium iodide crystal provide "activation centers" or luminescence centers that provide "easier" pathways for the return of the electrons from the conduction band of the crystal to the valence bands of atoms requiring electrons for electrical neutrality. Only a small amount of thallium impurity (0.1 to 0.4 mole %) is required in the sodium iodide crystal lattice to achieve the desired effect of making the scintillation process more efficient. The conversion efficiency of 13% is actually relatively high, and the crystals are internally transparent to the light photons so that they reach the photocathodes. The disadvantages of sodium iodide crystals are their fragility and the fact that they are also highly hydroscopic, necessitating hermetically sealed containers. In most applications the crystal is sealed on all sides by a thin aluminum cannister except on the photomultiplier tube side, which is covered by a quartz window to allow the scintillation photons to escape.

Other Detection Devices

A host of other radiation detection devices are used in nuclear medicine and radiology. These include photographic film, which is used in personnel film badges; semiconductors; thermoluminescent and ultraviolet fluorescent detection devices; and other chemical detectors useful for measuring cumulative radiation effects over long periods of time. They will not be discussed here.

GAMMA RAY SPECTROMETRY AND PULSE HEIGHT ANALYSIS

The energies and relative abundance of the ionizing radiations given off by each radionuclide are physical constants. The proportionality between the energy of a gamma ray and the output of the electrical pulse from the photomultiplier tube provides a means for distinguishing between gamma rays (or x-rays) of different energies. However, the spectrum of recorded energies is more complex than predicted from the decay scheme because of interactions both outside the NaI (Tl) scintillation detector and within the crystal itself. Recognizing the consequences of these interactions is important to the optimal use of counting and imaging instrumentation.

By convention the energy spectra from x-ray and gamma ray detection are plotted with energy on the x-axis and the relative number of events is plotted on the y-axis (Figure 2-2). The important relationships in gamma spectra will be illustrated for technetium-99m because it is the single most commonly used radionuclide in clinical practice.

Photopeak   In a perfect detecting system and with the complete absorption of the 140 keV gamma rays of Tc-99m in the detector, a single line would be recorded on the energy spectrum at exactly 140 keV. In practice the 140 keV *photopeak* is recorded as a bell-shaped curve centered at 140 keV (Figure 2-2). The gaussian distribution of recorded events is due to the statistical nature of the radiation detection process. Each step in the conversion of ionizing radiation to electrical current is subject to statistical fluctuation. Thus the light photons are given off with equal but random probability in all directions. Slightly different numbers of light photons impinge on the photocathode between different absorption events. The number of electrons dislodged is also subject to statistical fluctuation, as is the electron amplification at each dynode stage in the photomultiplier tube.

The energy resolution of a detecting system can be expressed by the spread in the photopeak. A frequently used measure is "full width at half maximum" (FWHM). This is defined as the energy range encompassed by the bell-shaped curve halfway down from the apex of the photopeak (Figure 2-2). A typical gamma scintillation camera might have an FWHM equal to 14 keV for detect-

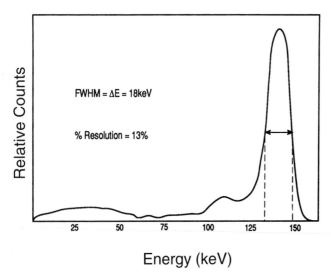

Energy (keV)

Fig. 2-2   Spectrum for technetium-99m in air. The figure illustrates the concept of "full width at half maximum" (FWHM). For the particular detector system illustrated the FWHM is 18 keV. The energy resolution of the detector system for Tc-99m is 13%.

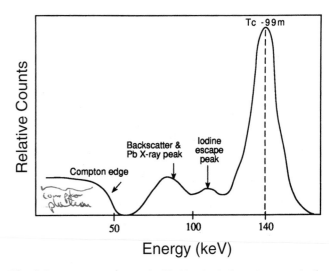

Energy (keV)

Fig. 2-3   Energy spectrum for Tc-99m in air for a gamma scintillation camera with the collimator in place. Note the iodine escape peak at approximately 112 keV. The 180° backscatter peak at 90 keV merges with the lead characteristic x-ray peaks. The Compton edge is at 50 keV.

ing Tc-99m. This can also be expressed as a percentage of the mean energy signal, and the detector would be said to have an energy resolution of 10% (14/140). Obviously the narrower the peak, the better the energy resolution of the detector, and the greater the ability to distinguish gamma rays with energies close to each other.

Iodine escape peak Photoelectric interactions occurring close to the edge of the sodium iodide crystal may result in the "escape" of iodine K-characteristic x-rays from the crystal. When this happens the corresponding x-ray energy of approximately 28.5 keV is not deposited in the crystal and will result in a small peak on the energy spectrum at 112 keV (i.e., 140 keV minus 28 keV) (Figure 2-3). This peak is referred to as the *iodine escape peak* and can be observed with a Tc-99m source in air but is typically not observed in in vivo settings, owing to the relatively much larger contribution from Compton-scattered photons from the patient in the recorded energy spectrum.

Compton valley, edge, and plateau Not every photon entering an NaI (Tl) crystal undergoes photoelectric absorption. If a primary photon undergoes a Compton-scattering interaction in the crystal with subsequent escape of the scattered photon, a smaller voltage pulse will be detected than those composing the photopeak. If we use the 140 keV gamma rays from technetium as the example, the maximum energy transferred to a recoil electron in the crystal occurs at the largest scattering angle (180°), which is 50 keV. This energy is referred to as the *Compton edge*. The energy from 0 to 50 keV is called the *Compton plateau* or *continuum* and corresponds to the energy deposited by photons that scatter from 0° to 180° before escaping the crystal (Figure 2-3). The portion of the energy spectrum between the Compton edge and the photopeak is the *Compton valley*. Some gamma rays undergo multiple Compton-scattering events before escaping from the detector crystal. These may be recorded in the region of the Compton valley. These energy relationships obviously differ for each radionuclide with differing photopeak energy.

Backscatter peak Another peak resulting from Compton-scattering occurs when primary gamma photons undergo 180° scattering outside the detector and are then completely absorbed. The scattering can take place either in front of the detector or behind it if a gamma ray has initially passed completely through the crystal without being scattered or absorbed. From the previous section, it is apparent that for Tc-99m the backscatter peak occurs at 90 keV (140 keV − 50 keV). (Figure 2-3).

Lead characteristic x-ray peak In most nuclear medicine applications, scintillation detectors are used in conjunction with lead collimators. The 140 keV primary photons of technetium are energetic enough to interact with the K shell electrons of lead. The resulting K-characteristic x-rays are in the range of 75 and 88 keV and are readily seen in the energy spectrum. The lead K-characteristic x-rays are readily absorbed in the sodium iodide crystal.

Coincidence or sum peaks The likelihood of two separate events taking place simultaneously in the sodium iodide crystal increases with the amount of radiation present. If two events occur close enough together in time, they can be recorded as a single event by the detector system. Two primary photons from Tc-99m that were detected in coincidence would appear at 280 keV on the energy spectrum. However, every combination of events is possible. That is, a primary photon can be detected in coincidence with a scattered photon of any energy or a lead characteristic x-ray, and so forth. For many detecting systems the ability to discriminate or resolve different discrete energies decreases with increasing amounts of radiation exposure because the likelihood of coincidence events increases.

Compton scatter in the patient The biggest single cause of degradation of clinical images is Compton scatter in the patient and the inability of contemporary imaging systems to completely discriminate primary from Compton-scattered photons. For the gamma scintillation camera, up to 35% of recorded events or even more are due to Compton-scattered photons. The energy spectrum for Tc-99m photons undergoing one scattering event in the patient ranges from 90 keV (i.e., 180° scattering angle) to just under the energy of the primary photon, 140 keV (Figure 2-4). In Tc-99m spectra

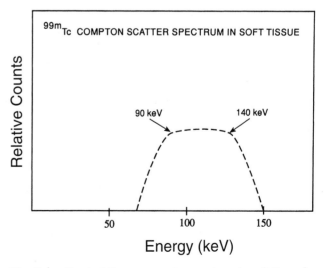

Fig. 2-4 Nominal Compton scatter spectrum in soft tissue for single scattering events. Note that Compton-scattered photons have energy less than 140 keV but can be recorded above this level because of the imperfect energy resolution of the gamma camera.

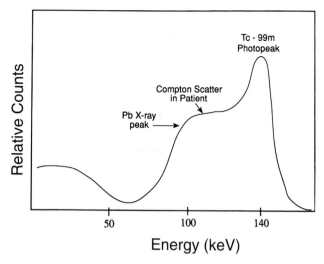

Fig. 2-5   The observed energy spectrum from a gamma scintillation camera with the Tc-99m activity in the patient. Note the loss of definition of the lower limb of the Tc-99m photopeak. This spectrum can be thought of as a sum of the spectra in Figures 2-3 and 2-4. This spectrum illustrates the difficulty of discriminating against Compton-scattered photons using pulse height analysis.

obtained with radioactivity in the patient, the lower limb of the primary photopeak merges into the events due to Compton scattering in the patient. This in turn merges with the lead K-characteristic x-ray peak (Figure 2-5).

IMAGING INSTRUMENTATION

The original instruments available for medical applications of radionuclides were handheld Geiger-Müller devices and simple scintillation probe systems. These systems did not allow spatial localization of radioactivity emanating from the body but did provide a means of crude overall counting. Early clinical applications in nuclear medicine were aimed at calculating the percentage uptake of radioiodine in the thyroid gland with these simple radiation detector systems.

Rectilinear Scanners

In the 1950s probe systems were adapted into electromechanical devices called *rectilinear scanners*. The geometric field of view of the probe was focused or restricted through the application of collimating devices, and the probes were mounted on mechanical transport systems to systematically traverse back and forth over an organ of interest. The original probe systems used calcium tungstate crystals, which rapidly gave way to sodium iodide crystals for the radiation detection step. By the 1960s rectilinear scanning systems were available with 3-inch, 5-inch, and 8-inch diameter detectors.

Gamma Scintillation Cameras

By the late 1960s the rectilinear scanners were progressively replaced by the gamma scintillation camera invented by Hal Anger and also known as the Anger camera. The gamma camera offers far more flexibility than the rectilinear scanner and has been developed into a very sophisticated series of imaging devices that permit dynamic and tomographic imaging, as well as conventional static planar imaging. In contemporary practice, gamma cameras have essentially completely replaced rectilinear scanners.

The major components of the gamma scintillation camera are illustrated in Figure 2-1. Perhaps the easiest way to understand the way gamma cameras work is to follow a photon through the entire radiation detection and spatial localization process, beginning with the origin of photons in the patient.

The patient as a source of photons   Ideally the flux of photons arriving at a radiation detector would be proportional to the number of photons emitted in the respective part of the body being imaged. This assumption would be valid only if the body part were a point source of radiation in air. This is clearly never the case in clinical practice, and a number of factors cause distortion of the photon flux reaching the gamma camera.

One may think of "good" photons as primary photons arising in the organ of interest and emitted parallel to the axis of the collimator field of view. These are the desired photons for creating the scintigraphic image. "Good" photons are reduced in number by attenuation and scatter, which decreases the information available for creating the image (Figure 2-6). In all clinical applications in nuclear medicine, many potentially useful photons are absorbed or scattered before they reach the detector.

Unwanted primary photons can arise from background radioactivity in tissues in front of or behind the structure of interest (Figure 2-6). These primary photons can travel directly to the detector and are then indistinguishable from photons arising in the body part of interest. They may be thought of as "bad" photons because they reduce image contrast and may distort quantitative data analysis. This kind of background activity due to primary photons is hard to correct. One major advantage of single photon emission computed tomography (SPECT) is the increase in image contrast due to reduction in background activity superimposed on object activity.

Another source of "bad" photons is primary photons arising from the organ of interest, which travel "off axis" toward the detector. Radiation is given off isotropically (i.e., with equal probability in all directions), and only a small fraction of the total emitted photons are useful for forming the image. A principal function of collimators is to absorb off-axis photons (Figure 2-7).

Compton scatter is a third source of "bad" photons. Photons originating in or adjacent to the organ of inter-

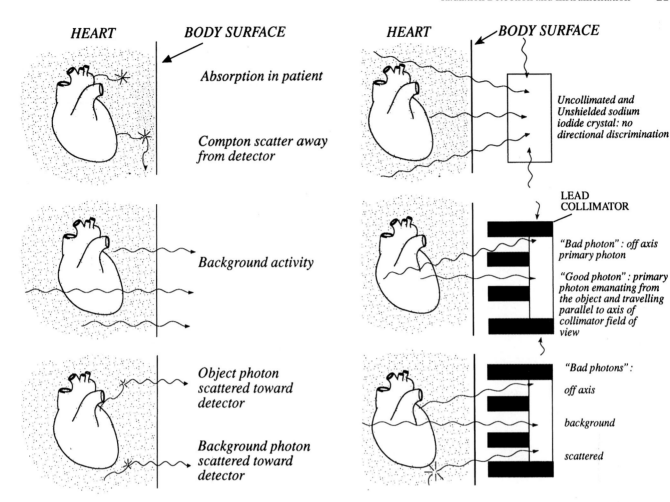

Fig. 2-6 The patient as a source of photons. The top schematic illustrates absorption and scattering of primary photons in the body. These never reach the detector. The middle schematic demonstrates background activity arising from in front, behind, and beside the organ of interest. The bottom schematic illustrates object and background photons scattered toward the detector.

Fig. 2-7 Schematic diagrams illustrating the interaction of photons arising in the patient with the detector and a simplified parallel hole collimator. The collimator provides *directional* discrimination for primary and scattered photons. It does not eliminate either background or scattered photons that travel toward the detector within the geometric acceptance field of view of the collimator. "Good" photons are primary (unscattered) photons that originate in the object and travel parallel to the axis of the collimator field of view. All other photons (i.e., background, scattered, off-axis) are undesirable in the image.

est can undergo scattering and subsequently travel toward the detector in a direction coincident with primary photons arising from another area of interest. Photons that undergo Compton scattering in the patient lose some of their energy and can be partially discriminated against by using pulse height analysis.

Collimators The collimator is the first part of the gamma scintillation camera potentially encountered by the photon after it leaves the patient. The purpose of the collimator is to define the geometric field of view of the crystal and specifically to define the desired direction of travel of gamma rays allowed to reach the crystal (Figure 2-7). The collimator discriminates against unwanted photons only on the basis of their direction of travel. The collimator does not distinguish between primary and scattered photons or between photons of different energies. The pulse height analyzer is used to discriminate

against scattered photons and other photons of unwanted energy that reach the detector.

There are four basic collimator types for gamma scintillation cameras—pinhole, parallel hole, converging, and diverging.

Pinhole collimators The geometric behavior of a pinhole collimator is similar to that of a pinhole camera (Figure 2-8). The field of view increases with distance, and the image is inverted. The principal use of the pinhole collimator in contemporary practice is in thyroid and parathyroid imaging. In this application, it offers the advantage of image magnification when the aperture-object distance is shorter than the distance from the detector to the aperture. The geometric magnification allows the resolution of objects smaller than the intrinsic resolution of the gamma camera. This is again particularly valuable for thyroid imaging, where lesions as small as 3 to 5 mm may be resolved. The pinhole collimator also offers great flexibility in patient positioning and is useful in obtaining oblique views of the thyroid. Pinhole collimators have also been used in pediatric patients to magnify small structures.

The major disadvantage of the pinhole collimator is poor count rate sensitivity. The usual pinhole aperture diameter is 3 to 6 mm. Any increase in this size to increase count rate results in a corresponding decrease in spatial resolution.

Parallel hole collimators The parallel hole collimator is the workhorse collimator in daily nuclear medicine practice (Figure 2-9). Typical collimators consist of lead foil with thousands of parallel holes or channels uniformly distributed. A number of terms are used to further characterize parallel hole collimators. The term *low-energy collimator* is used conventionally to refer to collimators designed for photons of the energy of Tc-99m (140 keV) or

[handwritten: Low energy collimators → ≤140 keV (eg. Tc-99m)]
[handwritten: Medium " " → < 400 keV (eg. Ga-67)]
[handwritten: High " " → > 400 keV (eg. I-131)]

lower. *Medium-energy* collimators are designed for radionuclides with gamma emissions lower than 400 keV, such as gallium-67 (multiple photopeaks at 93, 185, 300, and 395 keV). Although the principal gamma ray from I-131 (364 keV) falls in this energy range, the presence of several higher energy photons (>600 keV) in the decay scheme results in significant degradation and septal penetration artifacts with medium-energy collimators. *High-energy* collimators have been designed for I-131. These collimators have thicker septa than low-energy collimators.

Among low-energy collimators, designs are optimized for either sensitivity or resolution. For a given hole size and septal thickness, the thicker the collimator (i.e., the longer the holes), the higher is the spatial resolution and the lower the sensitivity. Longer holes of equal diameter have a smaller acceptance angle, resulting in loss of count rate sensitivity but an improvement in geometric or spatial resolution.

One useful way to think about parallel hole collimators is to look in detail at the geometry and characteristics of an individual hole. Conceptualized in this way, it is clear that the field of view of each hole becomes larger with increasing distance from the collimator face (Figure 2-10). Fields of view from adjacent holes begin to overlap, and geometic resolution is degraded. For this reason, it is important to position the organ of interest as close to the surface of the collimator as possible because that is where the resolution is best. Unlike pinhole collimators, image size is not affected by collimator-to-source distance with parallel hole collimators.

[handwritten: The closer the patient is to the collimator, the smaller the FOV, or the further, the ↑FOV & you will have many 2° photons contributing to your image.]

Crystal

image

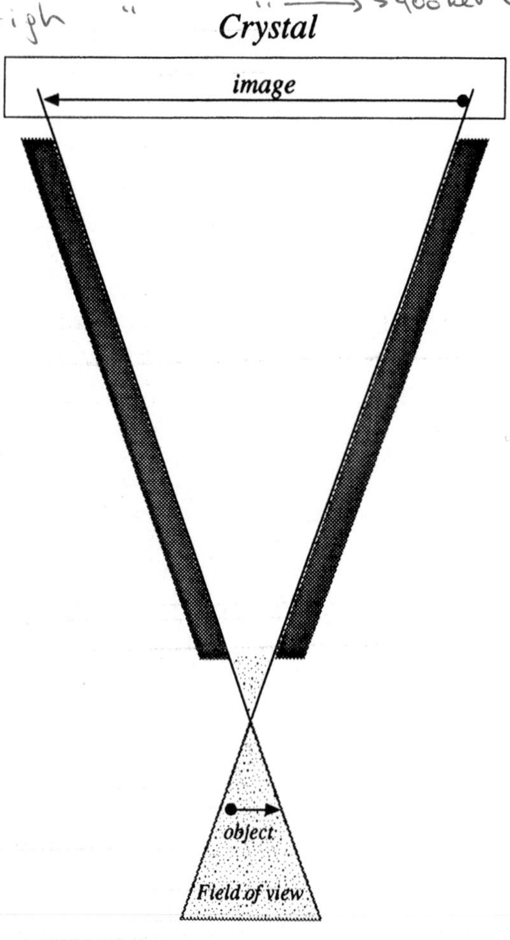

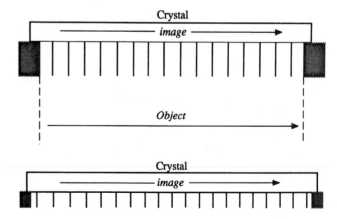

Fig. 2-8 Pinhole collimator. The image is inverted. The image is magnified if the distance from the aperture to the object is smaller than the distance from the aperture to the gamma camera crystal. The object is minified if its distance from the aperture exceeds the aperture-to-crystal distance. Spatial resolution and count rate sensitivity are inversely affected by aperture diameter.

Fig. 2-9 Schematic of two parallel hole collimators. The upper collimator with *longer* septa is designed to achieve higher resolution. Septal *thickness* and energy rating are the same.

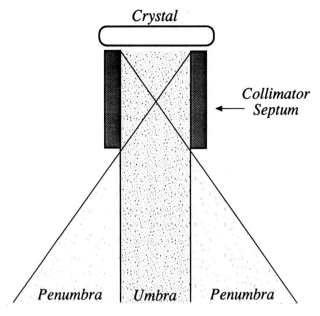

Fig. 2-10 Detail geometry of a single-hole collimator. The field of view increases with distance from the collimator face.

The physics of collimator design and response are quite complex. In essence there is a trade-off between spatial resolution and count rate sensitivity, and there is also a need to avoid excessive septal penetration. The need to minimize septal penetration defines the choice of septal thickness for a given energy (Table 2-1). The rule of thumb in collimator design is that fewer than 10% of recorded events should be due to septal penetration. The off-axis photons reaching the scintillation crystal by septal penetration degrade spatial resolution. However, thicker septa reduce sensitivity and observed count rate.

Converging and diverging hole collimators Converging hole collimators are used to magnify the image geometrically (Figure 2-11). They are applied especially in pediatric nuclear medicine where they have partially replaced pinhole collimators for this purpose.

Diverging collimators were popular before large field of view cameras became available (Figure 2-12). They permit a larger area of the body to be imaged than is possible with a parallel hole collimator. For example, a lung scan on a large patient is not feasible with a standard 10-inch-diameter field of view gamma camera but is readily accomplished with a diverging hole collimator.

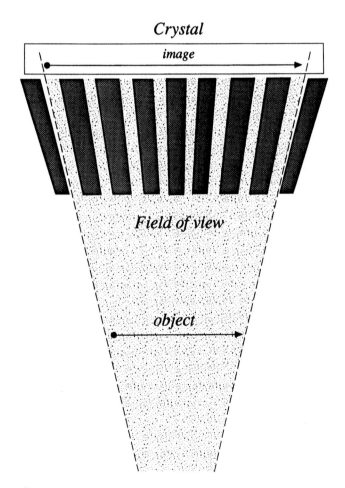

Fig. 2-11 Converging hole collimator. Objects are magnified.

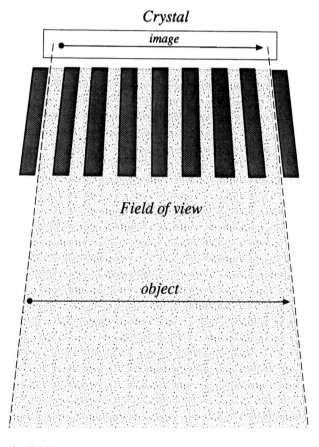

Fig. 2-12 Diverging hole collimator. Objects are minified.

The main drawback of converging and diverging collimators is distortion of the image. This occurs because each portion of the organ of interest is magnified or minified to a different extent, depending on how far the respective location is from the collimator.

Other special collimators In addition to these primary collimator designs a number of specialty use collimators have been described. Parallel slant hole collimators have found application in nuclear cardiology. A 30° caudal angulation is favored by some nuclear medicine physicians for separating the left atrium from the left ventricle in radionuclide ventriculography. Rotating slant hole collimators and multipinhole collimators have been used for limited angle emission computed tomography. More recently, special fan beam collimators have been designed for SPECT applications. These collimators have the advantage of higher geometric efficiency without loss of spatial resolution compared with parallel hole collimators.

Gamma ray detection: the sodium iodide crystal All modern gamma scintillation cameras use thallium-activated sodium iodide crystals as the radiation detector (Figure 2-1). The desired event in the camera crystal is the complete photoelectric absorption of a primary photon that reached the crystal by traveling parallel to the geometric axis of the collimator field of view from its origin in the organ of interest in the patient. The likelihood of a photoelectric interaction and complete energy absorption in the sodium iodide crystal is greater at low energies and decreases at higher energies where Compton scatter becomes progressively more likely (Table 2-1).

As discussed in the section on radiation detection the gamma ray energy is converted to light energy in the crystal. For every 140 keV technetium photon completely absorbed, approximately 4200 light photons are emitted, with an average energy of 3 eV. One of the limitations of lower energy gamma rays, including those from Tc-99m, is the limited number of light photons available for subsequent event localization. Higher energy photons potentially provide more light photons and better statistical certainty for event localization. This is counterbalanced by the greater likelihood of an initial Compton-scattering event in the crystal before a terminal photoelectric interaction. When multiple scattering events occur in the crystal before complete energy absorption, spatial resolution is reduced.

Signal processing and event localization The breakthrough concept in the design of the gamma scintillation camera is the use of an array of photomultiplier tubes behind the crystal for event localization. In the first commercial gamma camera, a 10-inch-diameter sodium iodide crystal was optically coupled to a hexagonal array of 19 3-inch-diameter photomultiplier tubes (Figure 2-13).

For each event, two kinds of signal processing are performed. First the output from all of the photomultiplier tubes is summed for the purpose of pulse height

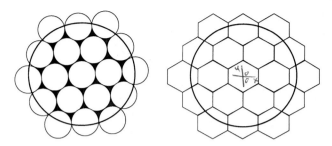

Fig. 2-13 Schematic demonstrating circular (*left*) and hexagonal (*right*) photomultiplier tubes. The tubes are arrayed using a hexagonal configuration so that the distance from each tube to all of its nearest neighbors is identical. The switch from round to hexagonal tubes allows more complete coverage of the gamma camera crystal.

analysis. This summed pulse is typically referred to as the Z pulse and is used to determine whether the detected event is within the desired energy range and should be accepted into the formation of the image or whether it is of lower or higher energy and should be discriminated against and rejected (Figure 2-1).

Simultaneously the output of each photomultiplier tube is looked at in a different way. Each tube may be thought of as having *x* and *y* coordinates in a Cartesian plane with the center of the central photomultiplier tube being the origin. Each photomultiplier tube then can be thought of as contributing either a positive or negative value for *x* and *y* positioning. The greatest number of light photons are collected by the photomultiplier tubes closest to the event, with lesser contributions from more remote tubes. The logic circuitry of the camera is used to compute the most likely coordinates of the event location in the crystal by adding together all of the *x* and *y* pulses from the 19 photomultiplier tubes (Figure 2-1).

Image recording If the Z pulse indicates that a primary photon has been absorbed, an *unblanking* signal is sent to the image recording device. On original cameras the recording system was an oscilloscope with a Polaroid camera or 35mm camera attachment. The *x* and *y* positioning signals provided the deflection coordinates for the cathode ray tube, and the event was recorded on film as a single flash of light from the screen. A typical image was created by recording 100,000 to 1,000,000 individual events.

In contemporary practice, most scintigraphic images are recorded on dedicated computer systems. An analog-to-digital converter is used to convert the *x*, *y* positioning signals into digital coordinates to be stored in computer memory.

Characteristics of Modern Gamma Scintillation Cameras

The original commercial gamma cameras had 10- to 12-inch-diameter crystals with a thickness of one-half inch. These cameras were designed in an era when I-131 (364 keV) was the most important radionuclide.

In the ensuing 25 years, crystal size and shape have changed. Large field of view cameras with 15-inch-diameter fields of view have become the standard. Square and rectangular sodium iodide crystals have been developed for special applications, including SPECT and whole body imaging.

A series of changes in the original gamma camera design has been aimed at improving spatial resolution. Crystal thickness in many cameras is now one-quarter inch. This crystal thickness is more suited to studies with lower energy radionuclides, such as Tc-99m and thallium-201. For Tc-99m with a 140 keV principal photon energy the loss in sensitivity between one-half inch and one-quarter inch thickness is only 6% (Table 2-1), while the spatial resolution is improved by 20%. For Tl-201 there is virtually no loss of sensitivity and the same 20% improvement in spatial resolution. However, for studies using gallium (93, 185, 300, 394 keV), indium-111 (172, 247 keV) or I-131 (364 keV), a better compromise may be a three-eighths inch thick crystal.

The number of photomultiplier tubes used in gamma cameras has been increased. The first step was to reduce tube diameter from 3 inches to 2 inches, which permitted 37 photomultiplier tubes to be used for a standard field of view camera. Contemporary large field of view cameras are available with 55, 61, 75, and even 91 tubes. Another advance in photomultiplier tubes is the hexagonal shaped photocathode, which allows the tubes to completely cover the crystal without leaving gaps between them (Figure 2-13). Light pipes have been replaced with "direct" coupling of the photomultiplier tubes to the crystal. The collection of more light photons reduces the statistical uncertainty in the (x, y) event localization logic circuitry.

An area that has received major attention over the years is field uniformity. The basic problem is that each photomultiplier tube behaves slightly differently and may "drift" in its performance over time. Field uniformity was not a major problem before SPECT but is now critical to avoid artifacts in SPECT images.

In addition to slight differences in photomultiplier tube response, there are subtle differences in the crystal itself and in the efficiency of the optical coupling of the photomultiplier tubes with the crystal. For this reason the energy spectrum that is collected from any one photomultiplier tube is different from all the other tubes (Figure 2-14). The observed energy spectrum from the overall camera is made up of a sum of the slightly different spectra from each tube. This could be dramatically demonstrated in older cameras by setting an asymmetric pulse height analyzer window over a photopeak to accentuate the differences in tube performance.

Although vendors have tried a number of approaches to match the performance characteristics of the photo-

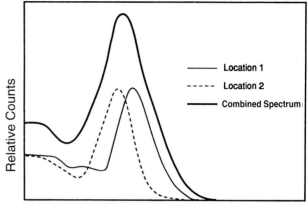

Fig. 2-14   Schematic illustrating slightly offset spectra from two different photomultiplier tubes or locations in the gamma camera crystal and the combined spectrum. Especially in older gamma scintillation cameras, a wide energy acceptance window was necessary to encompass the variations in response across the crystal.

multiplier tubes, problems persist. The current approach is to use computer correction of the response across the crystal. In effect, after the camera system is manufactured and tuned as well as possible, its actual performance relative to a known radioactive source energy and its imaging geometry are empirically mapped and correction factors are established for each small area of the detector. A uniform flood source of radioactivity is used, with the assumption that the count rate should be the same for each picture element or pixel in the image.

In the best contemporary cameras the recording of each event is corrected separately for location and energy. This kind of event-by-event correction permits the use of asymmetric windows. The advantage of an asymmetric window offset to the high side of the photopeak is reduction in scattered photons accepted in the image. However, unless energy correction is performed properly, the response across the image will vary depending on photomultiplier tube response. Events in areas of lower output tubes will be underrepresented in the image, while events in areas with higher output tubes will be overrepresented. Further advances from commercial vendors have led to automatic tuning systems and on-line adjustment systems for photomultiplier and overall system response.

Within the past 15 years there has been an explosion in the number and kinds of gamma cameras on the commercial market. Mobile cameras, whole body imaging systems, and cameras adapted to special nuclear cardiology applications are all available, as are camera systems with multiple detector heads for SPECT and whole body imaging.

Gamma Camera Quality Control

Gamma scintillation cameras are very complex devices with physical, mechanical, and electronic components. Malfunction or breakage of any of these can be catastrophic in system performance and may not be recognized from review of clinical images. For these reasons a number of rather comprehensive and sophisticated procedures have been developed over the years to ensure adequate camera performance. The ones used most often in routine clinical practice are summarized in Box 2-1. In addition to these the National Electrical Manufacturers Association has developed a comprehensive set of tests to measure camera performance.

Field uniformity One fundamental parameter that requires daily assessment is the uniformity response of the gamma camera across its entire field of view. A source of radioactivity of appropriate energy is used to test the camera response. Measurements made with the collimator in place are referred to as *extrinsic* and those made with the collimator off are referred to as *intrinsic*.

There are many variations on the specific methodology. For example, a uniform disk or flood source in a phantom can be used to measure extrinsic field uniformity. With this approach the radioactive source is placed at or on the surface of the gamma camera collimator. To measure intrinsic field uniformity a point source of radioactivity is positioned at the center of the crystal at a distance of 5 feet or more from the uncollimated crystal face. Typically, 1000k to 5000k counts are obtained to evaluate field uniformity for planar imaging.

For extrinsic field uniformity testing, most laboratories use either a phantom filled with a uniform solution of Tc-99m or a permanent disk source of uniformly distributed cobalt-57. The standard of practice is to obtain a flood image on each camera every day before it is used for clinical studies. In laboratories where it is more practical to obtain the daily flood image with the collimator in place, it is still useful to obtain an intrinsic flood image on a weekly basis and vice versa for laboratories that routinely acquire flood images without the collimator in place.

The image of the field uniformity examination should be carefully inspected. In a well-tuned camera with proper photomultiplier tube and correction circuitry performance the flood should provide a highly uniform appearance or only minor mottling with slightly increased intensity in regions corresponding to photomultiplier tubes (Figure 2-15). Photomultiplier tube drift or even the failure of a photomultiplier tube will be recognized as an area of decreased activity (Figure 2-16). Cracked crystals are readily identified, and even damage to a collimator can be detected. The soft lead in collimators is often protected by a covering but can still be subject to denting, with bending and distortion of the septa.

Spatial resolution and linearity The four-quadrant bar phantom is probably the most commonly used phantom for evaluating linearity and spatial resolution (Figure 2-15). Some authorities recommend this procedure daily, but with modern cameras a weekly basis is suitable.

The phantom is centered on the collimator face so that the center of the four-quadrant pattern corresponds to the center of the camera. A uniform Tc-99m flood source is then placed on the bar phantom. Four images are obtained at sequential 90° rotations between positions. Care must be taken not to position the bars on the

---

Box 2-1   Gamma Camera Quality Control Summary

PARAMETER	COMMENT
Daily	
Uniformity check	Flood field; intrinsic (without collimator) or extrinsic (with collimator)
Window setting	Confirm energy window setting relative to photopeak for each radionuclide used → how
Weekly	
Spatial resolution	Requires a "resolution" phantom (PLES, four-quadrant bar, orthogonal hole) and standardized protocol
Linearity check	Qualitative assessment of bar pattern linearity
Periodically (biannually or when a problem is suspected)	
Collimator performance	High count flood with each collimator
Energy registration	For cameras with capability of imaging multiple energy windows simultaneously
Count rate performance and count rate linearity	More important in cameras with "count skimming" or "count addition" correction circuitry
Energy resolution	Easiest in cameras with built-in multichannel analyzers
Sensitivity	Count rate performance per unit of activity

collimator in such a way that an interference or moiré pattern occurs (Figure 2-17).

Modern gamma scintillation cameras have excellent spatial resolution. When the spatial resolution check is made without the collimator in place, it is difficult to find a four-quadrant bar phantom with small enough bar spacing. An alternative is the *parallel-line equal-spacing* (PLES) bar phantom. When this device is used, only two images are necessary. Because signals from the photomultiplier tubes are processed through two essentially independent positioning circuits (*x* and *y*), it is possible for degradations to occur in a selective direction. Yet another alternative is the *orthogonal hole test pattern* (OHP). It is designed so that only a single image is required. Regardless of the phantom chosen, when trouble is suspected the procedure should be repeated with and without the collimator.

In a properly functioning camera, all groups of bars in the bar phantom pattern should appear straight and parallel (Figure 2-15). Some distortion is typically seen at the edge of the field of view. When the study is acquired on an analog CRT with direct film recording, it is very important to first calibrate the dot size and confirm the dot shape.

The spatial resolution of gamma cameras is often expressed as the full width at half maximum (FWHM) of a line spread function. A line spread function is obtained by first imaging a narrow line source of radioactivity on the collimator (extrinsic) or crystal face (intrinsic) and then determining a count profile or histogram perpendicularly across it. This histogram is called the *line spread function*. In an imaging system with perfect spatial resolution the line spread function would have a single spike

corresponding to the radioactive line source. In practice a bell-shaped curve is seen.

FWHM is simply the distance encompassed by the curve halfway down from its peak. This is the same kind

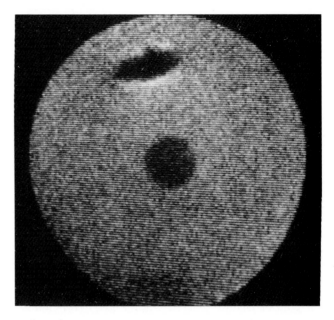

Fig. 2-16   Flood image from a camera with a nonfunctioning central photomultiplier tube and a crystal defect. (Courtesy KA McKusick, MD, and John Hergenrother, CNMT, Massachusetts General Hospital, Boston.)

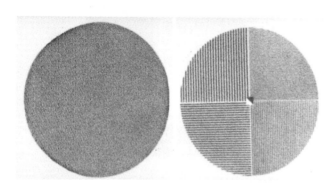

Fig. 2-15   Images of the flood source (*left*) and a four-quadrant bar phantom (*right*) from a well-tuned gamma scintillation camera with the collimator off. Note the slight mottling of the flood but no focal or localized areas of increased or decreased activity within the center of the field of view. The slightly increased activity along the rim is a common characteristic of gamma cameras seen on intrinsic flood images. The smallest bars are partially discernible on the bar phantom image. They have a spacing of 3 millimeters. Note also the good linearity of the bar images.

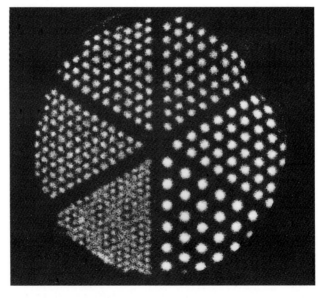

Fig. 2-17   Moire patterns are present in the three left sided triangles in an image of a "hot spot" phantom. Note the distortion especially in the lower left panel.

of measurement previously discussed for describing energy resolution. By analogy the narrower the peak, the better is the spatial resolution and therewith the ability to resolve objects close to each other. In modern gamma cameras, intrinsic resolution (collimator off) approaches 3 mm FWHM or less.

Clinical Use of the Gamma Scintillation Camera

Applying the gamma scintillation camera to clinical procedures requires the development of imaging protocols that define the diagnostic purpose, the radiopharmaceutical to be employed, patient preparation, and the imaging sequence. These issues will be discussed in the organ system chapters for the major scintigraphic studies. The protocols include selection of collimator, the timing of image acquisition following radiopharmaceutical administration, the number of counts to be obtained, and the actual images or views to be obtained.

One of the issues that falls between the cracks of quality control and clinical application of gamma cameras is the setting of the energy window. The most common approach is to use a symmetric window centered at the energy peak of the radionuclide label being used in the imaging procedure. For Tc-99m the most common approach is to use a 20% window centered at 140 keV. The acceptance range for this window is 126 keV to 154 keV. In gamma cameras with energy correction circuitry, it may be possible to set an asymmetric window to reduce Compton scatter. It may also be desirable to use a narrower window of 10% or 15% for higher resolution imaging. These latter approaches should be undertaken with caution for older gamma cameras because of the problems of nonuniform response across the crystal, which were discussed in some detail in a previous section.

The most conservative approach is to confirm the window setting for each radionuclide used during the course of a day and to actually confirm the window setting before imaging each patient. Setting the energy window ("peaking in the camera," "setting the peak") should be done with a radioactive source in air and *not* by using radioactivity in the patient. The spectrum from the patient includes scatter that can shift the perceived location of the photopeak.

Figure 2-18 illustrates four different window settings in the same patient. The top image was obtained with the optimal setting for the camera being used. The bottom three panels illustrate energy windows offset to the high and low sides of the photopeak, with consequent degradation of image quality. False positive and false negative interpretations may result because of artifacts and loss of resolution, respectively, with incorrect window settings. Occasionally the window is inadvertently

left at the setting for a Co-57 flood source (122 keV). Figure 2-19 illustrates the degradation of image quality in a Tc-99m diphosphonate bone study resulting from this.

Another practical problem of window setting occurs in cameras that image multiple photopeaks simultaneously. Care must be taken to ensure that the image data from the different photopeaks are correctly registered together on the clinical image. Figure 2-20 illustrates incorrect (left panel) and correct (right panel) multipeak registration for a Ga-67 flood image.

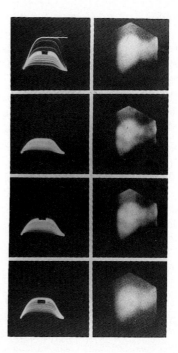

Fig. 2-18 Multiple images from the same subject obtained with different window settings. The *left-hand panel* of images illustrate the energy spectrum coming from the patient. The location of the energy window is indicated by the black rectangle superimposed over the spectral lines. The *top panel* illustrates a symmetric window centered at the photopeak. The *middle two panels* illustrate the energy window offset to the high side, and the *lower panel* illustrates the energy window offset to the low side. Note the loss of homogeneity in the liver in the two middle images with a geometric pattern of hot and cold areas owing to the location pattern of the photomultiplier tubes. Scatter is decreased, as indicated by the lower counts coming from the region of the heart, but the images are grossly misleading. On the bottom panel the image is degraded by excessive scatter and loss of spatial resolution. Note the blurring of the liver margin. (Courtesy KA McKusick, MD, and John Hergenrother, CNMT, Massachusetts General Hospital, Boston.)

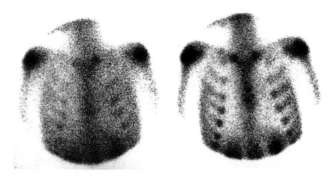

Fig. 2-19   The image on the *left* was obtained with a 20% window set at 122 keV, the energy of the cobalt-57 flood source. Note the dramatic improvement in image quality in the image on the *right*, which was obtained at the correct window setting for Tc-99m.

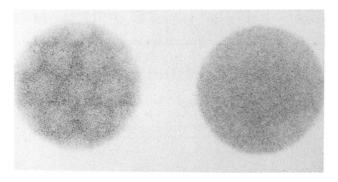

Fig. 2-20   Gallium-67 flood images obtained using multiple photopeaks. In the *left-hand panel* there are artifacts in the flood due to spatial misregistration. In the properly registered image on the right there is good uniformity. (Courtesy John Hergenrother, CNMT, Massachusetts General Hospital, Boston.)

COMPUTERS IN NUCLEAR MEDICINE

Computers in nuclear medicine were a curiosity until the development of multiframe gated blood pool imaging in the mid-1970s. Subsequently the computer has become a primary image acquisition and processing device and is frequently used for image management and to control film formatting, in addition to its integral role for dynamic studies and SPECT.

Creation of the Digital Image

The x and y pulses generated in the gamma scintillation camera logic circuitry define event location. In older cameras these pulses are in analog form and must be converted to digital form for computer processing. To accomplish this, an analog-to-digital converter is interposed between the gamma camera and the computer.

Some modern cameras convert the (x, y) signals to digital form within the camera's own electronic circuitry. The z pulse is still used in computer data acquisition to indicate that a particular event should be accepted for storage.

There are two fundamentally different modes of acquiring and storing digitized data—list (serial) mode and frame (histogram) mode. In the list mode approach, each pair of digitized (x, y) position signals is stored separately and sequentially in computer memory. The list is simply a line of data flowing into computer memory. If time information is desired, additional time markers are inserted into the list. Physiologic signals such as the R wave on the ECG can also be recorded (Figure 2-21).

The list mode approach offers great flexibility. For example, data from each cardiac cycle can be analyzed separately. If a particular beat was due to a dysrhythmia, the data from that beat can be excluded from the desired data from normal sinus beats. Or, data from beats caused by particular types of dysrhythmias can be analyzed separately. The major disadvantage of the list mode is that it requires a large amount of computer memory. It also requires additional time to process data into an image format.

In the alternative histogram or frame mode of data acquisition the digitized (x, y) pairs are used to locate the picture element they belong to. The image may be thought of as a grid or matrix superimposed on the analog data (Figures 2-22, 2-23). The x and y numbers determine which matrix element encloses the location of the original event. At the end of data collection, rather than having discrete information on each event, each matrix location has a number corresponding to the total events accumulated throughout the imaging period.

This mode is much more sparing of computer memory and has the further advantage that the data are immediately ready for display or analysis and no postprocessing or formatting is required. Physiologic signals can still be used to control data collection as in multigated cardiac studies.

The larger the matrix size, the better the potential spatial resolution but the longer the time required to achieve adequate counting statistics in each pixel. Most studies in current practice are obtained in a 64×64 or 128×128 matrix.

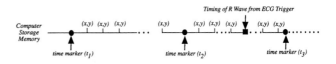

Fig. 2-21   Schematic of list mode data acquisition.

Analog Image With 6 x 6 Matrix Superimposed

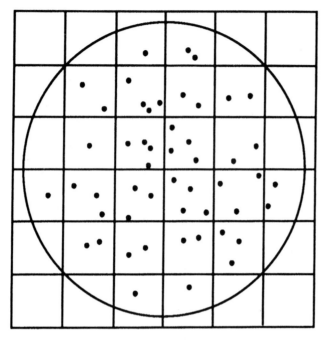

Fig. 2-22   Schematic of a matrix superimposed over a circular gamma camera field of view. The individual scintillation events are represented by dots. Each square within the matrix represents a picture element, or pixel. The number of events occurring within the picture element is recorded as a number in the digital image.

0	0	1	2	0	0
0	2.	4	2	2	0
0	1	4	4	2	0
1	3	3	4	3	2
0	2	2	2	3	0
0	0	1	1	0	0

Digital Image Matrix

Fig. 2-23   Digital image corresponding to schematic in Figure 2-22. Instead of individual scintillation events the total number of events is recorded for each picture element.

Data Analysis

Computer recording of image data greatly facilitates quantitative analysis. Specific types of analyses will be discussed in the respective organ system chapters. A recurring requirement in data analysis is the definition of a "region of interest." These regions can be defined by the computer operator or through the use of automated region of interest definition programs. The latter are often used to define the area of the left ventricle in calculating ejection fractions.

The computer can make various calculations on the pixels in regions of interest. In most applications the total count within the region is of most value. This kind of data analysis allows calculation of quantitative parameters such as the left ventricular ejection fraction or the percentage of the total glomerular filtration rate attributable to the left versus the right kidney, for example.

Data Display and Formatting

Clinics with contemporary computer systems frequently use them to archive image data and to control image formatting devices such as laser printers. The advantage of using the computer for this purpose as opposed to analog imaging or recording directly from the gamma camera CRT is that images may be windowed and centered to provide the optimum gray scale after the fact, and the same image data may be looked at with and without secondary image processing, including background subtraction or contrast enhancement. The computer is obviously invaluable for looking at dynamic data. This is most important in nuclear cardiology in viewing the beating heart, but it has value in the sense of time-lapse photography for other applications such as localizing the site of bleeding in gastrointestinal bleeding detection studies or assessing biliary dynamics during hepatobiliary imaging studies.

RADIONUCLIDE TOMOGRAPHY

Conventional or planar radionuclide imaging suffers a major limitation in loss of object contrast as a result of background radioactivity. In the conventional planar image, radioactivity underlying and overlying an object is superimposed on radioactivity coming from the object. The fundamental goal of all tomographic imaging systems is to more accurately portray the distribution of radioactivity in the patient, with improved definition of image detail. The Greek *tomo* means "to cut." Intuitively, tomography may be thought of as a means of "cutting" the body into discrete image planes.

Tomographic techniques have been developed for both single photon and positron tomography. Rectilinear scanners with focused collimators actually represent a crude type of tomography, for the count rate sensitivity is greatest in the collimator focal plane, and therefore more weight is given to radioactivity arising in that plane than in planes superficial or deep to it. However, this is not "true" tomography in the sense that there is still contribution from out-of-plane radiation in the image. The general class of restricted-angle or longitudinal (frontal) tomography shares this phenomenon. These systems are exemplified by multipinhole, rotating slant hole, and pseudo-random-coded aperture collimator systems. In-plane data are kept in focus, with blurring of out-of-plane data. Restricted-angle or longitudinal tomography is very analogous to conventional x-ray tomography where the relative position of the film and x-ray source remain constant for the desired image plane but move relative to each other in the overlying and underlying planes, thus blurring the out-of-plane structures.

A number of restricted-angle systems enjoyed a vogue in the late 1970s and early 1980s. These included the seven-pinhole collimator system and various kinds of rotating slant hole collimator systems. These systems have given way to rotating gamma camera systems. The rotating systems offer the ability to perform true transaxial tomography. The most important characteristic is that only data arising in the image plane are used in the reconstruction or creation of the tomographic image. Rotational SPECT shares this characteristic with x-ray computed tomography (CT) and positron emission tomography. This is an important characteristic because it offers the highest available image contrast compared to tomographic systems that merely blur the out-of-plane data.

Rotational SPECT

Various commercial systems are now available for performing rotational SPECT. The systems have found particular application for studies of the brain and heart. The most common approach to rotational SPECT is to mount one or more gamma camera heads on a special rotating gantry. Originally, systems used a single head but there are now systems commercially available with two, three, and even four heads. Multiple heads are

desirable because they allow more data to be collected in a given period of time. Rotational SPECT is "photon poor" compared to x-ray CT, and it is desirable both to collect as many counts as possible and to achieve imaging within the time frame of radiopharmaceutical pharmacokinetics. Thus a study of Tl-201 distribution in the heart must be accomplished before significant redistribution occurs. Multiheaded systems are a great advantage in this regard.

In addition to the special gantry that permits camera head rotation, other modifications have been necessary for rotational SPECT. Photomultiplier tube performance can be affected by gravitational and magnetic fields (Figure 2-24). These change depending on rotational angle, and subtle changes in photomultiplier tube energy response degrade images. Magnetic shielding of photomultiplier tubes reduces the problem.

Another modification of camera head design for rotational SPECT is shaping of the collimator and housing to facilitate rotation around the patient without making contact. Just as in conventional planar imaging, it is desirable to have the camera head as close to the object as possible. Collimator and camera head casing cutouts facilitate this. In advanced commercial systems the camera head can also be programmed to follow a body contour orbit around the patient and not just a circular orbit. This is accomplished by having the camera head move inward and outward from the patient, depending on the contour requirement perpendicular to the axis of rotation at each imaging location.

Rotational SPECT has highlighted the need to improve gamma camera system performance. Flood field

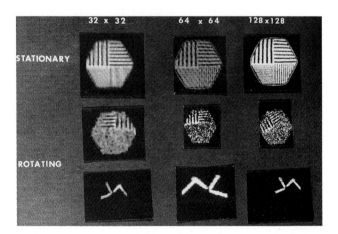

Fig. 2-24 Four quadrant bar phantom images obtained with the gamma camera stationary and during rotation. Note the degradation in bar phantom resolution in this early generation rotating SPECT system. (Courtesy KA McKusick, MD, and John Hergenrother, CNMT, Massachusetts General Hospital, Boston.)

nonuniformity is translated into tomographic images as major artifacts because it distorts the data obtained at each projection. Desirable characteristics for SPECT are an intrinsic spatial resolution of 3 mm, linearity distortion of 1 mm or less, uncorrected field uniformity within 3%, and corrected field uniformity within 1%.

All contemporary rotational SPECT systems have online uniformity and energy correction. Again, nonlinearities in photomultiplier tube energy response degrade both gamma camera energy resolution and spatial resolution. Degraded energy resolution is devastating, for 35% or more of recorded events can represent Compton-scattered photons. Poor energy resolution translates directly into degraded spatial resolution through reduced ability to reject scattered photons on the basis of pulse height analysis. It also degrades spatial resolution through decreased accuracy of determining x and y event localization coordinates.

Image data acquisition   Box 2-2 summarizes factors that must be considered in performing rotational SPECT. In addition to standard gamma camera quality control, it is important to confirm that the axis of rotation corresponds to the center of the matrix in the computer. Incorrect alignment results in a blurring of the image or a reduction in resolution and can even produce ring artifacts in the CT images.

Collimator selection is generally limited by the system vendor. For a given septal thickness and hole diameter, collimators with longer channels have higher resolution and lower sensitivity. Two special collimator options are available for imaging the brain: (1) angled collimators allow the camera head to be maintained closer to the patient, and (2) special fan beam collimators permit more of the camera crystal to be used for radiation detection.

In general, considerations for energy window settings are also similar for rotational SPECT and conventional imaging. If a gamma camera has sufficiently high perfor-

mance and good enough on-line correction circuitry, it may be feasible to use an asymmetric window. The window is offset to the high-energy side and may additionally be narrowed to 10% to 15%, versus the usual 20% for planar or SPECT imaging with older cameras.

The orbit selected will depend on the organ of interest and on whether the particular system being used offers noncircular orbit capability. An orbit should be chosen that keeps the gamma camera head as close to the organ of interest as possible, because resolution is best at the face of the collimator for parallel hole collimators.

For most clinical applications, matrix sizes of 64 × 64 or 128 × 128 are selected. For these matrices and a 15-inch-diameter large field of view camera the respective pixel sizes are roughly 6 × 6 mm and 3 × 3 mm. The exact pixel size will vary depending on the adjustment of the camera and the computer.

Angular sampling requirements can be looked at both theoretically and empirically. The most common angular sampling increment used clinically is around 6° with 60 to 64 projections in the data, for a 360° arc. For a given time period of data collection, multiheaded cameras offer the opportunity to collect either more angular projections or greater counting statistics in each image.

For cardiac studies, there has been a debate in the literature over the merits of 180° versus 360° rotation. A minimum of 180° is necessary for true transaxial tomography. Proponents of this approach argue that because the heart is close to the anterior chest wall, the available imaging time is best spent in a 180° arc from 135° left posterior oblique to 45° right anterior oblique. It should be noted again that overall imaging time is a factor with Tl-201, for it undergoes continuous internal redistribution. The 180° arc strategy has now been adopted for single-headed rotational SPECT systems. Multiheaded cameras render the 180° versus 360° question somewhat moot and provide more counting statistics in shorter time. For virtually all noncardiac applications, a full 360° acquisition is necessary for optimum results, whether single- or multiheaded systems are used.

Apart from the problem with tracers such as Tl-201 and Tc-99m-teboroxime that undergo rapid internal redistribution, the length of time devoted to each angular acquisition and for total imaging is a trade-off between counting statistics and the ability of the patient to cooperate with the procedure. It is desirable to keep total imaging time below 10 minutes for Tl-201 because of internal redistribution. For an agent such as Tc-99m-teboroxime, the imaging time must be even shorter, on the order of a few minutes. The biological half-life of Tc-99m-teboroxime in the heart is only 5 to 10 minutes.

For radiopharmaceuticals where the internal redistribution is not a factor, the major limitation in data acquisition is the ability of the patient to remain still. Within accepted limits for dosimetry and radiation exposure, the

---

Box 2-2   Image Acquisition Issues for Rotational SPECT

Center of rotation check
Collimator selection
Energy window selection
Orbit
Matrix size
Angular increment—number of views 180° vs. 360° rotation
Time per view
Total examination time
Patient factors

larger the administered dosage, the more counts are available. Although clinically accepted limits for administered radioactivity should never be exceeded, the radiation risk versus benefit must always take into account the likelihood of obtaining a diagnostic-quality image. The goal of obtaining higher counting statistics is meaningless if the patient moves so that data between the different angular sampling views are misregistered. Attempts have been made to register data after acquisition by using fiducial markers, but in practice this is cumbersome. To ensure patient compliance, it is worthwhile taking time during setup to position the patient comfortably. For scans of the head the patient's arms can be in a natural position at the sides. For rotational SPECT studies of the heart, thorax, abdomen, or pelvis, the arms typically are raised out of the field of view so that they do not interfere with the path of photons toward the detector. In all applications, it is important to keep the injection site out of the field of view to avoid artifacts resulting from residual or infiltrated activity (Figure 2-25).

Image processing and reconstruction Before initiating SPECT image reconstruction, it is useful to view the angular projections in a cinematic closed loop display. Excessive patient motion is readily detected in this

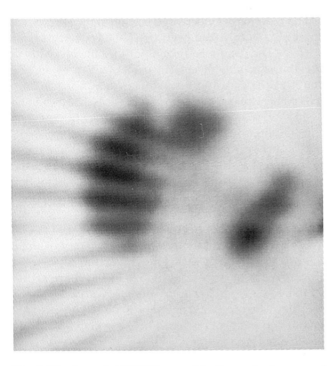

Fig. 2-25 Degraded SPECT image of the liver and spleen caused by focal activity at the injection site left in the field of view during imaging. The starburst artifact is due to backprojection of the hot spot activity across the image. In this particular case the degree of activity in the injection site could not be accommodated in the reconstruction algorithm.

way and attempts can be made to reregister the data. Some laboratories use radioactive marker sources placed on the patient to help in motion assessment. Cinematic displays also give a pseudo-three-dimensional quality to the data and can be very helpful in developing an overall orientation to structures in the field of view. Lesions such as hemangiomas of the liver are readily identified on such a display, for example.

In modern gamma cameras, corrections for field uniformity and linearity are performed event by event during imaging, and the center of rotation correction should be made before data acquisition. In a properly tuned system, no preprocessing corrections are necessary for these factors.

Each commercially available SPECT system takes a somewhat different and proprietary approach to the actual image reconstruction process. They have the use of backprojection and filtering in common. The concept of backprojection is that each pixel in the individual raw data images represents the cumulative activity from a ray projecting through the object, and perpendicular to the camera face. Simplistically, in backprojection the recorded values for each ray from all sampling angles are added together at their intersections in the tomographic image plane. That is, at each pixel in the tomographic image plane, rays from all of the angular projections intersect, and the count value given to the pixel is the sum of the values of all the rays intersecting at that point (Figure 2-26A,B). Although this is a gross oversimplification of the actual mathematics of backprojection, it provides an intuitive way for thinking about the process. "Hot spots" are associated with high count values in the backprojected rays intersecting at them (Figure 2-26A,B). Cold spots do not contribute to counts in the individual ray projections, and the value of the corresponding summation is less.

All reconstruction techniques make use of a special data processing technique called filtering. Filters are almost an art form in themselves and have been designed for enhancement of desired characteristics in the image such as background subtraction, edge enhancement, and suppression of statistical noise. Ramp filters are designed to reduce background activity but may cause ring artifacts. Low-pass filters selectively let through low frequencies and filter out high frequencies in the data; the opposite applies for high-pass filters. In practice, filters combining several features are typically used. Low-pass filters tend to smooth images, with resulting loss of resolution and edge definition. High-pass filters preserve resolution but tend to result in noisier images. Selection of a filter depends on the imaging study being performed and to some extent on observer preference. A balance between image contrast, resolution, and noise is sought (Figure 2-27).

Attenuation correction One of the special problems of SPECT is the attenuation of radiation in tissue.

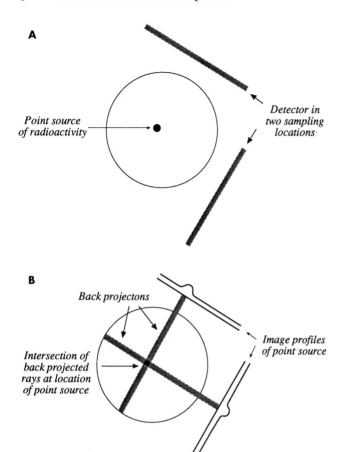

Fig. 2-26   **A**, Point source of radioactivity imaged from two projections. **B**, Simplified schematic of backprojection for two rays obtained at the different sampling angles. The respective counts for the rays are projected for each pixel along their paths. Note the summation at the point of intersection.

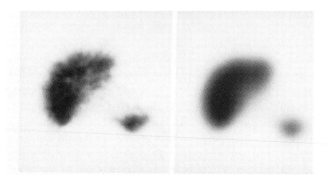

Fig. 2-27   Effect of different filters on the appearance of SPECT liver/spleen images. The filter on the left has resulted in excessive noise texture in the image. The filter on the right has over-smoothed the image, with loss of detail.

Radiation arising deeper within the subject is attenuated to a greater extent than more superficial activity. Even if the overall size of the subject and subject contour are known, it is not possible to directly correct for attenuation because the relative contribution along a projection ray from different depths is not known. However, after an initial reconstruction has been performed, some estimate of relative count rate is available from each point in the tomographic image. Corrections can then be made based on pixel location and the absorption factor in tissue for the gamma ray being used. For example, the half value thickness for the 140 keV photons of Tc-99m in soft tissue is 4.5 cm. In a "perfect" system an observed count at that depth would have to be doubled to correct for attenuation.

Transaxial and other views   One of the particular advantages of gamma camera rotational SPECT is that a volume of image data is collected simultaneously. This permits multiple tomographic slices to be obtained simultaneously with registration of the data between planes. In addition to the standard transaxial images, it is frequently useful to reconstruct other image planes that have special relevance to the organ of interest.

The resorting or reformatting approach is particularly valuable in cardiac imaging. The heart is variably oriented from patient to patient. In shorter subjects, it usually has a horizontal orientation and in taller subjects a more vertical orientation. Ideally, one would like to look at image planes both perpendicular and parallel to the long axis of the heart. This is readily accomplished with a volume data set. The computer operator defines the geometry of the long axis of the heart. The computer is programmed to resort the data to create cardiac long-axis and short-axis planes oblique to the transaxial slices. The optimum angulation is highly variable between patients, reflecting the differing orientations of their hearts.

Another very useful strategy is to reproject the tomographic data as a sequence of planar images having the same fields of view as the original angled sampling images. One advantage of using the reconstructed data is that overlying structures can be removed before the data are reprojected and selected features in the data can be emphasized. For example, in Tc-99m-pyrophosphate imaging of the heart the ribs can be subtracted from the three-dimensional data set before the data are reprojected. The ribs no longer obscure the cardiac activity. Another advantage of using reprojection versus tomographic images is to provide a better overall orientation of the heart in the chest.

Another important example is the reprojection of data from skeletal scintigrams. One strategy is to reproject the hottest point along each perpendicular ray. The reprojected images then emphasize areas of abnormally increased accumulation while again providing a better overall orientation of the abnormality to the skeleton.

Looking at individual transaxial tomograms can be very confusing without knowing where a lesion is relative to surrounding structures.

Quality assurance Rotational SPECT requires maximum gamma camera performance. All standard quality control procedures are observed, as well as several additional points (Box 2-3). The alignment of the detector, gantry, and imaging table is critical. In transaxial rotation the basic assumption is that the face of the collimator is truly perpendicular to the axis of rotation. If it is off-axis, the tilted field of view of the collimator will result in misregistered data.

The gamma camera–computer interface is also particularly critical in rotational SPECT. The pixel size must be carefully calibrated. Attenuation correction depends on depth estimates, and a change in pixel size will change distance and therefore attenuation correction factors. Pixel size is adjusted by the setting of the analog-to-digital converters and should be checked in both the x and y dimensions. Pixel width should be identical in the x and y directions. The y-axis determines slice thickness, and a difference in x and y pixel dimensions will create problems in reformatting image data into oblique planes. The importance of the center of rotation was discussed earlier. A shift in the performance of the analog-to-digital converters can result in movement of the center of rotation.

Uniformity corrections are critical in SPECT imaging. Detector non-uniformity results in bull's-eye or ring artifacts. The usual 1,000,000 to 5,000,000 count flood obtained for planar imaging is inadequate for uniformity correction in SPECT imaging. For large field of view cameras and a 64×64 matrix, 30,000,000 counts are acquired, or roughly 10,000 counts per pixel in the image to achieve the desired percent relative standard deviation of 1%.

$$\%SD = \frac{100}{\sqrt{10,000}} = 1\%$$

Acquiring this number of counts requires a significant amount of time. The temptation to use very large amounts of radioactivity should be avoided, because high count rates can be associated with changes in the performance of gamma camera electronics and can result in recording spurious coincidence events. The radioactivity in the flood itself must have a uniformity within 1% as well. Water-filled sources are subject to problems of incomplete mixing and introduction of air bubbles, as well as physical bulging of the container. Cobalt-57 sheet sources are more convenient and more reliable than water-filled sources for these reasons.

Positron Emission Tomography

Positron emission tomography (PET) is a special kind of tomography made possible by the unique fate of positrons. When positrons undergo annihilation by combining with negatively charged electrons, two 511 keV gamma rays are given off in opposite directions 180° apart. In PET imaging, instead of detecting single events, two detectors on opposite sides of the subject are used to detect these paired annihilation photons (Figure 2-28). PET imaging cannot be performed with conventional gamma cameras; specially designed instrumentation is required.

Instrumentation Instrumentation for PET has undergone several generations of development. Current clinical systems have multiple rings of detectors so that multiple tomographic planes over a continuous volume of tissue in the patient can be imaged simultaneously. Detectors on opposite sides of the patient are paired (Figure 2-28). Special circuitry allows detection of coincidence events from the two gamma ray photons given off by a single annihilation event. Thus the geometry of the detector ring defines a tomographic plane of interest. This detector geometry suppresses contribution from extraneous and scattered radiation. The detectors are also shielded from the sides to further reduce activity from outside the plane of interest. Even if such activity is not recorded as a coincidence event, it requires electronic processing and potential dead time in the system.

Box 2-3 Selected Quality Assurance Issues in SPECT

PARAMETER	COMMENT
Center of rotation	Center of rotation should match center of image matrix in the computer; look for horizontal shift on x-axis
Pixel size	x and y dimensions should be equal; any change in pixel size requires recalibration of attenuation correction factors
Uniformity	3M counts for routine intrinsic and extrinsic uniformity checks 30M counts for input for uniformity correction
Spatial resolution and linearity	Weekly per usual gamma camera quality control

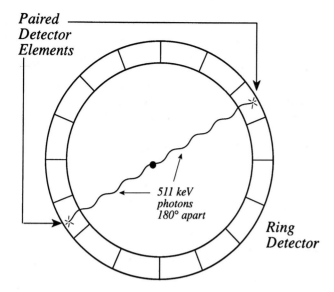

Paired Detector Elements

Ring Detector

511 keV photons 180° apart

Fig. 2-28 Simplified schematic of a ring detector system for positron emission tomography. The detection of two 511 keV annihilation photons is illustrated.

Similar to the history of x-ray CT and magnetic resonance imaging, the first ring PET scanners were designed for head imaging and had a typical diameter of 60 cm. The typical diameter for a body tomographic scanner is 100 cm.

The density and effective atomic number, Z, for NaI (Tl) crystals are not ideal for detecting the 511 keV gamma rays used in PET imaging. Bismuth germanate is approximately twice as dense, with an effective Z of 74, compared with an effective Z of 50 for NaI (Tl). Bismuth germanate detectors have been used extensively in PET imaging applications for this reason. Other detector materials that have found application include cesium fluoride and barium fluoride. These have much faster time resolution than bismuth germanate but are not as dense.

The spatial resolution of modern PET tomographs is excellent. Specialized experimental devices approach 3-mm resolution (FWHM) as measured by a line source in air. Resolution under clinical scanning conditions is superior to single photon planar or SPECT imaging.

The ultimate spatial resolution of PET is limited by two physical phenomena related to positrons and their annihilations. First, positrons are given off at different kinetic energies. Energetic positrons such as those given off in the decay of O-15, Ga-68, and Rb-82 may travel several millimeters in tissue before undergoing annihilation. Thus the detected location of the annihilation event is some distance from the actual location of the radionuclide. This travel in tissue degrades the ability to truly localize the biodistribution of the radioactive agent in the patient.

The second phenomenon is the noncolinearity of the annihilation photons. In addition to the energy equiva-

lent of the rest mass of two electrons, the annihilation event incorporates residual kinetic energies of the positron and the negative electron with which it combines. This results in a small deviation from true colinearity along a single ray. The angle by which the gamma rays depart from the theoretical 180° colinearity results in a 2- to 3-mm spatial uncertainty in event localization for head and body ring detectors used clinically.

Image reconstruction in PET uses many of the same principles as SPECT. Filtered backprojection and iterative reconstruction algorithms have both found application.

Attenuation correction and quantitative analysis A unique and important characteristic of PET imaging is the ability to correct for attenuation of the 511 keV gamma rays in tissue. The basis of this ability is the fact that attenuation and therefore coincidence detection of positron annihilation are independent of the location along a given ray between opposed detectors. The correction factor for each coincidence line can be determined empirically by performing a transmission scan. The observed count rate obtained along each ray during the actual scan is corrected by dividing it by the attenuation factor. This approach to attenuation correction assumes that the patient does not move between the transmission scan and the emission scan. The transmission scan must have sufficient counting statistics to avoid introducing statistical error into the data.

The ability to correct for attenuation improves the quality of PET images and permits absolute quantification of radioactivity in the body. Quantitative analysis is the basis for numerous metabolic, perfusion, and biodistribution measurements. For example, a therapeutic drug can be radiolabeled with a positron-emitting radionuclide. By knowing the specific activity of the radiolabeled drug and by being able to correct for attenuation, the absolute uptake and distribution of the drug can be quantitatively measured. Box 2-4 summarizes several of the important quantitative measurements used in applications of PET imaging.

Box 2-4 Selected Quantitative Measurements by Positron Emission Tomography

Regional (absolute) radionuclide localization
pH
Blood flow
Blood volume
Oxygen extraction fraction
Oxygen metabolism
Glucose metabolism
Receptor binding and occupancy

SUGGESTED READINGS

Croft BY: *Single-photon emission computed tomography,* Chicago, 1986, Year Book Medical Publishers.

Esser PD, editor: *Emission computed tomography: current trends,* New York, 1983, Society of Nuclear Medicine.

Freeman LM and Blauflox MD, editors: Positron emission tomography: part I, *Semin Nucl Med* 22:140-201, 1992.

Freeman LM and Blauflox MD, editors: Positron emission tomography: part II, *Semin Nucl Med* 22:210-288, 1992.

Hendee WR: *Medical radiation physics,* ed 3, St Louis, 1992, Mosby Yearbook.

Herman GT, editor: *Image reconstruction from projections: implementation and applications,* New York, 1979, Springer-Verlag.

Johns HE and Cunningham JR: *The physics of radiology,* ed 4, Chicago, 1983, Thomas Books.

Patton JA and Rollo FD: Basic physics of radionuclide imaging. In Freeman LM, editor: *Freeman and Johnson's clinical radionuclide imaging,* ed 3, New York, 1984, Grune and Stratton.

Phelps ME, Mazziotta JC, and Schelbert HR, editors: *Positron emission tomography and autoradiography: Principles and application for the brain and heart,* New York, 1986, Raven Press.

Reivich M and Alavi A, editors: *Positron emission tomography,* New York, 1985, Alan R Liss.

Rollo FD, editor: *Nuclear medicine physics, instrumentation and agents,* St Louis, 1977, CV Mosby.

Simmons GH: *The scintillation camera,* New York, 1988, Society of Nuclear Medicine.

Sorenson JA and Phelps ME: *Physics in nuclear medicine,* ed 2, Philadelphia, 1987, WB Saunders.

CHAPTER 3

Nuclear Pharmacy

The richness of diagnostic capability in nuclear medicine rests largely on the diversity of available radiopharmaceuticals. In some sense, the "best" radiopharmaceuticals are those that provide a true portrayal of the physiologic or pathologic system under investigation. The historical term "tracer" is actually a rather good one because it implies the ability to study or follow a process without disturbing the process. Radiopharmaceuticals have the highly desirable property that they do not perturb function, unlike some other types of diagnostic drugs, including iodinated x-ray contrast media, that have profound physiologic effects when administered intravascularly.

Most radiopharmaceuticals are a combination of a radioactive moiety that permits external detection and a biologically active moiety that is responsible for biodistribution. For a few agents such as the radioactive inert gases, the radioiodines, gallium-67, and thallium-201, the radioactive atoms themselves confer the desired localization properties and a larger chemical moiety is not required. Box 3-1 summarizes some of the important mechanisms of localization for radiopharmaceuticals used in clinical practice. Understanding the mechanism or rationale for the use of each agent is critical to understanding the normal and pathologic findings demonstrated scintigraphically. There is great flexibility in designing radiopharmaceuticals for specific diagnostic purposes because it is possible to radiolabel both naturally occurring molecules and synthetic molecules.

Radiopharmaceuticals for each major clinical application will be considered in detail in the discussion of the respective organ systems. This chapter presents some of the general principles of radiopharmaceutical production, radiolabeling, quality assurance, and dispensing.

TERMINOLOGY: RADIOPHARMACEUTICALS, RADIOCHEMICALS, AND RADIONUCLIDES

The terminology in nuclear pharmacy can be quite confusing. The term *radionuclide* refers only to the radioactive atoms. When a radionuclide is combined with a chemical molecule to confer desired localization properties, the combination is referred to as a *radiochemical*.

Box 3-1   Mechanisms of Radiopharmaceutical Localization

MECHANISM	APPLICATIONS/EXAMPLES
Compartmental localization	Blood pool imaging
	Direct cystography
Passive diffusion	Blood-brain barrier breakdown
(concentration dependent)	Glomerular filtration
	Cisternography
Capillary blockade	Arterial perfusion imaging
(physical entrapment)	
Physical leakage from a luminal	Gastrointestinal bleeding, detection of urinary tract or biliary system leak-
age	
compartment	
Metabolism	Glucose, fatty acids
Active transport	Hepatobiliary imaging, renal tubular function, thyroid and adrenal imaging
(active cellular uptake)	
Chemical bonding/adsorption	Skeletal imaging
Cell sequestration	Splenic imaging (heat-damaged RBCs), WBCs
Receptor binding/storage	Numerous PET applications, adrenal medullary imaging
Phagocytosis	Reticuloendothelial system imaging
Antigen/antibody	Tumor imaging

COMBINED MECHANISMS	APPLICATIONS/EXAMPLES
Perfusion and active transport	Myocardial imaging
Active transport and metabolism	Thyroid uptake and imaging

The term *radiopharmaceutical* is reserved for those radioactive materials that have met legal requirements for administration to patients or subjects. This often requires the addition of stabilizing and buffering agents to the basic radiochemical and requires approval in the United States by the Food and Drug Administration (FDA) before an agent is acceptable for routine clinical use.

The term *carrier-free* implies that a radionuclide is not contaminated by either stable or radioactive nuclides of the same element. The presence of carrier material can influence biodistribution and efficiency of radio-labeling. The term *specific activity* refers to the radioactivity per unit weight (mCi/mg). Carrier-free samples of a radionuclide have the highest specific activity. This term should not be confused with *specific concentration*, which is defined as activity per unit volume (mCi/mL).

PRODUCTION OF RADIONUCLIDES

All radionuclides in clinical use today are produced in either nuclear reactors or cyclotrons or other types of accelerators. Naturally occurring radionuclides have long half-lives and are heavy, toxic elements; they include uranium, actinium, thorium, radium and radon. They have no clinical role in diagnostic nuclear medicine.

Bombardment of medium atomic weight nuclides with low-energy neutrons in nuclear reactors results in neutron-rich radionuclides that typically undergo beta minus decay. This reaction is referred to as *neutron activation*. Since the daughter product is the same element, it is not possible to separate the radioactive and stable atoms, typically resulting in a low specific activity product with significant *carrier* from the original target material. Neutron activation of molybdenum-98 was the original production method used to obtain Mo-99 for Mo-99/Tc-99m generator systems.

Neutron bombardment of enriched U-235 results in fission products in the middle of the atomic chart. For example, Mo-99 is now obtained through such a fission reaction. The release of radioactive iodines in atomic bomb explosions and during accidents at nuclear power plants is a well-known phenomenon that can also be used for production purposes in a nuclear reactor.

Proton bombardment of a wide variety of target nuclides in cyclotrons or other special accelerators produces proton-rich radionuclides that undergo positron decay or electron capture. Tables 3-1 and 3-2 summarize the production source and physical characteristics of commonly used radionuclides in clinical nuclear medicine practice.

Table 3-1   Physical Characteristics of Radionuclides Used in Clinical Nuclear Medicine: Single Photon Radionuclides

Radionuclide	Principal Modes of Decay	Physical Half-life	Principal Photon Energy (keV) and Abundance (%)	Production Method
Mo-99	β−	2.8 d	740 (12) 780 (4)	Reactor
Tc-99m	IT	6 hr	140 (89)	Generator (Mo-99)
I-131	β−	8.0 d	364 (81)	Reactor
I-123	EC	13.2 hr	159 (83)	Accelerator
Ga-67	EC	78.3 hr	93 (37) 185 (20) 300 (17) 395 (5)	Accelerator
Tl-201	EC	73.1 hr	69 (73) Hg x-rays 81 (20) Hg x-rays 135 (2.5) 167 (10)	Accelerator
In-111	EC	2.8 d	171 (90) 245 (94)	Accelerator
Xe-127	EC	36 d	172 (26) 203 (7) 375 (17)	Accelerator
Xe-133	β−	5.2 d	81 (37)	Reactor

Table 3-2   Physical Characteristics of Radionuclides Used in Nuclear Medicine: Positron-Emitting (Dual Photon) Radionuclides

Radionuclide	Physical Half-life (min)	Positron Energy (MeV)	Range in Soft tissue (mm)	Production Method
C-11	20	0.96	4.1	Accelerator
N-13	10	1.19	5.4	Accelerator
O-15	2	1.73	7.3	Accelerator
F-18	110	0.635	2.4	Accelerator
Ga-68	68	1.9	8.1	Generator (Ge-68)
Rb-82	1.3	3.15	15.0	Generator (Sr-82)

RADIONUCLIDE GENERATORS

One of the practical issues faced in nuclear medicine is the desirability of using relatively short-lived agents (hours versus days or weeks) and at the same time the need to have radiopharmaceuticals delivered to hospitals or clinics from commercial sources. One way around this dilemma is the use of radionuclide generator systems. These sys-tems consist of a longer-lived parent and a shorter-lived daughter. This combination of half-lives allows for the logistics of shipping the generator from a commercial vendor while still being able to use a daughter product with a reasonable half-life for clinical applications. Although a number of generator systems have been explored over the years (Table 3-3), the most important generator is the Mo-99/Tc-99m system, which is ubiquitous in the practice of clinical nuclear medicine (Table 3-4).

Table 3-3	Radionuclide Generator Systems and Parent/Daughter Half-lives		
Parent	$T_{1/2}$	**Daughter**	$T_{1/2}$
Mo-99	66 hr	Tc-99m	6 hr
Rb-81	4.5 hr	Kr-81m	13 sec
Ge-68	270 d	Ga-68	68 min
Sr-82	25 d	Rb-82	1.3 min
Sn-113	115 d	In-113m	1.7 hr
Y-87	3.3 d	Sr-87m	2.8 hr
Te-132	3.2 d	I-132	2.3 hr

Table 3-4	Mo-99/Tc-99m Generator Systems	
	Parent Mo-99	**Daughter** Tc-99m
RADIONUCLIDES		
Half-life	66 hr	6 hr
Mode of decay	β^-	Isomeric transition
Daughter products	Tc-99m Tc-99	Tc-99
Principal photon energies	740 keV* 780 keV	140 keV (89%)
GENERATOR FUNCTION		
Composition of ion exchange column		Al_2O_3
Eluant		Normal saline (0.9%)
Time for elution to maximum daughter yield		23 hr

* The decay scheme for Mo-99 is actually very complex, with over 35 gamma rays of different energies given off. The listed energies are those used in clinical practice for radionuclidic purity checks.

MOLYBDENUM-99/TECHNETIUM-99m GENERATOR SYSTEMS

The historic production method of Mo-99 was a neutron activation reaction on Mo-98:

$$Mo\text{-}98\ (n,\gamma) \rightarrow Mo\text{-}99.$$

This production method results in low specific activity, requiring a large ion exchange column to hold both the desired Mo-99 and the carrier Mo-98 left over from the target material. The low specific activity column resulted in low specific concentrations of technetium-99m pertechnetate from generator elution due to the larger volume of eluant needed to completely remove the Tc-99m activity.

Mo-99 is now produced by the fission of uranium-235 (often referred to casually as "fission moly"). The reaction is:

$$U\text{-}235\ (n,fission) \rightarrow Mo\text{-}99.$$

After Mo-99 is produced in the fission reaction it is chemically purified and passed on to an anion exchange column composed of alumina (Al_2O_3) (Table 3-4). The column is typically adjusted to an acid pH to promote binding. The positive charge of the alumina binds the molybdate ions firmly.

The loaded column is placed in a lead container with tubing attached at each end to permit column elution. Commercial generator systems are autoclaved and the elution dynamics quality controlled before shipment.

Generator Operation and Yield

Figure 3-1 illustrates the relationship between Mo-99 decay and the in-growth of Tc-99m. Maximum buildup of Tc-99m activity occurs at 23 hours post elution. This is very convenient, especially if sufficient Tc-99m activity is available to accomplish each day's work. Otherwise the generator can be eluted or "milked" more than once a day. This is also illustrated in Figure 3-1. Fifty percent of maximum is reached in approximately 4.5 hours and 75% of maximum is available at 8.5 hours.

Although most attention is usually paid to the rate of Tc-99m buildup, it should also be remembered that Tc-99m is constantly decaying, with buildup of Tc-99 in the generator. Generators received after commercial shipment or generators that have not been eluted for several days over a weekend have significant carrier Tc-99 in the eluate. Because the carrier Tc-99 behaves chemically in an identical fashion to Tc-99m, it can adversely affect radiopharmaceutical labeling. Many labeling procedures require the reduction of Tc-99m from a +7 valence state to a lower valence state. If there is sufficient carrier Tc-99 in the eluate, complete reduction may not occur, with resultant poor labeling and undesired radiochemical contaminants in the final preparation.

There are two basic types of generator systems with respect to elution. "Wet" systems are provided with a reservoir of normal saline (0.9%) (Figure 3-2). Elution is accomplished by placing a special sterile vacuum vial on the exit or collection port. The vacuum vial is designed to draw the appropriate amount of saline across the column.

In "dry" systems, a volume-calibrated saline charge is placed on the entry port and a vacuum vial is placed on the collection port (Figure 3-3). The vacuum draws the saline eluant out of the original vial, across the column, and into the elution vial. Elution volumes are typically in the range of 5 to 20 mL, and partial elutions can be performed for add-on or emergency studies that come up in the course of a day (Figure 3-1).

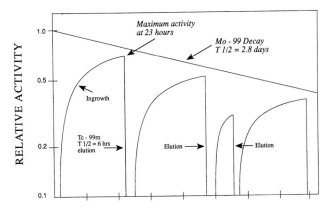

Fig. 3-1 Decay curve for molybdenum-99 and ingrowth curves for technetium-99m illustrating successive elutions including a partial elution. Relative activity is plotted on a log scale accounting for the straight line of molybdenum-99 decay.

"DRY" GENERATOR SYSTEM

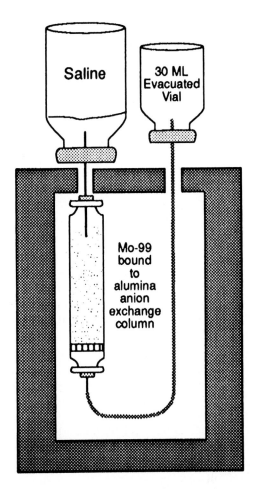

Fig. 3-3 Simplified schematic for a "dry" generator system.

"WET" GENERATOR SYSTEM

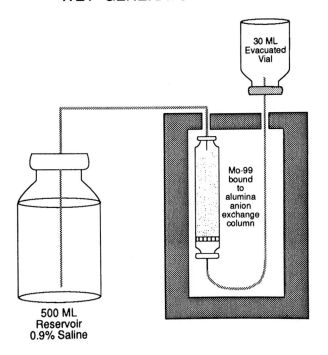

Fig. 3-2 Simplified schematic for a "wet" generator system.

From Figure 3-1 it is obvious that the amount of Tc-99m activity available from a generator decreases each day as a result of decay of the Mo-99 parent. In practice, the 2.8-day half-life of Mo-99 allows generators to be used for a week, although many larger nuclear medicine operations require two generator deliveries per week.

Quality Control

Although generators are rigorously quality controlled prior to commercial shipment, it is important that each laboratory perform quality control steps each time the generator is eluted (Table 3-5). These quality control steps are both good medical practice and necessary to meet various federal and JCAHO regulations and guidelines.

Radionuclidic purity The only desired radionuclide in the Mo-99/Tc-99m generator eluate is Tc-99m. Any other radionuclide in the sample is considered a radionuclidic impurity and is undesirable since it will result in additional radiation exposure to the patient without clinical benefit.

The most common radionuclidic contaminant in the generator eluate is the parent radionuclide, Mo-99. Technetium-99, the daughter product of the isomeric transition

Table 3-5 Purity Checks: Mo-99/Tc-99m Generator Systems

	Problem	Standard
Radionuclide purity	Excessive Mo-99 in eluant	< 0.15 μCi Mo-99/mCi Tc-99m *at time of dosage administration*
Chemical purity	Al$_2$O$_3$ from generator ion exchange column in elution	< 10μg/mL (fission generator) (aurin tricarboxylic acid spot test)
Radiochemical purity	Reduced oxidation states of Tc-99m (i.e., +4, +5, or +6 instead of +7)	95% of Tc-99m activity should be in +7 oxidation state

Table 3-6 Technetium 99m; Physical Decay Chart

Time (hr)	Fraction Remaining
0	1.000
1	.891
2	.794
3	.708
4	.631
5	.532
6	.501
7	.447
8	.398
9	.355
10	.316
11	.282
12	.251

Tc-99m physical half-life = 6.02 hours.

of Tc-99m, is also present but is not considered an impurity or contaminant. Although Tc-99 can be a problem from a chemical standpoint in radiolabeling procedures, it is not a problem from a radiation or health physics standpoint and is not tested for as a radionuclidic impurity. The half-life of Tc-99 is 2.1 × 10^5 years. It decays to ruthenium-99, which is stable.

The amount of Mo-99 in the eluate is subject to limits set by the Nuclear Regulatory Commission (NRC) and must be tested on each elution. Perhaps the easiest and most widely used approach is to take advantage of the energetic 740 keV and 780 keV gamma rays of Mo-99 with dual counting of the specimen. In brief, the generator eluate is placed in a lead container carefully designed so that all of the 140 keV photons of technetium are absorbed but approximately 50% of the more energetic Mo-99 gamma rays can penetrate. Adjusting the dose calibrator to the Mo-99 setting provides an estimate of the number of microcuries of Mo-99 in the sample. The unshielded sample is then measured on the Tc-99m setting and a ratio of Mo-99 to Tc-99m activity can be calculated.

The NRC limit is 0.15 μCi of Mo-99 activity per 1.0 mCi of Tc-99m activity in the *administered* dose (Table 3-5). Because the half-life of Mo-99 is longer than that of Tc-99m, the ratio actually increases with time. This is rarely a problem, but if the initial reading shows near maximum Mo-99 levels, either the actual dose to be given to the patient should be restudied prior to administration or the buildup factor should be computed mathematically. From a practical standpoint, the Mo-99 activity may be taken as unchanged and the Tc-99m decay calculated (Table 3-6). With modern generators, breakthrough is rare but unpredictable. When it does occur, Mo-99 levels can be far higher than the legal limit.

Chemical purity   Another routine quality assurance step is to measure the generator eluate for the presence of the column packing material, Al$_2$O$_3$. For fission generators the maximum alumina concentration is 10 μg/mL. Aurin tricarboxylic acid is used for colorimetric spot testing. The color reaction for a standard 10 μg/mL sample of alumina is compared with a corresponding sample from the generator eluate. Acceptable levels are present if the color is less intense than the color of the standard. The comparison is made visually and qualitatively. No attempt is made to measure the alumina concentration quantitatively. Aluminum levels in excess of this limit have been shown to interfere with the normal distribution of certain radiopharmaceuticals such as Tc-99m sulfur colloid (increased lung activity) and Tc-MDP (increased liver activity).

Radiochemical purity   The expected valence state of Tc-99m, as eluated from the generator, is +7 in the chemical form of pertechnetate (TcO$_4$−). The clinical use of sodium pertechnetate as a radiopharmaceutical and the preparation of Tc-99m-labeled pharmaceuticals, typically from commercial kits, is predicated on the +7 oxidation state. The U.S. Pharmacopeia standard for the generator eluate is that 95% or more of Tc-99m activity be in this +7 state. Reduction states at +4, +5, or +6 may be present and are detected by various thin-layer chromatography systems. In practice, problems with radiochemical purity of the generator eluate are not frequently encountered but should be considered if kit labeling is poor.

TECHNETIUM CHEMISTRY AND RADIOPHARMACEUTICAL PREPARATION

Technetium-99m has become the most commonly used radionuclide based on its ready availability, the favorable energy of its principal gamma photon, its favorable dosimetry with lack of primary particulate radiations, and its nearly ideal half life for many clinical imaging studies. On the other hand, technetium chemistry is challenging. In most labeling procedures technetium must be reduced from the +7 valence state. In current practice the reduction is usually accomplished with stannous ion.

The actual final oxidation state of technetium in many radiopharmaceuticals is either unknown or subject to debate. A number of technetium compounds are chelates, and others are used on the basis of their empirical efficacy without complete knowledge of how technetium is being complexed in the final molecule. One exception to the need to reduce technetium from the +7 oxidation state is in the preparation of Tc-99m sulfur colloid.

The details of individual technetium radiopharmaceuticals are discussed in the organ system chapters, including key points in preparation and the recognition of in vivo markers of radiopharmaceutical impurities. Box 3-2 summarizes the major Tc-99m-labeled agents that are used clinically.

The introduction of stannous ion for reducing technetium in radiolabeling procedures was a major break-through in nuclear medicine. Commercial kits contain a reaction vial with the appropriate amount of stannous ion, the nonradioactive pharmaceutical to be labeled, and other buffering and stabilizing agents. The vials are typically flushed with nitrogen to prevent atmospheric oxygen from interrupting the reaction. Figure 3-4 illustrates the sequence of steps in a sample labeling process. In brief, sodium pertechnetate is drawn into a syringe and assayed in the dose calibrator. After the proper Tc-99m activity is confirmed, the sample is added to the reaction vial. The amount of Tc-99m activity added for each respective product is determined by the number of patient doses desired in the case of a multidose vial, an estimate of the decrease in radioactivity due to decay between the time of preparation and the estimated time of dosage administration, and the in vitro stability of the product. The completed product is labeled and kept in a special lead-shielded container until it is time to withdraw a sample for administration to a patient. Each patient dosage is individually assayed prior to dispensing.

Excessive oxygen can react directly with the stannous ion, thereby leaving too little reducing power in the kit.

Box 3-2   Tc-99m Radiopharmaceuticals

AGENT	APPLICATION
Tc-99m-Sodium pertechnetate	Meckel's diverticulum detection
	Salivary gland scintigraphy
	Thyroid gland scintigraphy
	(Brain scintigraphy)
Tc-99m-Sulfur colloid	Liver/spleen scintigraphy (RES)
	GI bleeding detection
	Bone marrow scintigraphy
Tc-99m-Pyrophosphate	Acute myocardial infarction detection
	(Skeletal scintigraphy)
Tc-99m-Diphosphonate	Skeletal scintigraphy
Tc-99m-Macroaggregated albumin	Pulmonary perfusion scintigraphy
	Periperal and regional (e.g., liver) arterial perfusion scintigraphy
Tc-99m-Red blood cells	Radionuclide ventriculography
	GI bleeding detection
	Hepatic hemangioma detection
Tc-99m-Human serum albumin	Blood pool imaging (e.g., radionuclide ventriculography)
Tc-99m-DTPA (pentetate), (diethylenetriamine-pentaacetic acid)	Renal and urinary tract scintigraphy (GFR) (Brain scintigraphy)
Tc-99m MAG$_3$ (mercaptoacetyltriglycine)	Renal scintigraphy
Tc-99m-DMSA (dimercaptosuccinic acid)	Renal cortical scintigraphy
Tc-99m-HIDA and derivatives (hepatic iminodiacidic acid)	Hepatobiliary scintigraphy
Tc-99m-Sestamibi	Myocardial perfusion scintigraphy
Tc-99m-Teboroxime	Myocardial perfusion scintigraphy
TC-99m-HMPAO (hexamethyl propyleneamineoxime)	Cerebral perfusion scintigraphy

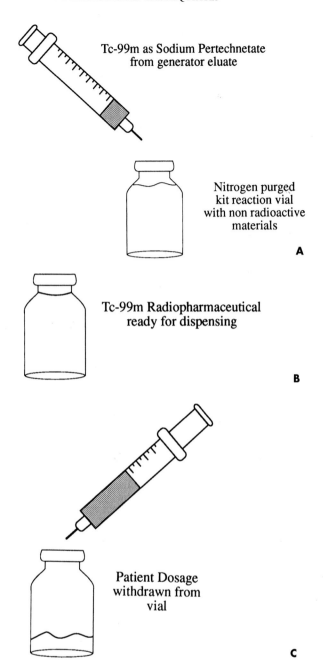

Tc-99m as Sodium Pertechnetate from generator eluate

Nitrogen purged kit reaction vial with non radioactive materials

A

Tc-99m Radiopharmaceutical ready for dispensing

B

Patient Dosage withdrawn from vial

C

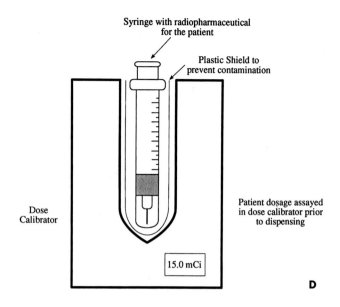

Syringe with radiopharmaceutical for the patient

Plastic Shield to prevent contamination

Dose Calibrator

Patient dosage assayed in dose calibrator prior to dispensing

15.0 mCi

D

Fig. 3-4   Selected steps in the preparation of a technetium-99m labeled radiopharmaceutical. **A**, Tc-99m as sodium pertechnetate is added to the reaction vial. **B**, The Tc-99m radiopharmaceutical is ready for dispensing. **C**, The patient dosage is withdrawn from the vial. **D**, Each patient dosage is measured in the dose calibrator prior to dispensing.

This can result in unwanted free Tc-99m-pertechnetate in the preparation. A less common problem is radiolysis after kit preparation. The phenomenon is seen when high amounts of Tc-99m activity are used. The kit preparations are usually designed so that multiple patient dosages can be prepared from one reaction vial.

QUALITY ASSURANCE OF TECHNETIUM-99m-LABELED RADIOPHARMACEUTICALS

The difficult nature of technetium chemistry highlights the importance of checking the final product for *radiochemical* purity. This term is defined as the percentage of the total radioactivity in a specimen that is in the specified or desired chemical form. For example, if 5% of the Tc-99m activity remains as free pertechnetate in a radiolabeling procedure, the radiochemical purity would be stated as 95%, assuming no other impurities.

For many agents, the presence of a radiochemical impurity can be recognized by altered in vivo biodistribution. However, it is obviously desirable to intercept the offending preparation before administration to a patient. To achieve this, a number of systems have been developed to assay radiochemical purity. The basic approach is to use thin-layer chromatography. There are many commercial products and variations available. In brief, radiochromatography is accomplished in the same manner as conventional chromatography, by spotting a sample of the test material at one end of a strip. A solvent is then selected for which the desired radiochemical and the potential contaminants have known migration patterns. The presence of the radiolabel provides an easy means of quantitatively measuring the migration patterns.

For soluble technetium radiopharmaceuticals, the presence of free pertechnetate and the presence of insoluble, hydrolyzed reduced technetium moieties are tested. For example, free pertechnetate migrates with the solvent front in a paper and thin-layer chromatography system using acetone as the solvent, while Tc-99m-diphosphonate and hydrolyzed reduced technetium remain at the origin (Figure 3-5). To selectively test for hydrolyzed reduced technetium, a silica gel strip is used with saline as the solvent. In this system both free pertechnetate and Tc-99m-diphosphonate move with the solvent front and, again, hydrolyzed reduced technetium stays at the origin (Figure 3-5). This combination of procedures allows each of the three components to be measured. Chromatography systems have been worked out for each major technetium-labeled radiopharmaceutical.

Elaborate systems are available to "read" the chromatography strips. Chromatographic scanners provide detailed strip chart recording of radioactivity distribution. In practice, the easiest way to perform chromatography is simply to cut the chromatography strip into two pieces that can be counted separately.

Chromatography is something of an art form, and a number of common pitfalls must be avoided. Inadvertently immersing the chromatography strip into the solvent past the location of the sample spot results in less migration than expected. Also, if spots are not allowed to dry before being used with organic solvents, spurious migration patterns will occur. On the other hand, excessive delay before starting the chromatogram can result in re-oxidation of the technetium in the sample; again, spurious results will be encountered.

OTHER SINGLE PHOTON AGENTS

Radioiodine-131 as sodium iodide was the first radiopharmaceutical of importance in clinical nuclear medicine. It was used exclusively for studies of the thyroid gland for several years in the late 1940s (Box 3-3). Subsequently I-131 was used as the radiolabel for a wide vari-

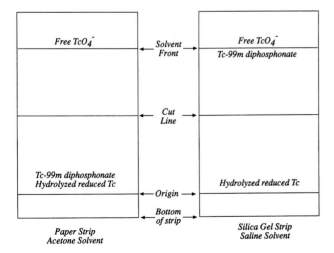

Fig. 3-5 Schematic of a two-part radiochromatography system for the quality control of Tc-99m diphosphonate.

Box 3-3	Radiopharmaceuticals for Single Photon Imaging (Non-Tc-99m)	
AGENT	**APPLICATION**
Tl-201 Thallious chloride	Myocardial perfusion scintigraphy
Ga-67 Gallium citrate	Inflammatory disease detection
	Tumor imaging
Xe-133 Xenon (inert gas)	Pulmonary ventilation scintigraphy
Xe-127 Xenon (inert gas)	Pulmonary ventilation scintigraphy
Kr-81m Krypton (inert gas)	Pulmonary ventilation scintigraphy
I-131 Sodium iodide	Thyroid scintigraphy Thyroid iodine uptake function studies Treatment of hyperthyroidism and thyroid cancer
I-123 Sodium iodide	Thyroid scintigraphy Thyroid iodine uptake function studies
I-131 Hippuran	Renal imaging and function studies
I-123 Hippuran	Renal imaging and function studies
In-111-labeled white blood cells	Inflammatory disease detection
In-111, I-131-labeled antibodies proteins and peptides	Wide variety of receptor binding and tumor localization studies
I-123 Iodoamphetamine	Cerebral perfusion scintigraphy

ety of radiopharmaceuticals, including human serum albumin, macroaggregated albumin, and a number of different antibodies, as well as agents for the kidney (hippuran) and multiple agents for adrenal scintigraphy (metaiodobenzylguanidine and labeled cholesterol derivatives). The disadvantages of I-131 include relatively high principal photon energy (364 keV), long half-life (8 days), and the presence of beta particle emissions. Radioiodine-131 remains an important agent in nuclear medicine practice for the treatment of hyperthyroidism and differentiated thyroid cancer. It also continues to be used for selected diagnostic applications, including antibody labeling and the labeling of adrenal agents.

The quality control of radioiodinated pharmaceuticals is important to reduce unwanted radiation exposure to the thyroid gland. In nonthyroid imaging applications of I-131 as a radiolabel it is common practice to block the thyroid gland with either Lugol's solution or with SSKI.

Whenever possible in contemporary practice, I-123 is substituted for I-131. It has a shorter half-life (Table 3-1) and its principal photon energy of 159 keV is better suited to imaging with the gamma scintillation camera. I-123 decays by electron capture, and the dosimetry is favorable compared to that of I-131. One limitation to the use of I-123 is its relatively high expense and limited availability owing to its short half-life of 13 hours. In some applications with radiolabeled antibodies and adrenal scintigraphy, it is desirable to image over a period of several days, which also represents a limitation of I-123 as compared to I-131.

Another versatile label that has found a variety of applications in clinical nuclear medicine is indium-111 (Box 3-3). Its principal photon energies of 172 keV and 245 keV are favorable compared to I-131. The 2.8-day half-life of In-111 permits multiday sequential imaging, which is commonly used in the evaluation of inflammatory disease (In-111-labeled white blood cells) and in imaging with antibodies.

The discovery that gallium-67 citrate localizes in tumors and inflammatory conditions was fortuitous. Different radionuclides of gallium were initially under evaluation as bone scanning agents. Soft tissue uptake in a patient with Hodgkin's disease was noted incidentally and led to the recognition of its utility as a tumor imaging agent and subsequently its utility for detecting areas of inflammation. In many respects, Ga-67 does not have favorable properties for clinical imaging. For example, the most abundant photon is the lowest energy (Table 3-1). Until gamma cameras became available that had the capability of imaging multiple photopeaks simultaneously, there was no ideal way to image Ga-67. In current practice it is common to bracket the lower three photopeaks (93 keV, 185 keV, 300 keV). Nonetheless, "downscatter" from the higher energies degrades the image data in the lower windows.

Other disadvantages of Ga-67 include slow clearance

from background tissues, necessitating delayed imaging at 24, 48, and even 72 hours or more in some applications. Early excretion (≤ 24 hours) through the kidneys and delayed excretion via the gut make imaging in the abdomen difficult. Care must be taken to interpret the scintigram with a full knowledge of the time following tracer administration at which the study was obtained. Laxatives may be required to clear confusing or obscuring activity from the colon.

Thallium-201 became clinically available in the mid-1970s as an agent for myocardial scintigraphy. Thallium behaves as a potassium analogue, with high net clearance (ca. 85%) in its passage through the myocardial capillary bed. This makes it an excellent marker of regional blood flow to viable myocardium. The major disadvantage of thallium as a radioactive imaging agent is the absence of an ideal photopeak for imaging. The gamma rays at 135 keV and 167 keV occur in low abundance (Table 3-1). In practice, the mercury x-rays at approximately 69 keV and 81 keV are used. The ability of the gamma scintillation camera to discriminate scattered events from primary photons is suboptimal at this energy. Literally from the time of introduction of Tl-201 into clinical practice there has been interest in the nuclear medicine community to find an alternative agent for myocardial perfusion imaging, preferably labeled with Tc-99m. Such agents are now available but have their own limitations, as discussed in the chapter on cardiac imaging.

The radioactive inert gases xenon and krypton are used for pulmonary ventilation imaging. Xenon-133 is a convenient agent to maintain in inventory due to its 5.2 day half-life. The major disadvantage of Xe-133 is the relatively low energy of its principal photon (81 keV). This low energy dictates the performance of ventilation scintigraphy prior to Tc-99m perfusion scintigraphy or the use of cumbersome subtraction techniques. Nonetheless, Xe-133 is still the most commonly used agent based on its ready availability and relatively low price compared to the alternative agents.

Xe-127 is theoretically superior to Xe-133 because of its higher photon energies (Table 3-1). Because its photon energies are higher than that of Tc-99m, it is possible to perform the ventilation portion of a ventilation/perfusion study after the locations of any perfusion defects are known. This allows the examination to be tailored to the findings in individual patients. The high cost of producing Xe-127 has kept it from wide use. For practical purposes, krypton-81m has never progressed beyond evaluation by a few dedicated clinical researchers. It has the potential advantage of allowing virtually continuous imaging. The short half-life of 13 seconds permits multiple views to be obtained without concern for retained activity.

A host of other radionuclides have been used over the years, but the radionuclides summarized in Table 3-1 are the most important in current practice.

RADIOPHARMACEUTICALS FOR POSITRON EMISSION TOMOGRAPHY

The physical characteristics of commonly used positron-emitting radionuclides are summarized in Table 3-2. There are now many dozens of radiopharmaceuticals described for positron emission tomography (PET) (Box 3-4). Carbon, oxygen and nitrogen are found ubiquitously in biological molecules. It is, thus, theoretically possible to radiolabel just about any molecule of biological interest. Fluorine-18 has the advantage of a longer half-life than C-11, N-13, or O-15 and has found use as a label for the glucose analogue F-18 fluorodeoxyglucose. This pharmaceutical has found widespread application in imaging of the brain, the heart, and a wide variety of tumors throughout the body. Tumors derive their energy from glucose metabolism, and the uptake of F-18 fluorodeoxyglucose is a marker of tumor metabolism and viability.

Rubidium-82 is available from a generator system with a relatively long-lived parent (Sr-82, 25 days) (Table 3-3). Rubidium is another potassium analogue and has found application for myocardial perfusion imaging. Its availability from a generator system obviates the need for an on-site cyclotron for production. One limitation of Rb-82 is the high energy (3.15 MeV) of its positron emissions. This high energy results in a relatively long average path in soft tissue before annihilation, degrading the ultimate spatial resolution available with the agent.

With the exception of Rb-82, the production of positron-emitting radionuclides and their subsequent incorporation into PET radiopharmaceuticals is both expensive and complex, requiring a cyclotron or other special accelerator and relatively elaborate radiochemical handling equipment. It is unlikely that PET facilities will become widely disseminated beyond major academic centers in the near future. However, radiochemists and radiopharmacists are expending effort to develop single photon agents based on mechanisms first studied using positron emitters. For example, there are now a number of single photon labeled receptor-binding agents and perfusion agents based on knowledge gained initially from PET radiopharmaceuticals.

Box 3-4 Selected Radiopharmacueticals for Positron Emission Tomography

PERFUSION AGENTS

    O-15 Carbon dioxide
    O-15 Water
    N-13 Ammonia
    Rb-82

BLOOD VOLUME

    O-15 Carbon Monoxide
    C-11 Carbon Monoxide
    Ga-68 EDTA

METABOLIC AGENTS

    F-18 Fluorodeoxyglucose
    O-15
    C-11 Acetate
    C-11 Palmitate
    N-13 Glutamate

TUMOR AGENTS

    F-18 Fluorodeoxyglucose

RECEPTOR-BINDING AGENTS

    F-18 Spiperone
    C-11 Carfentanil
    F-18 Fluoro-L-Dopa

DISPENSING RADIOPHARMACEUTICALS

Normal Procedures

The dispensing of radiopharmaceuticals is under a series of very exacting rules and regulations promulgated by the FDA and the NRC as well as state boards of pharmacy and hospital regulations. In brief, radiopharmaceuticals are prescription drugs that cannot be legally administered without being ordered by an authorized individual. It is incumbent upon the nuclear medicine physician and the radiopharmacy to confirm the appropriateness of the request, ensure that the correct radiopharmaceutical in the requested or designated amount be administered to the patient, and keep records of both the request and the documentation of the dosage administration.

Before any material is dispensed, all appropriate quality assurance measures should be carried out. These have been described in some detail for the Mo-99/Tc-99m generator system and Tc-99m-labeled radiopharmaceuticals. For other agents, the package insert or protocol for formulation and dispensing should be consulted to see what radiochromatography or other quality control steps must be performed prior to dosage administration. As a good standard of practice, quality control should always be performed even when not legally required.

Every dosage should be physically inspected prior to administration for the detection of any particulate or foreign material, for example, bits of rubber from the tops of multidose injection vials. Each dosage administered to a patient must be assayed in a dose calibrator. The administered activity must be within ±10% of the prescription request.

Special Considerations

Pregnancy and lactation The possibility of pregnancy should be considered in every woman of childbearing age referred to the nuclear medicine service for a diagnostic or a therapeutic procedure. Pregnancy alone is not an absolute contraindication to performing a nuclear medicine study. For example, pulmonary embolism is encountered in pregnant women, and ventilation-perfusion scintigraphy is a safe procedure. The radiation dosage is kept at a minimum. Neither of the radiopharmaceuticals employed (Xe-133, Tc-99m MAA) crosses the placenta in considerable amounts. On the other hand, radioiodine crosses the placenta. The fetal thyroid develops the capacity to concentrate radioiodine at approximately the 10th to 12th week of gestation, and there are documented cases of cretinism due to in utero exposure to radioiodine.

The management of women who are lactating and breast-feeding an infant is another special problem. The need to suspend breast-feeding is determined by the half-life of the radionuclide involved and the degree to which it is secreted in breast milk. Radioiodine is secreted, and conservatively, breast-feeding should be terminated altogether or for at least 3 weeks following administration of I-131 or I-125. The same recommendations hold for Ga-67 citrate and Tl-201 chloride. For technetium-labeled radiopharmaceuticals that are either cleared rapidly by the kidney or stay in the blood pool (Tc-99m pentetate, Tc-99m-labeled RBCs, Tc-99m diphosphonate), there is very little activity in breast milk, and nursing can resume after several hours. For other Tc-99m-labeled radiopharmaceuticals, nursing should be suspended for at least two half-lives (12 hours). In the United States, it is usually practical to simply discontinue breast-feeding if there is any question about exposure to the child.

Dosage selection for pediatric patients A number of approaches have been proposed for scaling down the amount of radioactivity administered to children. There is no one perfect way to do this because of the differential rate of maturation of body organs and the changing ratio of different body compartments to body weight. Empirically, body surface area correlates better than body weight for dosage selection. Various formulas and nomograms have been developed. Each laboratory should select a method and standardize its application.

Misadministration The definition and procedures for handling misadministrations of radiopharmaceuticals are defined in the Code of Federal Regulations (10 CFR-35). The code was revised in 1991, including the definition of a misadministration.

The occurrence of a misadministration as defined by NRC rules and regulations requires that specific administrative responses be performed by the respective radioactive material license holder in response to an incident. A misadministration is defined as follows:

A radiopharmaceutical dosage involving:
1. the wrong patient, or
2. the wrong radiopharmaceutical, or
3. the wrong route of administration, or
4. the administered dose differing from the prescribed dose when involving:
   Diagnostic doses other than iodine, and the patient effective dose equivalent exceeds 5 REM to the whole body, or 50 REM to any individual organ;
   Diagnostic doses of iodine, when the administered dose differs by more than 20% from the prescribed dosage and that difference exceeds 30 μCi;
   Therapy doses, when the administered dose differs by more than 20% of the prescribed dosage.

After a misadministration is recognized to have occurred, there are regulations guiding the reporting of the event and the management of the patient. The details are determined in part by the kind of material involved and the amount of the adverse exposure to the patient. All misadministrations must be recorded locally and, where appropriate, reported to the NRC. Complete records on each event must be retained and available for NRC review for 10 years.

Adverse reactions to diagnostic radiopharmaceuticals Adverse reactions to radiopharmaceuticals are much less common than adverse reactions to iodinated contrast media. Reactions are usually mild and, for the radiopharmaceuticals in use today, rarely fatal. The greatest concern is for agents containing human serum albumin. Also, preparations of Tc-99m-sulfur colloid have a gelatin stabilizer derived from animal protein. These agents can be associated with allergic reactions. Of concern in the future is the possibility of reactions due to the development of human antimouse antibodies (HAMA) following repeated exposure to radiolabeled antibody imaging agents. The concern over the development of HAMA and potential adverse consequences has been a factor in the delay in the FDA granting approval for radiolabeled antibodies, although the precedent has been set.

Radiation accidents (spills) In a busy nuclear pharmacy handling several dozen patient dosages a day as well as stock solutions of generator eluate with most materials in liquid form, it is not surprising to have an accidental spill of radioactive material from time to time. The spills are somewhat arbitrarily divided into minor and major categories, depending on the radionuclide and the amount spilled. For I-131, incidents involving activities up to 1 mCi are considered minor, and above that level major. For Tc-99m, Tl-201, and Ga-67, the threshold for considering a spill major is 100 mCi.

The basic principles of responding to both kinds of spills are the same. For minor spills people in the area are warned that the spill has occurred. Attempts are made to prevent the spread of the spilled material. Absorbent paper may be used to cover the spilled activity if the material is visibly identifiable. Minor spills can be cleaned up directly using appropriate technique, including disposable gloves and remote handling devices. All contaminated material is disposed of carefully, including contaminated gloves and other objects. The area is continually surveyed until the reading from a Geiger-Müller survey meter reads at background levels. All personnel involved should also be monitored, including their hands, shoes, and clothing. The spill should be reported to the institution's radiation safety officer.

For major spills the area is cleared immediately. Attempts are made to prevent further spread with absorbent pads and if possible the radioactivity is shielded. The room is sealed off and the radiation safety officer is notified immediately. The radiation safety officer typically directs the further response, including determination of when and how to proceed with cleanup and decontamination.

In dealing with both minor and major spills, an attempt is made to keep radiation exposure of patients, hospital staff, and the environment to a minimum. There are no absolute guidelines that provide a definitive approach to every spill. The radiation safety officer must restrict access to the area until it is safe for patients and personnel.

RADIATION DOSIMETRY

Radiation exposure to the patient represents a limitation on the amount of radioactivity that can be administered in the respective scintigraphic procedures performed in clinical nuclear medicine. In general, it is not possible to calculate the exact radiation dose that an individual patient receives from a nuclear medicine procedure. The amount of data necessary to calculate the actual radiation absorbed dose for a particular patient is not practical to acquire. It includes the percent localization of the administered dose in each organ of the body, the time course of retention in each organ, and the size and relative distribution of the organs in the body. This information can be obtained from biodistribution studies and pharmacokinetic studies in experimental animals during the development and regulatory approval process for the development of a new radiopharmaceutical. For each radiopharmaceutical, estimates of radiation absorbed doses are developed as part of the approval process for the radiopharmaceutical and may be taken as "average" or nominal levels of exposure.

In brief, the radiation absorbed dose to any organ in the body is dependent on biologic factors (percent uptake, biologic half-life) and physical factors (amount and nature of emitted radiations from the radionuclide). Radiation doses are typically given in rads (radiation absorbed dose). One rad is equal to the absorption of 100 ergs per gram of tissue. The formula for calculating the radiation absorbed dose is:

$$D(r_k \leftarrow r_h) = \tilde{A}_h S(r_k \leftarrow r_h)$$

The formula states that the absorbed dose in a region k due to activity from a source region h is equal to the cumulative radioactivity given in microcurie-hours in the source region ($\tilde{A}$) times the mean absorbed dose per unit of cumulative activity in rads per microcurie-hour (S). The cumulative activity is determined from experimental measurements of uptake and retention in the different source regions. The mean absorbed dose per unit of cumulative activity is based on physical measurements and is determined by the kind of radiations emanating from the radionuclide being used.

The total absorbed dose to a region or organ is the sum of the contributions from all source regions around it and from activity within the target organ itself. For example, in calculating the absorbed dose to the myocardium in a Tl-201 scan there is a contribution from radioactivity localizing in the myocardium and there are contributions from radioactivity in the lung, blood, liver, gut, kidneys, and general background soft tissues. The percentage uptake and the biological behavior of Tl-201 are different in each of those tissues. The amount of radiation reaching the myocardium is also different, depending on the geometry of the source organ and its distance from the heart. The formula is applied separately for each source region and the individual contributions are summed.

Factors that affect the dosimetry between patients include the amount of activity administered originally, the biodistribution in one patient versus another, the route of administration, the rate of elimination, the size of the patient, and the presence of pathologic processes. For example, for radiopharmaceuticals cleared by the kidney, radiation exposure will be greater in patients with renal failure. Another example commonly encountered is differing percentage uptakes of radioiodine in the thyroid depending on whether a patient is hyperthyroid, euthyroid, or hypothyroid. The complexity of the problem is further illustrated by the observation that turnover in hyperthyroid subjects may be more rapid than in euthyroid subjects, and therefore the cumulative activity (aggregate microcurie-hours) could paradoxically be less in the face of florid hyperthyroidism.

Estimates of radiation absorbed dose are provided in tabular form in the organ system chapters for each major radiopharmaceutical. The tables indicate the absorbed dose per unit of administered activity for selected organs.

QUALITY CONTROL IN THE NUCLEAR PHARMACY

Selected quality control procedures for Tc-99m-labeled radiopharmaceuticals and for Mo-99/Tc-99m generator systems were described earlier in this chapter. Considerations of radiochemical and radionuclidic purity also apply to other single photon agents and positron radiopharmaceuticals. For example, radiochemical purity is a special concern with radioiodinated agents because of the potential for uptake of free radioiodine in the thyroid. Additional quality control procedures in the nuclear pharmacy are aimed at ensuring the sterility and apyrogenicity of administered radiopharmaceuticals. It is also important to quality control the performance of the dose calibrator to ensure that administered activities are within prescribed amounts.

Sterility And Pyrogen Testing

Sterility implies the absence of living organisms; *apyrogenicity* implies the absence of metabolic products such as endotoxins. Because many radiopharmaceuticals are prepared just prior to use, it is impractical to do definitive testing before administering them to the patient. This doubles the need for careful aseptic technique in the nuclear pharmacy.

Autoclaving is a well-known means of sterilization. It is useful for sterilizing preparation vials and other handling utensils and materials but is not useful for any of the radiopharmaceuticals used in clinical practice. When terminal sterilization is required, various membrane filtration methods are used. Special small-pore filters with diameters smaller than microorganisms have been developed for this purpose. A filter pore size of 0.22μ is required to sterilize a solution. This size will trap bacteria, including small organisms such as *Pseudomonas.*

Sterility testing standards have been defined by the United States Pharmacopeia (USP). Standard media including thioglycollate and soybean caseine digest media are used for different categories of microorganism, including aerobic and anaerobic bacteria and fungi.

Pyrogens are metabolites of microorganisms or other contaminating substances that cause febrile reactions. They can be present even in sterile preparations. The typical clinical syndrome is fever, chills, joint pain, and headaches developing minutes to a few hours after injection. The pyrogenic reaction lasts for several hours and alone is not fatal.

The USP has established criteria for pyrogen testing. The historic method involved injecting pharmaceutical samples into the ear veins of rabbits while measuring their temperature response.

The current USP test uses limulus amebocyte lysate (LAL). The test is based on the observation that amebocyte lysate preparations from the blood of horseshoe crabs become opaque in the presence of pyrogens. The LAL test is more reliable, more sensitive, and easier to perform than the rabbit test.

Radiopharmaceutical Dose Calibrators

The dose calibrator is a key instrument in the radiopharmacy and is subject to quality control requirements. Four basic measurements are encompassed: accuracy, linearity, precision or constancy, and geometry.

Accuracy   *Accuracy* is measured by using reference standard sources obtained from the National Institute of Standards and Technology. The test is performed annually and two different radioactive sources are used. If the measured activity in the dose calibrator varies from the standard or theoretical activity by more than 10%, the device must be recalibrated.

Linearity   The *linearity* test is designed to determine the response of the calibrator over a range of measured activities. A frequently employed approach is to take a sample of Tc-99m pertechnetate and sequentially measure it during radioactive decay. Because the change in activity with time is a definable physical parameter, any deviation in the observed assay value indicates equipment malfunction—nonlinearity. An alternative approach is to use precalibrated lead attenuators with sequential measurements of the same specimen.

Precision or constancy   The *precision* or *constancy* test is designed to measure the ability of the dose calibrator to repeatedly measure the same specimen over time. A long-lived standard such as radium-226 can be used. The test is performed daily and observed values should be within 10% of the value for the reference standard.

Geometry   The *geometric* test is performed during acceptance testing of the dose calibrator. The issue is that the same amount of radioactivity contained in different volumes of sample can result in different measured or observed radioactivities. For a given dose calibrator, if readings vary by more than 10% from one volume to another, correction factors are calculated. For convenience, the correction factors are based on the most commonly measured volume of material, typically determined from day-to-day clinical use of the dose calibrator.

SUGGESTED READINGS

Chilton HM and Witcofski RL: *Nuclear pharmacy: an introduction to the clinical application of radiopharmaceuticals*, Philadelphia, 1986, Lea & Febiger.

Kowalsky RJ and Perry JR: *Radiopharmaceuticals in nuclear medicine practice*, Norwalk, Conn, 1987, Appleton & Lange.

Swanson DP, Chilton HM, and Thrall JH: *Pharmaceuticals in medical imaging*, New York, 1990, Macmillan.

CLINICAL
SCINTIGRAPHY

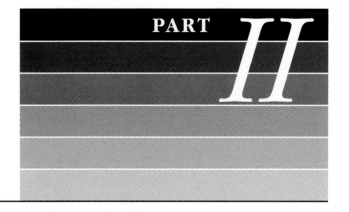

Cardiovascular System

Heart disease is the leading cause of death in the United States. Acute myocardial infarction (MI) claims over 600,000 lives per year and may strike without warning. Millions more people are at risk due to underlying coronary artery disease (CAD). A number of nuclear imaging procedures are available to aid in the diagnosis and management of heart disease; and collectively, nuclear cardiology procedures rival skeletal scintigraphy as the most commonly performed studies in nuclear medicine.

This chapter is divided into four principal sections that

address myocardial perfusion imaging (status of the myocardium and coronary perfusion), radionuclide ventriculography (status of heart function), cardiac positron emission tomography, and infarct-avid imaging (detection of acute MI).

The clinical utility of radiotracer studies of the heart must be considered in the context of other cardiac diagnostic procedures including echocardiography, contrast angiography, electrocardiography (ECG), and measurements of serum enzymes. The value of the scintigraphic studies comes largely from their noninvasiveness and their ability to accurately portray a wide range of functional and metabolic parameters.

MYOCARDIAL PERFUSION IMAGING

The single most important area of nuclear cardiology is the assessment of myocardial perfusion. Until recently the only radiopharmaceutical of clinical importance for this application was thallium-201 chloride. There are now two new classes of technetium-99m-labeled agents approved by the Food and Drug Administration (FDA) for clinical application, and there are several positron emitting agents available for perfusion imaging, including rubidium-82, which is also approved by the FDA.

There are numerous major and subtle differences between the different radiopharmaceuticals for myocardial perfusion imaging. However, the integrative concept is that the scintigram depicts two sequential events. First, tracer must be delivered to the myocardium. Second, there must be a viable, metabolically active myocardial cell present to localize the tracer. Thus, the scintigram may be thought of as a map of regional myocardial perfusion to viable myocardial tissue. If there is a decrease in relative regional perfusion, as is seen in hemodynamically significant CAD, or if there is a loss of cell viability, as is seen in MI, a cold area or photon-deficient lesion is depicted scintigraphically. All diagnostic patterns in the many diverse applications of myocardial perfusion scintigraphy follow from these simple observations.

Thallium-201 Chloride

Potassium is the major intracellular cation. Sodium-potassium homeostasis is maintained as an energy-dependent process involving the Na-K-ATPase pump. It is logical to consider potassium or a potassium analogue for myocardial perfusion imaging, and indeed, radionuclides of potassium, cesium, and rubidium have been evaluated. None is suitable for single photon imaging. Rubidium-82 is discussed below in the section on PET pharmaceuticals.

Thallium is a member of the III A series in the periodic table and behaves in its organ and tissue distribution much like potassium, although it is not a true potassium, analogue in a chemical sense. Thallium-201 has a physical half-life of 73 hours. It decays by electron capture to mercury-201. The photons available for imaging are mercury K-alpha and K-beta characteristic x-rays in the range of 69 to 83 keV (95% abundant) and thallium gamma rays of 167 keV (10% abundant) and 135 keV (3% abundant) (Table 4-1).

Mechanism of localization and pharmacokinetics
One of the principal advantages of Tl-201 for myocardial perfusion imaging is its high extraction fraction during transit through the myocardial capillary bed. Approximately 88% of thallium is extracted in the first pass through the coronary circulation under conditions of normal flow. At very high flow rates, the percent efficiency of extraction decreases, and at very low flow rates the percent extraction increases. However, over a wide range of flow rates the extraction is proportional to relative regional perfusion.

Blood clearance after intravenous (IV) injection of Tl-201 is rapid, with only 5% to 8% of the dose in blood 5 minutes after injection. Peak uptake in the myocardium occurs 10 to 20 minutes following injection. In normal subjects approximately 5% of the administered dose localizes in the myocardium. The scintigraphic images obtained early after injection reflect the blood flow conditions at the time of tracer administration. After initial uptake has occurred, thallium undergoes "redistribution" in the body. A dynamic changing equilibrium of Tl-201 exists between the myocardium and vascular pool. After initial uptake, Tl-201 leaves the myocardium and is partially replaced by circulating Tl-201 from the systemic pool, which is also undergoing constant recirculation and redistribution. Thus, several hours after initial tracer administration the scintigraphic images depict an equilibrated pattern. This is the basis of

Table 4-1	Thallium-201: Summary of Physical Characteristics and Dosimetry
PHYSICAL CHARACTERISTICS	
Mode of decay	Electron capture
Physical half-life	73 hr
Principal radiations (abundance)	
135 keV gamma rays	2.7%
167 keV gamma rays	10%
69-83 keV mercury x-rays	95%
DOSIMETRY*	
Organ	**rads/mCi**
Heart	0.5
Liver	0.55
Kidneys	1.2
Testes	0.5
Ovaries	0.5
Total body	0.2

*Modified from product information brochure for thallous chloride-201, *Du Pont Company*, Billerica, Mass.

the "stress-redistribution" imaging strategy that has been used in the detection of CAD and is discussed more fully below. Cold defects seen on early images may represent areas of significantly decreased flow or areas of myocardial scar without viable cells to fix the tracer. Defects on delayed or reinjection images depict scar. Areas demonstrating equilibration or "fill in" of activity represent viable myocardium rendered ischemic during exercise.

Technique   Numerous technical variations in the performance of Tl-201 myocardial perfusion imaging have been described, including types of equipment, imaging protocols, amounts and timing of tracer administration, and interventions. The choice of technique may in part be dictated by facilities and equipment available and details will differ from one institution to another. The following information is presented with this in mind. Important variations will be pointed out, but there is no one "correct" way to perform Tl-201 imaging and no one approach is overwhelmingly dominant in current practice.

Thallium-201 Myocardial Perfusion Scintigraphy: Rest Studies

Technique   The patient should be fasting. Direct IV injection is desirable to avoid drug-drug interactions and to minimize loss of tracer activity due to adsorption to IV tubing or adherence to venous structures being exposed to various medications (Figure 4-1). The usual package insert dosage recommendation is 1 to 2 mCi (33-74 MBq). However, this recommendation was based on the economics of Tl-201 when it was first approved by the FDA and not on either intrinsic radiation safety factors or ideal amounts for imaging. Most laboratories use 2.0 to 3.5 mCi (75-120 MBq) (Box 4-1).

Imaging is begun 10 minutes after injection. For planar imaging, a standard field of view camera or large field of view camera with a low energy, high resolution or all purpose collimator is used. A minimum of three views and preferably four views are obtained in the anterior, 35°- 40° left anterior oblique (LAO), 60°-70° LAO, and left lateral projections.

There are several choices for setting the energy window for the gamma camera. In one approach, a 20% to 25% window is centered at 80 keV. This window encompasses the K-beta series of mercury-201 x-rays. This asymmetric window setting on the mercury x-rays eliminates inclusion of scatter from the K-beta series into the energy

---

Box 4-1   Thallium-201 Myocardial Imaging: Protocol Summary

PATIENT PREPARATION AND FOLLOW-UP

Patients should ideally be fasting for 4 hrs.
ECG leads should be moved out of field of view.

DOSAGE AND ROUTE OF ADMINISTRATION

2-3 mCi (74-111 MBq) thallium-201 as thallium chloride.
Intravenous administration with patient upright, if
    possible.

TIME OF IMAGING

10 min post radiopharmaceutical administration.

PLANAR IMAGING

Use a low-energy, general-purpose, parallel hole collimator
    and a 20%-25% window centered at 80 keV. (A second
    30% window at 167 keV may also be used, if available.)
Obtain anterior, 35° LAO, 70° LAO, and left lateral views
    for 10 min each.
For rest redistribution studies, repeat the same views
    2-4 hr later.

**SPECT IMAGING ACQUISITION PARAMETERS (Elscint SP-4
tomographic camera)***

Use a general all-purpose collimator and a 10% window
    centered at 80 keV.
Patient position: Supine.
Rotation orbit: Circular or elliptical.
Matrix: 64 × 64 byte mode.
Arc and framing: 60 views/180°, 45° RAO, 135° LPO.

SPECT RECONSTRUCTION PARAMETERS*

Filter: Butterworth .35.
Attenuation correction: No.
Reconstruction technique: Filtered backprojection.
Images: Transaxial, short axis, horizontal long axis, and
    vertical long axis.

NOTE: Choice of SPECT acquisition and reconstruction parameters is highly influenced by equipment used. Protocols should be established in each nuclear medicine unit for available SPECT cameras and computers.

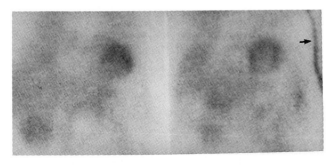

Fig. 4-1   Anterior (*left*) and left anterior oblique (*right*) thallium-201 scintigrams in a patient with a large apical and inferior myocardial infarction. The tracer was injected with the patient at rest. Note the retention of thallium in a vein in the left arm (*arrow*). Note also the uptake in the lung, liver, and abdominal viscera.

range of the K-alpha series and also reduces the contribution from lead characteristic x-rays generated by interactions in the collimator. The lead K-alpha series x-rays are in the 73 to 75 keV range. Thus, while it is tempting to use the entire mercury x-ray range to increase counting rates, the spatial resolution in the image is significantly degraded if this is done. Nevertheless, many clinics use a symmetric window to include all of the mercury x-rays. Even with modern correction circuitry this improves field uniformity and also improves counting statistics. If the gamma camera has an option for multiple windows, a second 20% window can be centered at 167 keV. This will increase the counting statistics by 10%.

Each view is obtained for 300k counts (standard field of view camera) to 500k counts (large field of view camera). An alternative is to obtain the anterior view first and subsequent views for the same length of time, or to image in each projection for a fixed length of time, typically on the order of 8 to 10 minutes.

For SPECT imaging, a general purpose or high-resolution collimator is used and the details of image acquisition are dictated by the particular SPECT system employed. Variations include continuous versus discontinuous data acquisition, length of acquisition, arc length, and shape of orbit. In current practice, laboratories with single-head cameras most often use a 180° arc length from a 45° right anterior oblique (RAO) position to a 135° left posterior oblique (LPO) position. Imaging is typically completed within 20 to 25 minutes to minimize internal redistribution of Tl-201 during the imaging sequence. Multiheaded SPECT systems lend themselves to 360° data acquisition and shorter imaging intervals. Noncircular orbits or body-contoured arc paths are desirable in theory to keep the camera head as close to the body surface as possible. Spatial resolution is degraded the farther the camera head is from the organ of interest.

Normal appearance of the thallium-201 scintigram Normal Tl-201 scintigrams obtained at rest should demonstrate uniform uptake of thallium throughout the left ventricular myocardium (Figure 4-2). In normal subjects the myocardium may appear thinner at the apex than in other portions of the ventricle. This pattern of apical thinning should not be misinterpreted as a pathologic defect. The valve planes also demonstrate absence of uptake, giving the heart a horseshoe or U-shaped appearance on long-axis SPECT views and on steep oblique and lateral planar views. The heart has a ring or donut appearance on short-axis SPECT views and a variably circular or ellipsoidal appearance on LAO planar views, depending on the patient's habitus and axial orientation of the heart in the chest.

Two special problems in imaging the left ventricle with Tl-201 have been described. First, in some women the overlying soft tissue of the breast causes attenuation of activity from the heart. This reduces the overall num-

ber of counts available for creating the image and can also result in spurious defects, especially along the lateral heart border. Images obtained in women should be carefully inspected for breast attenuation artifacts. Reimaging may be necessary with the breast held out of the field of view.

The second artifact is interposition of the diaphragm between the gamma camera and the heart on the left lateral view with the patient supine. Activity from the posterior lateral wall of the left ventricle can be attenuated, causing a spurious photon deficient defect. In planar imaging, the diaphragmatic artifact is minimized by placing the patient in the right lateral decubitus position.

In normal subjects at rest, the right ventricle typically is not seen by planar imaging. The demonstration of significant right ventricular activity suggests right ventricular hypertrophy. The right atrial appendage may be seen occasionally.

Thallium is taken up in all cellular, metabolically active tissues in the body with the exception of the brain. It does not cross the normal blood-brain barrier. Activity on resting studies is normally seen in the liver and gastrointestinal (GI) tract. Other structures accumulating significant thallium that may occasionally be in the field of view are the thyroid and salivary glands, the kidneys, and skeletal muscle. The lungs demonstrate variable degrees of uptake. Increased lung activity at rest has been linked to underlying lung disease, including interstitial and inflammatory processes, and increased uptake is frequently seen in smokers.

Diagnosis of myocardial infarction Studies obtained at rest are used for the diagnosis of acute MI, determination of infarct size (or, alternatively, determination of residual mass of viable myocardium), and to assess the results of therapeutic interventions such as angioplasty and thrombolysis (Figure 4-3).

The major advantage of Tl-201 imaging over Tc-99m pyrophosphate imaging for the diagnosis of MI is that the study is positive immediately post infarction. Areas of completed infarction are completely cold or photon deficient (Figures 4-1, 4-4). Areas of peri-infarct ischemia and edema also demonstrate diminished or absent tracer uptake.

When patients are imaged immediately post infarction the sensitivity of Tl-201 scintigraphy is very high, probably greater than 90% for transmural infarctions. This high sensitivity decreases with time as the peri-infarct edema and ischemia resolve. By 24 hours after the acute event, smaller infarctions may not be detectable, and the overall sensitivity is much lower, on the order of 60%.

A major limitation of Tl-201 scintigraphy in the diagnosis of acute MI is the inability to distinguish new from old lesions. Patients with sufficiently large healed infarctions resulting in scar formation may demonstrate cold defects indefinitely. Without the benefit of a baseline scan for comparison, a cold defect in the setting of new

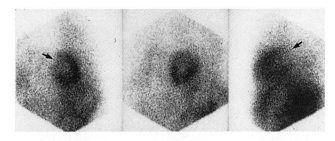

Fig. 4-2 Anterior, left anterior oblique, and left lateral views of a thallium-201 study obtained at rest in a normal subject. There is uniform uptake of thallium throughout the myocardium. Absence of tracer uptake in valve planes (*arrows*) gives the heart a horseshoe appearance on the anterior and left lateral views.

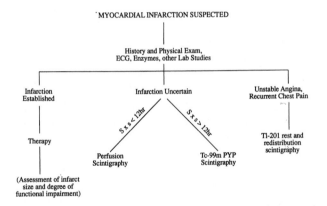

Fig. 4-3 Simplified schematic illustrating potential roles for scintigraphic imaging in suspected myocardial infarction.

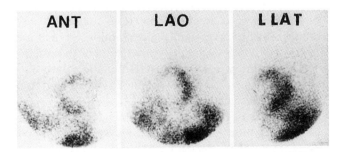

Fig. 4-4 Thallium-201 scintigraphy reveals a large anteroseptal infarction. Some 40% to 50% of the myocardium is involved.

chest pain is moot in such a patient. A conservative approach is to treat the patient expectantly as having had an acute MI until other tests, including ECG, serum enzyme determinations, or Tc-99m pyrophosphate scan, rule in or rule out this occurrence.

Insofar as half or even two thirds of patients admitted to coronary care units are subsequently found not to have sustained an acute MI, the use of thallium imaging to triage for CCU admission would appear to be very useful. Indeed, there have been strong proponents of this argument over the past decade and a half, but no general acceptance of the approach in practice. The reasons for this relate to several important limitations.

First, it is difficult logistically to maintain a 24-hour-a-day, 7-day-a-week capability to perform thallium scintigraphy on an immediate, emergency basis. Thus, the sequence of delays from the onset of chest pain to the arrival of the patient in the hospital through the conventional workup and assemblage of the nuclear medicine team makes it difficult and problematic to image in the most sensitive time window.

Second, thallium scintigraphy does not afford the ability to distinguish new from old infarctions. Also, physicians are frequently reluctant to transfer patients with chest pain to non-CCU or unmonitored beds until some period of observation is accomplished, even if MI cannot be established at the time of admission. The ideal agent for diagnosing acute MI would be positive immediately after the event and would distinguish new from old lesions. Such an agent is not yet available.

Risk stratification and prognosis following myocardial infarction The long-term prognosis of patients following MI has been a subject of intense interest clinically. Traditional evaluation has included assessment of Killip classification, the location of infarction, the presence of congestive heart failure, and a history of prior infarction. It is now well established that the size of the defect as demonstrated by Tl-201 scintigraphy is a predictor of patient outcome. This confirms the intuitive link between infarct size and long-term prognosis.

A number of scoring systems have been developed for both planar and tomographic studies to estimate the percentage of the myocardium involved by an acute infarction. In Silverman's study, patients with 40% or greater involvement of the left ventricle experienced a 92% mortality on follow-up over a period of 9 months (Figure 4-4). The mortality for patients with lesser involvement collectively was 7%. The exact percentages are probably less important than the general observation that there is a very positive correlation between infarct size and mortality.

Assessment of thrombolytic therapy Thallium-201 scintigraphy can be quite useful in assessing thrombolytic therapy, and a number of approaches have been described. In essence, prior to thrombolytic therapy, thallium scintigraphy can be used to demonstrate the ischemic areas of the heart and the watershed distal to the coronary thrombosis. Following successful clot lysis with reestablishment of perfusion, a post-therapy thallium scintigram is used to document the degree of reperfusion.

Although this paradigm seems rather straightforward, several pitfalls must be recognized. The most important is that the full significance of thallium accumulation as a predictor of long-term viability has not been established; and similarly, persistently diminished tracer activity may be due to edema and hemorrhage rather than failure to recanalize the affected vessel. Follow-up imaging 1 or 2 weeks after thrombolysis may be necessary to make the distinction in both cases.

The terms "stunned myocardium" and "hibernating myocardium" have been used to describe abnormal but still viable myocardium. Tissue in the affected watershed distal to a lysed thrombus may be viable and may accumulate Tl-201 (or other myocardial perfusion agent) in the time immediately following reperfusion. The uptake of thallium indicates viability, but the myocardial segment may be akinetic (stunned) and may not survive in the long run. Hibernating myocardium refers to severe, chronically ischemic tissue that is viable but appears cold on thallium imaging and nonfunctional on ventriculography or echography. PET imaging with F-18 fluorodeoxyglucose has been shown to detect such tissue and correctly indicate its viability.

There are a number of other less commonly indicated applications for resting Tl-201 myocardial scintigraphy. Patients with right ventricular hypertrophy due to pressure overload can demonstrate striking uptake in the right ventricular myocardium (Figure 4-5). Scintigrams in

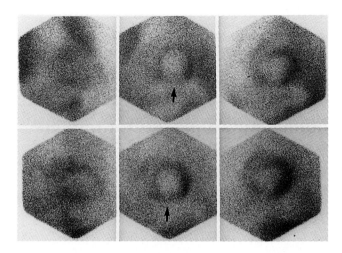

Fig. 4-6 "Rest-rest" thallium-201 scintigrams in a patient with acute chest pain. The *top row* illustrates decreased uptake in the septum, apex and anterior wall. There is marked uptake in the lung, compatible with congestive heart failure. On the delayed follow-up images, tracer has accumulated to a variable degree in all areas of abnormality. The inferoapical defect on the LAO view has filled in almost completely (*arrows*).

patients with cor pulmonale demonstrate enlargement of the right ventricle with lateral displacement and elevation of the left ventricular apex in the characteristic "right ventricular" pattern of cardiomegaly.

Occasional patients are encountered with unstable angina in whom rest and redistribution or delayed Tl-201 scintigraphy can be used to detect the ischemic tissue (Figure 4-6). Such a patient may be thought of as undergoing a natural stress test, and the patterns of early and delayed distribution have much the same significance as they do on a formal stress test. This also illustrates the potential for making a false positive diagnosis of MI in patients with acute chest pain.

Stress Thallium-201 Studies to Diagnose Coronary Artery Disease: Exercise Studies and Pharmacologic Interventions

A recurrent theme in nuclear medicine and in this book is the ability to extend the diagnostic capability of a nuclear imaging procedure by applying an interventional maneuver to alter organ function, often while testing functional reserve. Cardiac interventions in the form of various stress tests are the cornerstone of the diagnosis of CAD, and stress testing in conjunction with ECG was used for many years before nuclear cardiology was invented or became important.

The number of different approaches to cardiac exercise stress testing and their variations can be quite confusing. In essence, the rationale for all exercise stress testing in CAD is the same: to unmask critical CAD by increasing cardiac work and oxygen demand. Thus, the

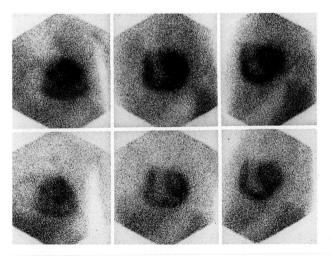

Fig. 4-5 Rest (*top*) and redistribution (*bottom*) thallium scintigrams in a patient with severe lung involvement by scleroderma. Note right ventricular hypertrophy and enlargement of the right ventricular cavity. The thickness and intensity of uptake in the right ventricular myocardium are equal to or greater than the thickness and intensity of uptake in the left ventricular myocardium.

physiologic rationale for the different exercise stress tests is the same, but the diagnostic end point is different, depending on the parameter(s) the test is designed to measure (Box 4-2).

With the traditional treadmill stress test, myocardial ischemia is detected by alterations in electrolyte flux across the ischemic cell membrane, which result in characteristic changes on the ECG. The ischemic cell membrane will not sustain a normal exchange of sodium and potassium. The classic ECG change is depression of the S-T segment. On Tl-201 myocardial scintigrams and scintigrams obtained with other perfusion agents, exercise-induced ischemia is manifested as a decrease in relative regional blood flow, which in turn is seen on the scintigram as a segmental photon-deficient or cold area. On exercise or stress radionuclide ventriculograms, myocardial ischemia is detected by assessing regional myocardial wall motion and global ventricular function. Ischemic myocardium does not contract normally. The hallmark of ischemia is the development of an exercise-induced regional wall motion abnormality. Also, the normal functional response to exercise is an increase in left ventricular ejection fraction. With significant myocardial dysfunction due to segmental ischemia, the ejection fraction fails to increase or even decreases in response to exercise-induced ischemia.

One of the important principles of all interventions is that the degree of stress must be sufficient to unmask underlying abnormalities. For cardiac stress testing by physical exercise, the adequacy of exercise is judged by how much the heart has to work. The blood pressure and heart rate provide an indication of the external work of the heart. They are monitored throughout exercise and recorded. Typically, patients achieving 85% of the age-predicted maximum heart rate ($220 - age = $ maximum predicted heart rate) are considered to have achieved adequate exercise to meet the rationale for exercise stress testing. Likewise, a "double product" is often calculated—the heart rate times the systolic blood pressure. A double product greater than 250,000 is another frequently used indicator of the adequacy of exercise achieved during stress testing.

As simple as this principle may seem, failure to achieve adequate exercise is probably the single most common reason for false negative stress tests. A number of the reasons for failure to achieve adequate exercise are summarized in Box 4-3. In many stress testing laboratories, 50% or less of patients tested achieve the levels noted above. This is always recorded as a qualification on the stress test report. That is, a negative test in the face of inadequate exercise or minimal exercise has much less significance than a negative test when adequacy criteria have been met.

Healthy subjects have tremendous coronary flow reserve, such that blood flow may increase three- to fivefold during exercise. However, flow reserve across a fixed mechanical stenosis is limited. If exercise is vigorous enough, myocardium in the watershed of a coronary artery with a hemodynamically significant stenosis can become ischemic. Lower blood flow to such an area than to surrounding normally perfused myocardium results in the delivery and localization of less Tl-201. This is seen on the scintigram as a cold defect in the poorly perfused area.

Coronary stenoses of up to 90% may not be associated with any observable perfusion abnormality or symptoms under baseline or resting conditions, and what percentage stenosis actually constitutes a hemodynamically critical lesion has been the subject of much study and debate. When the sensitivity of myocardial perfusion

---

Box 4-2   Rationale and End Point Measures in Exercise Testing

RATIONALE

Physical Exercise Increases Cardiac Work Load
Increased Work Increases Myocardial Oxygen Demand

Normal coronary arteries dilate and flow increases

Stenotic vessels do not dilate; flow reserve is limited
↓
Myocardial ischemia is induced

MANIFESTATIONS OF MYOCARDIAL ISCHEMIA

ECG: Ion flux across cell membrane is impaired by ischemia; electrical activity also changes and is manifested by S-T segment depression on the ECG.

Thallium-201 imaging: Relative decrease in regional flow is manifest as photon deficient area on scintigram.

Radionuclide ventriculography: Contraction of Ischemic myocardium is decreased and manifested by segmental wall motion abnormalities and a fall in global parameters, including ejection fraction.

Box 4-3   Reasons for Failing to Achieve Adequate Exercise

Poor general conditioning
Poor motivation
Arthritis, other musculoskeletal problems
Lung disease
Peripheral vascular disease
Medications (beta blockers, calcium channel blockers)
Angina
Dysrhythmia

imaging is assessed against cardiac catheterization as the gold standard, it is important to know what quantitative criterion was used. Most laboratories consider a coronary stenosis of 70% or greater as significant, based on the rapid fall-off of flow reserve augmentation ability above this level.

Technique The patient is prepared in the same way as for a standard treadmill exercise test. The patient should be fasting prior to the test, and at the discretion of the attending physician cardiac medication should be withdrawn. Box 4-4 summarizes some of the more important types of cardiac drugs and the length of time prior to exercise testing that they should be withdrawn to minimize residual effects. In some cases it will not be possible to discontinue the medications. If this is the case, it must be noted in the report, since medication effects can mask or prevent cardiac ischemia. A negative test while the patient is taking cardiac medications may augur well for the clinical course of the patient but is moot diagnostically.

In addition to a standard 12-lead ECG baseline evaluation and continuous monitoring during the treadmill test, an IV line with keep-open solution is placed so that it will not interfere with exercise. When the patient is judged to have achieved maximal exercise or near maximal exercise, Tl-201 is injected and flushed through the IV line. As with resting Tl-201 imaging, many laboratories use 3 to 3.5 mCi and, in current practice, may split the dose between an injection during stress and a reinjection at rest. This will be discussed in detail below.

After IV injection of Tl-201, the patient is asked to maintain exercise for another 30 to 90 seconds if possible. This ensures that the initial uptake of thallium in the heart will reflect the perfusion pattern at peak stress. Early discontinuation of exercise may result in a thallium distribution reflecting perfusion at submaximal rather than maximal exercise levels.

At one time, it was recommended that imaging be started immediately to avoid missing lesions that might "fill in" in the first minutes after initial tracer uptake. This unusual occurrence usually represented low-grade stenosis. Most nuclear medicine departments now wait 10 minutes to begin imaging, to allow the position of the heart to stabilize in the chest. Immediately after maximal exercise, patients are breathing deeply. The lungs are fully expanded and the diaphragm is down. As the patient returns to baseline, the diaphragm comes up in the chest and the heart moves cephalad. This "cardiac creep" is particularly bad when it occurs during SPECT imaging, since the position of the heart is slightly different in the angular views obtained sequentially during imaging. A compromise is to obtain a single planar image for 10 minutes while the patient's breathing stabilizes. The 40° LAO is the single best view from the standpoint of sensitivity of lesion detection. A SPECT study or standard multiview imaging then follows immediately.

For planar imaging, the same strategies are used as discussed for studies at rest (Box 4-1). A minimum of three and preferably four views are obtained. Imaging is either for time or counts, although most institutions acquire planar images digitally with computer systems and a time-based approach is more commonly used in current practice. The same considerations discussed above for resting SPECT studies also apply for SPECT following stress.

Although radiologists and nuclear medicine specialists do not commonly perform the stress portion of the thallium stress study, it is important to know the indications for terminating exercise. A brief summary is provided in Box 4-5. Most of the indications for stopping exercise are manifestations of ischemia.

Normal appearance of the stress thallium-201 scintigram Thallium-201 scintigrams obtained immediately post exercise or following pharmacologic stress intervention are strikingly different from those obtained

Box 4-4	**Cardiac Drugs That May Interfere with Stress Testing and Recommended Withdrawal Interval**
Beta blockers	72 hr
Calcium channel blockers	48-72 hr
Nitrates (long acting)	12 hr

Box 4-5 Indications for Terminating a Stress Test

Patient's request
Inability to continue because of fatigue, dyspnea, or faintness
Chest pain
Syncope, blurred vision
Pallor, diaphoresis
Ataxia
Claudication
Ventricular tachycardia
Atrial tachycardia or fibrillation
Onset of second- or third-degree heart block
S-T segment depression greater than 3 mm
Decrease in systolic blood pressure
Increase in systolic blood pressure above 240 mm Hg or in diastolic pressure above 120 mm Hg

at rest (Figures 4-7A, B; 4-8A, B). The target-to-background ratio is typically better. Right ventricular activity is frequently seen and routinely visualized on SPECT studies. During exercise, blood flow is diverted from the splanchnic bed, and less tracer activity should be seen in the liver and other abdominal structures. It is useful to assess the degree of uptake in the liver as an internal quality control check on the adequacy of exercise. Poorly exercised subjects will demonstrate higher than expected liver activity.

On delayed redistribution images and reinjection images the overall appearance of the heart is similar in

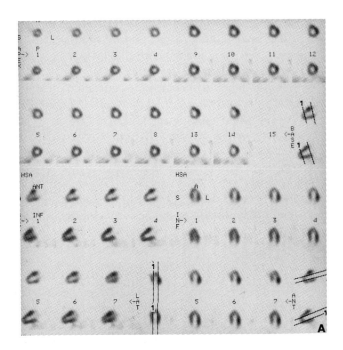

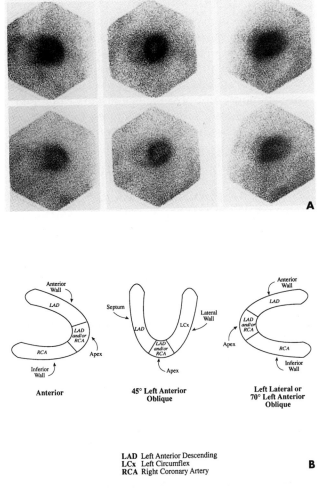

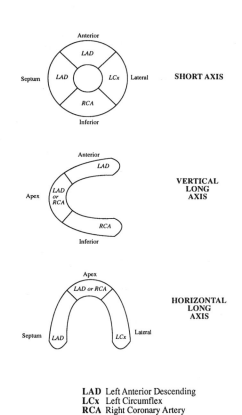

LAD Left Anterior Descending
LCx Left Circumflex
RCA Right Coronary Artery   **B**

Fig. 4-7 **A,** Normal stress thallium study with planar imaging. Immediate post-stress (*top*) and 3-hour delayed (*bottom*) thallium-201 scintigrams in a normal subject. The left ventricular myocardium-to-background ratio is excellent. There is distinct visualization of right ventricular uptake. On the immediate post-stress images, very little activity is seen on the region of the liver or other abdominal viscera. Some increase is seen on the delayed images. **B,** Line drawing illustrating the usual relationship between left ventricular wall segments and vascular supply as seen on anterior, LAO, and left lateral thallium-201 planar images.

LAD Left Anterior Descending
LCx Left Circumflex
RCA Right Coronary Artery   **B**

Fig. 4-8 Normal stress thallium study with SPECT imaging. **A,** Typical computer-generated display from a normal stress thallium-201 SPECT study. The top two rows for each slice orientation are the immediate post-stress images and the bottom two rows the delayed images. Short-axis (*top four rows*) vertical long-axis (*bottom left*), and horizontal long-axis views are typically used for interpretation. **B,** Line drawing of short-axis, vertical long-axis, and horizontal long-axis SPECT views illustrating the usual correlation of myocardial wall segments and vascular supply.

normal subjects to the immediate post-stress appearance. The myocardium-to-background ratio is usually decreased, and significantly more activity is seen in the liver and other abdominal structures.

The apical thinning phenomenon and pattern of activity at the valve plane described for studies obtained at rest also apply to exercise images (Figure 4-9).

Coronary artery disease The most frequent application of either exercise or pharmacologic stress thallium imaging is the diagnosis and management of patients with CAD. A diagnostic schema is presented in Table 4-2 that uses the appearance of the scintigrams on the immediate post-stress studies and the delayed or reinjection images to characterize people as (1) normal

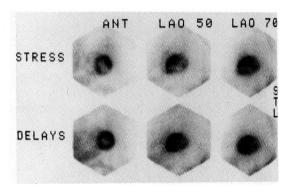

Fig. 4-9 Transient ischemia pattern, planar imaging. Post-stress planar thallium-201 images (*top row*) reveal a large inferoapical defect (*arrows*). The area of abnormality almost completely normalizes on the delayed images (*bottom row*). Note the low uptake in structures below the diaphragm immediately post stress, indicating a good level of exercise with subsequent fill-in on delayed images.

Table 4-2 Diagnostic Patterns: Myocardial Perfusion Imaging Post Stress Testing

Pattern on Immediate Post Stress Test Images	Pattern on Delayed or Reinjection Images	Diagnosis
Normal	Normal	Normal
Defect(s)	Normal	Transient ischemia
Defect(s)	Defect (unchanged)	Prior infarct with scar*
Defect(s)	Some normalization with areas of persistent defect	Transient ischemia and scar*
Normal	Defect	Reverse redistribution

*Delayed Tl-201 imaging may overestimate the presence and amount of infarcted area owing to incomplete redistribution.

(Figures 4-7, 4-8) (no defects noted on either image set), (2) having evidence of transient ischemia (Figures 4-9, 4-10) (defects on post-stress images that "fill in" on delayed images), or (3) having evidence of prior infarction (Figures 4-11, 4-12) (defects that remain "fixed" between the image sets). Patients may obviously have a combination of fixed and transient defects. The patterns apply to both planar and SPECT imaging.

An uncommon but vexing pattern is that of "reverse redistribution." Some patients demonstrate areas of apparent normal activity at the time of immediate post-stress test imaging that become abnormal at the time of delayed imaging. A number of hypotheses have been offered to explain this phenomenon. Theoretically, in patients with "balanced" multivessel disease there might be a differential rate of washout between normal and diseased areas. Another hypothesis is that an underlying area of scar is unmasked during washout. The finding has also been suggested to indicate subendocardial ischemia. However, the finding has been reported in patients without apparent hemodynamically significant CAD. A crisp statement of the significance of reverse redistribution is not possible at present. The findings should be noted and correlated with other information.

After initial assessment is made of the presence or absence of defects, a complete assessment of the Tl-201 stress study includes assessment of the size, location, and, when possible, the likely vascular distribution of the visualized abnormalities (Figures 4-7B, 4-8B). A useful approach to estimating size is to express defects as a percentage of the cardiac circumference.

Although the actual anatomy of the coronary circulation is variable in its details, the distribution of the major vessels is reasonably predictable (Figures 4-7B, 4-8B, 4-13). The left anterior descending coronary artery serves most of the septum and the anterior wall of the left ventricle. The left circumflex coronary artery serves the lateral and posterior walls. The right coronary artery serves the right ventricle, the inferior portion of the septum, and portions of the inferior wall of the left ventricle. The apex may be perfused by branches from any of the three main vessels. Defects in more than one coronary artery distribution area point to multiple-vessel disease.

In addition to the location and size of perfusion abnormalities in the myocardium, other factors should be assessed. Marked dilation of the left ventricular cavity is readily detected by comparing the images immediately after exercise with the delayed rest images (Figures 4-11, 4-14). Dilation may be a secondary indicator of ventricular dysfunction. Likewise, the amount of activity in the lung background should be carefully scrutinized. In normal subjects, lung background activity should be minimal. In patients experiencing left ventricular failure with increased left ventricular end-diastolic pressure and increased pulmonary capillary wedge pressure, lung uptake can be strik-

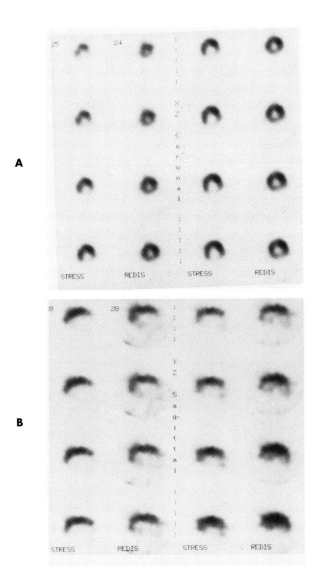

A

B

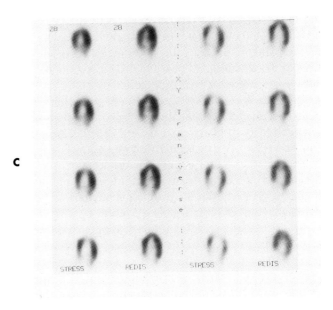

C

Fig. 4-10   Short-axis (**A**), vertical long-axis (**B**), and horizontal long-axis (**C**) images from a SPECT study in the same patient illustrated in Figure 4-9. The large inferoapical defect is appreciated on the short-axis and vertical long-axis views. The SPECT study shows the extent of the lesion. It also illustrates the value of obtaining tomographic reconstructions that "cut through" abnormal areas perpendicularly. It is very difficult to evaluate perfusion defects on tangential cuts due to partial volume effects and the lack of surrounding structures for anatomic localization. (Courtesy Merrill C. Johnson, M.D., Mount Auburn Hospital, Cambridge, Mass.)

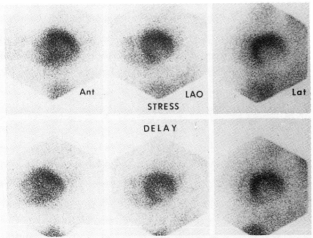

Fig. 4-11   Planar thallium-201 scintigrams post stress (*top row*) and with 2-hour delay (*bottom row*) reveal a fixed inferoapical defect. There is essentially no fill-in between the two sets of images. The ventricular cavity is slightly larger on the initial images, a common finding in patients with coronary artery disease.

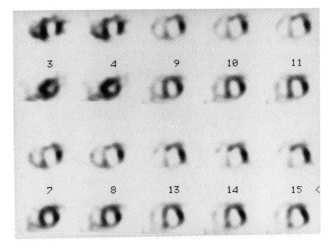

Fig. 4-12   Fixed defect pattern by SPECT imaging. The top two rows of short-axis images obtained immediately after stress testing reveal extensive abnormality in the septum and apical inferior area. The delayed images (bottom two rows) reveal an essentially identical pattern.

ing. Quantitatively, the ratio of lung activity to myocardial activity should be well below 0.5. Ratios at or above this level are abnormal and are secondary indicators of left ventricular dysfunction and possibly CAD. Lung uptake has also been reported in heavy smokers.

Quantitative analysis A number of techniques have been described for quantitative analysis of thallium scans obtained by both planar imaging and SPECT. These typically make use of a data set derived from normals that provides a reference for the expected range of relative regional uptake and rates of washout. A circumferential profile histogram is created from the patient's scintigram and compared with the reference standard (Figures 4-14A, B; 4-15).

In a particularly creative approach applied to short-axis SPECT tomograms, all of the circumferential profiles are presented for all of the slices in a two dimensional "bull's-eye" display. The display is generated by a polar mapping of nested sets of circumferential profiles obtained from the short-axis SPECT views, starting at the apex (Figure 4-16).

The merits of the various quantitative analysis techniques continue to be debated in the literature. Some of the pitfalls in using the approach include problems of misregistering the patient's study with the reference data set, using data sets generated from other laboratories on equipment different from that used in the patient's examination, and lack of uniformity in the amount of exercise or stress achieved. In particular, if washout criteria are used, the degree of initial stress and therefore the level of uptake of thallium in the heart directly affect the rate of washout. Higher levels of exercise are associated with more rapid washout. Following adequate exercise there should be a 30% to 40% decrease in thallium activity by 3 hours after tracer injection. Slower washout associated with lower levels of exercise could be misinterpreted quantitatively as abnormal.

Sensitivity and specificity The accuracy of stress thallium imaging has been studied in literally dozens of medical centers around the world. Reported sensitivities range from 60% to 95%. Specificity is variably reported

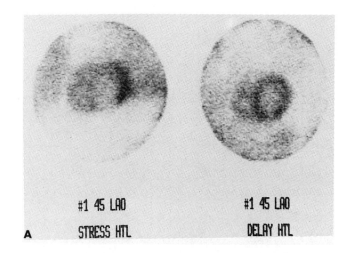

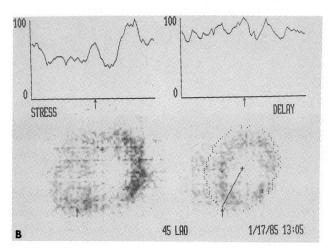

Fig. 4-14 **A**, Planar post-stress images in the LAO view reveal marked decrease in thallium-201 uptake in the septum and inferior wall, with dilatation of the left ventricular cavity. The delayed image reveals essentially complete normalization of myocardial uptake and reduction in left ventricular cavity volume. **B**, Transient defect with quantitative analysis using a circumferential profile technique. The maximum value along each of 60 rays from the center of the left ventricle is calculated and plotted clockwise as a histogram. The *arrow* on the image corresponds to the arrow on the x-axis of the histogram. Note the lower histogram values in the areas representing the inferoapical wall (to the right of the arrow) and the septum (to the left of the arrow). These areas demonstrate significant fill-in on the delayed image with corresponding normalization of the histogram values.

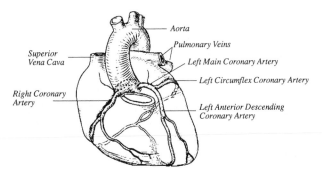

Fig. 4-13 Simplified line drawing illustrating the distribution of the main coronary arteries. Note the correlations with the wall segments for planar (Figure 4-7B) and SPECT (Figure 4-8B) images.

as 50% to 90%. These wide ranges in reported accuracy are due in part to differences in study populations. If patients with known multiple-vessel disease and prior MI are included in the study population, the sensitivity observed will be predictably high. On the other hand, if only younger subjects with suspected but not yet proven disease are studied, the sensitivity will be lower. Also, if the sensitivity is reported only for patients achieving adequate exercise, the sensitivity will be higher than if it is reported for all patients combined.

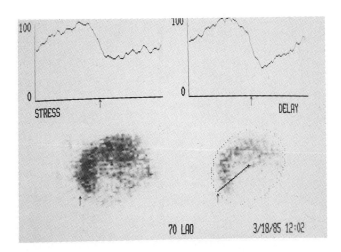

Fig. 4-15 Quantitative analysis of a fixed defect. Note failure of the curve to the right of the arrow to demonstrate significant normalization between stress and delay.

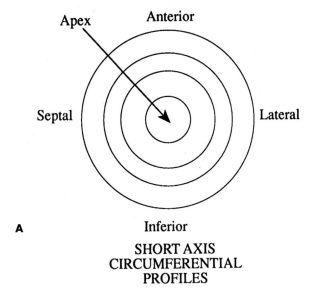

A

SHORT AXIS
CIRCUMFERENTIAL
PROFILES

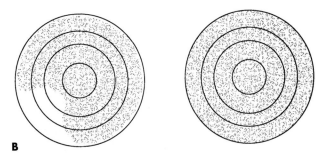

B

Fig. 4-16 **A,** Simplified schematic of the "bull's-eye" approach to quantitative analysis. The apex is represented at the center of the bull's-eye. Each concentric ring represents the next contiguous slice from the short-axis images. This allows the entire data set to be displayed as a single image. **B,** Schematic illustrating the appearance of a transient defect on the "bull's-eye" display. Post-stress imaging defects on three contiguous slices (*left*) normalize on delayed images (*right*).

Specificity is even more of a problem. Many institutions use the thallium scan as a decision point for performing cardiac catheterization and coronary arteriography. If only patients with abnormal or equivocal Tl-201 scans are sent to the catheterization laboratory, the specificity of the stress Tl-201 scan in the "proven" population will be predictably low.

In reading the literature, therefore, it is extremely important to determine in the Materials and Methods sections of an article exactly what patient population was studied, if the results of patients achieving adequate versus inadequate exercise were included, and whether patients with prior MI were included. In patients achieving adequate exercise and without prior MI or known CAD, a reasonable estimate of sensitivity is 85% to 90%. A figure for specificity is more difficult, for patients with normal thallium scans typically do not undergo arteriography. SPECT and quantitative analysis may increase observer confidence but have not been convincingly shown to improve overall study accuracy.

Risk stratification following myocardial infarction Another important application of stress thallium imaging is in the management and risk stratification of patients following acute MI (Figure 4-17). Some medical centers study patients prior to hospital discharge. The combined results of a treadmill ECG and a treadmill or dipyridamole stress thallium scan have become central to clinical decision making.

As indicated in the decision tree, if there is a single fixed defect (or no defect) and no ECG evidence of ischemia following adequate exercise, patients are treated conservatively. If the postinfarction thallium stress study demonstrates a reversible component contiguous to the site of infarction and a reversible or fixed defect remote from the infarct, residual ischemia or multivessel disease is highly likely. Patients with these findings are at much greater risk for subsequent cardiac events and death and

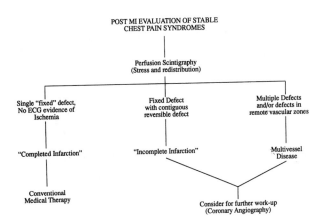

Fig. 4-17 Diagnostic scheme illustrating the incorporation of perfusion scintigraphy into an approach for stratifying risk after myocardial infarction.

warrant more aggressive management. It must be emphasized that the decision tree does not pertain to patients with unstable angina or other clinical manifestations of cardiac dysfunction such as congestive heart failure.

Assessment of therapy   Follow-up stress thallium imaging after coronary artery bypass graft (CABG) surgery or angioplasty provides an objective assessment of therapeutic effect on the coronary circulation. Successful surgery or angioplasty results in the elimination of transient defects due to exercise-induced ischemia. Surgery and angioplasty have no effect on scarred areas, and fixed defects should appear unchanged. If a patient experiences an infarction as a result of the therapeutic intervention, a previously transient defect may be converted into a fixed defect or there may be an entirely new defect as a result of the injury.

Later, when symptoms recur, as they do in a significant percentage of patients, the early post-therapy study serves as a useful baseline. The development of new or recurrent disease is readily detected on repeat thallium stress imaging.

In patients undergoing thrombolysis, myocardial perfusion studies are obtained under resting conditions as discussed above. After recovery, stress imaging is useful to determine outcome and detect any areas of residual exercise- or stress-induced ischemia.

Reinjection imaging   Beginning in the late 1970s and for over a decade thereafter, the most common stress Tl-201 protocol was to reimage the patient 3 to 4 hours after the initial post-stress images were obtained. These delayed images are supposed to depict the baseline or equilibrated perfusion pattern. It is now recognized that this approach overestimates the number of fixed myocardial defects (Figure 4-19). Imaging delayed up to 24 hours after tracer injection sometimes shows continued very slow redistribution. An alternative strategy is to administer a second injection of tracer at the time of delayed imaging (Figure 4-19). This need not be 3 hours later. The reinjection can be accomplished earlier, thereby shortening the overall length of the study for the patient. Many institutions are exploring combined thallium- and technetium-labeled myocardial perfusion agent studies to further streamline the study.

The rationale for reinjection imaging comes from the observation that 15% to 35% of ischemic segments do not fill in or normalize by 3 to 4 hours. If delayed imaging is relied on for distinguishing scar and ischemia, the number of fixed defects will be overestimated and the number of patients with stress-induced ischemia will be underestimated. This is a serious error, because it is the patients with transient ischemia who may benefit from surgery or angioplasty and who are at risk for ischemia-induced cardiac dysrhythmia and sudden death. There is a relationship between the degree of stenosis and the

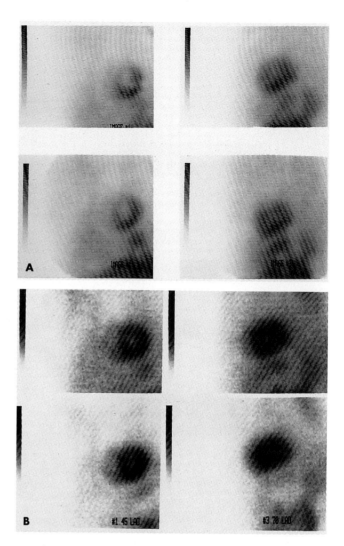

Fig. 4-18   **A**, Preoperative images from a stress thallium study reveal a transient defect in the septum and anterior wall. The top two images are the LAO and left lateral views, obtained immediately after stress, with corresponding delayed images on the bottom row. **B**, A repeat stress thallium study is normal postoperatively without evidence of ischemia.

rate of equilibration. Areas of severe narrowing appear to fill in more slowly.

Alternatives to leg exercise   One of the major attractions of the combined Tl-201-ECG stress test is the ease with which the nuclear medicine procedure is grafted onto the standard treadmill examination. The clinical information on exercise tolerance and the information from the ECG itself are valuable to the cardiologist, in addition to the information gained from the Tl-201 study. However, many patients are unable to achieve levels of exercise adequate to meet the underlying rationale of the exercise stress test. Cardiologists and nuclear medicine physicians have sought alternatives that might be applied in such patients.

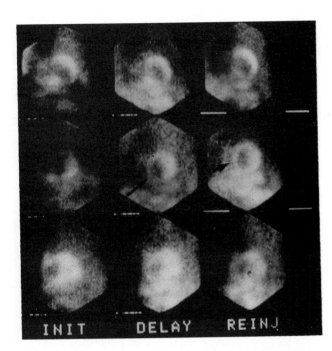

Fig. 4-19   Initial post-stress images reveal extensive defects in the septum and inferior wall. After a several-hour delay (*middle column*), extensive defects remain. Following reinjection (*right column*), all areas of the myocardium demonstrate some degree of uptake. The difference between the delay and reinjection images is most striking in the septum (*arrows*). (Courtesy H. William Strauss, M.D., Squibb Diagnostics, Princeton, NJ.)

Box 4-6   Alternatives to Leg Exercise in Cardiac Stress Testing

Isometric (handgrip) exercise
Atrial pacing
Esophageal pacing
Cold pressor testing
Ventricular stimulation; postextrasystolic potentiation
Pharmacologic stress: dipyridamole, adenosine, ergonovine, catecholamines ↳ *persantine*

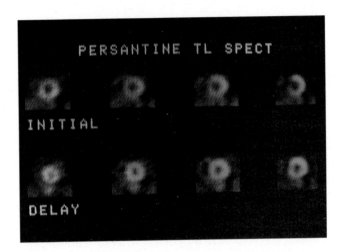

Fig. 4-20   Thallium-201 SPECT imaging following pharmacologic stress with persantine. A transient defect in the septum is demonstrated on these short-axis images. (Courtesy H. William Strauss, M.D., Squibb Diagnostics, Princeton, NJ.)

A number of alternative approaches are summarized in Box 4-6. Some of these have enjoyed brief popularity, including cold pressor testing. Other techniques such as isometric handgrip exercise have become useful as adjuncts in pharmacologic stress testing. Provocative testing with ergonovine has been used in patients with suspected Prinzmetal's angina. Ergonovine provokes coronary spasm that may not be elicited during standard exercise testing or other stress testing. This is certainly not a common indication and is somewhat dangerous, for the antidote for ergonovine-induced coronary spasm is intracoronary nitroglycerin.

Dipyridamole and adenosine pharmacologic stress The most important alternative to leg exercise is pharmacologic stress testing with dipyridamole and, more recently, adenosine. These agents are both potent coronary vasodilators capable of causing a four- to fivefold increase in flow in normal coronary arteries. They achieve this effect in basically the same way. Dipyridamole is an inhibitor of adenosine deaminase and, thus, acts by augmenting the effect of endogenous adenosine. In experience to date, both agents appear equal in their utility for diagnosing CAD (Figure 4-20).

Adenosine has the advantage of a very short plasma half-life. If patients experience symptoms, no antidote to the adenosine is necessary. Infusion is simply terminated. The action of dipyridamole, on the other hand, is more prolonged. The symptoms to watch for include chest pain (angina), nausea and vomiting, dizziness, headache, shortness of breath, and a drop in blood pressure. The antidote is IV aminophylline (125-250 mg) and may require repeating. In clinical experience, approximately 20% to 25% of patients undergoing dipyridamole pharmacologic stress testing experience chest pain. S-T segment depression is also noted in approximately 10% of cases. When using dipyridamole, some laboratories routinely administer 50 mg of aminophylline after tracer uptake is complete. In severe cases of angina, sublingual nitroglycerin is also administered.

The technical details for dipyridamole and adenosine protocols are significantly different due to their different half-times of pharmacologic effect. Both increase coronary flow on the order of 3.5 to 4.0 times. With dipyridamole, a "keep-open" IV line is started with 0.9% saline. The drug is infused at 0.14 mg/kg/min for 4 minutes (Box 4-7). Thallium-201 is injected IV 7 to 9 minutes after the start of infusion. Imaging is then begun 12 to 15 minutes

Persantine

Box 4-7   Dipyridamole Perfusion Scintigraphy: Protocol Summary

TIME FROM START OF INFUSION	PROTOCOL
Prior to start (min)	Obtain baseline ECG and blood pressure; report at 1-minute intervals
0-4	Administer dipyridamole IV, 0.14 mg/kg/min, for 4 minutes
7-9	Inject Tl-201 IV 7-9 minutes after **start** of infusion
12	Begin imaging at 12 minutes (5 minutes after Tl-201 injection)
10-12	Administer 50-100 mg aminophylline **slowly** by IV injection to reverse effects of dipyridamole

---

after the start of infusion. During the infusion and the interval before thallium injection, some departments also have the patient perform mild exercise such as handgrip isometric exercise or walking in place to augment the effect. Injection is ideally done with the patient standing or sitting to minimize splanchnic activity.

The protocol for adenosine is 140 ug/kg/min for 6 minutes. Thallium-201 is injected 3 minutes after the start of the adenosine infusion. Imaging is begun 5 minutes after tracer administration.

It is important to note that since both dipyridamole and adenosine are antagonized by methylxanthines, drugs containing them (such as theophylline) should be discontinued if possible for the time of study. Also, caffeine in coffee can antagonize dipyridamole and adenosine, and patients should fast prior to the study and imaging.

The dipyridamole and adenosine protocols are also used with the technetium-labeled myocardial perfusion agents and with PET agents.

Myocardial Perfusion Imaging With Technetium-99m-Labeled Agents

Attempts have been made for over a decade to develop technetium-99m-labeled myocardial perfusion imaging agents (Table 4-3). There are now two such agents available that have been approved for clinical use by the FDA. Although they share the Tc-99m label in

Table 4-3   Comparison of Tc-99m-Labeled Myocardial Agents and Thallium-201

	Tc-99m Agents	Tl-201
Energy	140 keV (ideal for gamma camera)	69-83 keV (Hg x-rays) (suboptimal for gamma camera)
First-pass studies of ventricular function	Possible with both agents	Not feasible
Gated imaging	Readily accomplished	Count rate marginal for gated imaging
Stress/rest imaging	Two injections required	May be accomplished with one dosage

Table 4-4   Comparison of Tc-99m Teboroxime and Tc-99m Sestamibi

	Tc-99m Teboroxime	Tc-99m Sestamibi
Myocardial extraction	> Tl-201	< Tl-201
Myocardial clearance	$T_{1/2} \sim$ 5-10 min	$T_{1/2} >$ 5 hr
Imaging time after injection	1-2 min	30-90+ min
Redistribution	Nil due to uptake; differential regional washout may cause scintigraphic appearance to change	Slight

common, their chemical and pharmacologic properties are quite different (Table 4-4). Both agents have been targeted by their respective developers for use in the diagnosis of CAD, but early experience suggests different strategies, and their widely different pharmacokinetics require completely different imaging protocols. The Tc-99m label confers favorable imaging characteristics for use with the gamma camera and dosimetry (Table 4-5).

Table 4-5   Dosimetry for Tc-99m Teboroxime and Tc-99m Sestamibi

	Tc-99m Teboroxime* (rad/mCi)	Tc-99m Sestamibi† (rad/mCi)
Heart wall	0.02	0.02
Liver	0.06	0.02
Kidneys	0.02	0.07
Gallbladder	0.10	0.07
Urinary bladder	0.03	0.07
Upper colon	0.12	0.18
Lower colon	0.09	0.13
Testes	0.01	0.01
Ovaries	0.04	0.05
Total body	0.02	0.02

*Modified from package insert, *Squibb Diagnostics*, Princeton, NJ.

†Modified from package insert, *Du Pont Radiopharmaceutical Division*, Billerica, Mass.

Technetium-99m teboroxime   Technetium-99m teboroxime is a neutral lipophilic agent from a class of compounds referred to as boronic acid adducts of technetium dioxime (BATO). Tc-99m teboroxime is avidly extracted from the blood during circulation through the myocardium. The extraction fraction is higher than that for Tl-201 (Table 4-4). At resting flow rates the extraction is 90% or better. The extraction fraction decreases with increasing flow but remains proportional to flow, so that the regional uptake and distribution of Tc-99m teboroxime is a suitable marker of regional myocardial perfusion.

Pharmacokinetics   The myocardial uptake and blood clearance of Tc-99m teboroxime are very rapid. The dominant component of blood clearance has a half-life of less than 1 minute. Myocardial clearance or washout is also extremely rapid, with a major component half-time on the order of 5 to 10 minutes. Early regional washout appears to be proportional to regional flow.

After initial clearance from the blood, the tracer is metabolized into complexes that do not show uptake in the myocardium. Therefore, significant redistribution does not occur with Tc-99m teboroxime, making it different in this respect from Tl-201. Changing patterns of Tc-99m teboroxime following initial uptake are due to differences in regional washout. The changing pattern for Tl-201 is due to both differential washout and reuptake.

The major route of excretion of Tc-99m teboroxime is the liver. Hepatic accumulation of tracer presents a significant problem in imaging. The inferior wall and apex of the heart can be obscured by uptake in the liver, and scattered photons from hepatic activity can also degrade the images of the inferior and apical wall segments. Peak uptake in the liver is delayed compared to peak uptake in the heart and is seen at approximately 6 minutes after tracer administration. The rapid clearance from the blood in the first 2 minutes with myocardial accumulation and the slightly delayed uptake in the liver dictate a narrow ideal time window for imaging between 2 and 6 minutes. During this time window the tracer distribution in the myocardium still reflects initial uptake.

Imaging technique   The accepted range for a single dose of Tc-99m teboroxime is 15 to 30 mCi (555-1,110 MBq) (Box 4-8). For combined rest/stress imaging in the diagnosis of CAD, a split dose of 35 to 50 mCi can be used (1,295-1,850 MBq).

All laboratories using Tc-99m teboroxime have modified their imaging protocols to allow for a very short interval between tracer administration and imaging. For planar imaging a useful strategy is to start in the anterior view, because liver overlap and interference are most problematic in this projection. Three-view imaging in the anterior, shallow LAO and steep LAO projections can be accomplished in less than 5 to 7 minutes. The count total is 300k to 500k per view. For rest/stress studies, the

---

Box 4-8   Tc-99m Teboroxime Imaging: Protocol Summary

PATIENT PREPARATION

Standard preparation and precautions for stress studies.

DOSE AND ROUTE OF RADIOPHARMACEUTICAL ADMINISTRATION

15-30 mCi (555-1,110 MBq) for single-dose study.
35-50 mCi (1,295-1,850 MBq) for rest/stress study.
Intravenous administration.

IMAGING PROTOCOL—PLANAR STUDIES

Use a high-resolution collimator and a 20% window centered at 140 keV.
Begin imaging 1-2 min after tracer injection.
Obtain the anterior view first, followed by 30° to 40° LAO and 70° LAO views.
Obtain 300k to 500k counts per view.
For computer acquisition, use a 64 × 64 or 128 × 128 matrix.
Total imaging time for all three views should be less than 10 min.
For stress/rest studies, wait 60 to 90 min before the second injection to allow myocardial clearance of the initial activity.

---

exercise portion of the procedure is accomplished first, with a repeat injection and repeat imaging 1.5 hours later to allow clearance of the initial dose of tracer from the heart.

An alternative approach to planar imaging is SPECT imaging. With multiheaded SPECT cameras, sequential tomograms can be obtained in 2 minutes. Modern triple-headed systems allow continuous data acquisition during rotation so that imaging time is not lost while the camera head moves from one position to another. Multiple sequential short acquisitions can be performed. The advantage of this approach is that imaging can be completed before significant hepatic uptake and the sequential images give some indication of myocardial clearance.

Clinical applications   The diagnostic accuracy of both planar and SPECT Tc-99m teboroxime imaging in the diagnosis of CAD is similar to that reported for Tl-201, with sensitivity and specificity both in the 80% to 90% range.

There is interest in using Tc-99m teboroxime for evaluating cardiac interventions. For example, the rapid clearance of Tc-99m teboroxime from the myocardium makes it a potentially ideal agent for assessing the effects of thrombolytic therapy. However, this agent is not widely used in current practice.

Technetium-99m sestamibi   Tc-99m sestamibi is a member of a chemical family referred to as isonitriles and is chemically hexakis 2-methoxyisobutyl isonitrile. The radiopharmaceutical Tc-99m sestamibi is a monovalent cation in which Tc-99m is surrounded by six isonitrile ligands.

Tc-99m sestamibi diffuses passively out of the blood and apparently localizes in mitochondria on the basis of their negative electrical potentials. The extraction fraction for Tc-99m sestamibi in the coronary circulation is lower than that of either Tc-99m teboroxime or Tl-201 (Box 4-4). At resting flows, the extraction is approximately half that of Tl-201. The maximum extraction decreases with increasing flow but remains proportional to flow. As with Tl-201, Tc-99m sestamibi underestimates flow at very high flows and overestimates flow at low flows.

Pharmacokinetics   Tc-99m is cleared from the blood fairly rapidly, with less than 5% of activity remaining in the blood at 10 minutes. Uptake in myocardium is also rapid but is somewhat obscured by activity in the lung and liver in the time immediately after tracer administration. However, the clearance half-time of Tc-99m sestamibi from the myocardium is quite long, in excess of 5 hours. There is minimal recirculation or redistribution of Tc-99m sestamibi after initial uptake in the heart so that there is a several-hour time window after tracer administration in which to accomplish imaging. Progressive clearance of liver and lung activity with excretion of the tracer through the kidneys and via the biliary system results in better myocardium-to-background activity ratios at 60 to 120 minutes than immediately after tracer administration. In current practice, imaging is initiated from 30 to 90 minutes after tracer administration.

Imaging technique   High-quality imaging with Tc-99m sestamibi can be accomplished by either planar or SPECT techniques (Box 4-9). With planar imaging, a dose of 10 mCi provides a sufficient count rate for imaging with a high-resolution collimator. Imaging is begun 60 to 90 minutes after tracer administration. The count rate is 750k to 1,000k counts obtained per image, with anterior, intermediate, and steep oblique views obtained. The high count rate afforded by Tc-99m sestamibi also permits the use of ECG gated image acquisition. The same computer program is used as for radionuclide ventriculography. The advantage of gated imaging is that the function of the myocardium may be evaluated by assessing wall thickening. Also, the "stop action" effect of gated imaging reduces blurring and improves spatial resolution in detecting perfusion defects.

Up to 30 mCi of Tc-99m sestamibi may be used for SPECT imaging. The time delay after tracer administration is the same as for planar imaging. Gated SPECT is feasible, especially if multiheaded SPECT systems are available. Some laboratories take advantage of the count rate available from the 10 to 30 mCi dose to perform first-pass radionuclide ventriculography. In this approach it is possible to assess both ventricular function and myocardial perfusion with a single dose of radiopharmaceutical.

Clinical applications   The single most important application is in the diagnosis of CAD. As with Tc-99m teboroxime, two injections of tracer are required for imaging the stress perfusion pattern and the baseline or resting perfusion pattern.

Techniques have been developed to accomplish the stress/rest procedure either as a 1-day study or on 2 different days. Since Tc-99m sestamibi has a long biological half-time in the myocardium, studies on the same day require

---

Box 4-9   Tc-99m Sestamibi Imaging: Protocol Summary

PATIENT PREPARATION

Follow standard preparation protocol and precautions for stress studies.

DOSE AND ROUTE OF RADIOPHARMACEUTICAL ADMINISTRATION

10-30 mCi (370-1,110 MBq), single dose.
Intravenous administration.

IMAGING PROTOCOL—PLANAR STUDIES

Use a high-resolution collimator and a 20% window centered at 140 keV.
Begin imaging 60-90 min after tracer injection.
Obtain anterior, 30°-40° LAO, and 70° LAO views.
Obtain 750k to 1,000k counts per view.
Consider ECG gating to evaluate questionable lesions.
For single-day rest/stress studies, give 10 mCi at rest and image at 60 min. Wait 4 hr, then give 20 mCi, with repeat imaging at 60 min.

IMAGING PROTOCOL—SPECT

One day rest/stress imaging:
   Rest: 8 mCi Tc-99m sestamibi; imaging begun at 60-90 min.
   Stress: 22 mCi Tc-99m sestamibi; imaging begun at 30-60 min.
Two day rest/stress or stress/rest imaging:
   22 mCi Tc-99m sestamibi for both studies.

SPECT ACQUISITION PARAMETERS (SIEMEN'S 7500 SPECT SYSTEM)*

Patient position: Supine.
Rotation: Counterclockwise.
Matrix: 64 × 64 word mode.
Image/arc combination: 64 views/180° degrees, 45°RAO, 135° LPO.

SPECT RECONSTRUCTION PARAMETERS*

Interslice filter.
Convolution filter: Butterworth.
   Rest: .4 cutoff.
   Stress: .4 cutoff.
Attenuation correction: No.
Oblique angle reformatting: Yes.

---

*The choice of SPECT acquisition and reconstruction parameters is highly influenced by the equipment used. Protocols should be established in each nuclear medicine unit for available cameras and computers.

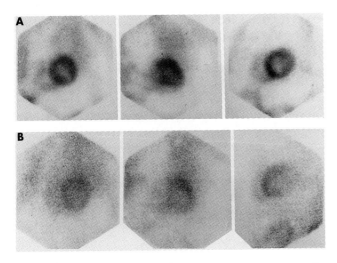

Fig. 4-21 **A,** Post-stress technetium-99m sestamibi images. The target-to-background ratio is extremely good. **B,** Corresponding thallium-201 images in the same patient. The myocardium is well visualized with both agents, but the count rate available with Tl-201 is less than with Tc-99m sestamibi.

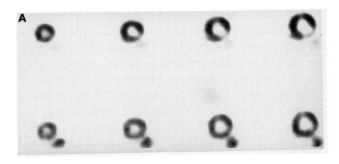

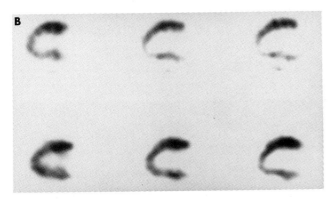

Fig. 4-22 Short-axis (**A**) and vertical long-axis (**B**) views of transient defect pattern on SPECT Tc-99m sestamibi scintigraphy. Immediate post-stress images (*top rows*) reveal an inferoapical defect. Significant uptake is demonstrated in the same area following repeat tracer injection at rest (*bottom rows*).

the use of a smaller initial dose followed by a larger dose. Different laboratories have chosen to do the stress portion or the resting portion of the procedure first. The initial

study is accomplished with 10 mCi Tc-99m sestamibi and the second study is obtained 3 to 4 hours later using 20 mCi. The image interpreter must take into account residual activity just as with reinjection thallium imaging. Another approach is to combine Tc-99m sestamibi with Tl-201 for a dual tracer approach. If thallium is used first for the resting procedure its lower energy does not interfere with subsequent imaging of Tc-99m.

The diagnostic criteria with Tc-99m sestamibi are the same as with thallium. Scintigrams in normal subjects should reveal no defects at either rest or exercise (Figure 4-21). Patients with prior MIs will demonstrate fixed abnormalities. Areas of exercise-induced ischemia will appear as defects on post-stress studies and will "normalize" on studies obtained with the tracer injected at rest (Figure 4-22).

As with early reports for Tc-99m teboroxime, the accuracy of the diagnosis of CAD with Tc-99m sestamibi appears comparable to that with Tl-201. There may be an accuracy advantage of SPECT imaging, but this remains to be proved.

RADIONUCLIDE VENTRICULOGRAPHY

The goal of radionuclide ventriculography is to evaluate global and regional ventricular function. Techniques are available to study both the right and left ventricles and may be categorized as either *first-pass* studies, in which all data collection occurs during the initial transit of a tracer bolus through the central circulation, or *equilibrium* studies, in which data are collected over many cardiac cycles using a tracer that remains in the blood pool. The principal advantages of radionuclide ventriculography over contrast ventriculography are the noninvasiveness of the nuclear imaging procedure, the ability to study all cardiac chambers simultaneously, and the ability to make repeated measurements over time or before and after an intervention.

Radiopharmaceuticals

Blood pool agents The pharmaceutical of choice for equilibrium gated blood pool imaging is technetium-99m-labeled red blood cells (Tc-99m RBCs). Labeling may be accomplished by any one of three different approaches—an in vivo approach, a modified in vivo approach, and an in vitro approach.

The original in vivo approach is the simplest. Cold stannous pyrophosphate is reconstituted with saline and injected directly IV. The dose is 15 mg/kg body weight. Fifteen to 30 minutes later, Tc-99m pertechnetate is also administered by direct IV injection. The pertechnetate diffuses across the RBC membrane, where it is reduced by the stannous ions administered previously. The Tc-99m label binds to the beta chain of hemoglobin.

Although the in vivo technique is very simple, the

labeling yield is less than ideal, on the order of 80% but frequently as low as 60% to 65%. Technetium-99m activity not labeled to RBCs can contribute to background and also reduces the number of counts available from the cardiac blood pool. In some cases the labeling fails dramatically due to drug-drug interactions or other causes of poor labeling (Box 4-10). Special care is taken not to inject through heparinized IV tubing. For these reasons many laboratories have adopted either the modified in vivo approach or the in vitro approach. Excessive gastric, thyroid, and soft tissue background activity suggests poor labeling with free Tc-99m pertechnetate.

In the modified in vitro approach, cold stannous pyrophosphate is again administered directly IV. After the 15- to 30- minute wait, 3 to 5 mL of blood is withdrawn through an IV line into a shielded syringe containing Tc-99m pertechnetate and a small amount of either acid-citrate-dextrose (ACD) solution or heparin. The blood is incubated at room temperature for at least 10 minutes. The syringe is agitated periodically and the syringe contents reinjected into the patient. The syringe is left attached to the IV line during the procedure so that the entire system is closed with respect to the patient's circulation. The labeling efficiency increases to approximately 90% in the modified in vivo approach.

In the in vitro approach, blood is first withdrawn from the patient and added to a reaction vial containing cold stannous chloride. The stannous ion diffuses across the red cell membrane. After incubation, sodium hypochlorite is used to oxidize excess extracellular stannous ion to prevent extracellular reduction of technetium-99m pertechnetate. A sequestering agent can also be added to remove extracellular stannous ion. Radioactive labeling is then accomplished by adding sodium pertechnetate. Tc-99m pertechnetate crosses the red cell membrane and is reduced by stannous ion in the cell. The mixture is incubated for 20 minutes. Labeling efficiency is on the order of 95% or greater. This approach is somewhat less convenient than the in vivo approaches but has the advantage of the highest labeling efficiency and is less subject to drug-drug interference to labeling and less subject to problems of excess or deficient stannous ion.

Another potential agent is Tc-99m-labeled human serum albumin (Tc-99m HSA). This agent is also typically prepared from a kit by adding Tc-99m pertechnetate containing human serum albumin and a reducing agent. The advantage of Tc-99m HSA is that it may be prepared ahead of time for administration of multiple doses. This facilitates studies in the CCU and whenever some urgency is required. Labeling efficiency is on the order of 90% for commercial kits, and satisfactory images of the blood pool can be obtained. The disadvantage of Tc-99m HSA is greater uptake in the liver with less activity available in the blood pool. The agent is also contraindicated in patients with histories of allergy to human albumin.

Pharmacokinetics One of the advantages of using Tc-99m-labeled red cells is that they circulate in the blood pool with essentially the half-life of the radiolabel. It is feasible to obtain multiple sequential studies during an interventional maneuver, and it is possible to reimage using the same dosage. By comparison, Tc-99m HSA demonstrates a progressive leakage or clearance from the intravascular space. Less than half of the original activity is available in the blood pool 4 hours after tracer administration. This still makes it feasible to perform multiple acquisitions during an interventional procedure such as stress ventriculography.

Dosimetry The dosimetry for Tc-99m RBCs is presented in Box 4-11.

Box 4-10   Causes of Poor Tc-99m Red Blood Cell Labeling

Drug-drug interactions	Heparin, doxorubicin, methyldopa, hydralazine, iodinated contrast media, quinidine
Circulating antibodies	Prior transfusion, transplantation, some antibiotics
Too little stannous ion	Insufficient to reduce Tc (VII)
Too much stannous ion	Reduction of Tc (VII) outside of RBC
Carrier Tc-99	Buildup of Tc-99 in the Mo-99/ Tc-99m generator due to long interval between elutions
Too short an interval for "tinning"	Not enough time for stannous ion to penetrate RBCs
Too short an incubation time	Not enough time for reduction of Tc (VII)

Box 4-11   Dosimetry for Tc-99m Red Blood Cells

ORGAN	TC-99M RED BLOOD CELLS* RAD/mCi
Blood	0.04
Liver	0.03
Spleen	0.11
Bladder Wall	0.02
Testes	0.01
Ovaries	0.02
Heart Wall	0.10
Total Body	0.015

*Data from package insert (Ultra To-g RBC™) Mallinckrodt Medical Inc., St. Louis, Mo.

First-pass agents All of the above agents may be administered by a bolus technique for first-pass imaging of the central circulation. Several other agents labeled with Tc-99m have also been used for first pass imaging. If only a single study is anticipated, Tc-99m as sodium pertechnetate may be used. The disadvantage of this approach is high residual background activity if multiple studies are required, as in a stress test. Technetium-99m sulfur colloid has the advantage of being rapidly cleared from the circulation, offering the ability to do multiple studies in succession. Likewise, Tc-99m DTPA has been used, although its blood clearance is less rapid than that of sulfur colloid.

Acquisition Techniques

First-pass studies First-pass studies are obtained by injecting a compact bolus of a suitable radiopharmaceutical IV. If a peripheral injection is used, the Oldendorf technique or a variation thereof is employed. The arm is held in a neutral position and a medial vein in the basilic system is used at the antecubital fossa. Use of veins in the cephalic system should be avoided, if possible, to prevent "hang-up" of the bolus at the thoracic inlet. Injections directly through central catheters placed in the superior vena cava provide the most compact boluses. A jugular approach is also sometimes used for interventional studies.

Details of data acquisition will depend on the computer system used. Data may be acquired either in rapid frame mode or by list mode, with or without ECG gating. Whichever approach is used, the goal is to obtain 16 to 30 frames per second while the bolus passes through the central circulation. In most patients, the total data acquisition time required is on the order of 30 seconds or less. In patients with congestive heart failure, bolus transit is delayed and conservatively, first-pass imaging is carried out for 60 seconds.

The patient may be placed in any position. Typically a right anterior oblique view at 20° to 30° angulation is chosen (Figure 4-23). This view best separates the right atrium and the right ventricle and is also one of the standard views of the left ventricle used during cardiac catheterization. This view is suitable for both quantitative and qualitative analysis of biventricular function.

The major advantage of the first-pass approach is that data are collected rapidly over a very few cardiac cycles. Therefore, ventricular function can be measured at peak stress during exercise ventriculography or other intervention. Right ventricular function is also easier to measure than on equilibrium gated blood pool studies, where there is usually overlap between the right and left ventricles in the RAO view and between the right atrium and the right ventricle in the LAO view.

The major disadvantage of the first-pass or first-transit approach is that counting statistics are low in each frame because of the count rate limitations of gamma scintillation cameras. Also, even with tracers that clear the blood, only a limited number of repeated measurements or views is possible. In current practice, equilibrium gated blood pool studies are performed much more frequently than first transit studies. A creative new approach made possible by the availability of Tc-99m-labeled myocardial perfusion agents is to obtain a first-transit ventriculogram and then obtain the myocardial perfusion image in a conventional manner.

Equilibrium gated blood pool studies The limited counting statistics available during any one cardiac cycle and the desirability of linking phases of the cardiac cycle to image data underlie the equilibrium gated blood pool approach to radionuclide ventriculography (RNV). In this approach, ECG leads are placed on the patient and a gating signal that triggers the R wave of the ECG is sent to the nuclear medicine computer system (Figure 4-24). The R wave is a useful marker because it occurs at the end of diastole and the beginning of systole. It is the largest electrical signal in the normal ECG and therefore is not only useful from a timing standpoint but is relatively easy to detect.

The cardiac cycle is divided into 16 to 24 frames in typical commercially available computer systems (Figure 4-25). Individual frame duration is approximately 40 to 50 msec. This frame rate is a compromise between temporal and statistical data sampling. Enough frames are needed to catch the peaks and valleys of the cardiac cycle (temporal sampling), but too many frames reduce counting statistics available in each one (statistical sampling).

During each heartbeat, data are acquired sequentially into the frame buffers spanning the cardiac cycle. With imaging of more than 100 to 300 cardiac cycles, sufficient counting statistics are obtained for valid quantitative analysis and reasonable spatial resolution. Studies at rest are obtained for 250,000 counts per frame. Studies obtained during exercise or other intervention are often obtained for somewhat fewer counts per frame in order to capture the peak effect of the stress (Box 4-12).

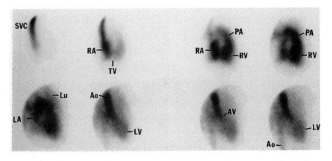

Fig. 4-23 First-pass radionuclide angiogram. Cardiac structures are sequentially visualized as the bolus passes through the right heart into the lungs and then returns to the left-sided structures. *SVC*, superior vena cava; *RA*, right atrium; *TV*, tricuspid valve; *RV*, right ventricle; *PA*, pulmonary artery; *LA*, left atrium; *Lu*, lung; *Ao*, aorta; *LV*, left ventricle; *AV*, aortic valve.

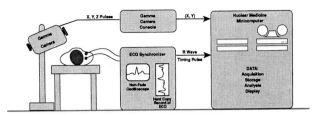

Fig. 4-24   Schematic of R-wave-gated radionuclide ventriculography acquisition. A special ECG synchronizer or gating device detects the R wave and sends a timing pulse to the nuclear medicine computer system. This timing pulse is used to sort incoming scintillation events into a sequence of frames that spans the cardiac cycle.

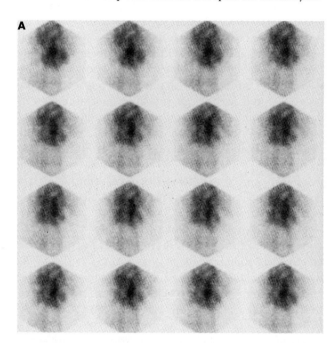

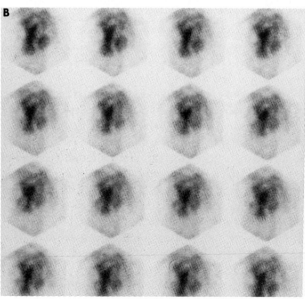

Fig. 4-25   R-wave-gated radionuclide ventriculograms in the anterior (**A**) and 45° left anterior oblique (**B**) views. In this study the cardiac cycle was divided into 16 frames. Note the change in size and count density of the cardiac chambers through the cardiac cycle.

Box 4-12   Equilibrium Gated Blood Pool Ventriculography: Protocol Summary

PATIENT PREPARATION AND PRECAUTIONS

Establish that patient is in normal sinus rhythm (less than 5%-10% PVCs).

DOSAGE AND ROUTE OF TRACER ADMINISTRATION

Tc-99m red blood cells, 10-20 mCi (370-740 MBq). Intravenous administration.

IMAGING PROTOCOL

Use a low-energy, general-purpose or high-sensitivity collimator and a 20% window centered at 140 keV.

Obtain 10° RAO (or anterior), mid-LAO, and left lateral views. Consider additional views (e.g., LPO) if clinical conditions warrant.

Use the gamma camera persistence oscilloscope to determine the optimum LAO position for separating left and right ventricular activity.

Obtain a minimum of 16 frames per cardiac cycle and use a frame duration of 50 msec or less.

Obtain 250k counts per frame for studies performed at rest (10-inch field of view camera).

Obtain 100k counts per frame in the optimum LAO view for studies obtained during an intervention (10-inch field of view camera).

The underlying assumption of R-wave gating is the presence of normal sinus rhythm so that data are added together from corresponding segments of the cardiac cycle over the entire time of the study (Figure 4-26). Any significant dysrhythmia degrades the quality of the data and renders quantitative analysis at least partially invalid.

A rhythm strip should be obtained in every patient prior to the injection of radioactivity to determine suitability for examination. For example, rapid atrial fibrillation with an irregular ventricular response is a contraindication to the study (Figure 4-26). Up to 5% to 10% premature ventricular contractions (PVCs) can be tolerated. Other problems with gating include spurious signals from skeletal muscle activity, giant T waves triggering the gating device, and artifacts from pacemakers. The pacemaker signal itself is usually a reliable trigger for gating, and high-quality studies may be obtained in patients with pacemakers.

Special computer techniques may be used to filter data from premature contractions and postextrasystolic beats but greatly increase the time needed to acquire a study. By the same token, elegant gated list mode data acquisition techniques have been developed to separately analyze the normal sinus beat, the premature contraction, and the postextrasystolic beat.

For studies at rest, multiple views are obtained to provide the most comprehensive evaluation of regional ven-

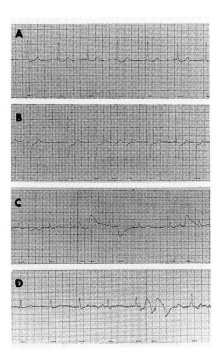

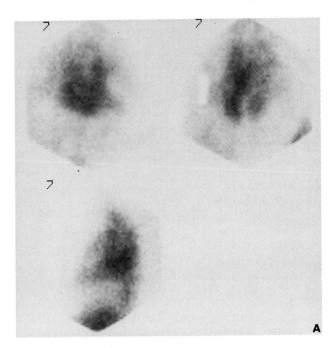

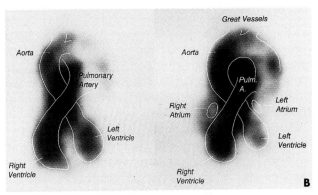

Fig. 4-26   ECG rhythm strips obtained from patients referred for gated radionuclide ventriculography. Panel **A** demonstrates the desired normal sinus rhythm. Excessive PVCs (**B**) or atrial fibrillation with irregular ventricular response (**C**) degrade image quality. Skeletal muscle artifacts can trigger the gating pulse in patients undergoing exercise (**D**). (From Brady TJ, Thrall JH, Clare JM, et al: Exercise radionuclide ventriculography: practical considerations and sensitivity of coronary artery disease detection, *Radiology* 132:697-702, 1979. Reproduced with permission.)

Fig. 4-27   **A,** End-diastolic images from a gated radionuclide ventriculogram. Anterior (*top left*), LAO (*top right*), and LPO (*bottom*) views are the most commonly performed. **B,** Line drawing over LAO end-diastolic (*left*) and end systolic (*right*) frames indicating position and relationships of major structures.

tricular wall motion. These views include a shallow 10° RAO, a 30° to 60° LAO, and an LPO (Figure 4-27). The exact angulation for the LAO view is determined empirically by moving the head of the gamma camera. The LAO angle that best separates the activity in the left and right ventricles is selected to facilitate calculation of the left ventricular ejection fraction and other quantitative and functional parameters. For studies obtained during exercise stress testing or other forms of stress intervention, the gamma camera head is left in the optimal LAO view, again to facilitate quantitative analysis of ejection fraction and other parameters.

Protocols for obtaining exercise RNVs are highly variable between institutions. Some departments measure the left ventricular ejection fraction at each stage of a graded exercise program designed to recapitulate graded treadmill stress. Other departments obtain a baseline study and a single repeat study during peak exercise. Exact exercise protocols are typically customized to the physical condition of the patient.

In addition to exercise stress, a number of other alternatives have been proposed, including cold presser testing, handgrip isometric exercise, atrial pacing, and pharmacologic stress. Unlike the success of pharmacologic intervention for myocardial perfusion imaging, none of the alternatives to leg exercise have proved efficacious for RNV.

Data Analysis and Study Interpretation

Qualitative analysis   Comprehensive analysis and interpretation of RNVs requires both qualitative and quantitative assessments (Box 4-13). Wall motion is typically analyzed by observing the RNV in a repetitive cinematic closed loop display on the computer screen. Wall motion is inferred from "shrinkage" of the ventricular activity from diastole to systole. Failure of activity to diminish or clear along the ventricular periphery is an indication of abnormal wall motion. Septal contraction is inferred from seeing the photon-deficient area between the right ventricular and left ventricular blood pools thicken during systole.

Complete absence of wall motion is termed *akinesis*. Abnormal areas demonstrating residual but diminished contraction are said to be *hypokinetic*. Areas demonstrating paradoxical wall motion—that is, an actual outward bulge during systole—are termed *dyskinetic*. If motion is still present but delayed compared to adjacent segments, the term *tardokinesis* is used.

In normal subjects all wall segments should contract, with the greatest excursion seen in the left ventricular free wall and apex. Areas of ventricular scar are typically akinetic or dyskinetic. Areas of ventricular ischemia are akinetic or hypokinetic. Tardokinesis may be seen secondary to ischemia or conduction abnormalities such as bundle-branch block.

The complete qualitative or visual analysis of the RNV includes an assessment of cardiac chamber size for all four cardiac chambers, assessment of regional wall motion and overall biventricular performance, and assessment of any extracardiac abnormalities such as aortic aneurysms or pericardial effusions that are in the detector's field of view. Accurate qualitative assessment requires some experience. The computer controls can be used to vary the speed of the cinematic closed loop display, which can be a visual cue for detecting more motion abnormalities. Only those portions of the ventricles not overlapped by other cardiac structures should be assessed on any given view. For example, on the anterior or shallow RAO view, there is usually some overlap of the right ventricle on the septum and inferior wall of the left ventricle.

In addition to visual analysis of regional wall motion, attempts have been made to use quantitative and functional or parametric images to detect abnormalities in regional wall motion. For example, regions of interest may be flagged along the ventricular perimeter to calculate regional ejection fractions. Fourier phase analysis and other parametric image analysis techniques will be described below.

Quantitative data analysis

Ejection fraction   The most frequently calculated quantitative parameter of ventricular function is the left ventricular ejection fraction (Box 4-13). This is defined as the fraction of the left ventricular end-diastolic volume expelled during contraction. The principle underlying the calculation is that the net left ventricular count rate at each point in the cardiac cycle is proportional to ventricular volume. The net ventricular counts are determined by flagging a region of interest over the left ventricle for each frame (Figure 4-28) of the cardiac cycle and a background region, typically taken as a crescent adjacent to the left ventricular apex (Figure 4-29). The background region of interest should not overlap activity emanating from the spleen. A background-corrected ventricular time–activity curve is then generated (Figure 4-29). End-diastole is taken as the frame demonstrating the highest counts and end-systole the frame with the fewest counts.

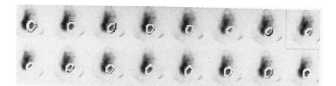

Fig. 4-28   In calculating the left ventricular ejection fraction a region of interest is defined over the left ventricle in each frame of the cardiac cycle.

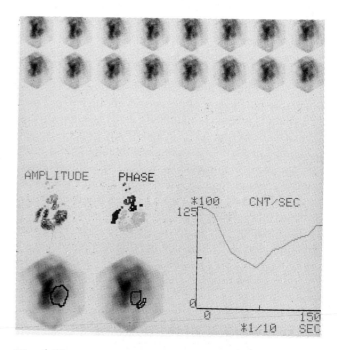

Fig. 4-29   Composite computer-generated display from the analysis of a gated radionuclide ventriculogram. The sequential LAO views are displayed across the top. The end-diastolic and end-systolic regions of interest are indicated, along with the crescent-shaped background region of interest (*bottom row*). Parametric images are displayed for amplitude and phase analysis along with the time–activity curve.

Ejection fraction is calculated as follows:

$$\text{Ejection fraction} = \frac{\text{End-diastolic count (net)} - \text{End-systolic count (net)}}{\text{End-diastolic count (net)}}.$$

The average ejection fraction in normal subjects is on the order of .65, with a range of .55 to .75. Many nuclear medicine departments use .50 as a cutoff for normal. (These fractions are also frequently given as percentages.) The accuracy of the ejection fraction calculation by RNV is considered very good, with numerous studies demonstrating good correlation with contrast-enhanced left ventriculography.

The time–activity curve should be inspected in each case as a quality control measure. Theoretically, the count values at the beginning and end of the curve should be identical. In practice, the trailing frames in late diastole usually have fewer counts, owing to slight variations in the length of the cardiac cycle, even in patients with normal sinus rhythm (Figure 4-30). In patients with frequent PVCs, the fall-off at the end of the curve is much greater. In atrial fibrillation with an irregular ventricular response there can be a marked fall-off because cardiac cycles of widely varying length are being added together. Quantitative analysis of gated data in cases with major dysrhythmias is not accurate.

Numerous other quantitative parameters have been proposed for calculation from equilibrium gated blood pool examinations (Box 4-13). None of these can be considered as well documented and validated as the left ventricular ejection fraction. Calculation of the right ventricular ejection fraction from equilibrium data is problematic due to overlap of chambers. Calculation of stroke volume and cardiac output requires correction of the left ventricular count rate for soft tissue attenuation. All proposed attenuation correction methods are subject

to error. Use of quantitative parameters other than the left ventricular ejection fraction is largely reserved for clinical research studies.

Rates of ventricular filling and emptying (dV/dt) (Figure 4-30) have found some utility in assessing drug therapy. For example, calcium channel blockers used in the treatment of idiopathic hypertrophic subaortic stenosis facilitate myocardial relaxation and thereby more rapid diastolic filling. Again, the measurement is used primarily in clinical research.

Fourier phase analysis Fourier phase analysis reduces four-dimensional data into a pair of two-dimensional images. These images portray cardiac contractility (amplitude) and contraction sequence (phase) (Figure 4-29). Simplistically, each pixel in the cardiac image can be considered to have its own cycle having an amplitude and a characteristic temporal relationship (i.e., phase) with respect to the R wave (Figure 4-31). The amplitude image (Figure 4-29) simply portrays the maximum net count variation for each pixel during the cardiac cycle. The phase image portrays the relative time delay from the R wave to the start of the cardiac cycle for that individual pixel.

If the complete cardiac cycle is taken as encompassing 360°, the atria and ventricles are 180° "out of phase" normally (Figure 4-32). Areas of the ventricle that contract slightly earlier in the cardiac cycle owing to the pattern of the electrical conduction down the septum and through the bundle branches are seen to be slightly out of phase with adjacent ventricular areas.

Wall motion abnormalities are portrayed on phase images as low-amplitude areas. Regions of paradoxical motion due to left ventricular aneurysms, for example, are 180° "out of phase" with the ventricle. Abnormal conduction patterns like those seen in Wolff-Parkinson-White syndrome or bundle-branch block cause affected areas to be slightly out of phase with adjacent portions of the ventricle owing to premature or delayed contraction.

Phase maps are often displayed in color to highlight the temporal sequences of cardiac chamber emptying. A dynamic display mode can be used to demonstrate the propagating wave front that sweeps across the ventricle during contraction, linking pixels with similar phase angles together.

Although Fourier phase analysis is very elegant, the studies require exceptionally well synchronized data to be useful for detecting conduction abnormalities. Amplitude and phase images are often presented automatically as part of computer analysis packages and are useful for cueing the observer to areas of abnormal wall motion.

Functional images Other functional images can also be created that are somewhat simpler to understand than Fourier phase analysis. The intensity of the computer display at each point in an image is determined by the number of scintigraphic events recorded at that point and in turn is proportional to the amount of radioactivity in the corresponding location. By subtract-

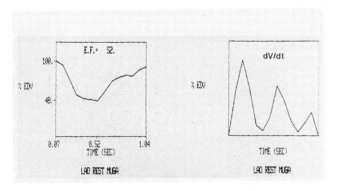

Fig. 4-30 Time–activity curve from the left ventricle (*left panel*) is used for calculation of the ejection fraction. The trailing end of the curve is slightly lower than the origin, due to variations in the time duration of the cardiac cycle. In this case rapid filling of the ventricle occurred immediately after systole, followed by slower filling (diastasis) and a late phase component ("atrial kick"). *Right-hand panel* depicts the rate of ventricular emptying and filling as the percentage of end-diastolic volume per second.

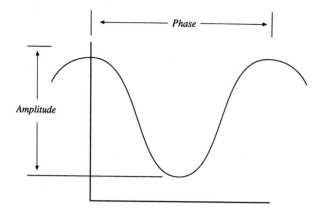

Fig. 4-31 Illustrated are the concepts of phase and amplitude. Each pixel has its own characteristic variation and count rate through the cardiac cycle and its own characteristic timing of the peaks and valleys of the amplitude change.

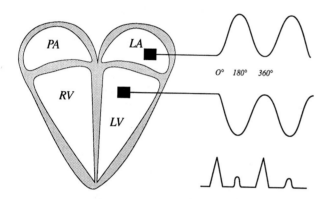

Fig. 4-32 Simplified schematic illustrating that the atria and ventricles are 180° "out of phase" with each other; that is, the ventricle fills while the atrium contracts.

ing the end-systolic image from the end-diastolic image point by point, a derived or functional image is created that portrays *regional stroke volume*. The stroke volume image may be further processed by dividing it point by point by the end-diastolic frame to create an "ejection fraction" image. In these images, akinetic wall segments correspond to areas of diminished or absent intensity.

In the paradox image the end-diastolic frame is subtracted from the end-systolic frame. In subjects with normal ventricular function, this leaves a void. In patients with areas of paradoxical ventricular wall motion, the systolic bulge is readily detected as an area of unsubtracted activity.

A complete analysis and interpretation of the RNV includes a qualitative visual assessment of the cardiac chambers and great vessels to assess their size and relationships. Visual assessment of the dynamic cinematic display is also used to analyze regional wall motion. Quantitative analysis includes at a minimum calculation of the left ventricular ejection fraction. For specific applications, other quantitative parameters such as left

and right ventricular stroke volume ratios, cardiac output, ventricular volume, and rates of ventricular filling and emptying may be also be calculated but require more sophisticated analysis and in some cases more sophisticated data acquisition techniques.

Clinical Applications

Acute myocardial infarction The hallmark of acute MI on RNV is the development of a wall motion abnormality in the region of the infarct (Figure 4-33) and a decrease in the global ejection fraction. The left ventricular ejection fraction may be decreased even in patients without clinical manifestations of congestive heart failure or other hemodynamic indicators of infarction.

The prognosis of patients following acute MI is directly linked to the degree of functional impairment. In most series, over 75% of patients with acute MIs have abnormal ejection fractions. The mean ejection fractions of those with uncomplicated infarcts is higher than in those who develop left ventricular failure or overt pulmonary edema. Patients showing a serial decline in ejection fraction have a significantly higher risk of mortality in the early postinfarction period.

In patients with inferior infarctions, the right ventricle should be carefully assessed in addition to the left ventricle. Right ventricular wall motion abnormalities may be seen in as many as 40% of patients with inferior infarctions. Right ventricular involvement is unusual in pure anterior infarctions. The finding of right ventricular involvement, particularly as an isolated or dominant finding, is significant in directing therapy. Therapy for right ventricular dysfunction includes volume loading to maintain left atrial filling pressure and thereby adequate left ventricular filling. Volume loading is usually contraindicated in left ventricular infarction.

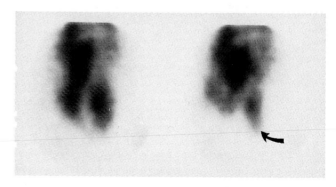

Fig. 4-33 Selected end-diastolic (ED) and end-systolic (ES) images from a patient with acute anteroapical myocardial infarction. The apex is akinetic (*arrow*). Note the good contraction of the right ventricle and the other portions of the left ventricle.

Radionuclide techniques are frequently applied after the acute phase of infarction to determine the presence of residual disease and the degree of functional impairment. Stress myocardial perfusion scintigraphy is more frequently employed for this purpose in contemporary practice than exercise RNV. The goal of both examinations is to detect myocardial segments at risk for future events. Sudden death following MI, either acute or delayed, is often due to arrhythmias arising from ischemic areas of the ventricle. Therefore, the prognosis and management of patients demonstrating no postinfarction ischemia are significantly different from that of patients with residual disease.

Coronary artery disease   Many patients with CAD have no clinical manifestations and have normal ventricular function at rest. Exercise-induced myocardial ischemia can be detected with RNV. The hallmark of ischemia is the development of a new wall motion abnormality during exercise stress testing that was not present at rest, and a failure of the ejection fraction to increase or even to decline in response to exercise (Box 4-14).

In patients able to achieve adequate levels of exercise, the technique is highly sensitive, on the order of 90%, for the detection of CAD. The major limitations of the technique are the inability of a significant percentage of patients to achieve adequate levels of exercise and the nonspecificity of an abnormal ventricular functional response to exercise stress. In Brady's series the overall sensitivity of RNV for CAD was 85%. In patients experiencing chest pain, S-T segment depression of at least 1 millimeter, or achieving a pressure-rate product greater than 250,000, the sensitivity was 94%. Twenty-five percent of the patients failed to achieve adequate exercise, and the exercise RNV was abnormal in only 62%.

The question of specificity is complex. In selected normal volunteers the specificity is very high, approaching 100%. However, when the test is applied in a broader cross-section of patients with noncoronary heart disease as well as coronary heart disease, specificity drops and has been reported as low as 55%. In current practice it is very difficult to assess the true sensitivity and specificity of noninvasive tests because the results are used to guide selection of patients for cardiac catheterization. This selection bias tends to make noninvasive tests look more sensitive and less specific than they really are because patients with abnormal tests are more frequently referred for the reference standard of cardiac catheterization than patients with normal results.

A decade ago, exercise stress RNV and stress Tl-201 myocardial perfusion imaging were competitive as the procedures of choice for the diagnosis of CAD. Myocardial perfusion imaging is the clear-cut winner in today's practice. It is far easier to perform and is easily grafted on to a standard treadmill stress ECG examination.

Box 4-15 lists some conditions other than CAD that result in abnormal response to exercise. These are all potential causes of false positive, abnormal test results, lowering the specificity of exercise RNV.

Evaluation following coronary artery bypass graft surgery   Exercise RNV has been used to evaluate the functional outcome of CABG surgery. Since resting studies are frequently normal prior to CABG, the comparison of interest is the pre- versus postoperative response to exercise stress. The literature consensus suggests that the majority of patients show improvement after surgery for both global ejection fraction and regional wall motion. Again, surgical efficacy can also be assessed with myocardial perfusion scintigraphy, and the ventriculographic approach is not frequently used.

Valvular heart disease   Patients with valvular heart disease may experience pressure overload, volume overload, or both. The response to pressure overload is concentric hypertrophy. The response to volume overload may be congestive heart failure, if it is acute, or dilation,

---

Box 4-14   Diagnostic Criteria for Exercise Radionuclide Ventriculography

NORMAL BASELINE

Resting ejection fraction greater than .50.
No regional wall motion abnormalities.
Normal ventricular chamber size.

NORMAL RESPONSE TO EXERCISE

Ejection fraction increases by .05 with continued normal regional wall motion.

ABNORMAL RESPONSE TO EXERCISE

Failure of ejection fraction to increase or an actual decrease, and/or development of a new wall motion abnormality with or without an increase in ventricular chamber size.

Box 4-15   Causes of Abnormal Ventricular Functional Response to Exercise

Hemodynamically significant coronary artery disease
Cardiomyopathy
Myocarditis
Valvular heart disease
Pericardial disease
Drug toxicity
Prior surgery or injury

if it is chronic and progressive. Radionuclide ventriculography allows assessment of ventricular size and ejection fraction. Because the ejection fraction is in part determined by preload, afterload, and heart rate, determination of the ejection fraction at rest cannot be used alone to assess myocardial contractility or functional reserve. Moreover, the diagnosis of CAD in patients with severe valvular abnormalities is problematic because abnormalities associated with valvular disease can cause both regional and global dysfunction.

The findings on RNV are essentially as would be predicted from observations at cardiac catheterization with respect to chamber size and function. One potentially very helpful measurement that is easier to determine with RNV than with contrast angiography is a calculation of stroke volume ratios for the left and right ventricles. With mitral insufficiency, for example, some of the blood is propelled antegrade and some regurgitates through the mitral valve during each left ventricular contraction. In normal subjects the stroke volume ratio between the ventricles should be 1.0, since all of the blood is propelled antegrade. Thus the stroke volume ratio provides a measure of the severity of regurgitation that can be followed sequentially and that has been shown to correlate with the clinical status of the patient.

The major limitation of the calculation of the stroke volume ratio from equilibrium blood pool studies is chamber overlap between the right and left ventricles and between the right ventricle and the right atrium. It is also difficult in many cases to establish the exact level of the pulmonic valve. For these reasons most investigators have established a normal cutoff at an LV/RV ratio of 1.5, or greater rather than 1.0.

Cardiomyopathy-myocarditis Cardiomyopathies are a diverse group of disorders. They may be classified as congestive, hypertrophic, or restrictive. In congestive cardiomyopathies the ventricles are typically enlarged and dysfunctional (Figure 4-36). The global ejection fraction is decreased and wall motion is uniformly poor, with the exception that there is frequently sparing of the septal and anterior basal segments.

The hallmark of the hypertrophic cadiomyopathies is asymmetric septal hypertrophy. Echocardiography is the diagnostic procedure of choice. The left ventricular chamber is typically small and the ejection fraction is above normal. Diastolic filling is abnormal due to poor compliance of the hypertrophied myocardium. Diastolic filling rates have been measured by RNV to assess response to therapy. Many patients improve with calcium channel blocker therapy.

Assessment of drug therapy The role of RNV has been studied extensively to assess the therapeutic effects of cardiac drugs and the toxic effects of noncardiac drugs. Studies of cardiac therapeutic drugs are not used in rou-

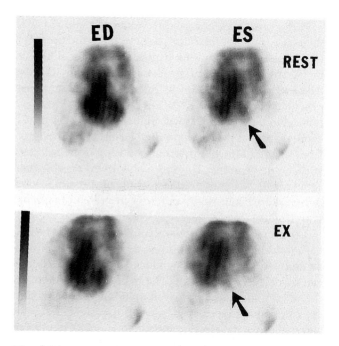

Fig. 4-34 Normal exercise radionuclide ventriculogram. Note the improved emptying of the left ventricle in response to exercise (*arrows*).

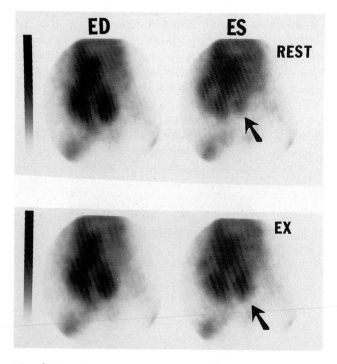

Fig. 4-35 Abnormal response to exercise in a patient with hemodynamically significant coronary artery disease. There is marked enlargement of the left ventricle at end-systole on the exercise study compared to the study obtained at rest (*arrows*).

tine clinical practice but are very valuable from a clinical research standpoint. Cardiac drugs studied by RNV in the literature include digitalis, nitroglycerin, aminophylline, propranolol and other beta blockers, isoproterenol, and calcium channel blockers among others. The functional outcome of thrombolytic therapy has been evaluated by RNV performed before and after thrombolysis.

Of perhaps more direct clinical applicability is the use of RNV to follow the cardiotoxic effects of noncardiac drugs. A well-studied drug in this regard is doxorubicin. Administration of doxorubicin (Adriamycin) in excess of 550 mg/m^2 results in cardiotoxicity in approximately one third of patients. However, in serial monitoring of drug response, as little as 350 mg/m^2 may result in toxicity, and some patients can tolerate significantly more drug than a nominal 550 mg/m^2. The recommendation of Alexander and co-workers is that the drug should be discontinued if there is a greater than 15% drop in ejection fraction during therapy. Functional recovery is poor.

Pulmonary disease   Most RNVs are obtained to assess left ventricular function. However, characteristic findings are seen in the right heart in patients with cor pulmonale. Right ventricular enlargement is readily detected, and in virtually all patients judged to have cor pulmonale on other grounds, the right ventricular ejection fraction is abnormal (Figure 4-37).

In patients with a new onset of dyspnea, the RNV can help differentiate left ventricular from pulmonary dysfunction. The demonstration of a normal left ventricular ejection fraction, wall motion, and chamber size strongly suggests a pulmonary etiology.

Congenital heart disease   Radionuclide ventriculography has not played a large role in the evaluation of patients with congenital heart disease. However, it is possible to detect shunts using the technique, and it is possible to calculate shunt index ratios for both left-to-right and right-to-left shunts.

For left-to-right shunts, the central circulation is studied using the first-transit technique. Early recirculation into the right ventricle is detected using a curve-fitting technique.

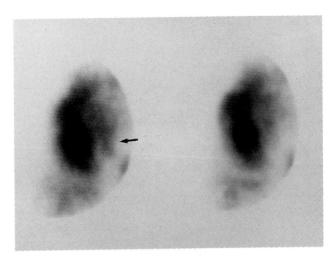

Fig. 4-37   Radionuclide ventriculography in a patient with cor pulmonale demonstrates an unusually dilated right ventricle with poor contraction between end-diastole (*left*) and end-systole (*right*). The left ventricle is small and contracts normally (*arrow*).

In brief, the lung transit curve (Figure 4-38A) is modeled by a mathematical function called a gamma variate (Figure 4-38B). The contribution to the time–activity curve from recirculation is taken as the difference between the total area under the time–activity curve minus the area under the gamma variate fit (Figure 4-38C). It is possible to detect shunts as small as 20% using this approach.

Right-to-left shunts may be detected using Tc-99m-labeled macroaggregated albumin. The ratio of tracer in the lung to tracer gaining access to the systemic circulation provides a measure of the severity of shunting. Right-to-left shunts are generally given as a relative contraindication to the use of macroaggregated albumin, owing to the theoretical risk of embolizing the capillary bed of the brain. In practice this has not been a problem, but great caution and care are needed in preparing the material and using this approach.

POSITRON EMISSION TOMOGRAPHY STUDIES OF THE HEART

Positron emission tomography (PET) affords superior spatial resolution compared to single photon imaging and also offers a wide variety of physiologically and biochemically useful radiopharmaceuticals. PET is available in a limited number of institutions but provides a horizon for the future of nuclear cardiology.

The three most important radiopharmaceuticals in current practice are rubidium-82, nitrogen-13 ammonia, and F-18 fluorodeoxyglucose (FDG). Rb-82 is obtained from a strontium/rubidium generator. N-13 and F-18 are obtained from cyclotron production.

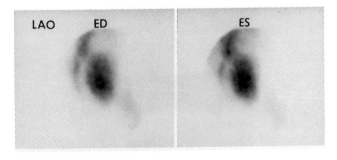

Fig. 4-36   Markedly enlarged left ventricle with poor contraction in a patient with long-standing congestive cardiomyopathy.

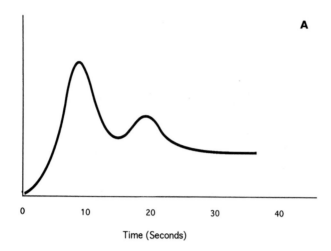

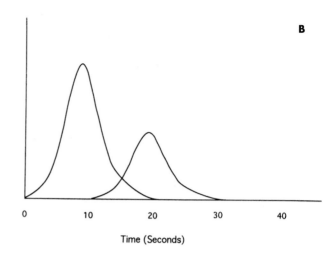

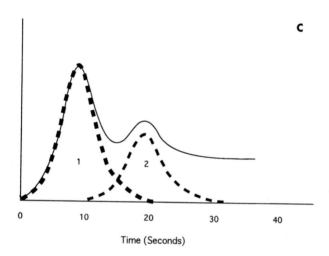

Fig. 4-38   A, Time–activity curve obtained from a region of interest over the lungs in a patient with a left-to-right shunt. The second peak is due to early recirculation of tracer through the left-to-right shunt. **B,** The relative contributions from the initial transit and the shunt are determined from a curve-fitting technique. **C,** This figure illustrates the initial time–activity curve and the two mathematically fitted curves. The shunt ratio (Q_p/Q_s) is calculated from the areas under these curves.

Rb-82 and N-13 ammonia are markers of myocardial perfusion. FDG is a marker of myocardial glucose metabolism.

The scintigraphic appearance and diagnostic criteria for Rb-82 and N-13 ammonia studies are analogous to findings on Tl-201 myocardial perfusion scans (Figures 4-39, 4-40). The same rest-stress paradigms and interventional protocols may be used, although the short half-lives strongly favor pharmacologic stress versus exercise. The reported sensitivity of PET in the diagnosis of CAD is on the order of 95%. The specificity reported in the early literature is also at the level of 95% or better. This specificity should be regarded with caution, since early reports under clinical research protocols frequently use normal volunteers to determine specificity, which is very different from determining specificity in a more broadly chosen cross-section of patients with and without CAD.

An additional advantage of the PET technique for perfusion imaging is the ability to actually calculate perfusion per gram of myocardial tissue. This offers the ability to determine myocardial functional reserve and to aid in the distinction between severely ischemic and nonviable tissue.

Another method of assessing myocardial viability is the combined use of a perfusion tracer and FDG (Figure 4-41). Under normal conditions, 85% of the energy needs of the heart are met through fatty acid metabolism. Areas of ischemia switch preferentially to glucose metabolism. A characteristic pattern of markedly reduced perfusion demonstrated by Rb-82 or N-13 ammonia coupled with preserved or even increased accumulation of FDG (Figure 4-42) indicates ischemic but viable myocardium (Table 4-6). Early studies indicate that myocardial wall segments failing to show uptake of a perfusion agent but demonstrating FDG uptake prior to coronary artery bypass surgery show improved function after surgery in over half of cases. Necrotic myocardial tissue does not demonstrate FDG accumulation. Areas demonstrating no FDG accumulation show improvement in less than 5% of cases.

Following MI, PET studies are useful for distinguishing viable myocardium from myocardial scar. Routine Tl-201 perfusion scintigraphy appears to overestimate the number of fixed defects indicating scar. An increased uptake of FDG after surgery is a predictor of contractile function recovery. Early experience also suggests that half of segments with diminished perfusion following infarction but with FDG uptake maintained will improve functionally.

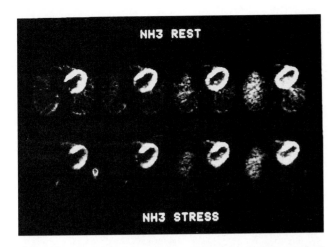

Fig. 4-39   Rest and stress nitrogen-13 ammonia studies in a normal subject. Uptake is uniformly good throughout the left ventricular myocardium. Faint uptake is also visualized in the right ventricular myocardium (images are in standard computed tomography format).

Table 4-6   Diagnostic Patterns for Combined PET Perfusion and FDG Imaging

	Perfusion (NH₃, Ab)	Glucose Metabolism (FDG)
Normal myocardium	+	+
Ischemic myocardium (severe, chronic)	↓ or −	+
Necrotic myocardium or scar	−	−

INFARCT-AVID IMAGING

Radiopharmaceuticals

In the early 1960s, mercury-203 chlormerodrin was shown to localize In acutely infarcted myocardium. Subsequently a variety of agents have been shown to have the same property. Many of these have been labeled with Tc-99m, including tetracycline, gluceptate, medronate, and pyrophosphate. The current agent of choice for infarct-avid imaging is Tc-99m pyrophosphate. This radiopharmaceutical has been shown empirically to be superior to Tc-99m diphosphonate for this specific application.

An alternative approach to infarct-avid imaging is the use of radiolabeled antimyosin antibodies. Indium-111-labeled antimyosin localizes avidly in areas of acute MI. The Fab fragment is used. Infarcted areas are clearly visible by 24 hours after injection. However, the optimal interval between injection and imaging is 48 hours, and an FDA-approved agent is not available in the United States.

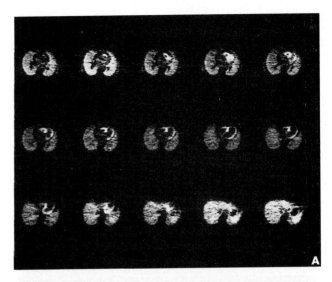

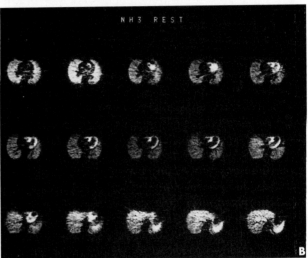

Fig. 4-40   **A,** Stress myocardial perfusion study obtained with nitrogen-13 amonia and persantine. The patient has an extensive defect in the anterior and apical wall (images are in standard computed tomography format). There is significant uptake in the lung, which is frequently seen with N-13 amonia. **B,** Corresponding rest study reveals a smaller anteroapical defect, indicating that the patient has both fixed and transient abnormalities.

Tc-99m Pyrophosphate

Preparation and pharmacokinetics   Technetium-99m-labeled pyrophosphate is prepared in the same way that the Tc-99m-labeled bone imaging agents are prepared. Sodium pertechnetate from a generator is added to a vial containing pyrophosphate and stannous ion Sn (II) as the reducing agent. The technetium-99m forms a chelate with the pyrophosphate molecule. The labeling process is susceptible to the adverse effects of oxygen, with the potential for formation of colloidal impurities and/or reduction in labeling efficiency with the presence of free pertechnetate. Colloidal impurities are recognized by excessive uptake in the liver, and free pertechnetate is recognized by uptake in the thyroid gland, salivary glands, GI tract, and excessive vascular and soft tissue background activity. In clinical practice it is important to avoid introduction of air into multidose vials; and, as with the skeletal agents, it is desirable to use the prepared radiopharmaceutical within 2 or 3 hours.

The pharmacokinetics of Tc-99m pyrophosphate are essentially the same as for Tc-99m diphosphonate. Clearance from the vascular space is rapid, with less than 8% to 10% remaining in the circulation after 3 hours. Skeletal uptake is on the order of 40% to 50% of the injected dose, and the cumulative urinary excretion at 24 hours is approximately 60%. In the early experience with Tc-99m pyrophosphate, imaging was begun 1 hour after tracer administration. In current practice, most departments wait 3 to 4 hours after tracer administration to allow more complete clearance from the blood. Radioactivity retained in the circulation contributes to background activity in the cardiac blood pool. This activity can be confused with myocardial uptake and potentially result in false positive interpretations of Tc-99m pyrophosphate images. A further delay to allow more complete clearance should be considered in this circumstance.

Mechanisms of localization Following cell death in acute MI there is an influx of calcium and the formation of various calcium phosphate complexes. These microcrystalline deposits act as sites for Tc-99m pyrophosphate uptake. Some binding may also occur on denatured macromolecules. Also, the status of the peri-infarction circulation is important in tracer uptake. Some residual blood flow is necessary to deliver the tracer to the infarct area and surrounding tissue. The tracer then diffuses into the necrotic tissue and is bound. The highest uptake of Tc-99m pyrophosphate is at the periphery of infarctions. In large infarctions, with neither direct flow nor diffusion to the central area, no tracer is delivered, and a characteristic ring or donut pattern is seen due to activity around the margin of the damaged area (Figure 4-43).

Technique Technetium-99m pyrophosphate infarct-avid studies are most commonly performed in the CCU with a mobile gamma scintillation camera. Fifteen to 25 mCi (555–925 MBq) is administered IV, with imaging begun 3 to 4 hours later. A high-resolution collimator should be used, and most departments acquire three or four views, including the anterior, 35° LAO, 70° LAO, and left lateral views. At least 500k counts are obtained. An alternative is the acquisition of a 500k anterior view and subsequent imaging for the same length of time in the other views (Box 4-16).

The optimum time to apply the procedure is 24 to 48

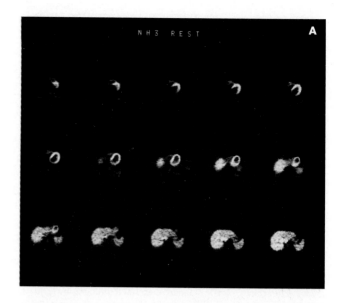

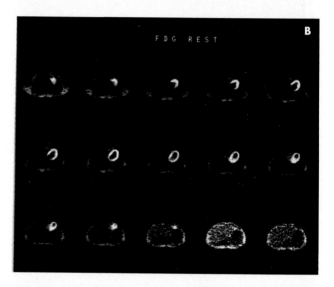

Fig. 4-41 Combined nitrogen-13 ammonia (**A**) and fluorine-18 (FDG) (**B**) imaging in a patient at rest and without significant coronary artery disease. The patterns of uptake are concordant.

hours after acute infarction. Earlier or more delayed imaging may be indicated by the clinical situation. For patients able to be transported to the nuclear medicine department, SPECT imaging should be considered. This technique offers greater image contrast, allowing detection of smaller abnormalities and also more exact anatomic localization of infarcts (Figure 4-44).

If initial images reveal diffuse activity in the region of the heart, further delay can be helpful to allow more complete clearance of tracer from the blood pool. If a comparison of early and further delayed images reveals a decrease in skeletal-to-heart activity, it suggests residual

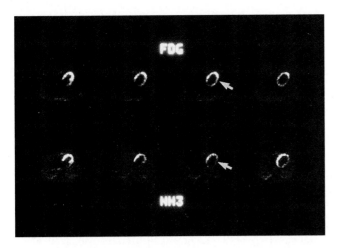

Fig. 4-42   Combined N-13 amonnia and F-18 FDG imaging in a patient with severe myocardial ischemia. Note the decreased perfusion in the lateral wall on the N-13 amonia study in an area showing preserved F-18 FDG uptake (*arrows*).

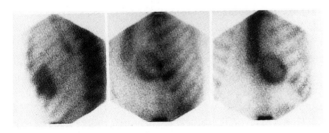

Fig. 4-43   Technetium-99m pyrophosphate scan in a patient with a huge anterior myocardial infarction. Uptake is greatest at the periphery of the infarct, producing a donut appearance on the LAO (*middle*) and anterior (*right*) views.

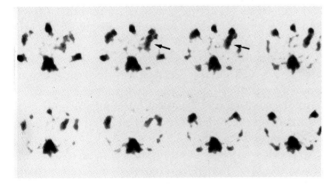

Fig. 4-44   SPECT imaging with Tc-99m pyrophosphate. A large area of abnormal uptake is clearly delineated (*arrows*).

blood pool background. On the other hand, if the activity becomes more focal or increases relative to surrounding skeleton, it points to a myocardial etiology.

Normal appearance of the Tc-99m pyrophosphate scintigram   Technetium-99m pyrophosphate is an avid bone seeker. In normal subjects and in patients without MI, the sternum and ribs should be clearly seen, with no focal or diffuse activity in the region of the heart. Faint residual activity is often seen in the cardiac blood pool.

Time Course of Scan Positivity Following Acute Myocardial Infarction

One of the major limitations of Tc-99m pyrophosphate imaging for diagnosis of acute MI is the delay between the time of infarction and the time of scintigram positivity. Significant uptake becomes demonstrable at 12 hours after infarction. Maximum localization occurs at 48 to 72 hours. Thereafter, uptake begins to diminish as healing in the infarcted area occurs and, in uncomplicated cases, the scintigram reverts to normal by 14 days.

Scintigraphic Patterns in Acute Myocardial Infarction

The classic scintigraphic pattern in MI is a focal area of increased tracer uptake corresponding to the affected

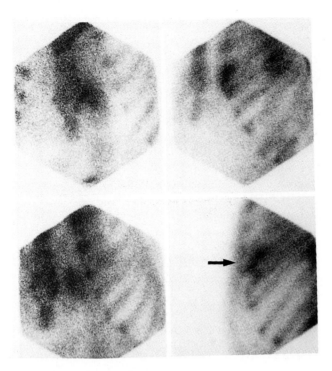

Fig. 4-45   Large anterior wall infarction. Note the convex anterior configuration on the lateral view (*arrow*).

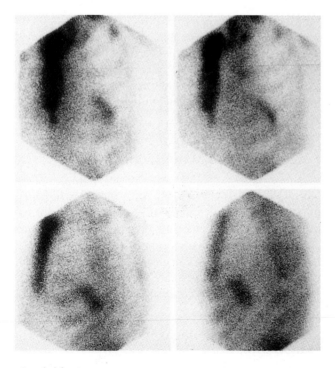

Fig. 4-46   Lateral wall infarction. Uptake is greater than rib uptake and not quite equal to sternal uptake.

region of the heart. It is useful to grade the degree of uptake. One grading system assigns zero to a normal study, 1+ to faint uptake, possibly due to residual blood pool activity, 2+ to uptake equal to rib intensity, and 3+ to uptake greater than rib intensity. The degree of diagnostic confidence increases with the relative grade of uptake and with focal versus diffuse activity.

In addition to the presence of an abnormality, a complete interpretation includes an assessment of location and size. Location is inferred from comparison of the relationship of the abnormal uptake to the skeletal structures on the multiple views obtained from different angles. Anterior infarctions are seen en face on the anterior view and project just behind the sternum on the lateral view (Figures 4-43, 4-45). Lateral wall infarcts appear as vertical curvilinear lesions on the anterior view (Figure 4-46). With progressive obliquity the area of abnormality moves either closer to the sternum (anterolateral infarcts) or farther from the sternum (posterolateral infarcts). Inferior wall infarctions are concave upward and may have a characteristic "lazy 3" configuration if they involve the inferior portion of the septum and right ventricle.

As noted, large infarctions, most frequently in the anterior wall of the left ventricle, may exhibit a donut pattern of increased uptake resulting from absence of tracer in the center of the infarct area (Figure 4-43). This pattern is associated with a poor clinical prognosis; it is typically seen only with quite large infarctions.

There have been numerous attempts to use the Tc-99m pyrophosphate scan to estimate infarct size. Studies have shown that the volume of distribution of abnormal tracer uptake is a relatively good indicator of the area of tissue damage but not a good indicator of the intensity or completeness of tissue damage, since ischemic tissue is frequently interspersed with cords of infarcted myocardium because of interdigitating blood supply and collaterals. Experimental data suggest that a minimum of 3 grams of tissue must be infarcted for scintigraphic detection.

The sensitivity of Tc-99m pyrophosphate scintigraphy is very high, on the order of 95%, for transmural or Q-wave infarctions. The sensitivity for subendocardial infarctions is difficult to establish but is significantly less, probably on the order of 65% for planar Tc-99m pyrophosphate scintigraphy.

The true specificity of the study is difficult to establish due to the lack of an ideal reference standard for ruling out MI. In the early literature, the specificity was reported to be over 90% in the majority of series.

Numerous potential causes of false positive Tc-99m pyrophosphate scans have been reported. Some of the more important are summarized in Box 4-17. False positive studies may result from diffuse activity in the cardiac blood pool that is misinterpreted as emanating from the myocardium. Uptake in areas of chest wall trauma, nec-

Box 4-17   Causes of False Positive Tc-99m Pyrophosphate Infarct-Avid Studies

FOCAL

Old myocardial infarction (persistent positivity)
Calcification (valvular, pericardial)
Ventricular aneurysm
Costal cartilage calcification

DIFFUSE

Myocarditis
Pericarditis
Cardiomyopathy
Amyloidosis
Radiation therapy
Persistent blood pool activity
Doxorubicin (Adriamycin) therapy

rotic skeletal muscle due to prior cardioversion, and in calcifications in or near the heart account for most false positives (Figures 4-47, 4-48). Calcifications in the costal cartilage are occasionally associated with uptake. Old or chronic conditions with mature calcification take up less tracer than do evolving abnormalities.

Several conditions can result in diffusely increased myocardial uptake of Tc-99m pyrophosphate. The most dramatic is amyloidosis (Figure 4-48). The tip-off to amyloid as the etiology is visualization of the entire myocardium, including the right ventricle, with quite good myocardium-to-background ratio. Myocarditis, postradiation injury, and doxorubicin cardiotoxicity are all reported causes of diffusely increased myocardial uptake.

Technetium-99m pyrophosphate scintigrams may remain abnormal for weeks or months after an MI. Those that continue to show uptake for more than 3 months are called *persistently abnormal*. Patients in this category are at higher risk for future MIs and are more likely to have ongoing angina.

Clinical Applications and Utility

The major limitation of Tc-99m infarct-avid scintigraphy is its delayed positivity following the onset of symptoms. In most patients the diagnosis is established from the history, physical examination, ECG, and serum enzyme determinations before the ideal time window for Tc-99m pyrophosphate imaging. The study is not a routine test in suspected acute MI.

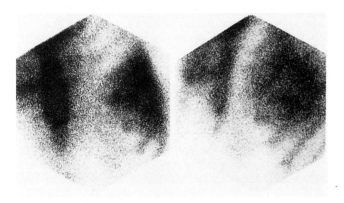

Fig. 4-47   After repeated cardioversion, there is marked uptake in the skeletal muscles of the chest wall. No abnormal uptake is seen in the region of the heart.

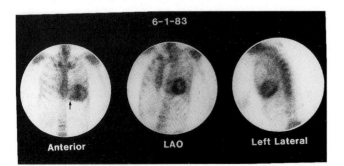

Fig. 4-48   Cardiac amyloidosis. Note uptake of Tc-99m-pyrophosphate throughout the left ventricular myocardium. There is also subtle uptake in the right ventricular myocardium (*arrow*). (From Brown ML, Muroff LR, Mettler FA, Gottschalk A, Thrall JH: Nuclear radiology correlative imaging panel, *RadioGraphics* 5:457, 1985.)

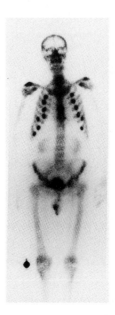

Fig. 4-49   Following cardiac arrest and resuscitation there are multiple rib fractures. Note increased uptake of technetium-99m pyrophosphate.

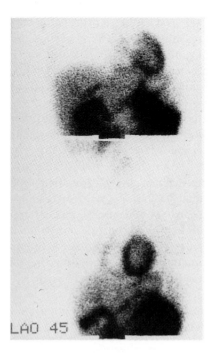

Fig. 4-50   Iodine-123-labeled fatty acid imaging in a volunteer subject affords excellent visualization of the left ventricle and demonstrates some right ventricular uptake.

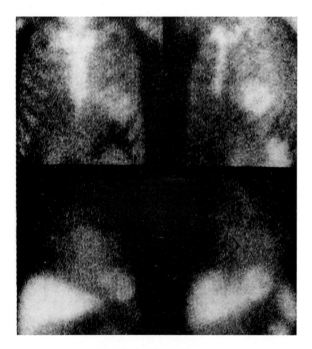

Fig. 4-51   Images in the top row were obtained with technetium-99m pyrophosphate and demonstrate a large area of uptake in an acute myocardial infarction. The bottom two images were obtained with indium-111-labeled antimyocin antibody and demonstrate uptake in the same area. (Courtesy Tsunehiro Yasuda, M.D., Massachusetts General Hospital, Boston.)

Box 4-18   Clinical Settings Where Tc-99m Pyrophosphate Scintigraphy May Have Clinical Utility

Suspected infarction in a patient with left bundle-branch block
Delay in diagnosis; enzymes past expected peak
Post cardioversion
Post major surgery or trauma
Subendocardial (non-Q-wave) infarction versus ischemia
Baseline ECG abnormal due to prior myocardial infarctions
Right ventricular infarction

The main utility of the Tc-99m pyrophosphate study is when the diagnosis of MI is uncertain (Box 4-18). If there is a delay in diagnosis, serum enzyme levels and ECG changes may already have returned to normal. Following surgery or major trauma there may be "spillover" into the MB fraction, making determination of serum creatine kinase isoenzymes problematic. In patients with left bundle-branch block it can be difficult to assess Q waves, and the Tc-99m pyrophosphate study can add to the diagnostic certainty.

OTHER RADIONUCLIDE TECHNIQUES FOR STUDYING THE HEART

A number of experimental radiopharmaceuticals have been used to study the heart. Radiolabeled fatty acids with either single photon or positron-emitting radiolabels have been studied. As noted earlier, 85% of the energy needs of the heart are normally met by fatty acid metabolism. It has been hoped that radiolabeled fatty acids could be used to measure this important metabolic parameter. Several radiolabeled fatty acids have yielded excellent images of the heart, but there is still controversy regarding the significance of the metabolic information provided (Figure 4-50). Metabolic turnover is inferred from the clearance of pharmacokinetics in the myocardium.

Radioiodinated metaiodobenzylguanidine has been used to study the adrenergic status of the heart. The heart is richly innervated, and MIBG has been used to provide some interesting insights. Uptake of MIBG is blocked in patients taking drugs like guanethidine and cocaine that compete for uptake into the presynaptic storage vesicles of the adrenergic system. Decreased uptake is seen following MI and in diabetics with denervated hearts. Some patients with cardiomyopathies also exhibit diminished or absent uptake. A clinical role has not been established for MIBG.

A more promising agent from a clinical standpoint is

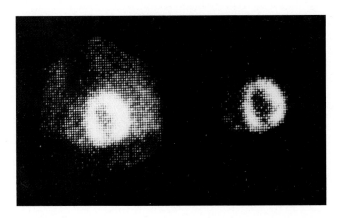

Fig. 4-52   Myocardial scintigram obtained with I-131 metaiodo-benzylguanidine in a normal volunteer subject. The tracer is taken up in presynaptic storage vesicles in the adrenergic nervous system. Cocaine abusers and diabetics with cardioneuropathy have decreased uptake.

radiolabeled antimyosin antibody. This agent is available commercially in Europe but has not yet been approved for clinical use in the United States. The tracer localizes in areas of acute MI (Figure 4-51). The Fab fragment is radiolabeled with In-111 or Tc-99m. The sensitivity for detecting acute MI is quite high, over 85% in reported series. A major disadvantage is the slow pharmacokinetics of antimyosin antibody, which means that optimum imaging cannot be accomplished for many hours after radiopharmaceutical administration. False positive studies may also be seen in patients with myocarditis.

The heart continues to be a fertile ground for the development of additional new radiopharmaceuticals, again with both single photon and positron labels. Metabolic, antibody-binding, and receptor-binding agents are all under active development in laboratories around the world (Figure 4-52).

SUGGESTED READINGS

Bonte FJ, Parkey RW, Graham KD et al: A new method for radionuclide imaging of myocardial infarcts, *Radiology* 110:473, 1974.

Brady TJ, Thrall JH, Lo K, and Pitt B: The importance of adequate exercise in the detection of coronary heart disease by radionuclide ventriculography, *J Nucl Med* 21:1125, 1980.

Braunwald E and Rutherford JD: Reversible ischemic left ventricular dysfunction: evidence for the "hibernating myocardium," *J Am Coll Cardiol* 8:1467, 1986.

Freeman LM and Blaufox MD, editors: Cardiovascular nuclear medicine, *Semin Nucl Med*, vol 21, 1991.

Gerson MC, editor: *Cardiac nuclear medicine*, New York, 1987, McGraw-Hill.

Gould KL, Westcott RJ, Albro PC, and Hamilton GW: Non-invasive assessment of coronary stenoses by myocardial imaging during pharmacologic coronary vasodilation; II Clinical methodology and feasibility, *Am J Cardiol* 4:279, 1978.

Guiberteau MJ, editor: *Nuclear cardiovascular imaging*, New York, 1990, Churchill Livingstone.

Khaw A, Gold HK, Yasuda T et al: Scintigraphic quantification of myocardial necrosis in patients after intravenous injection of myosin-specific antibody, *Circulation* 74:501, 1986.

Marcus ML, Schelbert HR, Skorton DJ, and Wolf GL, editors: *Cardiac imaging*, Philadelphia, 1991, WB Saunders.

Schelbert HR: Current status and prospects of new radionuclides and radiopharmaceuticals for cardiovascular nuclear medicine, *Semin Nucl Med* 27:145, 1987.

Schwaiger M and Hutchins GD: Evaluation of coronary artery disease with positron emission tomography, *Semin Nucl Med* 21:210, 1992.

Silverman KJ, Becker LC, Bulkley BH et al: Value of early thallium-201 scintigraphy for predicting mortality in patients with acute myocardial infarction, *Circulation* 61:996, 1980.

Skeletal System

Skeletal scintigraphy is the first or second most frequently performed imaging procedure in most nuclear medicine departments in the United States. The singular advantages of skeletal scintigraphy are its high sensitivity in detecting early disease and the ease of surveying the entire skeleton quickly, at reasonable expense. Most broadly, the uptake of skeletal seeking radiotracers depicts osteoblastic activity and regional blood flow to bone. Any medical condition that changes either of these factors in a positive or negative way can result in an abnormal skeletal scintigram.

The major limitation of skeletal scintigraphy is its nonspecificity. Any cause of altered bone formation will result in abnormal tracer localization. In the vast majority of cases, the diagnostic significance of the scintigraphic findings comes from the clinical context and not the image findings alone.

RADIOPHARMACEUTICALS

The first clinically important radiopharmaceutical for skeletal imaging was strontium-85 (Table 5-1). This radionuclide is an analogue of calcium and an avid bone seeker. Limitations of Sr-85 include higher than ideal gamma photon energy (514 keV) and a long half-life (65.1 days), resulting in a high radiation absorbed dose. Imaging had to be delayed for 2 days to allow background clearance. The tracer is also excreted partially in the gastrointestinal (GI) tract. This frequently required cleansing enemas to remove background activity.

Strontium-87m enjoyed a brief vogue in the 1960s. This tracer is obtained from an yttrium-87 parent in an

Table 5-1   Characteristics of Selected Skeletal–Seeking Agents

Radionuclide	Physical Half-life	Principal Mode of Decay	Principal Photon Energy (keV)	Usual Dosage (mCi)
Sr-85	65 d	Electron capture	514	0.1 - 0.25
Sr-87m	2.8 hr	Isomeric transition	388	3-10
F-18	1.8 hr	Positron	511	3-10
Tc-99m MDP	6.0 hr	Isomeric transition	140	15-25

yttrium-87/strontium-87m generator system. Strontium-87m has a short half-life (2.8 hours), decays by isomeric transition, and has a more favorable energy (388 keV) compared to Sr-85. Neither Sr-85 nor Sr-87m is used in current practice. The beta emitter, strontium-89, has been used for the therapy of skeletal malignancy in the treatment of bone pain.

Fluorine-18 is an avid bone seeker and is an analogue of the hydroxyl ion found abundantly in the calcium hydroxyapatite crystals of bone. Fluorine-18 was the agent of choice for skeletal imaging prior to the development of Tc-99m-labeled bone imaging agents. Fluorine-18 decays by positron emission (97%) and has a half-life of 1.8 hours (Table 5-1). The available photons for imaging have an energy of 511 keV. This tracer is enjoying a modest renaissance in institutions with cyclotrons and positron emission tomography (PET) scanners but is not widely available commercially.

The modern era of skeletal imaging began with the invention of Tc-99m-labeled polyphosphate in 1971. As discussed throughout this book, Tc-99m is a desirable label with its reasonable 6-hour half-life, 140 keV principal photon, and availability from the Mo-99/Tc-99m generator system. Rapidly after the description of Tc-99m polyphosphate, a family of Tc-99m label compounds were developed. In current practice the agents of choice are in the chemical class of diphosphonates (Figure 5-1). These agents are characterized by the organic P-C-P structure. Subtleties of uptake and pharmacokinetics are controlled by the R groups attached to the central carbon atom. The diphosphonates are preferred over the closely related Tc-99m-labeled pyrophosphate radio-

pharmaceutical. The diphosphonates demonstrate superior clearance from the circulation and from background soft tissues due to less protein binding.

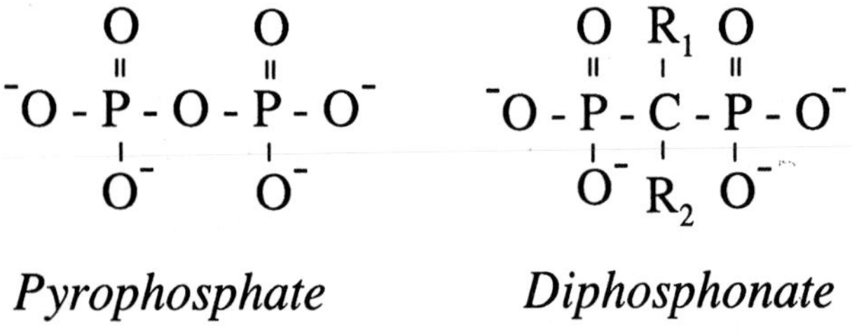

Preparation of Tc-99m-Labeled Bone Imaging Agents

Technetium-99m labeled bone agents are prepared by the addition of sodium pertechnetate (NaTcO$_4$) obtained from a Mo-99/Tc-99m generator system to a vial containing the respective diphosphonate (or pyrophosphate) compound and stannous ion, Sn(II), a reducing agent. Technetium-99m forms a chelate with the diphosphonates. Successful labeling requires sufficient Sn(II) to reduce Tc(VII) to effect the chelation. If oxygen is

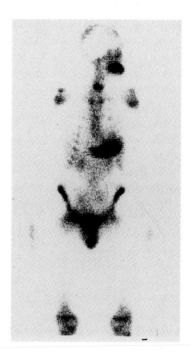

Fig. 5-2   Free pertechnetate in the radiopharmaceutical preparation has resulted in uptake in the stomach, the thyroid gland, and the oropharynx. By the usual time of imaging at 2 to 4 hours after tracer administration, free pertechnetate has cleared from the salivary glands, accounting for the activity in the oropharynx and the absence of salivary activity.

Pyrophosphate   *Diphosphonate*

Fig. 5-1   Chemical structures of pyrophosphate and diphosphonate.

allowed into the vial, Sn(II) is hydrolyzed, with the potential formation of colloidal impurities that can result in liver and other reticuloendothelial uptake in vivo, degrading images of the skeleton. Moreover, if the available Sn(II) is hydrolyzed, the labeling efficiency is compromised, resulting in free pertechnetate, which also degrades in vivo images by uptake in the soft tissues, thyroid gland, salivary gland, and stomach (Figure 5-2). In clinical practice it is important to avoid introduction of air into multidose vials and it is desirable to use the radiopharmaceutical within 2 or 3 hours of preparation.

Pharmacokinetics After Intravenous Administration of Tc-99m-Diphosphonate

The Tc-99m-labeled skeletal radiopharmaceuticals distribute rapidly throughout the extracellular fluid (ECF) space (Figure 5-3). Uptake in bone is also rapid and by 2 to 6 hours after tracer injection represents approximately 50% of the injected dose. Net clearance from the body is via the kidneys, primarily by glomerular filtration. By 24 hours 50% to 60% of the injected dose has been excreted in the urine of patients with normal renal function. The skeleton-to-background tissue ratio improves with time, and the selection of imaging time is based on a compromise between clinical convenience, decay of the radiolabel, and target-to-background ratio. In practice, most nuclear medicine departments begin imaging 2 to 3 hours after tracer administration. By then the blood level is 3% to 5% of the injected dose.

Mechanisms of Tracer Localization

The mechanism of radiostrontium and radiofluorine localization is straightforward. They are analogues respectively of calcium and hydroxyl ion and bind avidly to hydroxyapatite crystals in bone. The mechanism of uptake of the Tc-99m phosphorus-containing com-

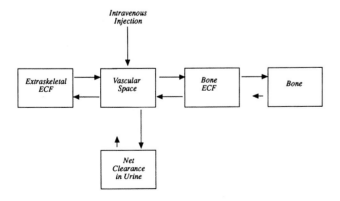

Fig. 5-3 Schematic diagram of technetium-99m diphosphonate distribution. Clearance from the extracellular fluid space and the vascular space is necessary for optimum visualization of the skeleton.

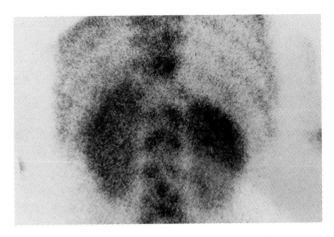

Fig. 5-4 Complete destruction of the L-1 vertebral body with corresponding photon defficient or cold lesion.

pounds is less well understood. For Tc-99m diphosphonates it is felt that adsorption is primarily to the mineral phase of bone, with little binding to the organic phase. The uptake is significantly higher in amorphous calcium phosphate than in mature crystalline hydroxyapatite, which helps explain the avidity of the tracer for areas of increased osteogenic activity.

Another clinically important factor in regional tracer distribution is local blood flow. More radiopharmaceutical is delivered to hyperemic areas. The coupling of disease processes with both increased blood flow and increased osteogenesis for many types of lesions results in higher tracer uptake than in unaffected parts of the skeleton.

Decreased tracer localization is seen in areas of reduced or absent blood flow (bone infarction) and in areas where the skeleton has been destroyed to the point that no bone matrix elements are present for uptake to occur. This is seen in some aggressive metastases (Figure 5-4). Cold areas are often referred to as "photon deficient."

Dosimetry

Estimates of the radiation absorbed doses for the total body and selected organs are provided in Table 5-2. The radiation dose to the bladder wall, the ovaries, and the testes is dependent on the frequency of voiding. The provided estimates assume a 2-hour voiding cycle. Significantly higher doses can occur with infrequent voiding, and before patients are allowed to leave the imaging clinic they are reminded to continue frequent voiding. As usual, administration of radiopharmaceuticals to pregnant women should only be done if clearly needed on a risk versus benefit basis. Technetium-99m is excreted in breast milk, and formula feedings should be substituted for several days.

Table 5-2   Tc-99m Diphosphonate: Radiation Absorbed Dose

Organ	Radiation Absorbed Dose (rads/20 mCi)
Whole body	0.13
Skeleton	0.70
Marrow (red)	0.56
Kidneys	0.80
Bladder (2-hr void)	2.60
Ovaries (2-hr void)	0.24
Testes (2-hr void)	0.16

Modified from package insert, Du Pont Radiopharmaceutical Division, Billarica, MA.

Box 5-1   Skeletal Scintigraphy: Protocol Summary for Whole Body Survey

PATIENT PREPARATION AND FOLLOW-UP

Patient should be well hydrated.

Patient should void immediately prior to study.

Frequent voiding after the procedure (reduces radiation dose to bladder wall).

Remove metal objects (jewelry, coins, keys) prior to imaging.

DOSAGE AND ROUTE OF ADMINISTRATION

20 mCi Tc-99m diphosphonate (adult dose, standard).

IV injection (site selected to avoid known or suspected pathology).

Adjust dosage for pediatric patients.

TIME OF IMAGING

Begin imaging 2-4 hr after tracer administration.

PROCEDURE

Obtain anterior and posterior views of the entire skeleton.

Obtain a minimum of 1,000k counts per view for whole body imaging systems.

Obtain 300k-500k counts per image if multiple spot views are used.

Use the highest resolution collimator that permits imaging in a reasonable length of time.

Obtain high count (1,000k) spot views or use SPECT for more detail.

TECHNIQUE

Technical details vary from department to department and include variations for special purposes that will be discussed in this chapter (Box 5-1). For whole

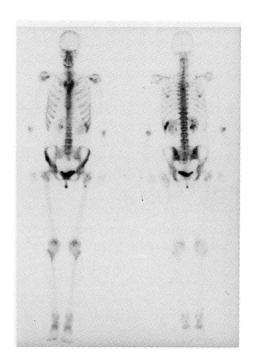

A

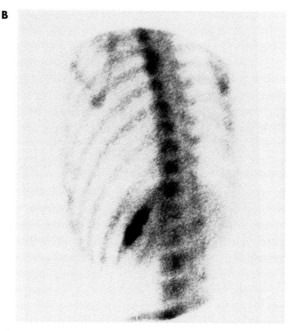

B

Fig. 5-5   A, Anterior and posterior whole body images obtained in a patient with carcinoma of the breast. Whole body images have the advantage of depicting the entire skeleton in a single view. Note the abnormal uptake in one of the left lower posterior ribs. **B,** High count density spot view of the left posterior ribs. The location and appearance of the lesion are better delineated in the spot view.

body surveys, the most common application, most departments use 20 mCi (740 MBq) of Tc-99m diphosphonate and begin imaging 2 to 3 hours after intravenous (IV) administration of the radiopharmaceutical. Dynamic imaging immediately following injection is performed in cases of suspected osteomyelitis versus cellulitis.

Imaging is accomplished with a gamma scintillation camera equipped with a low-energy, all-purpose or high-resolution collimator. For contemporary large field of view cameras, either a spot view or whole body approach may be used. Whole body imaging has the advantage of providing anatomic continuity of image data (Figure 5-5A). Spot views provide significantly higher resolution, and the highest quality bone scintigrams are obtained with high count (1,000k) regional spot views. A frequently used compromise is to obtain an initial whole body survey followed by high resolution, high count supplementary spot views of suspicious or symptomatic areas (Figure 5-5A,B). Patients are asked to empty their bladders immediately before imaging, and care is taken to avoid contamination of the skin or clothing, which may result in misinterpretation of urinary contamination as a soft tissue or skeletal lesion.

Special imaging techniques include dynamic scanning for the differential diagnosis of skeletal versus soft tissue disease, single photon emission computed tomography (SPECT) for high-contrast regional imaging, and computer recording of images for quantitative analysis. Magnification imaging with a pinhole collimator or converging collimator can be very helpful in children and has been used in evaluation of the hip for osteonecrosis.

CLINICAL APPLICATIONS

Normal Appearance of the Skeletal Scintigram

The appearance of the normal skeletal scintigram changes dramatically from infancy to childhood, adolescence, and mature adulthood. In the early neonatal period skeletal tracer uptake is not as avid as it is even a few months later. For example, little activity is seen in the sutures of the skull in the first months of life, and the differentiation of increased activity in growth centers is also less in the first few months than by age 6 months. Contamination of skin and clothing is a special problem in infants because the radiopharmaceutical is excreted in the urine.

A striking feature of the growing skeleton is the marked uptake of radiopharmaceutical in growth centers (Figure 5-6). These are hotter than surrounding bone. The observation applies to all epiphyseal and apophyseal growth centers and the sutures in the skull until their closure. The degree of uptake in the growth centers is a reflection of relative metabolic activity. The three "hottest" centers in order are the distal femur, proximal tibia, and proximal humerus (Figure 5-6)—also the order of relative occurrence of osteosarcoma in this age group! The amount of metabolic or growth activity is paralleled by the likelihood of malignant transformation.

In the normal adult, growth center activity becomes

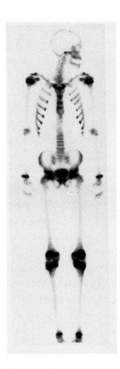

Fig. 5-6   Anterior whole body view in a growing adolescent. Note the increased uptake in growth centers. This study is a particularly nice example of increased activity at the anterior rib ends, the sternal ossification centers, and the growth centers in the shoulders.

Box 5-2   Reported Causes of Bilaterally Increased and Decreased Renal Visualization on Skeletal Scintigrams

INCREASED UPTAKE

Urinary tract obstruction
Chemotherapy (doxorubicin, vincristine, cyclophosphamide)
Nephrocalcinosis
Hypercalcemia
Radiation nephritis
Acute tubular necrosis
Thalassemia

DECREASED UPTAKE

Renal failure
Metastatic disease–superscan
Metabolic bone disease–superscan
Paget's disease
Osteomalacia
Hyperparathyroidism
Myelofibrosis–superscan
Nephrectomy

equal to activity in adjacent bone. Tracer uptake is greatest in the axial skeleton (spine and pelvis), with relatively less intense uptake in the extremities and skull. Background activity is normally seen in the soft tissues. The kidneys are routinely visualized in normal subjects and should have less intensity than the adjacent lumbar spine. If the kidneys are of equal or greater intensity, a renal abnormality or concomitant drug therapy should be suspected (Box 5-2).

A number of normal variants must be recognized for correct scintigraphic interpretation. The skull frequently presents an uneven or variable activity along its margin, probably due to slight variations in calvarial thickness. Bilaterally increased radionuclide concentration in the frontal area with thinning at the midline may be due to hyperostosis frontalis interna. In slightly oblique views of the skull, a flame shaped or triangular area of activity is frequently seen projecting from the base of the skull just posterior to the orbit where the sphenoid ridge meets the calvarial structures. Sutural activity is not discretely seen in adults.

The anterior aspect of the mandible may appear as a "hot spot" on lateral views of the skull. The projected bone mass of the mentum is greater in this view than the rami. The laryngotracheal cartilages are usually seen in adults, probably related to some degree of calcification. The thyroid gland will also avidly accumulate unbound pertechnetate, resulting in superimposed activity in the same general region.

Some mild diffuse asymmetry in paired joints is frequently seen in adults. The phenomenon is most common in the shoulders and correlates with handedness. This normal variant appearance should be distinguished from focal asymmetry involving only part of the joint.

In high-resolution scintigrams, the sternal-manubrial joint is frequently visualized as a focal hot spot. In the growing skeleton, sternal ossification centers can be confused with abnormal uptake, but these centers should not be seen in the adult.

Increased activity at the costochondral junction is abnormal in adults but is routinely seen in children and adolescents (Figure 5-6). Increased uptake in a limited number of rib ends is usually due to trauma. Increased uptake at the costochondral junction in adults is seen in some types of metabolic bone disease.

Some asymmetry is frequently seen in the sacroiliac joints, especially in patients with scoliosis or abnormal gait. Scoliosis can also result in subtle rotation of the pelvis with apparent asymmetry of the ala iliae, especially on anterior views. Asymmetric activity in the sacroiliac joints and pelvic structures should be interpreted with caution in patients with scoliosis.

Interpretation of uptake in the spine itself is potentially difficult in patients with marked scoliosis. The pedicles appear asymmetric. The altered weight-bearing results in remodeling and degenerative changes that can produce confusing patterns of tracer activity.

The normal spinal curvatures cause the vertebrae at different levels of the spine to be at different distances from the face of the collimator, with corresponding differences in the amount of interposed soft tissues. For example, the lower lumbar spine generally appears hotter on the anterior view than the area of the thoraco-lumbar junction due to the normal lumbar lordosis, which brings the spine forward, with less intervening soft tissue.

Although the marked uptake in the epiphyseal-metaphyseal area is not seen in adults, the ends of the long bones continue to demonstrate greater uptake than the diaphyses. This is due to the greater bone volume and more avid uptake of radiopharmaceutical in cancellous than compact bone.

In women, activity in the breast should reflect general soft tissue activity. Focal or asymmetric breast activity is not normal and may indicate breast disease. Following mastectomy, the ribs on the operative side appear hotter due to loss of soft tissue and less attenuation.

Metastatic Disease

The most common clinical application of skeletal scintigraphy is in the evaluation of patients with extraskeletal primary malignancies for the presence of metastatic disease. The different kinds of information sought are summarized in Box 5-3. In many patients, the presence or extent of skeletal metastasis directly influences treatment decisions and prognosis. Bone pain and pathologic fractures are common management problems in patients with skeletal metastatic disease for which bone scintigraphy plays a role.

Pathophysiology: Basis of scintigraphic and radiographic detection   Nonosseous neoplasms gain access to the skeleton by three mechanisms: (1) direct extension, (2) retrograde venous flow, and (3) via the arterial circulation after venous or lymphatic access. For epithelial tumors the initial seeding of metastatic deposits via

---

Box 5-3   Skeletal Imaging: Applications in Patients with Extraskeletal Malignancies

Initial staging: Metastatic skeletal survey.
Protocol monitoring: Response to chemotherapy and decision to change therapy.
Radiation therapy treatment field planning and response to radiation therapy.
Detection of areas at risk for pathologic fracture.

the arterial circulation is typically in the red marrow. This helps explain the predominance of metastatic lesions in the axial skeleton. In normal adults, the red marrow is distributed to the bones of the axial skeleton, including the cranium, and the proximal portions of the femurs and humeri. Over 90% of skeletal metastatic lesions from most epithelial tumors are found in this distribution, with only a small percentage outside of red marrow-bearing areas.

As metastatic lesions grow in the marrow space, the surrounding bone remodels through osteoclastic (resorptive) and osteoblastic (depositional) activity. The relative degree of bone resorption and deposition elicited is highly variable among the different types of tumors and sometimes even between different locations for the same tumor. The relationship between the two remodeling processes determines whether a metastatic deposit will appear as predominantly lytic or sclerotic or will exhibit a mixed pattern radiographically.

Radionuclide bone scintigrams are very sensitive for detecting the altered local metabolism in areas of skeletal remodeling associated with metastatic deposits. On the other hand, a 30% to 50% change in bone density is required before small lesions can be detected radiographically.

These observations are reflected in a characteristic sequence of image findings for skeletal scintigrams and standard radiographs. Early in the natural history of the metastatic lesion, both the skeletal scintigram and standard radiograph are normal. As the metastases grow, bone remodeling results in increased skeletal metabolism and increased tracer localization; the scintigram becomes abnormal and the radiograph remains normal. As the process continues, net calcium content and skeletal trabecular architecture change; the scintigram remains abnormal and the standard radiograph also becomes abnormal. This sequence occurs over a period of weeks to months.

If healing occurs as a result of therapy, the bone scintigram may revert to normal while the radiograph typically remains abnormal, although there are occasional exceptions. If the cancerous process is very indolent or diffusely lytic, the skeletal scintigram may fail to reveal an abnormality. This is due in turn to a failure to alter bone metabolism or local blood flow sufficiently to produce a focally detectable lesion. Multiple myeloma is a notorious cause of false negative skeletal scintigraphic studies on this basis.

It is also important to realize that the skeletal tracers do not localize mainly in the cancerous tissue per se but in the remodeling, metabolically active bone surrounding or being invaded by the metastatic tissues. This is well illustrated in Figure 5-7, which shows the growth of a metastatic lesion in the calvarium. The circular rim of increased tracer uptake is in the reactive bone surrounding the cancerous tissue. As the cancer enlarges, the rim is displaced

A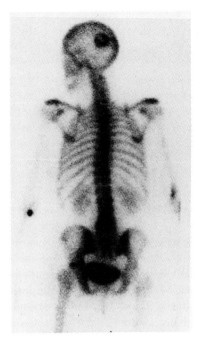

B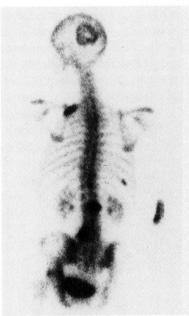

Fig. 5-7 **A,** Initial skeletal scintigram in a patient with multiple skeletal metastases, including the skull. Note the intense uptake in the calvarial lesion with a small area of decreased uptake centrally. **B,** Several months later the metastatic disease had progressed in both the axial skeleton and the calvarium. The overall diameter of the skull lesion increased, with a much larger central photon-deficient area. The increased uptake is in bone at the margin of the metastatic lesion.

as bone is completely destroyed. The central cancerous tissue is photon deficient without tracer uptake.

Magnetic resonance imaging (MRI) has suggested a new approach to the early detection of skeletal metastases. The intense, uniform signal from marrow fat is

Box 5-4	Scintigraphic Patterns in Metastatic Disease

Solitary focal lesions
Multiple focal lesions
Diffuse involvement (superscan)
Photon-deficient lesions ("cold" lesions)
Normal (false negative)
"Flare" phenomenon (follow-up studies)
Soft tissue lesions (tracer uptake in tumor)

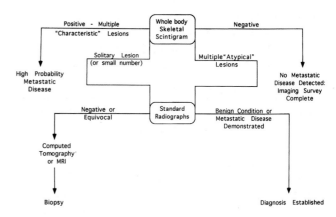

Fig. 5-8   Simplified algorithm for the workup of patients with suspected skeletal metastasis.

altered by metastatic lesions. It has been demonstrated in a number of studies that early lesions in the marrow can be detected before they elicit a sufficient osteogenic response to be detected by scintigraphy. The major problems in the use of MRI for this application are the difficulty in surveying the entire skeleton and the frequent presence of incidental benign defects or heterogeneity in marrow fat unrelated to metastatic disease, making the specificity of the observation problematic.

Although bone scan is significantly more sensitive than standard radiography as a survey technique, the actual difference in sensitivity depends on the stage of disease being evaluated. In early disease, the sensitivity of the bone scintigram is severalfold greater and the sensitivity is also significantly greater on a per lesion basis. However, if all patients with metastatic disease are considered, including patients with advanced disease, the relative superiority is less because both types of examinations are positive in a higher percentage of cases. The accuracy of skeletal scintigraphy will never be precisely known, due to the lack of a reference standard for comparison. The sensitivity for detecting metastatic disease is often quoted as high as 95% or above.

Scintigraphic patterns   The scintigraphic patterns encountered in skeletal metastatic disease are summarized in Box 5-4, and a decision tree or algorithm for the workup of patients with proven nonosseous primary tumors is provided in Figure 5-8. The point of entry in the algorithm is the whole body bone scintigram. If the examination is positive and characteristic for metastatic disease, the screening workup is complete. The classic, "typical" pattern that provides the most diagnostic certainty is the presence of multiple focal lesions distributed randomly throughout the axial skeleton (Figure 5-9).

However, a number of other conditions may also result in multiple scintigraphic abnormalities (Box 5-5). A key feature in recognizing nonmetastatic causes for multifocal scan abnormalities is the pattern of distribution. For example, in both Cushing's syndrome and osteomalacia, there is frequently a disproportionate number of rib lesions (Figure 5-10A,B) as compared to other areas. In

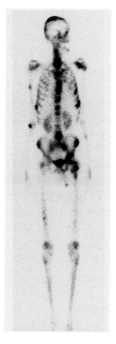

Fig. 5-9   Anterior whole body scintigram in a patient with widely distributed metastatic disease. There are lesions in the spine, ribs, sternum, and upper and lower extremities.

patients with osteoporosis, dorsal kyphosis and patterns of associated fractures such as the H type fracture of the sacrum provide clues to the correct diagnosis.

Skeletal scintigrams in older subjects almost routinely reveal evidence of osteoarthritis. This is generally recognized by its characteristic locations. The uptake can be quite intense and is not necessarily closely related in degree to current symptoms. Involvement of both sides of a joint is often seen and is not characteristic of metastatic disease. Medial and lateral compartment arthritis in the knee, changes in the hands and wrists (especially at the base of the first metacarpal), and changes in the

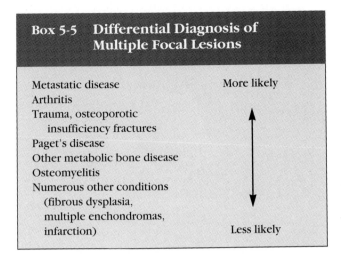

Box 5-5   Differential Diagnosis of Multiple Focal Lesions

Metastatic disease   More likely
Arthritis
Trauma, osteoporotic
     insufficiency fractures
Paget's disease
Other metabolic bone disease
Osteomyelitis
Numerous other conditions
     (fibrous dysplasia,
     multiple enchondromas,
     infarction)   Less likely

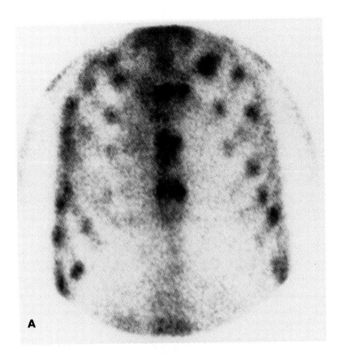

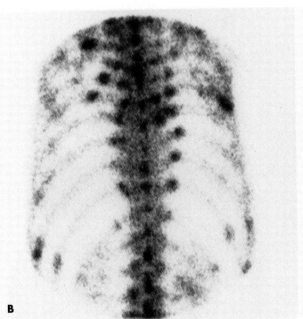

Fig. 5-10   Anterior (**A**) and posterior (**B**) views from a skeletal scintigram obtained in a patient with osteomalacia. The patient was referred to the nuclear medicine service to rule out metastatic disease. The unusually large number of rib lesions alerted the nuclear medicine physician to suspect metabolic bone disease.

shoulder are extremely common scintigraphic findings. Degenerative changes in the lower lumbar spine can pose a special problem because of the high incidence of both metastatic disease and degenerative disease in this location. The pattern of scintigraphic abnormality must be assessed with caution. Degenerative changes typically involve the facet joints and vertebral end-plates with hypertrophic spurring. Metastatic disease more typically involves the pedicle and body of the vertebra. The spatial resolution of conventional bone scintigrams often is not sufficient to make these distinctions. Modern SPECT imaging should be considered in difficult cases.

Trauma is a frequent cause of multiple lesions, and patients should be routinely questioned for history of trauma. In the ribs there is often a characteristic vertical alignment of fractures due to the mechanism of injury in falls or automobile accidents. This nonrandom pattern would not be expected in metastatic disease. Displaced fractures can be recognized by their structural deformity, but otherwise a healing fracture and a metastatic lesion may appear the same scintigraphically. Persistently positive skeletal scintigrams from old trauma are a major interpretative problem. The issue is discussed in more detail later in the chapter.

Multifocal osteomyelitis can simulate metastatic disease, but from a practical clinical standpoint it is not frequently present as an incidental and unsuspected problem in the cancer patient. Conversely, Paget's disease of bone is relatively common in the cancer age group, and it may be impossible on the bone scintigram to differentiate Paget's disease from metastatic disease in specific lesions. Paget's disease can be suspected from its characteristic patterns of involvement and the extreme intensity of tracer uptake. In particular, involvement of a hemipelvis, a long portion of a long bone, and expansion of osseous structures all point to Paget's disease. Osteoporosis circumscripta causes a very characteristic rim

pattern of activity in the skull but may also be difficult to distinguish from metastasis. Radiographic correlation is frequently required when the differential diagnosis rests between Paget's disease and metastatic disease.

Multiple infarctions with reactive bone causing increased tracer uptake can also mimic skeletal metastatic disease. This pattern is most commonly seen in patients with sickle cell anemia and is rarely a practical problem. It is recognized from the history and the presence of other characteristic changes on the bone scan.

Solitary lesions Scans showing either solitary scintigraphic abnormalities or a small number of lesions pose special problems in interpretation and have been the subject of several major clinical studies (Figures 5-8, 5-11). The potential for diagnostic error results from the frequency with which incidental benign conditions involve the skeleton and are detected on bone scintigraphy. When a solitary lesion is encountered, it is important to proceed in a systematic fashion, using an algorithm such as the one presented in Figure 5-8. Frequently, standard radiographs will confirm the presence of either a metastatic deposit or a benign condition, ending the diagnostic evaluation. If standard radiographs are normal or equivocal and the presence or absence of metastatic disease is important to clinical decision making, further imaging should be carried out and, if necessary, biopsy (Figure 5-12).

The most common cause of solitary benign abnormalities is degenerative arthritis followed by healing fracture. Other benign bone lesions including monostotic Paget's disease, enchondroma, frontal osteoma, fibrous dysplasia, and osteomyelitis can also be the cause of solitary abnormalities.

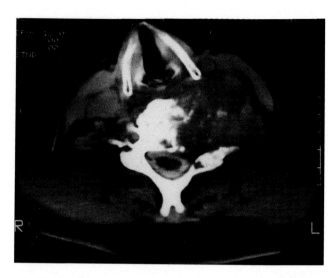

Fig. 5-12   CT scan obtained at the level of a scintigraphic abnormality reveals extensive destruction of the corresponding vertebral body and a clinically palpable soft tissue mass in the neck.

Location and pattern are important scintigraphically. Lesions in the anterior rib ends are rarely due to metastases. This is a location subject to trauma, and the costochondral junction can be quite positive scintigraphically with no radiographic abnormality following even minor trauma. Conversely, 40% to 80% of proven solitary lesions in the spine are shown to be metastatic in origin.

In Brown's summary of his own experience with bone scintigraphy in a pediatric population, combined with other large series from the literature, solitary abnormalities were due to malignancy approximately in 55% of cases. However, rather than attempting to assign an overall probability of malignancy or a specific probability for each anatomic area, it is more important simply to recognize the potential pitfall presented by the solitary lesion and have a systematic approach to it.

Superscan Another scintigraphic pattern that can cause interpretative problems for the unwary is the "superscan." In some patients with breast cancer and prostatic cancer, the entire axial skeleton becomes diffusely and rather uniformly involved with metastatic disease. If the involvement is uniform enough, the scan may appear deceptively normal (Figure 5-13). There are a number of clues that provide a tip-off, including unusually good bone-to-soft tissue background ratio, absent or faint visualization of the kidneys, and an increase in the ratio of uptake in the axial versus appendicular skeleton. One helpful rule to avoid being fooled by uniform tracer uptake is to review at least one radiograph in every patient undergoing bone scintigraphy. Virtually all patients have had chest radiographs or other studies so that sufficient correlative information is available to avoid this uncommon diagnostic pitfall.

Flare phenomenon Another potentially perplexing

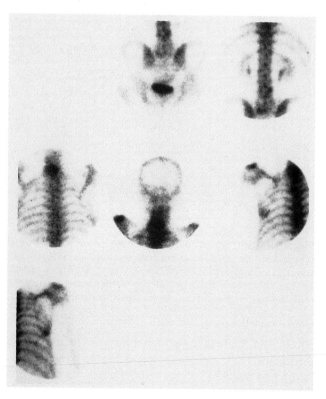

Fig. 5-11   Posterior spot views obtained in a patient with suspected metastatic disease. Note the solitary area of abnormally increased uptake in the lower cervical spine.

pattern is seen in evaluating follow-up bone scans in patients undergoing cyclic chemotherapy. In some patients who have a good response to chemotheraphy, the bone scan appears to paradoxically worsen, with a "flare" of increased activity (Figure 5-14). The hypothesis to explain the flare phenomenon is that as lesions begin to heal following therapy, there is an osteoblastic response, resulting in increased activity on the scintigram. Some patients may experience pain in these areas following the onset of chemotherapy, further confusing the issue clinically. When these lesions are followed radiographically, healing with increased sclerosis is seen over 2 to 6 months. The flare phenomenon reinforces the fact that tracer uptake is not in tumor tissue but in the surrounding bone.

Other patterns   Some metastatic lesions elicit a predominantly resorptive or destructive response in bone. Areas of the skeleton that are completely replaced by metastatic tumor or that are purely lytic radiographically may appear as "cold" or photon-deficient lesions on bone scan (Figure 5-4). Therefore, the focal absence of

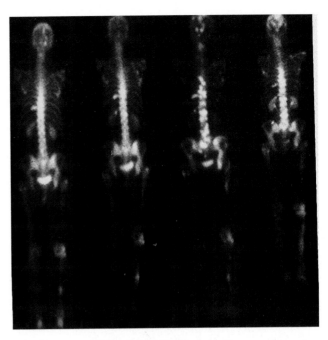

Fig. 5-14   The flare phenomenon demonstrated in sequential posterior whole body scintigrams obtained over a period of 10 months in a patient with carcinoma of the breast undergoing chemotherapy. Note the increased intensity of uptake in the skull, spine, and pelvis, especially between the second and third images in the sequence. The scintigram appears worse, but the patient was improving clinically, with reduced bone pain and radiographic evidence of healing.

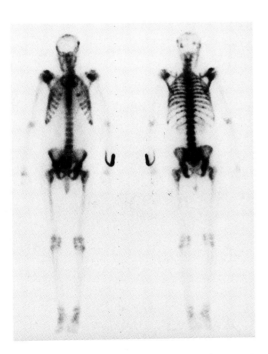

Fig. 5-13   "Superscan" obtained in a patient with prostatic carcinoma. In this case there is enough nonuniformity of uptake to easily recognize the abnormality. Note the increased skeletal-to-soft tissue uptake ratio, the axial-appendicular disproportion in uptake, and the very faint visualization of the kidneys. The bladder is well visualized, indicating that failure to see the kidneys is not due to absent excretion of tracer through them. Rather, the uptake in the skeleton is so intense that the kidney activity is below the threshold for recording on the film.

expected normal tracer uptake should be sought on bone scintigrams, as well as areas of focally increased uptake. The photon-deficient area is often bordered by a rim of increased uptake (Figure 5-7).

A more difficult problem is the scintigraphic detection of some lesions that are characterized by a permeative pattern radiographically. As noted in the discussion on pathophysiology, if the neoplastic process is indolent or causes no reactive bone formation, the scan may falsely appear normal. This is a particular problem with round cell tumors and multiple myeloma. If all sites of involvement are considered, the sensitivity of the bone scan in multiple myeloma is low, although studies in the literature suggest that the majority of patients will have some abnormality, often related to pathologic fractures. The combination of bone scintigraphy and radiographic bone survey yields the best results.

Scintigraphy in specific tumors   The mnemonic "lead kettle," or Pb KTL, is useful for remembering the common nonosseous tumors that metastasize to bone: cancers of the *p*rostate, *b*reast, *k*idney, *t*hyroid, and *l*ung. In particular, carcinomas of the prostate, lung, and breast are among the most common causes of cancer and death from cancer.

Carcinoma of the prostate   Demographic factors

and aging of the population have resulted in more cases of carcinoma of the prostate being seen in clinical practice. Until the introduction of prostate-specific antigen (PSA), the skeletal scintigram was considered the most sensitive technique for detecting metastatic disease. Compared with scintigraphy, alkaline phosphatase testing is only half as sensitive an indicator of skeletal metastatic disease, and radiographs are normal in approximately 30% of cases with abnormal scintigrams. The likelihood of an abnormal skeletal scintigram correlates positively with clinical stage. In early Stage I disease, 5% or fewer patients have abnormal scintigrams.

Prostatic cancer and breast cancer are the two tumors most frequently associated with both the superscan and the flare phenomenon (Figures 5-13, 5-14). Serial imaging is useful in following response to therapy, and lesion regression can be quite dramatic. The flare phenomenon is obviously seen when the timing of the follow-up scan corresponds to osteoblastic healing. The majority of patients dying with prostatic cancer have skeletal metastases. These are often dramatic and extensive. When they coalesce to involve essentially the entire axial skeleton, the superscan appearance is seen scintigraphically.

The intensity of uptake in prostatic carcinoma can be confused with Paget's disease. This is especially true when there is contiguous spread to involve a hemipelvis.

Carcinoma of the breast   Carcinoma of the breast has reached almost epidemic proportions in the United States. The historic lifetime incidence of one in 11 or 12 women developing carcinoma of the breast has now increased to an estimated lifetime incidence of one in nine. Mammographic screening is used to make the diagnosis early, but a large number of woman still present with advanced clinical stage disease and must be evaluated for skeletal metastases.

It is now recognized that the yield on skeletal scintigraphy for Stage I disease is low, probably less than 3% to 5%. Early literature on this topic had reported much higher early-stage scan positivity, but in retrospect there were many false positive interpretations because of failure to critically evaluate solitary lesions and consider benign causes of abnormal tracer uptake.

Because of the low yield in early-stage disease, there has been controversy about when to use skeletal scintigraphy in the management of breast cancer. In some institutions, the study is performed in all patients preoperatively. Others reserve the test for patients with clinical Stage II and III disease and in the routine follow-up of patients with positive nodes, who are at higher risk of developing skeletal metastatic disease. Conversion from scan negative to scan positive is a bad prognostic sign. A reasonable approach to newly diagnosed patients is to image those who have skeletal pain, those with Stage II or III disease, those whose chemotherapy protocols require scintigrams, and those with a history of other malignancy.

In addition to arterial dissemination of metastases, patients with carcinoma of the breast may experience local invasion in the ribs or, via the substernal nodes, into the sternum. As noted above, both the superscan pattern and the flare phenomenon can be seen in carcinoma of the breast. Skeletal metastates are often widely disseminated. Soft tissue metastases from carcinoma of the breast may accumulate sufficient tracer to be visualized (Figure 5-15).

Following mastectomy, the ipsilateral ribs appear relatively more intense than the contralateral ribs. This has been explained on the basis of loss of intervening soft tissue with reduced attenuation. There may be secondary blood flow effects due to healing in the mastectomy bed. This pattern is seen less frequently with the decline in popularity of the radical mastectomy.

Carcinoma of the lung   Lung cancer remains the leading cause of cancer death in men and is a rapidly increasing cause of cancer death in woman. Although up to 50% of patients dying of primary lung cancer have osseous metastases at autopsy, there is again incomplete agreement on when to use skeletal scintigraphy. If a curative operative attempt is anticipated, the workup should be aggressive. Skeletal scintigraphy, mediastinal and adrenal computed tomography, and mediastinoscopy with biopsy are performed. However, if treatment is palliative

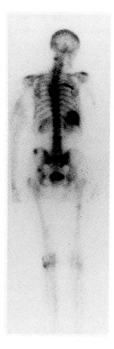

Fig. 5-15   Posterior whole body scintigram from a patient with widely disseminated carcinoma of the breast. There are multiple skeletal metastases. There is intense uptake in a soft tissue metastasis in the liver. This projects just superolateral to the right kidney.

with evidence of local invasion or mediastinal metastases, there is obviously less utility in surveying the skeleton.

Metastatic spread of lung cancer to bone can occur either by direct invasion or through arterial metastases. It is common to see involvement and even complete destruction of adjacent ribs. Although the distribution of arterially disseminated metastases is still predominantly to red marrow-bearing areas, tumor emboli may reach the distal portions of the extremities. Appendicular involvement relatively early in the course of disease is more common with aggressive lung cancers than cancer of the breast or prostate.

Characteristic periosteal uptake is seen in lung cancer patients who develop hypertrophic osteoarthropathy (Figures 5-16, 5-17) The scintigram typically shows parallel uptake along the medial and lateral margins of long bones commonly restricted to the diametaphyseal area. Although the long bones of the extremities, including those in the hands and feet, are most frequently thought of, the patella, scapula, skull, and clavicle can also be involved. The classic appearance is for the "double stripe" or "parallel track" activity to be fairly uniform. It can also be patchy with skip areas.

Other tumors of epithelial origin. A number of other extraosseous tumors metastasize to bone. Renal cell carcinoma and thyroid carcinoma are classically included in the differential diagnosis of lesions that frequently metastasize to bone. However, these are far less common tumors than cancers of the breast, lung, and prostate. Whole body survey for metastatic disease is usually accomplished with radioiodine-131 for differentiated thyroid cancer.

Gastrointestinal tract and gynecologic cancers do not commonly metastasize to bone early in their courses. Late-stage disease involves bone by direct extension. The success of chemotherapy, including regional chemotherapy, in controlling GI tract tumors has led to an increase in cases with skeletal involvement owing to longer survival and control of the local and regional metastases that usually cause death before bone metastases are manifest.

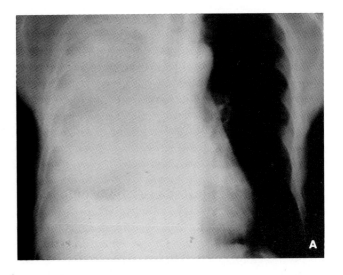

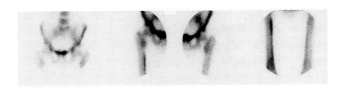

Fig. 5-16   Anterior spot views of the pelvis and femurs in a patient with carcinoma of the lung. Note the increased uptake along the medial aspects of the femurs, greater on the right than the left. This corresponds to periosteal new bone due to hypertrophic osteoarthropathy.

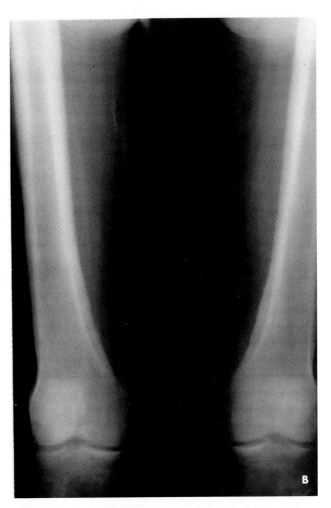

Fig. 5-17   **A,** Corresponding chest radiograph from the patient in Figure 5-16. The entire right hemithorax is Opacified as a consequence of the tumor. **B,** Radiograph of the femurs reveals characteristic periosteal new bone bilaterally on both the medial and lateral aspect of the femoral shaft.

Neuroblastoma Neuroblastoma is a tumor of neural crest origin and is the most common solid tumor in children that metastasizes to bone. As with adult epithelial tumors, radionuclide skeletal scintigraphy is far more sensitive than radiography for detecting bone involvement. On a lesion-by-lesion basis, radionuclide scintigraphy is twice as sensitive as skeletal radiography. The characteristic pattern of skeletal involvement is multifocal activity in the metaphyses. However, involvement in the skull, vertebrae, ribs, and pelvis is also common. Early, symmetric involvement may be difficult to diagnose scintigraphically because of the normal high intensity of uptake in the ends of growing bones.

A unique characteristic of neuroblastoma is the avidity of Tc-99m diphosphonate for the primary tumors. Approximately 30% to 50% of primary tumors can be demonstrated scintigraphically. Occasionally the diagnosis of neuroblastoma is made in children undergoing radionuclide imaging to evaluate another condition. Particular attention should be paid to the abdomen.

Extraskeletal uptake in soft tissue neoplasms A number of common soft tissue neoplasms exhibit variable degrees of skeletal-seeking tracer uptake in both the primary tumor and soft tissue metastases. The mechanism of localization is not well understood but is thought to be a combination of tumor calcification and binding to macromolecules. The degree of uptake and the consistency with which it is seen are not sufficient to use the Tc-99m-labeled bone agents as primary tumor imaging agents, although this has been explored for carcinoma of the breast.

Tumors most frequently imaged, in addition to carcinoma of the breast, are carcinoma of the lung, metastatic carcinoma of the colon in the liver, melanoma, and neuroblastoma (Figure 5-15).

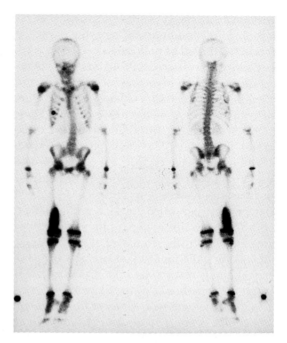

Fig. 5-18 Anterior and posterior whole body scintigrams in a patient with osteosarcoma of the right distal femur. The degree of tracer accumulation in the lesion is striking. Note also the "watershed" phenomenon with increased tracer accumulation in all of the bones of the right lower extremity above and below the lesion. The increased blood flow induced by the osteosarcoma results in increased tracer delivery to the entire limb. This extended or augmented pattern of uptake adds to the difficulty in using the skeletal scintigram to determine the margins of primary bone tumors. (The focal activity over the right ribs is a marker.)

Primary Bone Tumors

Uptake of skeletal-seeking radiopharmaceuticals in primary bone tumors is avid and frequently striking (Figures 5-18, 5-19). However, skeletal scintigraphy is not commonly used in the workup of patients with osteosarcoma or other primary bone neoplasms because the radionuclide technique does not answer the questions the orthopedic surgeon must address. The skeletal scintigram does not accurately portray the tumor margins in bone, nor does the scintigram allow assessment of soft tissue extent. Plain radiographs, CT, and MRI are better for making these determinations (Figures 5-20, 5-21). Although most primary bone tumors are monostotic, occasional polyostotic involvement will be missed without a whole body survey of some kind.

There may be a role for skeletal scintigraphy if metastases are suspected. Skeletal scintigraphy is capable of demonstrating soft tissue, pulmonary, and skeletal meta-

static lesions (Figure 5-22). It must be emphasized, however, that the value of scintigraphy is for surveying the entire body. If metastases are suspected in a given area, a higher resolution technique is employed. Thus, pulmonary metastases are typically evaluated with CT, not scintigraphy.

The effectiveness of modern multimodality therapy for primary bone tumors has changed the pattern of metastatic disease. As patients are living longer, more are developing osseous metastases than was the case historically. Skeletal scintigraphy retains its utility for whole body survey studies for this indication.

Studies of primary tumors have led to at least one important observation about skeletal tracer uptake. Many tumors elicit marked hyperemia. The increased blood flow is not restricted to the tumor itself but affects the entire watershed distribution of regional flow, most

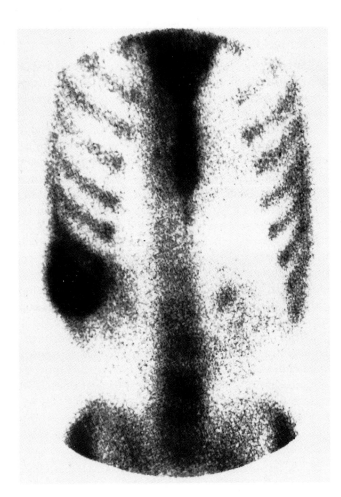

Fig. 5-19   Anterior spot view of a patient with a primary chondrosarcoma arising from the right anterior ribs.

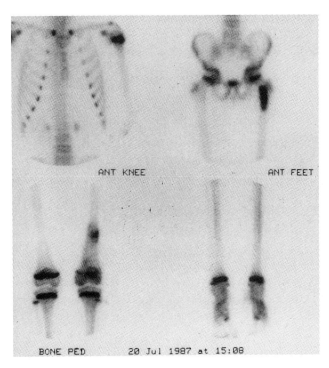

Fig. 5-20   Anterior spot views in a patient with osteosarcoma of the left distal femur and a metastatic lesion in the left proximal femur.

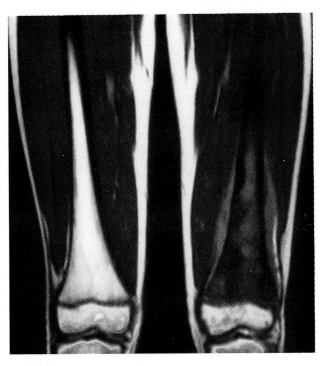

Fig. 5-21   Coronal view from an MRI study of the patient in Fig. 5-19. The MRI study provides superior anatomic information about the osseous and soft tissue extent of the tumor. However, the MRI study missed the second lesion in the proximal femur.

characteristically involving an entire extremity (Figure 5-18). Thus, markedly increased tracer uptake is seen in adjacent structures. The augmented or extended uptake pattern can be seen in other hyperemia-inducing lesions, including fractures, osteomyelitis, and nerve injuries resulting in reflex sympathetic dystrophy syndrome.

Multiple myeloma   The most common primary malignant disease to involve bone is multiple myeloma. Myeloma is really a disease of the red marrow space and the most frequently involved skeletal structures are the vertebrae, pelvis, ribs and skull.

On skeletal radiographs, the only finding in myeloma may be osteopenia. Unless there is an associated fracture or focal lesion such as a plasmacytoma, skeletal scintigrams are often normal. MRI is an excellent modality for evaluating the marrow space for areas of involvement.

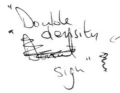

"Double density sign"

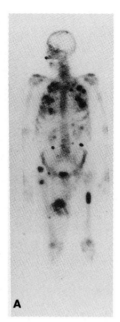

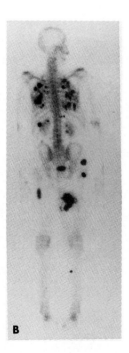

A

B

Fig. 5-22 Anterior (**A**) and posterior (**B**) whole body scintigrams in a patient with an extraosseous osteosarcoma arising in the right medial thigh area. The lesion is widely disseminated with skeletal metastases, soft tissue metastases, and pulmonary metastases. This study is a dramatic example of the ability of skeletal scintigraphy to survey the entire body. (Courtesy David A. Parker, M.D., Toledo, Ohio.)

Benign Bone Tumors

Osteoid osteoma Osteoid osteomas are often associated with excruciating bone pain that classically is greater at night. They are most common in adolescents and young adults.

Skeletal scintigraphy, especially with SPECT, is highly sensitive for detecting osteoid osteomas. They can be very difficult to find by standard radiography, especially in the spine. The most common location of occurrence is the femur (Figures 5-23, 5-24). In the spine, the posterior elements are usually affected rather than the vertebral body. Some surgeons have used intraoperative scintigraphic probes to help localize osteoid osteomas which in many cases are not immediately apparent from inspecting the surface of the bone. Recently it has become possible to treat osteoid osteomas percutaneously using either radiofrequency-induced injury to cause the lesion to involute or image-guided curettage.

Other benign bone tumors Osteochondromas, chondroblastomas, and enchondromas demonstrate a spectrum of abnormalities on skeletal scintigraphy. In some cases the scintigram is normal or near normal. In other cases there can be striking uptake, especially for osteochondromas and chondroblastomas. Enchondromas rarely demonstrate striking uptake unless secondarily involved by fracture.

Skeletal Trauma

Skeletal trauma is extremely common and presents both an opportunity and a problem in skeletal scintigraphy. The opportunity arises in the ability of skeletal scintigraphy to demonstrate abnormalities early after direct trauma or early in the course of a process such as stress fracture (Figures 5-25, 5-26). The problem comes in recognizing the effects of skeletal trauma when using

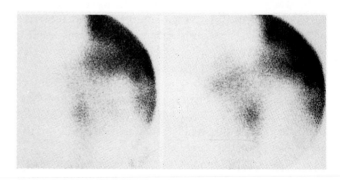

Fig. 5-23 Internal and external rotation pinhole spot views of the proximal femur in a patient with suspected osteoid osteoma. An area of abnormally increased uptake is seen just lateral to the lesser trochanter.

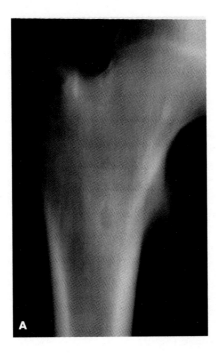

skeletal scintigraphy for another purpose, such as the detection of metastatic disease.

Detection of fractures   The time course of scintigraphic positivity after trauma is important in consideration of skeletal imaging to detect fractures and in understanding the problem of persistent positivity that could contribute to a false positive diagnosis of metastatic disease. According to data provided by Matin, approximately 80% of fractures can be visualized by 24 hours after trauma. The earliest scintigraphic appearance is diffusely increased uptake, most likely due to hyperemia at the fracture site. By 3 days, 95% of fractures are positive; in patients under the age of 65, essentially all fractures are positive by this time. Advanced age and debilitation are factors contributing to nonvisualization or delayed visualization of fractures. Maximum fracture positivity occurs 7 or more days post trauma, and delayed imaging in this time frame is recommended in difficult or equivocal cases.

The length of time it takes a fracture to return to normal scintigraphically is highly dependent on the location and degree of damage to the skeleton. Some 60% to 80% of nondisplaced uncomplicated fractures will revert to normal in 1 year and over 95% in 3 years (Table 5-3). However, there are many documented instances of displaced fractures remaining positive indefinitely, and involvement of a joint by posttraumatic arthritis causes prolonged positivity. A careful history is important. All patients undergoing metastatic skeletal survey should be routinely questioned concerning prior trauma. In a prospective study by Kim, nearly half of patients being evaluated for skeletal metastatic disease reported previous fractures. Twenty-six percent of the fracture sites

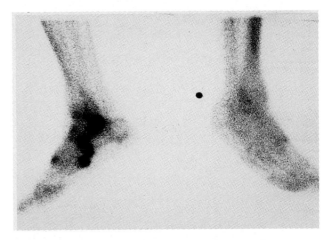

Fig. 5-25   Skeletal scintigram in a patient who had sustained direct trauma to the right foot and ankle reveals multiple focal areas of abnormal tracer accumulation. Each of these areas was subsequently demonstrated radiographically to correspond to a fracture.

Fig. 5-24   **A,** Conventional tomograph of the right proximal femur reveals a characteristic radiolucent nidus surrounded by sclerotic bone. **B,** Specimen radiograph confirms the complete excision of the nidus.

were positive at the time of scintigraphic examination, including 16 (16%) of 98 sites where the time post trauma was greater than 5 years (Table 5-3). Structural deformity and posttraumatic arthritis were the most common reasons for prolonged positivity.

Iatrogenic trauma Iatrogenic trauma to either the skeleton or soft tissues may be manifest scintigraphically. Again, the key to correct interpretation is an accurate history. Craniotomy typically leaves a rim pattern at the surgical margin that may persist for months postoperatively.

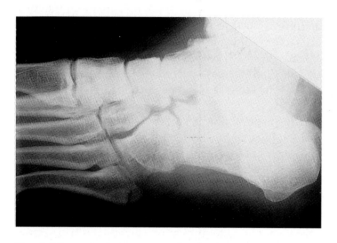

Fig. 5-26 Radiograph of the patient in Figure 5-25 illustrating fractures of the base of the fifth metatarsal and lateral cuneiform.

Rib retraction during thoracotomy can elicit periosteal reaction and increased uptake without actual resection of bone being involved. Bone resections are recognized as photon-deficient areas, although small laminectomies are usually not appreciated scintigraphically.

The pattern in bone grafting depends on the timing postoperatively. Intercalary grafts will demonstrate increased uptake at the apposed bone ends, with gradual fill-in of tracer activity as the graft is revitalized. In pedicle grafts or grafts where microvascular anastomoses are made, tracer uptake should be visualized immediately and if not seen may indicate loss of bone viability.

Areas of the skeleton receiving curative levels of ionizing radiation (typically 4,000 rads or greater) characteristically demonstrate decreased uptake within 6 months to 1 year following therapy. The threshold for the effect is on the order of 2,000 rads. The mechanism is probably on the basis of decreased osteogenesis and decreased blood flow to postirradiated bone. The hallmark scintigraphically is a geometric pattern of regionally decreased tracer uptake (Figure 5-27). Some observers have reported an actual increase in uptake immediately after therapy, but the mechanism is not known.

Athletic injuries

Stress fractures Normal bone is constantly remodeling. Bone resorption and deposition are balanced (Table 5-4). When the skeleton is placed under stress, due to a change in activity or repetitive activity, the rate of remodeling increases. Lamellar bone is remodeled into stronger osteonal bone. If resorption and deposition remain balanced, the skeleton adapts to the new demands being made on it. However, if the rate of

| Table 5-3 | Skeletal Scintigraphy in Trauma: Time Course Post Fracture for Return to Normal |

PERCENT NORMAL, BY INTERVAL NON-MANIPULATED CLOSED FRACTURES*

	1 yr (%)	3 yr (%)
Vertebrae	59	97
Long bone	64	95
Ribs	79	100

ALL FRACTURES†

	% NORMAL		
	<1 yr	2-5 yr	>5 yr
All sites	30%	62%	84%

*Modified from Matin P. The appearance of bone scans following fractures, including immediate and long term studies, *J Nucl Med* 20: 1227-1231, 1979.

†Modified from Kim HR, Thrall JH, Keyes JW Jr: Skeletal scintigraphy following incidental trauma, *Radiology* 130:447-451, 1979.

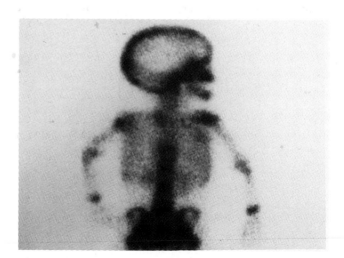

Fig. 5-27 Posterior view of a child following radiation therapy to the upper thoracic spine. Note the sharply marginated cutoff in the midthoracic region with greatly diminished uptake in the treated area compared to the lower thoracic spine and the lumbar spine.

Table 5-4   Sequence of Findings in Stress Reaction

	Clinical Findings	X-Ray	Scintigram
Normal (resorption = replacement)	−	−	−
Accelerated remodeling (res. > rep.)	±	−	+
Fatigue (res. >> rep.)	+	±	+++
Exhaustion (res. >>> rep.)	++	+	++++
Cortical fracture	++++	++++	++++

Modified from Roub LW, et al: Bone stress: a radionuclide imaging perspective, *Radiology* 132:431-438, 1979.

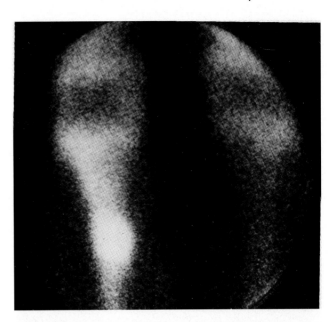

Fig. 5-28   Anterior spot view in a military recruit with exercise-induced pain in the right proximal tibia. The scintigram reveals intensely increased uptake in an oval configuration with a long axis parallel to the shaft of the tibia. The increased activity above and below the focal lesion is probably due to watershed hyperemia. (Courtesy G. E. Geslien, M.D.)

resorption sufficiently exceeds the rate of replacement, cortical bone is weakened and may be buttressed by periosteal and endosteal new bone. The final result of imbalance between resorption and replacement is a stress fracture (Table 5-4).

From the foregoing, it is clear that a "stress fracture" is not necessarily an all-or-none phenomenon. It is probably more useful to think of a continuum of injury from early periosteal reaction to overt fracture. In fact, in cases diagnosed and treated early, a discrete fracture line may never develop. If skeletal scintigraphy is performed early enough and the patient's activity is changed appropriately, radiographs may never show an abnormality. If the process is allowed to continue to the point of overt fracture, healing is predictably on the order of several months or more, compared to the several weeks required for healing of an early stress reaction.

Skeletal scintigraphy is exquisitely sensitive to the remodeling process and is typically abnormal 1 to 2 weeks or more prior to the appearance of radiographic changes in stress fractures (Table 5-4). The characteristic scintigraphic appearance is that of intense uptake at the fracture site. The configuration is oval or fusiform with the long axis of increased uptake parallel to the axis of the bone (Figures 5-28, 5-29).

Shin splints   The term "shin splints" is applied generically to describe patients with stress-related leg soreness. In nuclear medicine, the term is now used to describe a specific combination of clinical and scintigraphic findings. Patients complain of mild to moderate exercise-induced pain along the medial or posteriomedial aspect of the tibia. This is associated with corresponding increased tracer uptake on the scintigram, typically involving greater than one third of bone length and involving the middle to distal tibia (Figure 5-30). Most cases are bilateral although not necessarily symmetric. The radionuclide uptake is of only mild to moderate intensity and does not have the focal aspect seen with true stress fractures. The etiology is thought to be microperiosteal tears at points of periosteal stress. The stress may be mediated by Sharpey's fibers through their connection to muscle and bone.

The clinical significance of the shin splint pattern is quite different from that of the stress fracture pattern. Unless there is a focal component to the tracer uptake, the shin splint pattern is not predictive of further injury.

A perhaps mechanistically related phenomenon is activity-induced enthesiopathy. The term itself simply refers to a disease process at the site of tendon or ligament attachment to bone. In athletes, repeated microtears with subsequent healing reaction can result in increased tracer uptake at corresponding locations. Osteitis pubis and plantar fasciitis are examples, as are Achilles tendinitis and some cases of "pulled" hamstring muscles. A periosteal reaction develops at the site of stress, resulting in increased skeletal tracer localization.

Rhabdomyolysis   Another athletic injury that is seen in this day of marathons and triathalons is rhabdomyolysis (Figure 5-31). The localization of skeletal tracers in exercise-damaged skeletal muscle is probably similar to the localization in damaged myocardium. Calcium buildup in damaged tissue provides a site for radionuclide deposition.

The scintigraphic pattern reflects the muscle groups

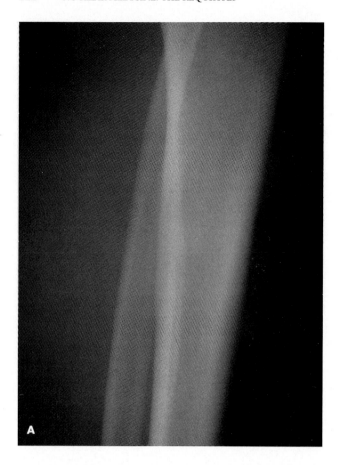

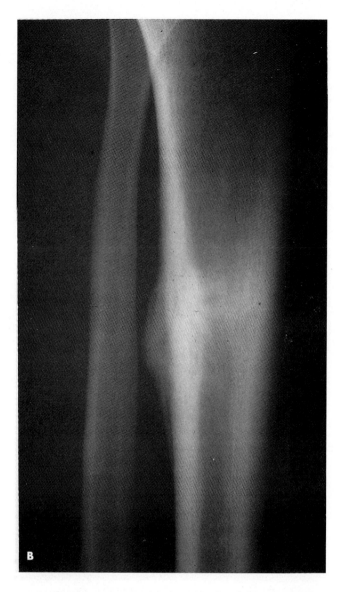

Fig. 5-29 **A,** Radiograph obtained at the same time as the scintigram of the patient in Figure 5-28. The examination does not reveal an acute abnormality. **B,** Follow-up radiograph obtained 2 weeks later shows both periosteal and endosteal changes consistent with stress fracture.

undergoing injury. In marathon runners the most striking uptake is usually in the muscles of the thigh. The time course of scintigraphic positivity appears to be similar to that for acute myocardial infarction. Matin has described a pattern of maximum positivity 24 to 48 hours following injury, with resolution by 1 week.

Child abuse The generally high sensitivity of skeletal scintigraphy would seem to make it an ideal survey test in cases of suspected child abuse. In actual practice,

the sensitivity is somewhat disappointing. This probably relates to the timing of injury in relation to scintigraphy. Older fractures may have healed scintigraphically, and calvarial fractures in young children have been reported to be missed by skeletal scintigraphy. In child abuse, radiographic skeletal survey is more sensitive than bone scintigraphy because of its ability to demonstrate old fractures. Scintigraphy should be reserved for cases of suspected child abuse where radiographs are unrevealing.

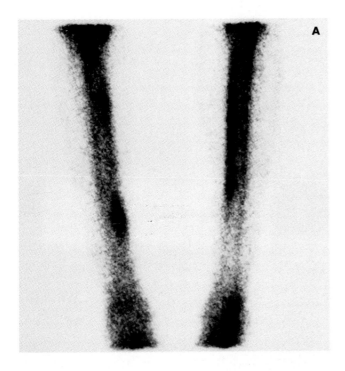

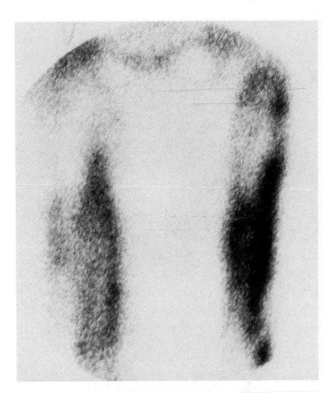

Fig. 5-31 Anterior view of the thighs in a patient who had recently competed in a marathon reveals bilateral soft tissue uptake compatible with rhabdomyolysis.

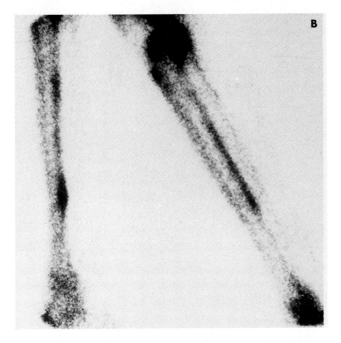

Fig. 5-30 Anterior (**A**) and lateral (**B**) views of a patient demonstrating the classic finding in shin splints of increased tracer uptake along the posteromedial aspect of the tibia on the left. There is a similar pattern on the right, but with the addition of a focal area distally suspicious for stress fracture.

Bone Infarction—Osteonecrosis

There are numerous causes of bone necrosis (Box 5-6). The appearance on skeletal scintigraphy is highly dependent on the time course of the process. With acute interruption of the blood supply, newly infarcted bone appears cold or photon-deficient scintigraphically. In the postinfarction or healing phase there is increased osteogenesis and increased tracer uptake at the margin of the infarcted area. Skeletal scintigrams can show intensely increased tracer uptake during the healing period (Figures 5-32, 5-33).

Legg-Calvé-Perthes disease Legg-Calvé-Perthes disease most commonly affects children between the ages of 5 and 9 years, with a predominance in boys (4:1 to 5:1). It is a form of osteochondrosis and results in avascular necrosis of the capital femoral epiphysis. The mechanism of injury is not known except that the vascular supply of the femoral head is thought to be especially vulnerable in the most commonly affected age group.

The best scintigraphic technique for detecting the abnormality in the femoral head is to use some form of

Box 5-6   Causes of Aseptic Bone Necrosis

Trauma (accidental, iatrogenic)
Drug therapy (steroids)
Hypercoagulable states
Hemoglobinopathies (sickle cell disease and variants)
Post radiation therapy (orthovoltage)
Caisson disease
Osteochondrosis (pediatric age group; Legg-Calvé-
    Perthes disease)
Polycythemia
Leukemia
Gaucher's disease
Alcoholism
Pancreatitis
Idiopathic

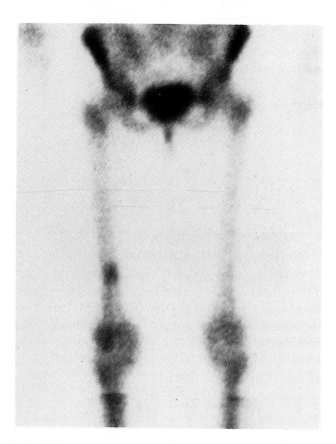

Fig. 5-32   Anterior view of the lower extremities demonstrating focally increased uptake in the distal right femoral diaphysis during the healing phase of bone or bone marrow infarction.

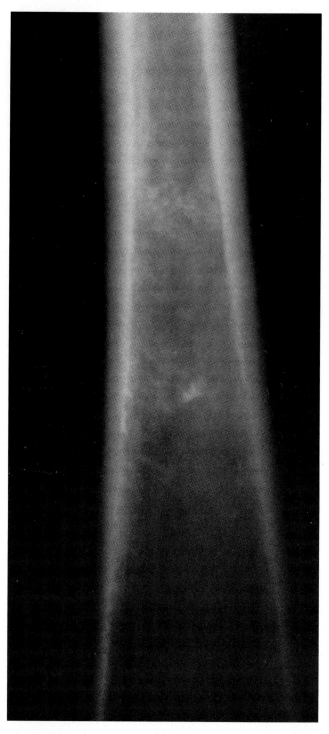

Fig. 5-32   Anterior view of the lower extremities demonstrating focally increased uptake in the distal right femoral diaphysis during the healing phase of bone or bone marrow infarction.

magnification and to image in the frogleg lateral projection. Classically, in patients imaged early in the course of the disease, before healing has occurred, there is a discrete photon-deficient area in the upper outer portion of the capital femoral epiphysis with a lentiform configuration (Figures 5-34 to 5-37).

As healing occurs, increased uptake is first seen at the margin of the photon-deficient area, and gradually the scintigram demonstrates filling in of activity. In severe cases, the femoral head never reverts to normal. Increased tracer uptake is seen for a prolonged period—of many months or more.

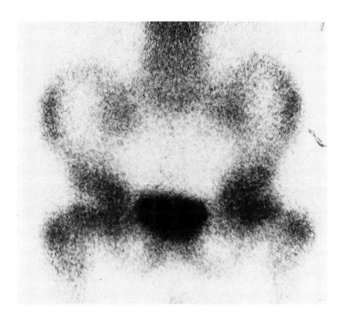

Fig. 5-34   Anterior view of the hips and pelvis in a patient with suspected Legg-Calvé-Perthes disease. There is distinct asymmetry with decreased uptake in the superior and lateral aspect of the right femoral epiphysis.

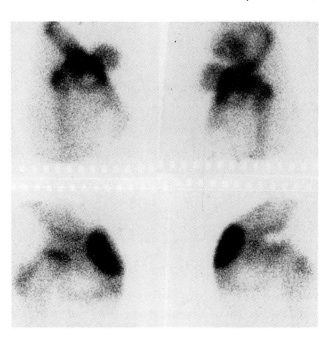

Fig. 5-36   The benefit of pinhole magnification is demonstrated from a comparison of the top two images, obtained with a standard parallel hole collimator, and the bottom two images, obtained with a pinhole collimator (same patient). The characteristic lentiform area of decreased uptake is seen on the left.

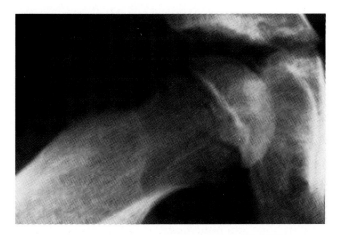

Fig. 5-35   Radiograph corresponding to the scintigram in Figure 5-34 is essentially normal without evidence of deformity or abnormal density of the epiphysis.

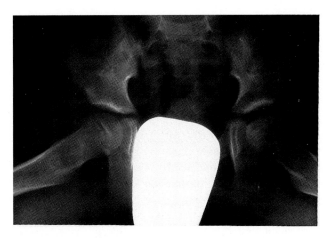

Fig. 5-37   Radiographs corresponding to the scintigrams in Figure 5-36 reveal deformity of the left femoral epiphysis with flattening, increased density, and increased distance between the epiphysis and the acetabulum.

Currently MRI is being explored as an alternative to scintigraphy in the diagnosis of avascular necrosis. MRI is very sensitive to changes in marrow fat, but in children the hematopoietic elements dominate in the marrow of the proximal femurs. MRI appears to be superior for making the diagnosis of avascular necrosis in adults.

The issue has not been settled for children.

Steroid-induced osteonecrosis   Another entity that may be confusing on skeletal scintigraphy is drug-induced, especially steroid-induced, osteonecrosis. Intuitively, one would think that areas of osteonecrosis would appear photon-deficient on skeletal scintigraphy. However, in

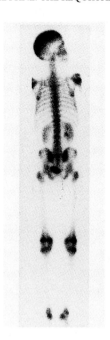

Fig. 5-38   Posterior whole body scintigram in a young adult man with sickle cell anemia. There is markedly increased uptake in the calvarium due to the expanded marrow space. There is also greater than expected uptake in the knees, and the overall skeletal uptake is striking compared to background soft tissues.

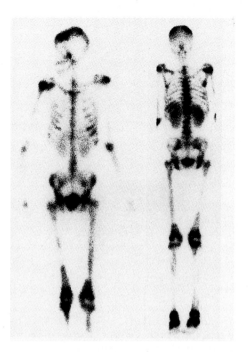

Fig. 5-39   Anterior and posterior whole body views of a patient with sickle cell anemia. Note increased calvarial uptake with relative thinning at the midline. There is prominent skeleton-to-soft tissue uptake. The kidneys appear large, and there is intense uptake in the spleen. There is a greater than expected uptake for an adult subject in the knees and ankles. Note the photon-deficient areas in the right femur due to bone/bone marrow infarction.

the vast majority of cases, increased uptake is demonstrated scintigraphically. Although the pathogenesis of steroid-induced osteonecrosis is still being debated, it is a chronic process manifested by microfractures and repair. The net effect most often seen scintigraphically is increased tracer localization.

Sickle cell anemia   Skeletal scintigrams in patients with sickle cell anemia have a number of characteristic features that suggest the diagnosis (Figure 5-38). In the skull, the expanded marrow space results in bilaterally increased calvarial uptake of tracer. In the extremities, there is usually greater relative uptake compared to the axial skeleton than is seen in normal subjects. This increased uptake may be related in some way to the persistence of hemopoietic elements throughout the extremities, including the hands and feet, of patients with sickle cell anemia. As noted earlier, in normal adults the red marrow extends only to the proximal portions of the femurs and humeri. The overall skeleton-to-background ratio is usually very good and is further accentuated by the increased appendicular uptake.

In many patients with sickle cell anemia, the kidneys appear somewhat larger than normal, which may be related to a defect in the ability to concentrate urine. It is not unusual to see avid accumulation of skeletal tracer in the spleen, presumably due to prior splenic infarction and calcification (Figure 5-39).

Patients with sickle cell anemia are subject to infarctions in bone and bone marrow. If the involvement is primarily in the marrow space, the skeletal scintigram may be normal acutely but typically demonstrates increased uptake during the healing phase, beginning within a few days of the acute event (Figure 5-40).

Bone marrow scans (Tc-99m sulfur colloid) are very sensitive for detecting bone marrow infarction and are positive immediately following the acute event (Figure 5-41). Affected areas fail to accumulate tracer and are seen as cold or photon-deficient areas. The confounding problem in making the diagnosis of acute bone marrow infarction is the almost invariable presence of chronic marrow defects from prior bone marrow infarctions in the majority of patients with sickle cell anemia. Thus,

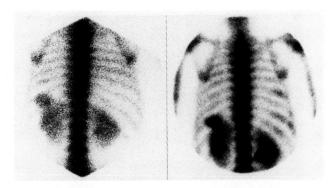

Fig. 5-40   Posterior views obtained at the time of onset of acute chest pain (*left*) and several days later (*right*) in a patient with sickle cell anemia. Note uptake in the spleen on both images. Typically, once the spleen is visualized scintigraphically it remains positive. The initial image reveals no abnormality in the ribs. The follow-up image demonstrates increased uptake, particularly in the right ribs, associated with healing of infarctions.

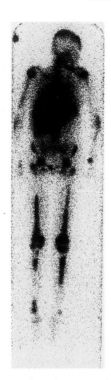

Fig. 5-41   Technetium-99m sulfur colloid bone marrow scan in a patient with sickle cell anemia. Note intense uptake in the liver. The uptake in the bone marrow extends throughout the upper and lower extremities. There are numerous focal defects indicating marrow infarctions. It is not possible to distinguish new from old abnormalities with one examination.

the significance of a photon-deficient area on marrow scanning is somewhat uncertain unless a recent baseline study is available for comparison.

In a patient with sickle cell anemia presenting with skeletal pain, the most important differential diagnosis is between bone or bone marrow infarction and osteomyelitis. The treatment of the former is hydration and general support, whereas osteomyelitis requires IV antibiotics. Unfortunately, increased uptake in an area of pain in a patient with sickle cell anemia can be due to either a healing marrow infarction or acute osteomyelitis. For this reason, the skeletal scintigram has not proved to be terrribly helpful alone in the management of patients with sickle cell anemia. Other agents such as indium-111-labeled white blood cells or gallium-67 citrate are probably better for establishing the presence or absence of osteomyelitis in these patients. Bone marrow scans with Tc-99m sulphur colloid are also not useful for making the distinction since both marrow infarction and osteomyelitis result in destruction of the phagocytic cells responsible for tracer localization.

Osteomyelitis

Acute hematogenous osteomyelitis typically begins by seeding of the infectious organism in the marrow space. Extension of the untreated process from the medullary cavity is through Volkmann canals horizontally and in the Haversian canal system axially. The skeletal scintigram is almost invariably abnormal by the time there are clinical symptoms. Increased tracer uptake is the typical finding (Figure 5-42).

In children, *Staphylococcus aureus* is the most common organism and is probably responsible for 50% or more of cases. The skeletal infection, is often associated with some other staphylococcal infection, often of the skin. Enteric bacteria and *Streptococcus* are also important pathogens.

Osteomyelitis may involve any skeletal structure. In adults, the axial skeleton is affected more often than the extremities (Figures 5-43, 5-44). When vertebrae are involved, the organisms may be carried through the perispinous venous plexus, producing involvement at

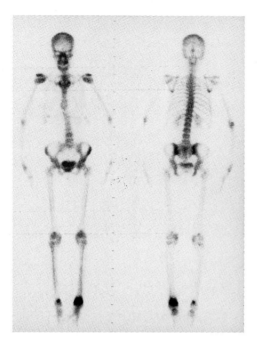

Fig. 5-42 Anterior and posterior views in a patient with acute osteomyelitis of the distal left tibia showing strikingly increased uptake. Note in addition the subtly increased uptake in the skeletal structures adjacent to the lesion, most likely due to regional hyperemia induced by the osteomyelitis.

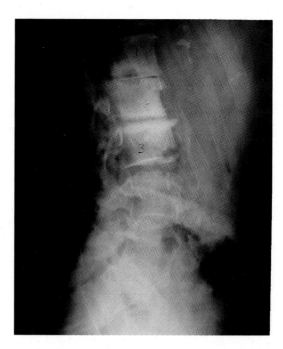

Fig. 5-44 Radiograph corresponding to the scintigram in Figure 5-43 shows destructive and sclerotic changes involving the L-2 vertebral body and adjacent portions of L-1 and L-3. The process has involved the intervertebral disks, with loss of height in the disk space.

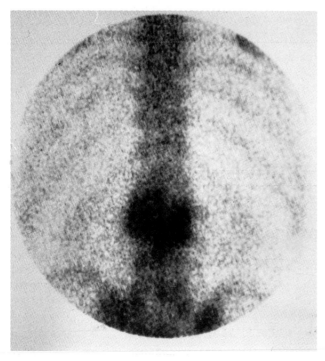

Fig. 5-43 Posterior spot view in an adult patient with spinal osteomyelitis. Note intensely increased uptake in the midlumbar region involving more than one level.

multiple levels. An exception to the axial involvement in adults is seen in diabetics, in whom the feet are often involved. However, the infection often begins in the soft tissues with extension to bone.

In some patients, especially children, increased pressure in the marrow space or thrombosis of blood vessels results in paradoxically decreased tracer uptake and a cold or photon-deficient lesion. Organisms most commonly responsible for this pattern are coagulase-positive *Staphylococcus aureus* and *Streptococcus*.

Numerous studies in the literature document the superior sensitivity of skeletal scintigraphy compared to conventional radiography in the diagnosis of acute hematogenous osteomyelitis. False negative scintigraphic studies are unusual but have been reported in young children, especially infants under the age of 1 year. Other causes of false negative examinations are imaging very early in the course of disease and failure to recognize the significance of cold or photon-deficient areas.

Three-phase scintigraphy Dynamic, or three-phase, imaging is a special technique employed in the differential diagnosis of cellulitis and osteomyelitis. This is an important differential diagnosis in diabetics, who have a high incidence of both problems. The distinction is clinically important because of the therapeutic implications of prolonged treatment when osteomyelitis is diagnosed.

The technique for dynamic scanning is summarized in Box 5-7 and the key diagnostic criteria in Box 5-8. Cellulitis typically demonstrates delayed or venous phase hyperemia with increased uptake diffusely on the blood pool images and clearance of tracer on delayed images without focally increased uptake in bone (Figure 5-45). The typical appearance of osteomyelities is early or arterial hyperemia with both focally and possibly dif-

---

Box 5-9   Other Lesions that can Mimic Osteomyelitis on Three-Phase Skeletal Scintigraphy

Osteoarthritis
Gout
Fracture
Stress fracture
Osteonecrosis (healing)
Charcot joint
Osteotomy
Reflex sympathetic dystrophy syndrome

Box 5-7   Three-Phase Skeletal Scintigraphy: Protocol Summary

RADIOPHARMACEUTICAL DOSAGE AND ROUTE OF ADMINISTRATION
Standard tracer and dosage are used and given as a bolus injection.

PROCEDURE
The gamma camera is positioned prior to radiopharmaceutical administration immediately over the site of suspected pathology.

FLOW PHASE
Dynamic 2-5 sec images are obtained for 60 sec after bolus injection (30 sec in children).

BLOOD POOL AND TISSUE PHASE
Acquire immediate, static images for time (5 min) or counts (300k).

SKELETAL PHASE
Acquire delayed 300k-1,000k images at 2-4 hr.

Box 5-8   Three-Phase Skeletal Scintigraphy: Interpretive Criteria

Osteomyelitis: *Arterial* hyperemia, progressive focal skeletal uptake with relative soft tissue clearance; In children, a focal cold area may be seen if osteomyelitis is associated with infarction.
Cellulitis: Venous (delayed) hyperemia, persistent soft tissue activity. No focal skeletal uptake (may have mild to moderate diffusely increased uptake).
Septic joint: Periarticular increased activity on dynamic and blood pool phases that persists on delayed images. Less commonly, the joint structures will appear cold if pressure in the joint causes decreased flow or infarction.

---

fusely increased uptake of tracer on the blood pool images and progressive focal accumulation in the involved bone at delayed imaging (Figure 5-46). While the technique has been shown useful in distinguishing cellulitis from osteomyelitis, the pattern described for osteomyelitis is not specific. The same sequence of image findings can be seen in neuropathic joint disease, gout, fracture, and rheumatoid arthritis, among other conditions (Figures 5-47, Box 5-9).

Prosthesis evaluation Numerous attempts have been made to use skeletal scintigraphy in the evaluation of patients following total joint replacement or implantation of other metallic prostheses. The distinction between component loosening and infection is critical in guiding management.

The findings on skeletal scintigraphy are not specific enough to reliably make the distinction between loosening of a prostheses and infection (Figure 5-48). Reactive bone around a loose prosthesis may be indistinguishable from increased tracer uptake secondary to osteomyelitis. Classically, in cases of a loose prosthesis there is increased uptake in the region of the greater and lesser trochanters and at the tip of the prosthesis. This is presumably due to remodeling of bone in response to movement of the prosthesis. In osteomyelitis there is increased activity in the bone surrounding the prosthesis.

The differential diagnosis is better made with tracers such as indium-111-labeled WBCs and either contrast or radionuclide arthrography. In one approach, a skeletal scintigram is first obtained with Tc-99m diphosphonate, followed by a radionuclide arthrogram using a radionuclide with higher energy than Tc-99m. Images with the two different tracers can be superimposed on each other so that skeletal anatomic landmarks can be correlated with tracer distribution on the arthrogram. If a prosthesis is firmly in place, the tracer (or radiographic contrast medium) cannot flow around it and is confined to the joint space. With prosthesis loosening, the tracer is readily detected outside of the joint space. For example, with a loose femoral component, tracer may be seen all the way to the tip.

The best combination of sensitivity and specificity for detecting an infected prostheses is offered by In-111-labeled white blood cells. This tracer localizes in areas of infection and not in areas of remodeling or reactive bone. The two pitfalls in the use of In-111-labeled white blood cells are the difficulty in distinguishing cellulitis from septic arthritis and some false negative examinations in chronic osteomyelitis.

A

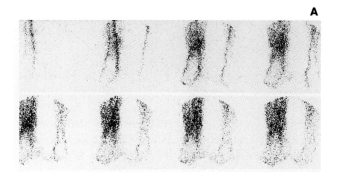

B

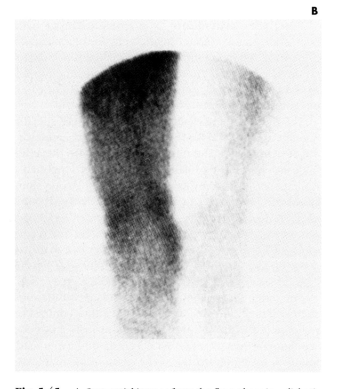

Fig. 5-45 **A**, Sequential images from the flow phase in a diabetic patient diagnosed with cellulitis. Note marked hyperemia in the region of the ankle and the visualized portion of the leg. **B**, Follow-up blood pool images revealed diffusely increased activity in the areas corresponding to the hyperemia. No focal abnormality was demonstrated on follow-up late-phase imaging.

Metabolic Bone Disease

A number of metabolic conditions can result in marked abnormalities on bone scintigrams. Although these do not represent important clinical indications for bone scintigraphy, they may be encountered incidentally in other applications, most importantly during metastatic skeletal survey. Hyperthyroidism, primary hyperparathyroidism, renal osteodystrophy, osteomalacia, and hypervitaminosis D can all result in generalized increased tracer uptake throughout the skeleton that has some features in common with the superscan seen in metastatic disease (Figure 5-49). These features are an increased skeleton-to-soft tissue ratio and faint or absent visualization of the kidneys. Involvement of the long bones of the extremities and increased periarticular uptake are features that distinguish scans in these conditions from the superscan of metastatic disease.

Another striking feature occasionally seen in metabolic bone disease is "beading" of the costochondral junction akin to the rachitic rosary (Figure 5-49). A number of other features are seen in some of the metabolic bone diseases. For example, in primary hyperparathyroidism and renal osteodystrophy, extraskeletal uptake may be seen in the lungs and stomach (Figure 5-50). In osteomalacia, pseudofractures are frequently seen and demonstrate avid radiopharmaceutical uptake (Figure 5-10).

Osteoporosis Osteoporosis is an increasingly common problem with the aging of the population. Skeletal scintigraphy does not have a role in the diagnosis of osteoporosis but is very useful in surveying the entire skeleton for osteoporotic insufficiency fractures. These may actually be asymptomatic, and the ability to survey the entire skeleton is advantageous. Compression fractures of the spine are very common (Figure 5-51). Sacral insufficiency fractures are also common. Sacral fractures are often difficult to diagnose radiographically. The most common pattern is the H pattern with a horizontal band of increased uptake across the body of the sacrum and two vertical limbs of activity in the sacral alae (Figure 5-52). Several pattern variations exist, including asymmetry of the alar activity. Less severe fractures may show only horizontal linear uptake.

Paget's Disease

Paget's disease of bone involves the skeleton focally. The scintigraphic appearance is striking, with intensely increased tracer localization (Figure 5-53). The expansion of bone demonstrated radiographically is not well assessed by scintigraphy, owing to the lower resolution of the technique, but is certainly suggested on the images (Figure 5-53). The pelvis is the most commonly involved site, followed by the spine, skull, femur, sca-

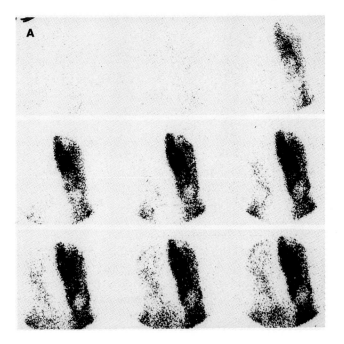

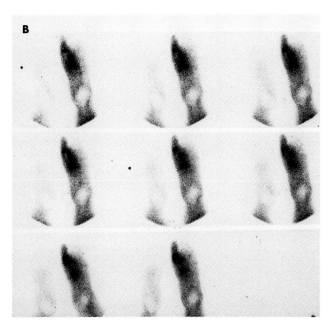

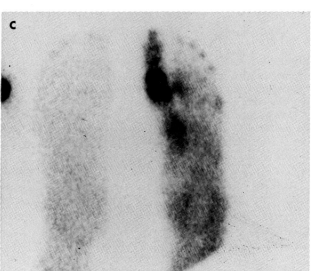

Fig. 5-46 **A**, Sequential dynamic images in a middle-aged diabetic male with osteomyelitis. Note the intense arterial phase hyperemia. **B**, Blood pool images already reveal localization in skeletal structures. **C**, Delayed static images reveal intense focal accumulation in multiple areas of the great toe and distal first and second metatarsals.

pula, tibia, and humerus. The increased uptake is seen both in the early resorptive or lucent phase of the disease and in the proliferative or sclerotic phase. In osteoporosis circumscripta there is a characteristic rim of increased uptake bordering the lesion.

Bone Dysplasias

Numerous bone dysplasias demonstrate increased skeletal tracer uptake (Figures 5-54, to 5-56). Fibrous dysplasia is the most commonly encountered of these and may be monostotic or polyostotic. The degree of increased tracer uptake is typically very high, rivaling that seen in Paget's disease. Distinguishing features are the younger age of the patient and the different pattern

of involvement. When Paget's disease involves a long bone, it invariably extends to at least one end of the bone. Fibrous dysplasia frequently does not involve the end of the bone. Other dysplasias associated with increased tracer uptake are listed in Box 5-10.

Arthritis

Skeletal scintigraphy is a sensitive marker of both osteoarthritis (Figure 5-57) and rheumatoid arthritis. Numerous attempts have been made over the last two decades to develop scintigraphic techniques for staging the severity of arthritis and assessing response to therapy. These have been largely unsuccessful, and skeletal scintigraphy is not commonly used to evaluate arthritis
Text continued on p. 126.

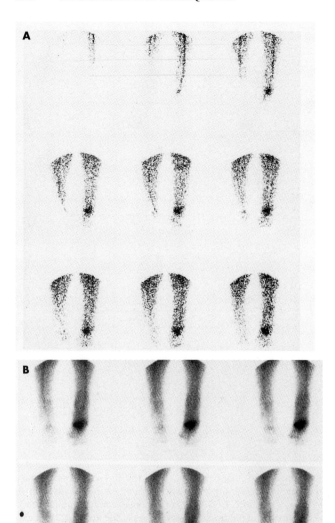

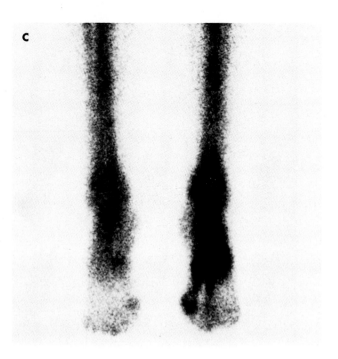

Fig. 5-47   **A**, Sequential dynamic images in a patient subsequently shown to have foot and ankle fractures. There is focal arterial hyperemia on the left. **B**, Multiple images from the blood pool phase confirm hyperemia in the region of the left foot and ankle. **C**, Delayed static images demonstrate intensely increased uptake in the left foot and ankle. The distinction between osteomyelitis and fracture cannot be made from the three-phase skeletal study alone but requires clinical and radiographic correlation.

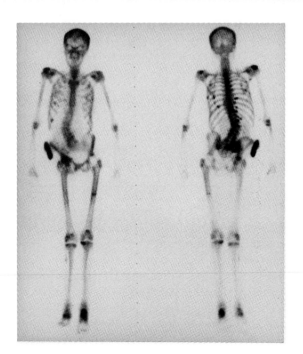

Fig. 5-48   Anterior and posterior whole body images in a patient with severe scoliosis and skeletal metastases from carcinoma of the breast. The patient has a left femoral prosthesis, subsequently shown to be loose. Note the increased uptake at the tip of the prosthesis and the subtly increased uptake in the region of the trochanters, especially the greater trochanter. Note also the intensely increased uptake in the right femoral head due to dysplastic and degenerative arthritic changes.

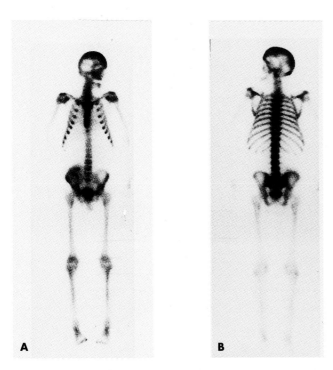

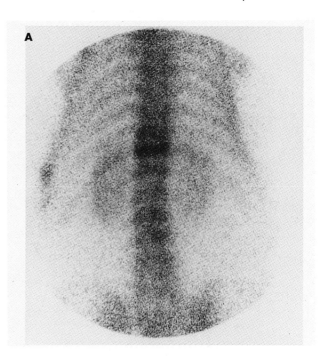

Fig. 5-49   Anterior (**A**) and posterior (**B**) whole body images in a patient with renal osteodystrophy. There is a striking increase in the skeletal-to-soft tissue ratio of uptake. The patient's native kidneys had failed, and there is a renal transplant in place in the right iliac fossa. The anterior rib ends are especially prominent.

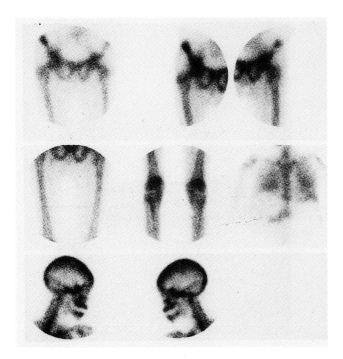

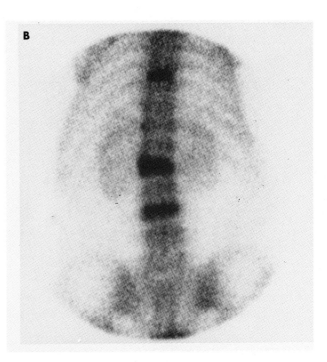

Fig. 5-50   Multiple spot views in a patient with hyperparathyroidism. The anterior view of the lungs and upper abdomen (*middle right image*) reveals diffuse uptake in both lungs and the stomach.

Fig. 5-51   Surveillance images obtained several months apart. **A**, The initial study revealed a single vertebral compression fracture due to osteoporosis involving the lower thoracic spine. **B**, A subsequent study revealed healing with normalization of uptake in the abnormality seen on the earlier image. Three new compression fractures are demonstrated in the mid-dorsal spine and the lumbar spine.

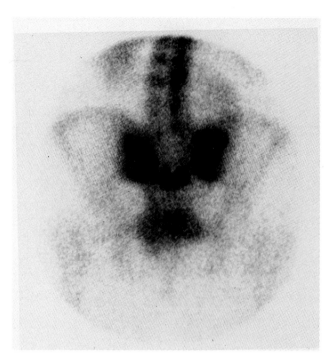

Fig. 5-52   Posterior spot view from a patient with osteoporosis. Note the H type insufficiency fracture with a horizontal band of increased uptake across the body of the sacrum and bilaterally increased uptake in the sacral alae.

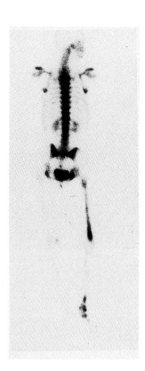

Fig. 5-54   Posterior whole body image from a patient with melorheostosis. There is intensely increased uptake in a somewhat patchy distribution involving the right femur.

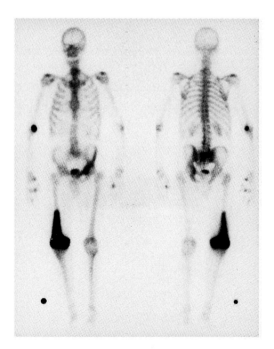

Fig. 5-53   Anterior and posterior whole body images in a patient with Paget's disease involving the right distal femur and the left hemipelvis. The uptake is extremely intense, with the appearance of bony expansion. The observation about expansion must be made with caution owing to the extreme intensity of uptake and "blooming" of the recorded activity.

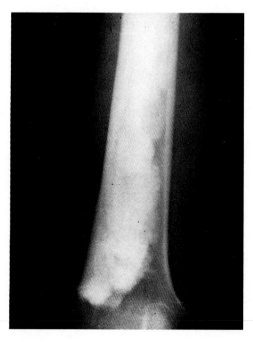

Fig. 5-55   Spot view of the distal femur from the patient in Figure 5-54 reveals the characteristic intensely sclerotic lesion of melorheostosis, often characterized as having the appearance of dripping candle wax.

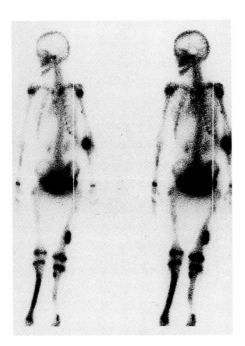

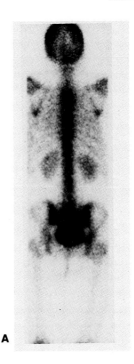

Fig. 5-56   Two anterior views at different intensities in a patient with osteogenesis imperfecta. Note the deformity of the tibia with increased uptake throughout the right tibital shaft. There are focal areas of abnormal uptake in the left femur and left proximal tibia. The increased uptake at the left elbow is the injection site.

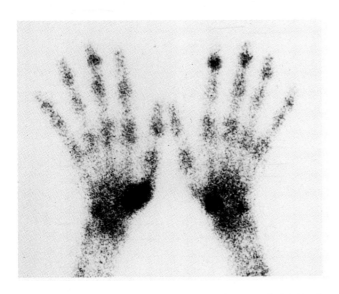

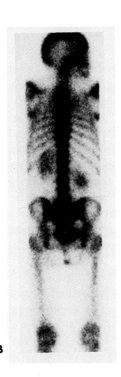

Fig. 5-57   Characteristic appearance of osteoarthritis in the hands and wrists. There is increased uptake involving multiple distal interphalangeal joints. Note the particularly intense uptake at the base of the first left metacarpal, a very characteristic place of involvement for osteoarthritis.

Fig. 5-58   Posterior images obtained several months apart in a patient with lung cancer. The initial image (**A**) is unremarkable. The follow-up image (**B**) reveals downward displacement of the right kidney. The nuclear medicine physician suggested the possibility of an adrenal metastasis, which was subsequently demonstrated by computed tomography.

in current clinical practice. The major importance of arthritis is its ubiquitous presence in the elderly and therewith the likelihood of encountering increased focal uptake in patients undergoing metastatic surveys. Arthritis in the extremities is typically not a problem. Special care must be taken in assessing the lower lumbar spine because of the common occurrence of both osteoarthritis and metastatic disease in this location.

Extraskeletal and Genitourinary Findings

A number of causes of nonosseous uptake of skeletal radiopharmaceuticals are routinely encountered in clinical practice. They often offer the opportunity to make an additional diagnosis, and the extraskeletal distribution of tracer should be inspected in every case (Figure 5-58).

A number of normal or normal variant causes of extraskeletal tracer uptake were discussed in the section on the appearance of the normal scintigram. The thyroid cartilage, calcifications in blood vessels, and calcified costal cartilages can all demonstrate uptake.

The kidneys and bladder should be seen in normal subjects. Many genitourinary tract abnormalities are diagnosed incidentally by skeletal scintigraphy (Figures 5-59, 5-60). Renal tumors and cysts are readily seen if large enough. Displacements of the kidney including crossed renal ectopia and horseshoe kidney are also readily visualized. The cause of renal enlargement or abnormally small kidneys may not be apparent on skeletal scintigraphy but the findings should be noted for further workup.

Dystrophic calcifications in the soft tissues as well as acute injury to myocardium and skeletal muscle can show avid uptake. Patients with cardiac amyloidosis can demonstrate striking uptake in the heart. Myositis ossificans avidly accumulates skeletal-seeking tracers (Figures 5-61, 5-62). The condition may develop following direct injury to muscle or as a consequence of paralysis. The maturity of the process can be assessed scintigraphically based on the relative uptake of tracer over sequential studies. As the process matures, the degree of uptake diminishes. Skeletal imaging has been used to help time surgical intervention, which is best done after the lesion matures.

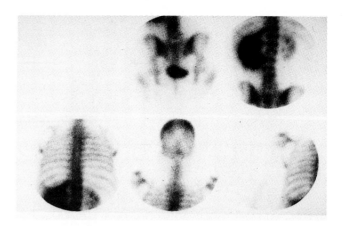

Fig. 5-59 Posterior spot views in a patient with breast cancer reveal an abnormal accumulation of tracer in the region of the left kidney. The appearance suggests obstruction and possible extravasation of urine around the left kidney.

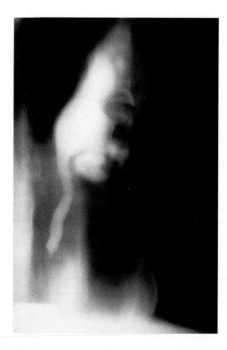

Fig. 5-60 Corresponding nephrotomogram of the left kidney in the patient in Figure 5-59 reveals complete obstruction of the left ureter due to a metastatic lesion. There is pyelotubular backflow and extravasation accounting for the scintigraphic appearance.

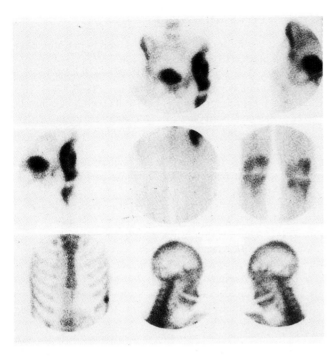

Fig. 5-61   Multiple anterior spot views in a patient with an acute spinal cord injury reveal intense accumulation of tracer in the region of the left hip and proximal thigh. The location and intensity of the uptake strongly suggest the presence of myositis ossificans.

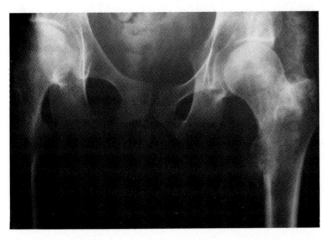

Fig. 5-62   Radiograph corresponding to the scintigram in Figure 5-61 reveals exuberant soft tissue calcification indicative of myositis ossificans.

BONE MARROW SCINTIGRAPHY

Bone marrow scintigraphy is not important in current practice but does have a small number of indications. The procedure is most commonly performed with Tc-99m sulfur colloid, which localizes in the reticuloendothelial elements of the red marrow.

In patients with sickle cell anemia, bone marrow imaging demonstrates the extent of marrow expansion into the extremities (Figure 5-41). In most normal subjects the marrow is confined to the proximal thirds of the femurs and humeri. In patients with hemoglobinopathies the marrow uptake is typically seen throughout the appendages. Marrow imaging is highly sensitive for detection of bone marrow infarction and can also define the extent of involvement. The major limitation is not being able to distinguish new from chronic infarctions. Moreover, areas involved by osteomyelitis will demonstrate defects on marrow imaging, so that the technique is not useful in distinguishing infarction from osteomyelitis. In current practice, marrow imaging is used in some institutions in conjunction with In-111-labeled WBCs to diagnose osteomyelitis.

Marrow imaging has also enjoyed a vogue for the diagnosis of aseptic necrosis of the hip. Marrow elements are lost in the necrotic area. Although the technique is fairly sensitive, it has given way to MRI.

MEASUREMENT OF BONE MINERAL

A number of methods have been developed to quantitatively measure bone mineral mass. All of the techniques are based on the differential absorption of photons in bone versus soft tissue and calibration of percent absorption against calcium-containing reference standards.

The simplest technique is single photon absorptiometry (SPA). In this technique a photon source, typically iodine-125, is collimated and scanned across the radius and/or calcaneus. These sites are selected to minimize soft tissue, for there is no way to correct for soft tissue attenuation in the SPA technique.

Dual-photon absorptiometry (DPA) again uses a collimated photon source that is scanned over the skeletal part of interest. It is a more flexible technique because the soft tissue attenuation can be corrected based on the differential absorption of the beam at different energies. The dual-photon absorptiometry technique typically uses gadolinium-153 with photon energies between 40 and 100 keV. Areas frequently studied by DPA include the lumbar spine and both the neck and the intertrochanteric region of the femur.

More recently, bone densitometry measurements have been made using either dedicated x-ray densitometer devices or special quantitative computed tomography (QCT) algorithms. Single- and dual-energy techniques have been described for both x-ray and QCT. The advantage of the x-ray technique is higher photon flux compared to SPA and DPA instruments. Radiation exposure is essentially identical for dual-energy x-ray densitometry and DPA.

The main advantage of QCT is the ability to separately measure cortical and trabecular bone. Dual-energy QCT has the advantage of allowing correction for fat in the marrow space, compared to single-energy QCT. Both techniques are quite flexible with respect to body part examined. In contemporary practice, dual-energy x-ray absorptiometry and variations of QCT are considered superior to the isotope-based methods.

The main application of bone mineral measurements is in the evaluation of patients with osteoporosis to establish baseline diagnostic measurements and to follow the course of therapy. Primary osteoporosis has been divided into two subtypes. Type I or postmenopausal osteoporosis is related to decreased estrogen secretion after menopause. Type II or senile osteoporosis is presumably due to age-related impaired bone metabolism.

Risk factors for osteoporosis include female sex, caucasian or Asian race, smoking, chronic alcohol intake, and a positive family history. Early menopause, long term treatment with corticosteroids, or any one of a number of nutritional disorders including malabsorption are also risk factors. Obesity is protective.

Acknowledgments

Portions of this chapter appeared in a slightly different form and are reprinted with permission from Thrall JH, Ellis BI: Skeletal metastases, *Radial of Clin North Am* 25:1155-1170, 1987.

SUGGESTED READINGS

Brown ML: Significance of the solitary lesion in pediatric bone scanning, *J Nucl Med* 24:114-115, 1983.

Charkes ND, Young J, and Sklaroff DM: The pathologic basis of the strontium bone scan, *JAMA* 206:2482, 1968.

Chilton HM, Francis MD, and Thrall JH: Radiopharmaceuticals for bone and bone marrow imaging. In Swanson DP, Chilton HM, and Thrall JH, editors: *Pharmaceuticals in medical imaging*, pp 537-563, New York, 1990, Macmillan.

Corcoran RJ, Thrall JH, Kyle RW et al: Solitary abnormalities in bone scans of patients with extraosseous malignancies, *Radiology* 121:663-667, 1976.

Fogelman I, editor: *Bone scanning in clinical practice*, London, 1987, Springer-Verlag.

Freeman LM and Blaufox MD, editors: Nuclear orthopedics, *Semin Nucl Med* 18:78-161, 1988.

Kim H, Thrall JH, and Keyes JW Jr: Skeletal scintigraphy following incidental trauma, *Radiology* 130:447-451, 1979.

Martin P: The appearance of bone scans following fractures including immediate and long-term studies, *J Nucl Med* 20:1227-1231, 1979.

McNeil BJ: Value of bone scanning in neoplastic disease, *Semin Nucl Med* 14:277-286, 1984.

Roub LW, Gamarman LW, Hanley EN et al: Bone stress: a radionuclide imaging perspective, *Radiology* 132:431-438, 1979.

Shirazi PH, Rayudu GVS, and Fordham EW: Review of solitary ^{18}F bone scan lesions, *Radiology* 112:369-372, 1974.

Shirazi PH, Rayudu GVS, and Fordham EW: [18]F bone scanning: review of indications and results of 1500 scans, *Radiology* 122:361, 1974.

Silberstein EB, editor: *Bone scintigraphy*, Mount Kisco, 1984, Futura.

Tofe AJ, Francis MD, and Harvey WJ: Correlation of neoplasms with incidence and localization of skeletal metastases: an analysis of 1355 diphosphonate bone scans, *J Nucl Med* 16:986, 1975.

Woolfenden JM, Pitt MJ, and Durie BGM et al: Comparison of bone scintigraphy and radiography in multiple myeloma, *Radiology* 134:723-728, 1980.

Pulmonary System

The single most important application of pulmonary scintigraphy is the evaluation of patients with suspected pulmonary embolism (PE). This frequently fatal condition continues to defy clinical diagnosis at the bedside and is all too often first diagnosed at postmortem examination. Some authorities have estimated the annual incidence of PE in the United States at over 650,000 cases per year, with over 100,000 deaths. The mortality from untreated significant PE is on the order of 30%. This mortality is greatly reduced by treatment with anticoagulants and other therapies, including vena cava filter placement. The combination of nonspecificity of clinical presentation and the potentially high mortality from untreated PE have created an ongoing need for noninvasive testing. Although pulmonary angiography has been and remains the reference standard for the definitive diagnosis of PE, it is expensive, invasive, and not without its own morbidity and mortality. The contemporary approach to the diagnosis of PE requires the judicious melding of clinical observations, application of ventilation/perfusion scintigraphy, and selective referral for pulmonary angiography.

There are a number of less common indications for pulmonary scintigraphy that merit brief discussion. These include quantitative analysis of relative lung perfusion prior to lobectomy or pneumonectomy, and studies in patients with adult respiratory distress syndrome.

VENTILATION SCINTIGRAPHY

Ventilation and perfusion in the lung are coupled in many conditions and not linked directly together in others. The finding of "concordant" versus "discordant" ventilation and perfusion abnormalities thus becomes pivotal in the differential diagnosis of combined ventilation/perfusion (V/Q) studies. The findings from ventilation studies lend additional specificity and significance to the patterns identified on perfusion studies.

Radiopharmaceuticals

Radioactive gases Two classes of radiopharmaceuticals are used for ventilation imaging, radioactive gases and radioaerosols. The radioactive gases include xenon-133, xenon-127, and krypton-81m. The most widely used of these agents is Xe-133 (Box 6-1). Its half-life is 5.27 days, which makes it relatively easy to distribute and keep in stock in nuclear medicine pharmacies. It is available in either a single-dose or multidose vial form from commercial vendors.

A major drawback to the use of Xe-133 is the relatively low 81 keV energy of its principal photon. This low energy makes it difficult to perform Xe-133 ventilation studies after a perfusion study with a technetium-99m agent. There is significant compton scatter from the 140 keV principal gamma of Tc-99m into the Xe-133 window. This "downscatter" potentially obscures abnor-

Box 6-1   Xenon-133: Summary of Physical Characteristics and Dosimetry

I. PHYSICAL CHARACTERISTICS

Mode of decay	Beta minus
Physical half-life ($T_{1/2}$)	5.2 days
Photon energy	81 keV
Abundance	36.5%

II. DOSIMETRY*: XENON-133 GAS ADMINISTERED BY INHALATION

ORGAN	RADS/30 mCi
Lungs	0.25
Whole body	0.0027

*Modified from product information brochure for Xenon-133 Gas, Dupont Radiopharmaceutic Division, Billerica, MA.

malities on the Xe-133 study and significantly degrades the image. Even with subtraction techniques, images are degraded. Therefore, Xe-133 ventilation scintigraphy is typically performed first in combined V/Q imaging.

Xe-127 has a physical half-life of 36.4 days and three usable photons at 172 keV, 203 keV, and 375 keV, respectively. These energies are higher than that of Tc-99m, and therefore Xe-127 can be readily used following the perfusion portion of the V/Q examination. The advantage of this is the flexibility in selecting the ideal view or projection in which to perform ventilation scintigraphy, based on the results of the perfusion scintigram. Despite this theoretical advantage, Xe-127 has not become widely used, owing to its greater cost compared with Xe-133.

Krypton-81m is obtained from a rubidium-81/krypton-81m generator system. The physical half-life of the Ru-81 parent is 4.6 hours and the generator system is good for only 1 day for all practical purposes. The lack of general commercial availability, the high cost, and the logistical impracticality of daily generator replacement have kept Kr-81m from becoming clinically important.

There are some definite theoretical advantages to using Kr-81m. The generator can be continuously eluted. This feature, coupled with the short, 13-second half-life of Kr-81m, allows multiple views to be readily obtained. Also, the principal photon energy of Kr-81m is 190 keV, which readily permits ventilation studies following perfusion scintigraphy with Tc-99m-labeled agents.

Over the time frame of ventilation scintigraphy, the radioactive gases remain within the bronchoalveolar space. Sequential images during inhalation, steady-state breathing, and exhalation or washout depict the overall and regional dynamics of ventilation. It should be noted that a small amount of the radioactive gas equilibrates

across the alveolar-capillary membrane with blood and is carried throughout the body in the systemic circulation. Xenon is relatively fat soluble, and a significant accumulation may be seen in the liver in patients with fatty infiltration (Figure 6-1).

Radioaerosols   As an alternative to radioactive gases for ventilation studies, various radioaerosols may be used. Radioaerosols depict the distribution of ventilation during the inhalation phase. The inhaled aerosol is deposited on the lining of the bronchoalveolar spaces, so that subsequent imaging shows the regional patterns of ventilation. An advantage of the aerosol technique is the ability to image in multiple views or projections following administration of a single dose of radiotracer.

A number of radioaerosols have been tried for ventilation imaging. The current agent of choice is Tc-99m pentetate (DTPA). Commercial nebulizers are available that provide particles of appropriate size. The ideal aerosol particle size is in the range of 0.1 to 0.5 microns. Particles smaller than this may simply be inhaled and then exhaled. Particles greater than 2 to 3 microns tend to settle out on large airways, including the trachea and bronchi. This effect has the potential of obscuring the alveolar distribution in adjacent portions of the lung. In the ideal preparation, the particles penetrate the lung without significant deposition in the large airways.

Another approach with radioaerosols has used Tc-99m-labeled carbon particles. The agent has been called "technegas" and is in some sense a "pseudogas". The particles are very small (0.005 microns) and do not settle out in the lung.

Because the radioaerosols typically use the same Tc-99m radiolabel as the pulmonary perfusion agents, the relative doses are adjusted to minimize the "cross-talk" or interference between radioactivity from the two different portions of the examination.

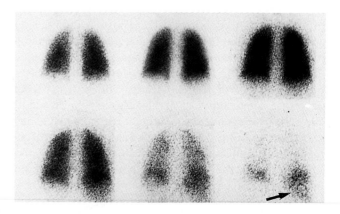

Fig. 6-1   Posterior view of a xenon-133 ventilation study. There is delayed washout of xenon at both lung bases as well as significant xenon uptake in the region of the liver (*arrow, bottom right image*).

Technique

Radioactive gases   Ventilation studies with Xe-133 are ordinarily performed first during combined V/Q imaging. A large field of view gamma camera with a low-energy all purpose collimator is used. A 20% energy window is centered at 81 keV. The usual adult dose of Xe-133 is 10 to 20 mCi (370 to 740 MBq) (Box 6-2).

A high-quality ventilation scan requires patient cooperation. The study is accomplished in three phases, the single-breath or wash-in phase, the equilibrium phase, and the washout phase. Severely tachypneic, or uncooperative or unresponsive patients may require modifications of the standard protocol or an alternative approach with a radioaerosol.

The patient is placed for a posterior view. Patient orientation should be the same as subsequently used for the perfusion portion of the study. Some laboratories routinely perform both parts of the study with the patient supine. Others favor a sitting position if the patient can tolerate it. The sitting position is generally better because it permits a fuller excursion of the diaphragm and facilitates obtaining oblique views during the washout phase. Also, chest radiographs are ordinarily obtained with the patient upright, and the best correlative information comes from comparisons in like positions.

To begin the study, the patient is asked to take in and hold a single maximal deep inspiration. The breath is taken through a mouthpiece attached to a Xe-133 delivery apparatus. An initial image is obtained for 100,000 counts (100 k).

The next phase of the study is the equilibrium phase. Typically, two images are obtained for 90 seconds each, beginning after the initial breath image is completed. During this time, the patient continues to breathe a mixture of air and xenon. When Kr-81m is used a true equilibrium is never achieved because the short 13-second half life does not allow complete penetration of the alveolar spaces.

The third phase of the examination is composed of multiple washout images. The valve on the xenon delivery apparatus is shifted from the delivery reservoir to a xenon-trapping device while the patient breathes room air. Three or four sequential 45-second washout images are obtained. As an option, additional 45-second images are obtained in both the 45° left posterior and right posterior oblique projections, followed by a final 45-second posterior view. The sitting position greatly facilitates oblique views. The patient is placed on a backless chair with a swivel seat that allows rapid positioning for the oblique images. It should be noted that many patients referred for V/Q scintigraphy will not be comfortable in or able to maintain a sitting position and the same sequence may be obtained with the patient supine and the camera under the imaging table. The oblique views are then obtained by helping the patient roll onto a 45° bolster.

Studies with Xe-127 may be performed using the same protocol. As discussed above, there is flexibility in choosing the imaging view or projection and also in choosing the sequence of the ventilation and perfusion portions of the examination. The rapid clearance of xenon from the lung after the delivery apparatus is switched to room air allows imaging in multiple views if sufficient radioactive gas is available.

Radioaerosols   For studies with radioaerosols, the radiopharmaceutical is placed in a special nebulizer system. The patient is asked to breathe through the mouthpiece of the delivery system until sufficient radioaerosol is delivered to the lungs. This may require several minutes. Because only 5 to 10% of the radioactivity in the nebulizer is delivered to the lung, 25 to 75 mCi of Tc-99m-pentetate is placed in the nebulizer. The goal is to deliver enough radioaerosol to the lung so that 150,000 to 250,000 count images may be obtained in 1 to 2 minutes.

The views obtained in radioaerosol studies should be the same as those obtained for the perfusion phase. Most nuclear medicine clinics obtain anterior, posterior, right and left lateral, and both posterior 45° oblique views. The right and left 45° anterior obliques may also be readily obtained. The Tc-99m-DTPA aerosol remains in the lung, with a biological half-life approaching 1 hour. This is more than enough time to accomplish multiple view imaging.

> **Box 6-2   Xenon-133 Ventilation Scintigraphy: Protocol Summary**
>
> **PATIENT PREPARATION**
> None.
>
> **DOSAGE AND ROUTE OF ADMINISTRATION**
> Xenon-133 20 mCi (370 MBq) adult dosage by inhalation.
>
> **PROCEDURE**
> Use a wide field of view camera with a parallel-hole all-purpose collimator and a 20% window centered at 81 keV.
> The patient is seated (if possible) with the camera positioned in the posterior view.
> First-breath (wash-in) phase: The patient exhales fully and is asked to take a maximal inspiration and hold it long enough, if possible, to obtain 100k counts.
> Equilibrium phase: Obtain two sequential 90-second images while the patient breathes normally.
> Washout phase. Obtain three sequential 45-second posterior images and then LPO and RPO images and a final posterior image.

PERFUSION SCINTIGRAPHY

Radiopharmaceuticals

The diameter of red blood cells is approximately 7.7 microns. Larger-diameter particles introduced into the bloodstream proximal to the pulmonary capillary bed will lodge in the pulmonary capillaries and precapillary arterioles. If mixing has been adequate to prevent laminar flow effects, the resulting distribution of radioactivity is a very accurate map of regional perfusion in the lung. Numerous particulate agents, both biodegradable and nonbiodegradable, have been studied experimentally and clinically for perfusion scintigraphy. The first studies in humans were obtained with radioiodinated (I-131) macroaggregated albumin.

The two agents providing the most clinical experience are Tc-99m-labeled human albumin microspheres (Tc-99m-HAM) and Tc-99m-labeled macroaggregated albumin (Tc-99m-MAA). Human albumin microspheres (HAM) are prepared by heating albumin in an oil emulsion and selecting particles of the appropriate size from the resulting microspheres. In suitable preparations, over 95% of the microspheres are in the range of 10 to 40 microns. The ability to control the size range is a distinct advantage of HAM preparations. However, HAM preparations are not currently available commercially in the United States, and Tc-99m-MAA has become the dominant agent.

In current practice, MAA preparations contain particles ranging in size from a few microns to 90 to 100 microns. The majority (60 to 80%) of MAA particles in commercial preparations are in the 10 to 30 micron range.

In commercial preparations, a vial is supplied that contains MAA with stannous ion. Tc-99m as sodium pertechnetate is added to the reaction vial, resulting in rapid labeling of the MAA particles.

Following intravenous (IV) injection into a peripheral vein, the radiolabeled particles travel through the right atrium and right ventricle, where thorough mixing occurs. They are then filtered or trapped in the pulmonary vascular bed. In areas of absent or decreased perfusion, correspondingly fewer particles are delivered and trapped, resulting in relatively photopenic or "cold" areas.

The clearance of Tc-99m-MAA from the lung is primarily due to a physical, mechanical degradation of the particles. As particles are fragmented they may initially lodge in smaller branches of the pulmonary circulation, but eventually they gain access to the systemic circulation, where they are phagocytized in the reticuloendothelial system and further degraded. The biological half-life of current Tc-99m-MAA preparations in the lung is 2 to 3 hours. Of historic interest is the somewhat longer biological half-life of HAM of 4 to 6 hours, probably due to the spherical configuration of these particles and

therefore a lower susceptibility to fragmentation. The dosimetry for Tc-99m MAA is summarized in Table 6-1.

Because any particles reaching the systemic circulation will lodge in the capillary beds of critical organs of the body, right-to-left shunts are a relative contraindication to the use of Tc-99m-MAA. Following injection of this radiopharmaceutical in patients with shunts, the brain, heart, kidneys, and other structures are readily visualized (Figure 6-2). Although this sounds alarming in theory, it is remarkably well tolerated in practice. Substantial clinical experience has been obtained in using various macroaggregates of albumin to quantitatively assess the degree of right-to-left shunting by measuring radioactivity trapped in the lung versus the amount of activity gaining access to

Table 6-1	Dosimetry for Technetium-99m-labeled Macroaggregated Albumin	
Organ		**Dose (Rads/4 mCi)**
Lungs		0.88
Bladder wall		0.12
Testes		0.024
Ovaries		0.030

Modified from product information brochure for Macrotec, Squibb Diagnostics, Princeton, NJ.

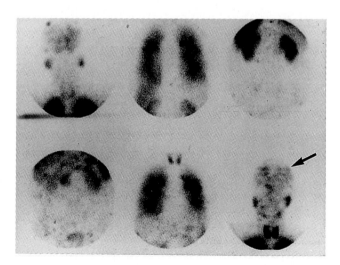

Fig. 6-2 Technetium-99m-MAA scintigrams in a patient with right-to-left shunts in the lung. Note the uptake in the brain (*arrow, lower right hand image*). Free pertechnetate would not be taken up in the cerebrum. There is also marked uptake in the salivary glands, thyroid, kidneys and other abdominal viscera. (From Bank ER, Thrall JH, Dantzker DR: Radionuclide demonstration of intrapulmonary shunting due to cirrhosis. *AJR*; 140:967-969, 1983. Reproduced with permission.)

the systemic circulation. Also, investigators around the world have injected radiolabeled particles directly into many organs to assess relative regional blood flow, with an apparently wide margin of safety. Nonetheless, the possibility of right-to-left shunt should be borne in mind when performing this study.

From time to time, when activity is seen outside the lungs, the question arises as to whether it is due to right-to-left shunting or to free Tc-99m-pertechnetate in the radiopharmaceutical preparation. The distinction can be readily made by imaging the brain. Tc-99m-pertechnetate and other nonparticulate potential radiocontaminants do not cross the blood-brain barrier or localize in the brain. Shunted Tc-99m-MAA will lodge in the cerebral circulation (Figure 6-2).

Another important consideration is the number of radiolabeled particles comprising the diagnostic dose. Administering too small a dosage of particles does not result in a statistically valid distribution pattern in the capillary bed. On the other hand, injecting too many particles could theoretically obstruct a hemodynamically significant portion of the pulmonary circulation. Empirically, a minimum of 60,000 particles is required to meet statistical distribution criteria. In practice, an upper limit of 400,000 particles is observed. Because it is estimated that there are over 280 billion pulmonary capillaries and 300 million precapillary arterioles, administration of even 400,000 particles should result in obstruction of only a very small fraction of the cross-section of the normal vascular bed. The margin of safety is quite large in normal subjects and in most patients undergoing evaluation. Caution is still advised, including the use of the minimum number of particles in patients with pulmonary hypertension who may have significantly fewer remaining pulmonary capillaries than normal.

Another special situation requiring caution is pregnancy. When PE is a clinical consideration in pregnant patients, the minimum radiation dose is always figured on a risk-versus-benefit basis. However, with perfusion imaging it is still necessary to deliver the minimum of 60,000 particles. To get the right balance between the amount of radioactivity and the number of particles, the amount of Tc-99m-pertechnetate added to the reaction vial may have to be adjusted. Also, because the commercially available kits provide for multiple doses, the ratio of radioactivity to particles changes continuously after the initial labeling. This should be borne in mind in making these calculations.

Technique

The usual dose of Tc-99m MAA for pulmonary perfusion imaging is 2 to 5 mCi (Box 6-3). The dose is administered IV and should be given slowly over several respiratory cycles. The patient should be encouraged to

---

Box 6-3   Tc-99m-MAA Perfusion Scintigraphy: Protocol Summary

PATIENT PREPARATION AND PRECAUTIONS

Right-to-left shunts are a relative contraindication.
Pregnant women: Adjust dosage and observe requirement for a minimum of 60,000 particles.
Pulmonary hypertension: Reduce number of particles to 60,000.

DOSAGE AND ROUTE OF ADMINISTRATION

Tc-99m-MAA: 4.0 mCi (148 MBq) adult dosage.
Intravenous administration over several respiratory cycles with the patient supine.

PROCEDURE

Use a wide field of view gamma camera with a low-energy, high-resolution or all-purpose collimator and a 20% window centered at 140 keV.
Obtain anterior, posterior, right lateral, left lateral, and right and left lateral posterior oblique images (anterior oblique images are optional).
Obtain 500k-750k counts per image.

---

breathe deeply. The injection should be made with the patient supine to foster even distribution of particles cephalocaudally in the lung. If the particles are injected with the patient sitting or standing, a basilar predominance can occur.

Once the injection is complete, imaging may begin immediately. The patient position for imaging should be the same as that selected for the ventilation portion of the study. A large field of view gamma scintillation camera equipped with an all-purpose or high-resolution collimator is used. A 20% window is centered at 140 keV. Images are obtained in the anterior, posterior, right and left lateral, and both 45° posterior oblique views. The 45° anterior oblique images are also frequently obtained. A minimum of 500,000 counts per image are recommended.

Some laboratories image the more normal lung in the lateral view for 500,000 counts and the contralateral, more abnormal lung for the same time as was required for the initial lateral view. The rationale is to recognize and avoid misleading patterns due to shine-through of activity from right to left or vice versa. For example, the right lateral view in a patient without a right lung can appear surprisingly normal due to shine-through from the left! The combined count- and time-based approach alerts the observer to the true differences in right lung versus left lung activity.

Care is taken during the venipuncture not to withdraw blood into the syringe. Occasionally a small clot will form in the syringe when this happens. Adherence of Tc-99m-MAA particles to the clot results in a spurious hot spot in the lung due to reinjection of the small clot. Also, the syringe should be agitated just prior to injection to avoid sedimentation or settling out and aggregation of particles. The particles should be injected through a 23-gauge or larger needle to prevent fragmentation during dose administration.

CLINICAL APPLICATIONS

Appearance of the Normal Ventilation Scintigram

In normal subjects the initial breath or wash-in image reveals homogeneous distribution of radioxenon. In subjects taking an effective deep breath, the distribution is fairly complete. In the equilibrium phase the appearance is again homogeneous, with the full outline of the lungs now demonstrated. The spine attenuates activity in the midline and appears as a linear photopenic area separating the left and right lungs. In some thin subjects a relative photopenia is also seen on the left side, corresponding to the projected area of the heart (Figure 6-3A).

During the washout phase there is a progressive and uniform decrease in activity from the lungs. The half-time of washout should be 2 minutes or less and the last washout image should have faint or no discernible activity. In some otherwise normal subjects, washout may appear delayed as a result of the subject's inability to breathe comfortably through the mouthpiece of the delivery apparatus. The left and right posterior oblique images should not reveal any focal accumulations at the time they are obtained.

In some subjects discernible activity accumulates in the right upper quadrant of the abdomen in the area of the liver. When significant accumulation occurs, it is ordinarily due to fatty infiltration of the liver (see Figure 6-1). Distribution of radioaerosols is similar to initial breath xenon studies. In radioaerosol studies, activity may be seen in the larger airways, and swallowed activity is sometimes seen in the stomach (Figure 6-4).

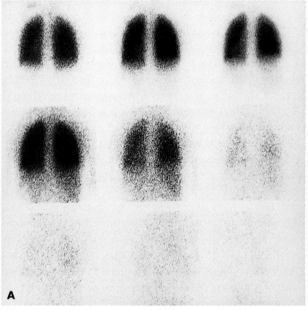

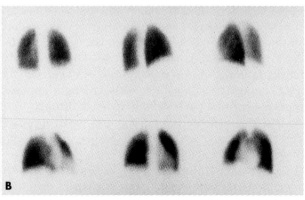

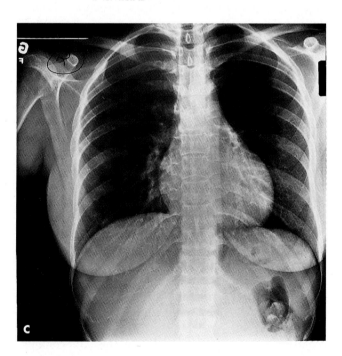

Fig. 6-3   **A**, Normal ventilation study obtained with xenon-133. The initial-breath (*left*) and equilibrium images are in the *upper row*, followed by the sequential washout images in the *middle* and *lower rows*. There is uniform distribution of xenon with no evidence of air trapping. Minimal activity is seen in the region of the liver. **B**, The corresponding technetium-99m-MAA study also demonstrates homogeneous distribution of tracer activity throughout the lungs. The defect due to the cardiac structures is clearly seen. No focal abnormalities are demonstrated. **C**, Corresponding chest radiograph reveals fully expanded lungs with no cardiovascular or pulmonary abnormalities.

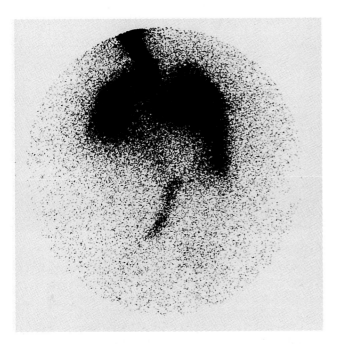

Fig. 6-4 Technetium-99m-DTPA aerosol study reveals intense uptake in the trachea and midabdominal activity due to swallowed radiopharmaceutical in the stomach.

Appearance of the Normal Perfusion Scintigram

The scintigram in healthy subjects should show homogeneous, uniform distribution of tracer throughout the lungs (Figure 6-3B). The hilar structures are frequently perceived as photopenic areas corresponding to the large airway and vascular structures in the hilum. The area of the heart is obviously photopenic on the anterior view and results in variable degrees of apparent regionally decreased activity on other views, depending on the habitus of the patient. Again, in thin subjects a cardiac "defect" may be seen on the posterior view, and an area of decreased activity corresponding to the heart is frequently seen on the left lateral view.

The spine and sternum effectively attenuate activity in the midline, resulting in a separation of the left and right lungs.

The pulmonary outline on the perfusion images commonly appears slightly smaller than on the ventilation images. This is most likely due to the lower spatial resolution on the ventilation study (lower photon energy and fewer counts).

The location of the diaphragms, the size of the heart, and the size of hilar defects should correspond to the location and appearance of these structures as seen on chest radiographs (Figure 6-3C). Camparison with the chest radiographic findings is most useful when the radiograph has been obtained with the subject in the same position as for the perfusion and ventilation images. This is another

reason for performing all three examinations with the subject upright if possible. Again, the upright position usually results in better excursion of the diaphragm and fuller expansion of the lungs than the supine position.

The perfusion images should always be scrutinized for extrapulmonary activity that may indicate either a right-to-left shunt or a radiopharmaceutical contaminant in the preparation. Uptake in the thyroid and stomach typically indicates free pertechnetate. Uptake in the liver indicates colloidal impurities, and uptake in the brain indicates right-to-left shunting as described in the discussion of radiopharmaceuticals.

Pulmonary Embolism

By far the most important indication for V/Q imaging is suspected PE. This condition in many respects is a medical "orphan." Patients come from every service in the hospital, and the majority of physicians initially encountering patients with PE do not have special expertise in its diagnosis or management. PE is not the province of any medical specialty. In many institutions the radiologist serves as the de facto expert because all patients undergoing diagnostic evaluation go through the nuclear medicine or angiography laboratories for study. This creates an opportunity for the radiologist to become a key person in the diagnosis and management of patients with PE.

Clinical presentation The signs and symptoms of PE are highly variable from patient to patient and are generally nonspecific. The majority of patients have tachypnea and dyspnea. Other common signs and symptoms are cough, pleuritic pain, and tachycardia. Patients are frequently apprehensive. Less common findings are hemoptysis and wheezing. Severe symptoms, including hypotension and syncope, are even less common. The classic triad of dyspnea, pleuritic chest pain, and hemoptysis is not encountered very frequently.

Chest radiographic findings and laboratory findings are also frustratingly nonspecific. Radiographically, local oligemia may be observed in the area distal to an occluding PE. This may involve an entire lung if the clot is proximal and is referred to as Westermark's sign. In patients with pulmonary infarction, a characteristic pleural based, wedge-shaped density can be seen (Hampton's hump). When infarction is present, there is frequently a small pleural effusion. Large pleural effusions are not characteristic of PE. An increase in the size of the main pulmonary artery and cardiomegaly may be seen in some cases. After PE resolves, there may be permanent parenchymal scarring; characteristically a linear density that extends to the pleural surface is seen.

The majority of patients have abnormalities in serum enzymes, and classically the oxygen pressure (PO_2) is low. Because patients tend to hyperventilate, this is associated with a respiratory alkalosis. The majority of patients also probably have electrocardiographic abnormalities, but these are transient and may or may not be detected.

A number of associated clinical conditions are thought to predispose to PE. These include recent surgery (within 3 months), immobilization, thrombophlebitis, and underlying malignancy or some other cause of a hypercoagulable state. In women, the use of estrogen has been considered a risk factor.

Diagnosis   Over the years a number of diagnostic schemes have been developed that incorporate information from chest radiographs as well as ventilation and perfusion studies to arrive at probability estimates for PE. If PE were the only condition affecting pulmonary perfusion, the diagnosis would be straightforward. However, innumerable pulmonary and cardiac conditions may distort normal pulmonary perfusion. The chest radiograph and ventilation study are used to help identify the possible presence of these alternative nonembolic causes of perfusion abnormality. As a corollary observation it is fair to say that the more extensive the preexisting pulmonary morbidity, the harder it becomes to rule- in or rule- out superimposed PE.

Terminology   A special set of terms has been developed to facilitate the use of the diagnostic schemes employed in the interpretation of V/Q scans. The diagnostic schemes require correct application of the concepts embodied in this special terminology.

The first concept is that of the matched versus mismatched perfusion defect (Box 6-4). A perfusion defect is said to be *matched* if there is a corresponding ventilation abnormality. The ventilation abnormality either may be the absence of ventilation in the corresponding area, as might be seen in pleural effusion or secondary to tumor, or may reflect altered ventilatory dynamics, as might be seen in chronic airways disease with both delayed wash-in and delayed washout.

A *V/Q mismatch* refers to an area of abnormal perfusion that demonstrates normal ventilation. The concept also applies to a comparison of the perfusion scintigram with the chest radiograph. In most diagnostic schemes a perfusion defect that is substantially larger than a corresponding radiographic or ventilatory abnormality is still considered to be mismatched.

The distinction of whether a given perfusion defect is matched or mismatched is fundamental. Typically, matched defects are due to nonembolic causes. Acute PE classically results in V/Q mismatch. That is, there is a perfusion defect due to the embolus blocking blood flow, but ventilation remains normal because there is no corresponding blockage in the airway.

The next important concept embodied in the diagnostic terminology is the difference between a *segmental* and a *non-segmental defect* (Box 6-5). Perfusion defects due to blockage of the pulmonary arterial tree

Box 6-4	Concept of Ventilation/ Perfusion Match and Mismatch
V/Q match:	Both scintigrams are abnormal in the same area; defects are of equal size.
V/Q mismatch:	*Abnormal* perfusion in an area of *normal* ventilation.

Box 6-5	Terminology for Ventilation/ Perfusion Scintigraphy

A) **SEGMENTAL DEFECT**

Caused by occlusion of a branch of the pulmonary artery. Characteristically wedged-shaped and pleural based. Conforms to the segmental anatomy of the lung.
- Large segmental defect: >75% of a lung segment.
- Moderate segmental defect: 25%-75% of a lung segment.
- Small segmental defect: <25% of a lung segment.

B) **NONSEGMENTAL DEFECT**

Does *not* conform to segmental anatomy and/or does not appear wedge-shaped.

should reflect the branching or arborization of the pulmonary circulation in its classic segmental pattern (Figure 6-5). Thus, a classic *segmental defect* corresponds to one or more bronchopulmonary segments, is wedge shaped, and is pleural based. The term *non-segmental defect* is reserved for abnormalities that do not correspond to the pulmonary segments, are not pleural based, and do not have the classic wedge shape. Causes of nonsegmental defects are summarized in Box 6-6. Many of the conditions resulting in nonsegmental defects are apparent radiographically, such as pleural effusion and tumors.

Assessment of the size of a given defect and determination of the number of defects present in each category are also important to the correct application of the clinical diagnostic schemes. By convention, a defect is considered *large* if it equals more than 75% of the size of a lung segment, *moderate* if it is between 25% and 75% of the size of a lung segment and *small* if it is less than 25% of the size of a lung segment. It is useful to have a diagram of the segmental anatomy of the lungs available for reference when interpreting V/Q studies (Figure 6-6).

Finally, the complexity of interpretation of combined ventilation and perfusion studies has led to the use of probability categories rather than the simple assignment of positive or negative. If no abnormalities are demon-

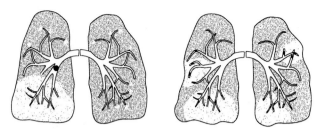

Fig. 6-5 Schematic diagram illustrating the branching pattern of the pulmonary arteries. Emboli may be due to larger, more proximal clots as illustrated in the left-hand schematic, or to showers of smaller clots lodging more distally. In either case the resulting defects should be pleural based and correspond to the segmental anatomy of the lung.

Box 6-6   Causes of nonsegmental defects

Pacemaker artifact
Tumors
Pleural effusion
Trauma
Hemorrhage
Bullae
Cardiomegaly
Mediastinal and hilar adenopathy
Atelectasis
Pneumonia
Aortic ectasia or aneurysm

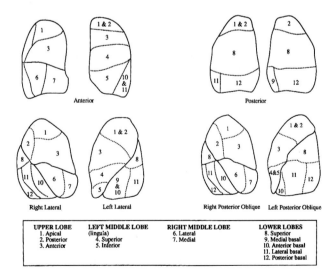

UPPER LOBE	LEFT MIDDLE LOBE	RIGHT MIDDLE LOBE	LOWER LOBES
1. Apical	(lingula)	6. Lateral	8. Superior
2. Posterior	4. Superior	7. Medial	9. Medial basal
3. Anterior	5. Inferior		10. Anterior basal
			11. Lateral basal
			12. Posterior basal

Fig. 6-6 Segmental anatomy of the lung. There is significant variability between patients. Also, the segments have variable size, which must be borne in mind in assessing relative defect size.

---

strated, the combined study is considered normal. Depending on the number, size, and combined patterns of demonstrated abnormalities, abnormal studies are classified in the different diagnostic schemes as *low* probability, *intermediate* probability (also referred to as *indeterminate*), or *high* probability.

Diagnostic criteria Numerous diagnostic schemes employing the terminology and probability categories described above have been proposed over the years. The criteria summarized in Box 6-7 are modified from those used in a multi-institutional study of the accuracy of V/Q scintigraphy sponsored by the National Institutes of Health, the Prospective Investigation of Pulmonary Embolism Diagnosis (PIOPED). The original PIOPED criteria were derived from the literature and drew heavily on the work of Dan Biello. The scheme represented in Box 6-7 differs from the original PIOPED criteria based on an analysis of how the original criteria performed. For

---

Box 6-7   Modified PIOPED Criteria for Combined-Study Interpretation

HIGH PROBABILITY: >80%

• *Two* or *more large mismatched segmental defects* without a radiographic abnormality (or the perfusion defect is substantially larger than the radiographic abnormality).
• Any combination of mismatched defects equivalent to the above (two moderate defects = one large defect).

INTERMEDIATE PROBABILITY (INDETERMINATE): 20%-80%

• One moderate mismatched segmental defect with a normal radiograph.
• One large and one moderate mismatched segmental defect with a normal radiograph.
• Difficult to categorize as high or low probability.
• Not meeting the stated criteria for high or low probability.

LOW PROBABILITY: <20%

• Nonsegmental perfusion defects (e.g., small pleural effusion with blunting of costophrenic angle, cardiomegaly, elevated diaphragm or enlargement of the aorta, hila, or mediastinum).
• Any perfusion defect with a substantially larger radiographic abnormality.
• Matched ventilation and perfusion defects with a normal chest radiograph.
• Small subsegmental perfusion defects.

NORMAL

No perfusion defects.

example, in the original criteria, a single moderate mismatched V/Q defect with a correspondingly normal radiograph had been considered low probability but is now included as intermediate probability in the criteria presented in Box 6-7, based on the PIOPED experience (Figure 6-7). It is also important to note that the number of combinations of diagnostic findings in the intermediate (indeterminate) category exceeds any practical ability to enumerate them individually. This is accounted for in the criteria by the observation that if an abnormal study does not meet the criteria for high or low probability, it should be considered indeterminate. It cannot be emphasized enough that the specific criteria in different published diagnostic schemes are highly variable, particularly in separating low probability from intermediate probability studies.

The scintigraphic hallmark of PE is a perfusion defect corresponding to a bronchopulmonary segment that exhibits normal ventilation, with no abnormality on chest radiograph (or a radiographic abnormality that is *much* smaller than the perfusion defect). When two or more such large segmental defects or their equivalent are seen, the likelihood of PE is over 80% to 85% (Figures 6-8, 6-9).

At the other end of the spectrum, when the perfusion study is completely and unequivocally normal, without a segmental or other defect, the likelihood of PE is less than 5% and the likelihood of significant morbidity or mortality from PE is probably less than 1% (see Figure 6-3).

In the experience of most investigators studying PE, if a patient has a limited number of matched abnormalities in ventilation and perfusion but the radiograph of the respective area is normal, the probability of PE is still low, on the order of 5% to 15% or 5% to 20% (Figures 6-10, 6-11).

Practical approach to ventilation/perfusion scintigram interpretation   The complexity of interpreting V/Q studies, including the integration of information from the chest radiograph, warrants a rigorous systematic approach. This is not a study that can or should be interpreted hastily. An approach used successfully in a number of institutions is as follows:

First, the chest radiograph is reviewed and all abnormalities are recorded. Ideally, the radiograph should be obtained at the same time as the V/Q study and with the patient in the same position. The most common chest radiographic abnormalities in patients with PE are pleural effusion, an elevated hemidiaphragm, and atelectasis. Oligemia (Westermark's sign) and opacities associated with pulmonary infarction are less common; enlargement of the pulmonary artery is also less common. Although large pleural effusions are rarely caused by PE, they can obscure significant portions of the pulmonary parenchyma, and large effusions often render V/Q scintigraphy indeterminate. Other frequent findings

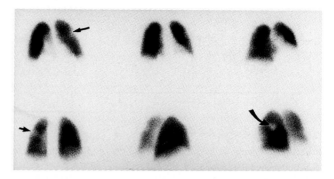

Fig. 6-7   Perfusion study with technetium-99m-MAA reveals a single moderate defect in the left lung (*arrows*). The ventilation study and chest x-ray were normal. Under the original PIOPED criteria this study would have been characterized as indicating a low probability of pulmonary embolism. This is now characterized as having intermediate probability.

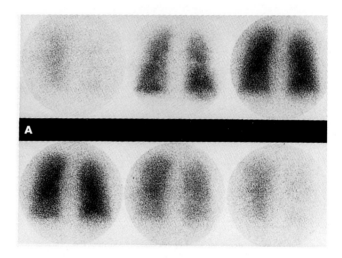

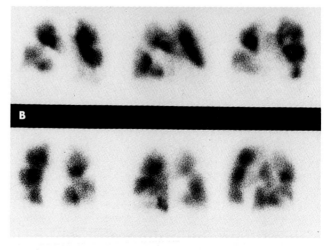

Fig. 6-8   **A,** Posterior ventilation study with Xenon-133. There is some delay in wash-in due to the patient's dyspnea. The distribution of xenon is uniform, without focal retention. **B,** Corresponding technetium-99m-MAA perfusion study reveals multiple bilateral large segmental sized wedge shape pleural based defects. This pattern fits the high probability diagnostic category.

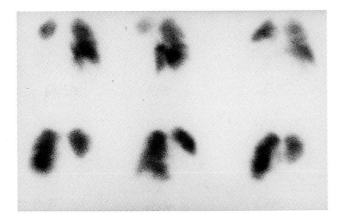

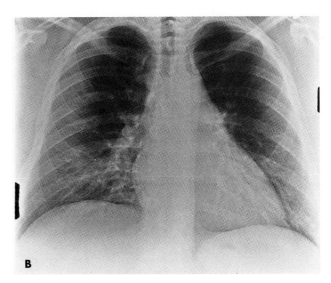

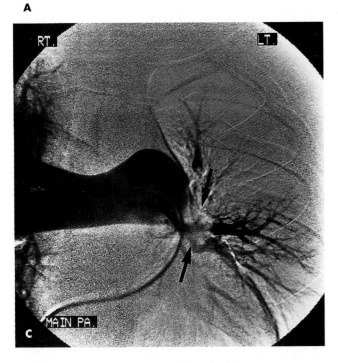

Fig. 6-9 **A**, High-probability study. Technetium-99m perfusion study reveals absence of activity in the entire left lower lobe and left middle lobe (*arrows*). There is also a moderate-sized segmental defect at the right base and a small defect in the region of the right middle lobe. The xenon-133 ventilation scan was normal. **B**, A corresponding chest radiograph reveals no focal abnormalities. There are no secondary signs of embolism, including pleural effusion, oligemia, or apparent hilar enlargement. **C**, Pulmonary arteriogram with an injection in the main pulmonary artery reveals extensive clot in the left-sided circulation (*arrows*). Some contrast is seen distal to the clots, which do not completely occlude the involved arteries in this case.

due to intercurrent disease in the population of patients referred for suspected PE include cardiomegaly, pulmonary parenchymal opacities, hilar enlargement, and signs of airways disease. Occasionally a pneumothorax is seen and may account for the patient's clinical signs and symptoms.

After review of the chest radiograph, all segmental or subsegmental perfusion defects are identified on the perfusion scan and are recorded by location. The ventilation scan is then reviewed in the area of each perfusion defect. The number and location of V/Q mismatches are recorded, and each is, in turn compared with the corresponding area on the chest radiograph. If there is no radiographic explanation for the perfusion defect and if the ventilation scan is normal, these mismatch areas are all candidates for sites of PE. Some authorities assign high probability in the face of one or more large segmental sized

mismatches. The PIOPED criteria (see Box 6-7) require two segmental-sized defects or their aggregate equivalent.

If no mismatches are demonstrated or if only small subsegmental mismatches are seen, attention is turned to seeing whether the study can be categorized as low probability or less. Again, specific criteria differ between authorities, but areas of V/Q match and no corresponding radiographic abnormalities have empirically been associated with a low probability of PE (see Box 6-7).

If the study cannot be categorized as high probability, low probability, or normal, it is by definition indeterminate, and the various radiographic, perfusion, and ventilation abnormalities are described for documentation in the report.

Approaching the diagnosis in this way keeps the observer from pingponging back and forth between abnormalities. Adhering to institutionally agreed-upon

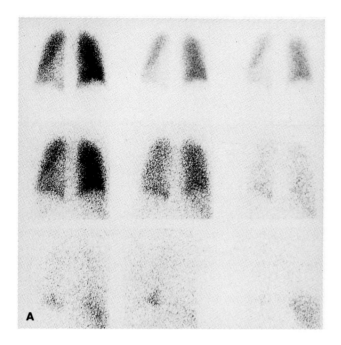

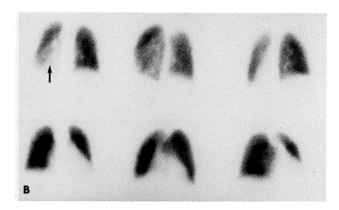

Fig. 6-10   **A**, Xenon-133 ventilation study reveals an area of delayed washout at the left medial base. Incidental note is also made of activity in the liver. **B**, Corresponding technetium-99m-MAA perfusion study reveals a perfusion defect in the medial aspect of the left base on the posterior view corresponding to the area of ventilation abnormality (*arrow*). The chest radiograph was clear in this area of matched ventilation and perfusion defects. This pattern indicates a low probability of pulmonary embolism.

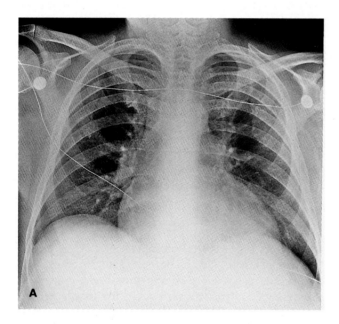

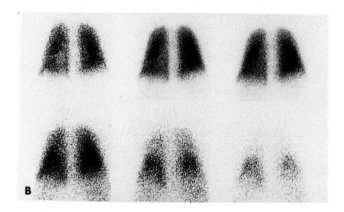

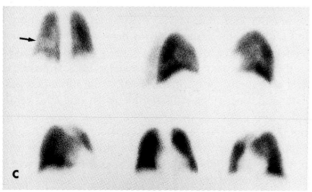

Fig. 6-11   **A**, Chest radiograph reveals some cardiomegaly and blunting of the right costophrenic angle. The lungs are clear without focal opacities. **B**, Ventilation study with xenon-133 reveals good distribution on the initial-breath image and equilibrium images (*top row*). The washout images reveal significant delay in clearance from the lung bases bilaterally. **C**, Corresponding technetium-99m-MAA perfusion study reveals a large area of relatively decreased perfusion in the left lower lobe (*arrow*) and a smaller area at the right base in the general region of the ventilation abnormalities. The combination of matched ventilation and perfusion defect with no corresponding radiographic abnormality indicates a low probability of pulmonary embolism.

diagnostic criteria makes the results of the V/Q study more reliable and more meaningful to the clinician receiving it than a less organized approach or even a *gestalt* approach.

Accuracy of ventilation/perfusion scintigraphy   In the PIOPED trial the specificity of a V/Q study with a high probability was 97%. However, only 41% of patients shown by angiography to have PE had a high-probability pattern scintigraphically. In a way, this is a disappointingly low sensitivity, but it must be remembered that V/Q scintigraphy is not a test of PE per se but a test of lung function. By setting the threshold for a high-probability interpretation at the level of two or more large segmental mismatches, the specificity is kept high at the expense of sensitivity. If the criteria were relaxed, for example, to require only one large mismatch or one large and one moderate mismatch for assignment of high

probability for PE, the sensitivity for detecting PE would go up, but at the expense of specificity (Figures 6-12, 6-13). The high specificity allows us to recommend that in the appropriate clinical setting, a high-probability interpretation provides sufficient diagnostic certainty that the clinician begin anticoagulation without resorting to pulmonary angiography. Patients with significant risk factors for anticoagulation may still require angiography.

The percentage of patients with angiographically demonstrated thromboemboli and intermediate-probability study interpretations in the PIOPED series was 33%. When both clinical outcome and angiographic findings were used, the occurrence of PE in the low probability and the normal/near-normal interpretive categories was 12% and 4%, respectively.

One of the unique features of the PIOPED study was a complete clinical evaluation of each patient before the

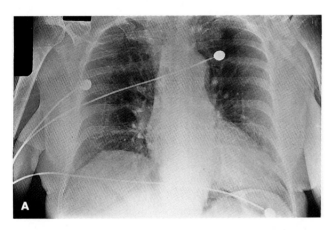

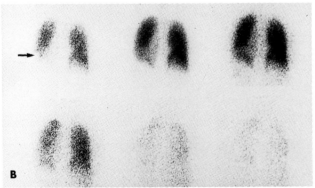

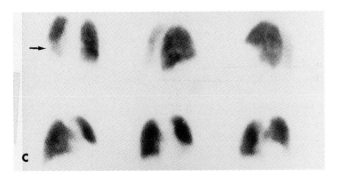

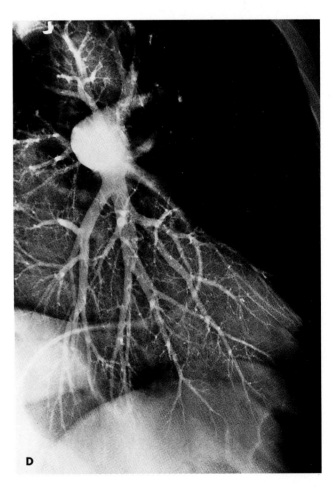

Fig. 6-12   **A,** Chest radiograph reveals cardiomegaly and is otherwise unremarkable. **B,** Ventilation study reveals some delayed wash-in at the left lung base (arrow) but no air trapping. **C,** Corresponding perfusion study reveals a large defect at the left lung base in the posterior view (*arrow*) that was felt to be more extensive than could be accounted for by the ventilation study. With both "matched" and "mismatched" areas, the study was interpreted as of intermediate probability. **D,** subsequent pulmonary arteriogram revealed no evidence of emboli.

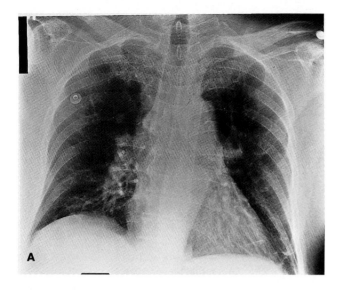

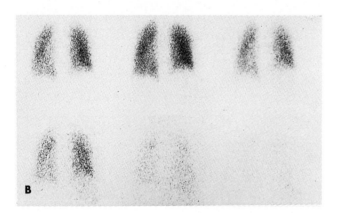

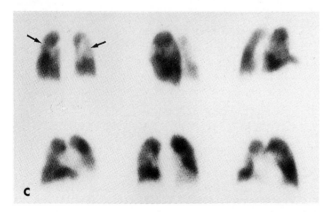

Fig. 6-13   **A,** Chest radiograph reveals some scarring at the left base and prominence of the right hilum. **B,** Corresponding ventilation study is essentially normal. **C,** The perfusion study reveals a large segmental abnormality involving the entire superior segment of the right lower lobe (*arrow*) and a moderate sized segmental defect on the left (*arrow*). The combination of one large and one moderate segmental mismatch places this study in the intermediate probability category.

patient underwent scintigraphy or angiography. Each patient was assigned a "clinical science" probability of having PE. When the clinical probabilities were compared with the scan-based probabilities the results were quite striking. Of patients with a high-probability scintigraphic interpretation and a high clinical probability of having PE, 96% were shown to have PE by angiography. On the other hand, when the clinical probability was low and the scintigraphic interpretation was normal or near-normal, only one (<2%) of 61 patients was found to have PE by angiography. These observations are remarkable and illustrate the absolute importance of interpreting test results in the clinical context.

Another important observation from the PIOPED study is the low likelihood of an adverse clinical outcome in patients with low probability and normal scintigraphic patterns. There were 150 patients followed up for at least 1 year who had either a low-probability or normal/near-normal scan but who did not undergo angiography. In no patient was there an adverse event or readmission to the hospital for suspected PE. Some of them may well have had small PE but none received anticoagulant therapy, and the clinical course was unremarkable. This finding adds strength to several other studies in the literature that suggest a benign clinical course in low-probability cases.

Differential diagnosis   A list of differential possibilities for V/Q mismatch are provided in Box 6-8. These are all potential causes of false positive interpretations. One of the most vexing is chronic PE with incomplete resolution of clot and incomplete restoration of pulmonary perfusion. Whenever an old examination or baseline

Box 6-8   **Conditions Associated With Ventilation/Perfusion Mismatch**
Acute pulmonary embolism
Chronic pulmonary embolism
Other causes of embolism (drug abuse, iatrogenic)
Bronchogenic carcinoma (other tumors)
Mediastinal or hilar adenopathy with obstruction of pulmonary artery or veins
Hypoplasia of pulmonary artery
Swyer-James syndrome (some cases)
Post radiation therapy
Vasculitis

study is available for comparison, it should be consulted to avoid this pitfall. In one large study assessing the sensitivity and specificity of V/Q scintigraphy and in which observers were blinded to prior history and prior test results, chronic PE was the most common cause of false positive interpretations. Unfortunately, in clinical practice, many patients coming for evaluation have not undergone prior scintigraphic studies. Clinical history can help avoid this kind of misinterpretation.

Data on the time course of resolution of PE are disappointingly scarce in the literature. This is probably due to the fact that most studies have been retrospective. Sequential follow-up V/Q scans are generally not obtained on a routine basis. Factors favoring early, complete resolution are small size of the emboli, no preexisting or intercurrent comorbidity, and younger patient age. Small emboli in otherwise healthy young subjects may resolve in 24 hours. Large emboli in older patients with underlying lung disease may never resolve completely (Figure 6-14). It is also important to note that the pattern of perfusion defects may change even without recurrent emboli. As large proximal clots break up, either spontaneously or secondary to therapy, they may relodge more peripherally.

The large vascular structures of the lung, especially the pulmonary veins, are relatively compressible compared to the larger bronchi. Hilar tumors, either primary or metastatic to the lung, may obstruct these vessels, with resultant decrease in regional perfusion. This pattern can mimic PE unless a mass is discernible on the chest radiograph.

Common conditions resulting in matched V/Q abnormalities are summarized in Box 6-9 (Figure 6-15). In patients with asthma, bronchoconstriction results in a reflex decrease in perfusion. The classic pattern on V/Q scintigraphy is multiple matched ventilation and perfusion defects. In patients with congestive heart failure, variable degrees of perfusion abnormality are seen that are due to both pulmonary congestion and pleural fluid. In areas of blebs and bullae, destruction of the lung

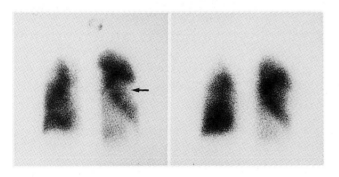

Fig. 6-14   Initial (*left*) and 2-month follow up (*right*) anterior perfusion studies in a patient with pulmonary emboli. The large defect in the left midlung (*arrow*) on the original study has undergone significant but not complete resolution.

Box 6-9	**Conditions Typically Associated With V/Q Matched Abnormalities**

Chronic obstructive pulmonary disease (COPD)
Bronchitis, bronchiectasis
Blebs, bullae
Congestive heart failure
Pulmonary edema
Pleural effusion
Asthma
Pulmonary trauma, hematoma
Inhalation injury
Mucous plugs
Bronchogenic carcinoma (other tumors)

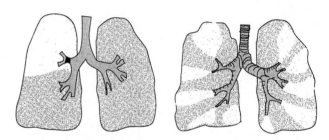

Fig. 6-15   Ventilation abnormalities may be due either to obstructions in larger airways, as might be caused by bronchogenic carcinoma or mucous plugs, or to constriction of smaller bronchi, as may be seen in asthma (*right*).

parenchyma results in absent perfusion. During the wash-in phase of the ventilation study, the corresponding areas demonstrate decreased tracer distribution. During equilibration the radioactive xenon can gain access to the bullae, with evidence of trapping and delayed clearance on the washout phase of the ventilation study. Obviously, on ventilation studies performed with radioaerosols, bullae are seen as cold areas. In patients with chronic bronchitis, and bronchiectasis there is an actual destruction of the bronchial walls, with decreased perfusion in the affected area. There is correspondingly decreased ventilation with delayed washin and air trapping with delayed clearance (see Figure 6-11).

Special signs   A number of special signs have been recognized that can aid in the interpretation of V/Q studies. The *stripe sign* refers to a margin of radioactivity between a perfusion defect and the pleural surface of the lung. Because the pulmonary circulation branches progressively toward the pleural surface, most pulmonary emboli result in pleural based and wedge-shaped defects. The presence of interposed activity (the stripe) suggests a parenchymal abnormality such as pulmonary hemorrhage or other fluid accumulation rather than PE.

The *swinging heart* sign refers to unusually large cardiac defects seen on lateral views when the patient has been imaged lying down and turned to the right and left sides for the lateral views. The heart has a certain mobility in the chest and may displace or compress lung tissue, resulting in this somewhat confusing appearance.

Fluid in the pleural space can be difficult to recognize if patients are imaged in the supine position. Fluid that layers out between the lung and the gamma camera results in increased attenuation of activity. If the fluid is unilateral, a uniform difference in intensity between the two lungs is seen (Figure 6-16). Unless the cause is rec-

ognized, this can be quite confusing, for the asymmetry is seen only on the dependent view. Likewise, if the patient is imaged in the upright position, a subpulmonic collection of fluid may be missed if radiographic/scintigraphic correlation is not carried out carefully. Fluid in the interlobar fissures causes curvilinear perfusion defects (*fissure sign*) that may or may not have corresponding radiographic findings (Figure 6-17).

Patients with pacemakers have easily recognizable imaging defects. The pacemakers have clear-cut borders and do not correspond by shape or location to pulmonary segments, nor are they seen as defects on orthogonal views (see Figure 6-16). Smaller defects may be seen if electrocardiographic monitoring leads are left on the patient.

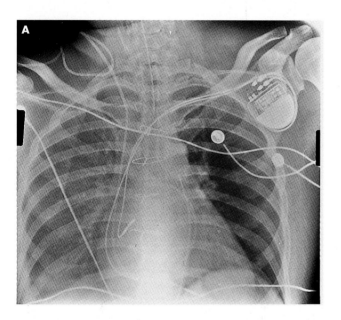

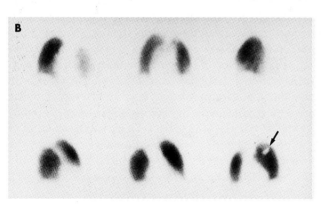

Fig. 6-16   **A**, Chest radiograph reveals the uniformly greater density in the right lung compared to the left lung due to fluid layering out posteriorly with the patient supine. The patient has a pacemaker in place in the left axilla. **B**, Corresponding technetium-99m-MAA perfusion study reveals uniformly decreased activity in the right lung in the posterior view. Apparent activity between the two lungs is equal in all other views, tipping off the observer to the explanation for the discrepancy in the posterior view. Note also the well-defined defect due to the pacemaker (arrow).

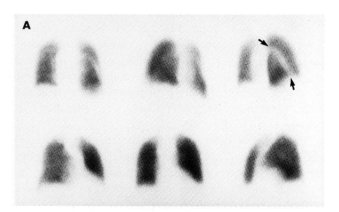

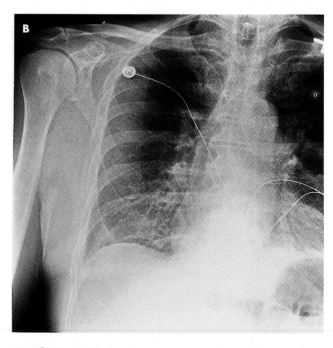

Fig. 6-17   **A**, Technetium-99m-MAA perfusion scan reveals a curvilinear defect in the area of the major fissure of the right lung (*arrows*) ("fissure sign"). The study is otherwise unremarkable. **B**, Corresponding chest radiograph reveals blunting of the right costophrenic angle but provides no indication of the extensive fluid accumulation in the fissure.

Other Applications of Ventilation/Perfusion Scintigraphy

A number of other clinical applications have been suggested for V/Q scintigraphy. None of these has approached the importance of evaluating patients with suspected PE. In some institutions, patients undergoing lung resection are studied by quantitative V/Q imaging. The percentage of overall ventilation and perfusion to each lung can be determined. For example, if a patient has an apparently operable lung carcinoma on one side but poor overall lung function, an estimate of the remaining postoperative lung function can be critical in making the decision to operate. In patients undergoing unilateral lung transplantation, quantitative imaging is useful for monitoring the function of the transplanted lung (Figures 6-18, 6-19).

Detection of venous thrombosis Although the major thrust of this chapter is the diagnosis of PE, the search for their origin is also a clinical objective. Sub-

stantial advancements have been made over the past decade in the development of new techniques for detecting venous thrombi. The traditional radiographic test is contrast venography. This procedure has the shortcoming of being somewhat cumbersome to perform, and it may actually result in phlebitis due to stasis of contrast media in patients with significant venous compromise. Also, contrast venography does not permit the diagnosis of pelvic venous thrombosis.

Some nuclear medicine clinics take advantage of the dosage administration process for pulmonary perfusion scanning to do a combined radionuclide venogram and perfusion study. The radiopharmaceutical is administered through a vein in the foot and forced into the deep system through application of a tourniquet above the ankle. Interpretation below the knee is problematic due to the number of deep veins and in the inability to resolve them as individual structures scintigraphically. However, above the knee, radionuclide venography is very sensitive in demonstrating venous thrombosis. In addition to demon-

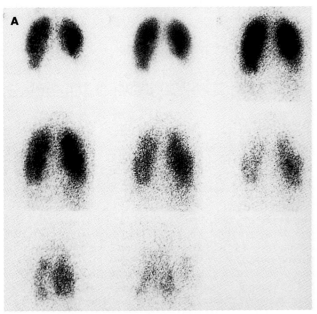

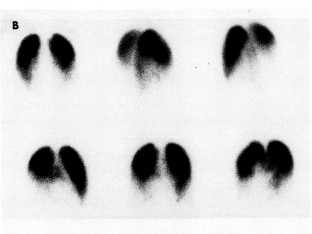

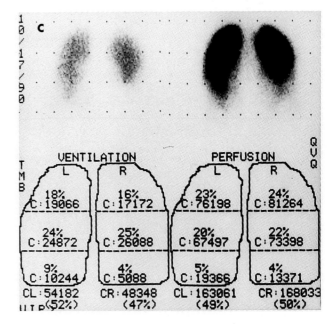

Fig. 6-18 **A,** Xenon-133 ventilation study in a patient with α_1-antitrypsin disorder. There is extensive ventilation abnormality at the lung bases bilaterally with delayed wash-in and air trapping. **B,** Corresponding Tc-99m perfusion study reveals fairly symmetrical perfusion deficits at both lung bases. **C,** Preoperative quantitative analysis of relative right versus left lung ventilation and perfusion reveals essentially symmetric function.

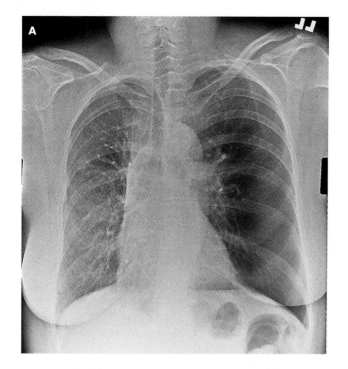

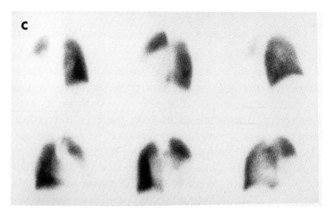

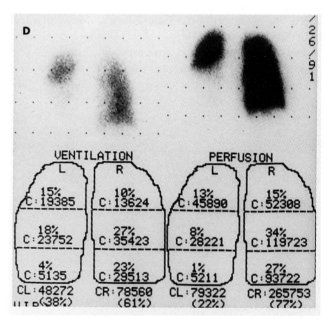

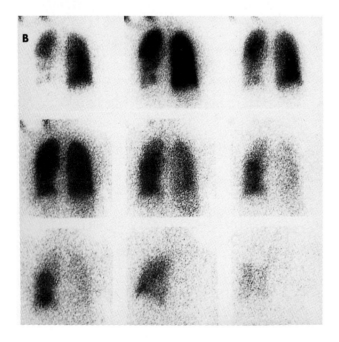

Fig. 6-19 **A,** The patient with the α_1-antitrypsin deficiency underwent right lung transplantation. Postoperative chest radiograph reveals hyperlucency of the left lung compared to the transplanted right lung. **B** Postoperative ventilation study reveals continued ventilation abnormality in the native left lung and normal ventilatory dynamics in the transplanted right lung. **C,** Corresponding perfusion study reveals essentially normal homogeneous perfusion on the right with marked abnormality on the left. **D,** Postoperative quantitative analysis of ventilation and perfusion confirms the improved function on the right. Sixty-one percent of the ventilation and 77% of the perfusion is accounted for by the right lung.

strating venous obstruction (Figure 6-20), the key diagnostic findings are the presence of collaterals and focal accumulations of Tc-99m-MAA at the trailing end of thrombi (Figure 6-21). The radionuclide technique also has some utility in the iliac external and inferior vena caval systems. The dilutional effects that hamper contrast venography are not a problem in the same way. Abnormalities in the external iliac veins and vena cava can be demonstrated.

The technique obviously does not provide information about the internal iliac veins.

A number of new radionuclide techniques have also been described. Antifibrin monoclonal antibodies labeled with a variety of radionuclides, including Tc-99m, have shown some promise. The advantage of the antifibrin technique is the ability to positively identify thrombi, owing to direct uptake of the radiopharmaceu-

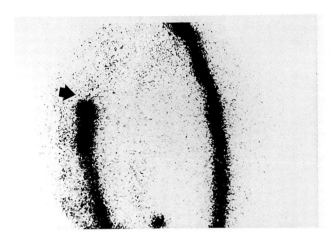

Fig. 6-20 Radionuclide venogram demonstrates venous obstruction on the right due to thrombus (*arrow*).

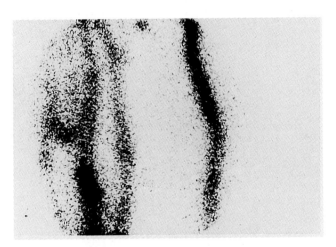

Fig. 6-21 Radionuclide venogram demonstrates extensive collateralization indicating obstruction of the deep venous system.

tical. Although early experience suggests that sensitivity is greater in the thigh, the technique also has applicability below the knee. It is likely that further advances in "hot spot" radionuclide imaging techniques for detection of thrombi will continue. Various radiolabeled peptides are also being tested.

In the past five years a number of new approaches to thrombus detection using ultrasound have been introduced. The most comprehensive use color Doppler imaging in conjunction with various compression techniques to assess the integrity of the venous system. Thrombosed veins are not compressible and exhibit altered flow patterns. The technique is best applied above the knee because of difficulty in identifying the venous structures in the calf.

Adult respiratory distress syndrome The rate of clearance of aerosolized Tc-99m-DTPA is significantly affected by the presence of various pulmonary diseases. The clearance half-time is approximately 80 minutes in healthy subjects. In patients with adult respiratory distress syndrome the clearance is more rapid. This appears to be due to more rapid diffusion of Tc-99m-DTPA across the air space epithelium to the pulmonary circulation. Other conditions associated with more rapid clearance include cigarette smoking and alveolitis. More rapid clearance is also seen in hyaline membrane disease in infants. A clear-cut clinical utility has not been established for the application of the technique, although it has been suggested that serial studies could be used to guide therapy and assess its efficacy.

SUGGESTED READINGS

Alavi A and Palevsky HI, editors: Nuclear Medicine's role in thromboembolic disease, *Semin Nucl Med,* 1991.

Alderson PO and Martin EC: Pulmonary embolism: diagnosis with multiple imaging modalities, *Radiology* 164:297-312, 1987.

Alderson PO, Rujanavech N, Secker-Walker RH et al: The role of 133Xe ventilation studies in the scintigraphic detection of pulmonary embolism, *Radiology* 120:633-640, 1976.

Bedont RA and Datz FL: Lung scan perfusion defects limited to matching pleural effusions: low probability of pulmonary embolism, *AJR* 145:1155-1160, 1985.

Biello DR, Mattar AG, McKnight RC et al: Ventilation-perfusion studies in suspected pulmonary embolism, *AJR* 133:1033-1037, 1979.

Biello DR, Mattar AG, Osei-Wusu A et al: Interpretation of indeterminate lung scintigrams, *Radiology* 133:189-194, 1979.

Carson JL, Kelley MA, Duff AH et al: The clinical course of pulmonary embolism: one year follow-up of PIOPED patients, *N Engl J Med* 326:1240-1245, 1992.

Carter WD, Brady TM, Keyes JW et al: Relative accuracy of two diagnostic schemes for detection of pulmonary embolism by ventilation-perfusion scintigraphy, *Radiology* 145:447-451, 1982.

Gottschalk A, Juni JE, Sostman HD et al: Ventilation-perfusion scintigraphy in the PIOPED study; Part I Data collection and tabulation, *J Nucl Med* 34:1109-1118, 1993.

Gottschalk A, Sostman HD, Coleman RE et al: Ventilation-perfusion scintigraphy in the PIOPED study; Part II Evaluation of the scintigraphic criteria and interpretations, *J Nucl Med* 34:1119-1126, 1993.

Lee ME, Biello DR, Kumar B et al: "Low probability" ventilation-perfusion scintigrams: clinical outcomes in 99 patients, *Radiology* 156:497-500, 1985.

PIOPED Investigators: Value of the ventilation/perfusion scan in acute pulmonary embolism: results of the prospective investigation of pulmonary embolism diagnosis (PIOPED), *JAMA* 263:2753-2759, 1990.

Sostman HD and Gottschalk A: A prospective validation of the stripe sign in ventilation-perfusion scintigraphy, *Radiology* 184:455-459, 1982.

Infection and Inflammation

Nuclear medicine has played an important role in the diagnosis and localization of infection since the early 1970s, when gallium-67 was first noted to have an infection-seeking property as well as tumor avidity. Methods for in vitro labeling of leukocytes were actively investigated in the late 1970s, and In-111 oxine was approved for this purpose in the mid-1980s.

The use of labeled white blood cells (WBCs) for infection imaging has been a major clinical advance. Although In-111 oxine–labeled leukocytes are now widely available and used for localizing infectious and inflammatory processes, this method has limitations, among them a long preparation time, poor count rate due to the low allowable administered dose, and relatively high splenic dosimetry. Therefore, Tc-99m-labeled infection-seeking radiopharmaceuticals have been actively sought. A number of new Tc-99m-labeled radiotracers with various mechanisms of uptake are under investigation and may become available for clinical use (Tables 7-1, 7-2). To date, none of the radiopharmaceuticals available for imaging infection can differentiate nonpyogenic inflammation from infection.

Table 7-1   Status of FDA Approval of Infection Imaging Radiopharmaceuticals

APPROVED
Ga-67 citrate
In-111 oxine-labeled leukocytes
Tc-99m HMPAO-labeled leukocytes
Tc-99m albumin colloid

INVESTIGATIONAL
Nonspecific polyclonal IgG antibodies
Monoclonal antibodies
Chemotactic peptides
Tc-99m nanocolloid

Table 7-2   Mechanisms of Localization of Infection-Seeking Radiopharmaceuticals

Radiopharmaceutical	Mechanism
Gallium-67 citrate	Vascular permeability, binding to lactoferrin
Radiolabeled leukocytes	Diapedesis and chemotaxis
Polyclonal IgG antibodies	Increased vascularity, non immunologic
Monoclonal IgG antibodies	Antibody-antigen binding on leukocytes
Chemotactic peptides	Bind to leukocyte surface
Tc-99m albumin and nanocolloids	Enhanced vascular permeability

---

GALLIUM-67 CITRATE INFECTION IMAGING

Although developed as a bone-seeking radiopharmaceutical and initially used clinically as a tumor imaging agent, Ga-67 citrate's ability to localize at the site of infection became quickly appreciated in the early 1970s, and this tracer subsequently became the mainstay of infection scintigraphy for over a decade. It still has clinical utility.

Mechanism of Uptake

Ga-67 is cyclotron produced, with a half-life of 78 hours, and biological behavior in many ways similar to that of the ferric ion. It binds to iron-binding molecules, including transferrin, lactoferrin, ferritin, and siderophores.

After injection, Ga-67 citrate dissociates and binds to transferrin in the blood, which transports it to the site of inflammation or infection. Localization depends on a number of factors, the importance of which may differ in different clinical situations. *Adequate blood supply* is a primary requisite for localization. The Ga-67–tranferrin complex is delivered to an inflammatory site as a result

of the *increased vascular permeability* of the capillaries. Although *bacterial uptake* and *binding to leukocytes* occur, they do not seem to be major mechanisms of localization. On the other hand, the neutrophil does play an important indirect role.

After migration to a site of infection, neutrophils degranulate, depositing large amounts of lactoferrin. Physiologically, lactoferrin traps free ferric ions, which inhibit bacterial growth. Ga-67 localizes at the site of inflammation by binding to the lactoferrin, since Ga-67 has a higher affinity for lactoferrin than for the transporting protein, transferrin.

Imaging Characteristics

From an imaging standpoint, Ga-67 is not optimal. It emits four photopeaks ranging from 91 keV to 394 keV (Table 7-3). The lower energy photons result in a high percentage of scatter relative to usable photons, and the higher energy photons are difficult to collimate and not efficiently detected by present-day thin gamma camera crystals. To maximize sensitivity, two and, if the camera permits, three photopeaks should be used. The lower ones are used (91-93, 185, and, if possible, 300 keV) because of their greater relative abundance.

Dosimetry

The target organ of Ga-67 is the large intestine (0.90 rads/mCi) and the whole body absorbed dose is 0.26 rads/mCi (Table 7-4).

Methodology

For infection imaging, the usual administered dose of Ga-67 is 5 mCi, with pediatric doses of 40 μCi/kg. Imaging is routinely performed at 48 hours (Box 7-1), although images obtained 6 to 24 hours after injection may occasionally be useful for early detection of an abscess. Early images can also be helpful for interpreting abdominal images obtained 48 to 96 hours after tracer injection. Activity within the abdomen not present at 24 hours but seen at 48 hours is not likely to represent a site of acute infection but rather normal bowel clearance. Further delayed imaging, laxatives, and enemas can help confirm this. Controversy exists regarding the utility of routine use of laxatives and enemas to facilitate bowel clearance. Besides not always being effective, vigorous bowel cleansing may produce mucosal irritation and inflammation, which can result in increased Ga-67 uptake.

Normal Distribution

The organ with the greatest Ga-67 uptake is the liver. Much less uptake occurs in the spleen. The next greatest

Table 7-3   Physical Characteristics of Ga-67 and In-111

Radionuclide	Half-life (hr)	Photopeaks (keV)	Relative Abundance of Photons per 100 Disintegrations (%)
Ga-67	78	91 and 93 keV	41
		185	23
		300	18
		394	4
In-111	67	173 keV	89
		247	94

Table 7-4   Radiation Dosimetry (rads) for Ga-67 Citrate and In-111-Labeled WBCs

ORGAN	Ga-67 (5 mCi)*	In-111 WBCs (500 μCi)*	Tc-99m HMPAO (10 mCi)*
Bladder wall			2.8
Large intestine	4.5		3.6
Liver	2.3	2.66	1.5
Bone marrow	2.9	1.99	1.6
Spleen	2.7	20.00	2.2
Ovaries	1.4	0.20	0.3
Testes	1.2	0.014	1.9
Total body	1.3	0.370	0.3

Modified from IRCP Publication No. 53, MIRD Report No. 2, and the In-111 oxine package insert, Mallinckrodt, Inc., St. Louis.

*Doses in parentheses indicate administered activity.

Box 7-1   Gallium-67 Imaging: Protocol Summary

PATIENT PREPARATION

No recent barium contrast studies.

RADIOPHARMACEUTICAL

Ga-67 citrate, 5 mCi, injected IV.

INSTRUMENTATION

Camera: Large field-of-view gamma camera.
Photopeak: 20% window over 91-93, 185, and 300 keV photopeaks.
Collimator: Medium (or high) energy.

IMAGING PROCEDURE

Whole body imaging including head and extremities, unless the site of suspected infection is localized to one site, e.g., to rule out infection of a hip prosthesis.
500k count spot images of anterior chest; the remaining whole body images for equal time.
Images at 24 hr: Abdomen and site of suspected infection. Imaging at 48 hr: Anterior and posterior images of the chest, abdomen, and pelvis; anterior view of the head.
Delayed abdominal imaging at 72-96 hr as needed to differentiate intra-abdominal infection from normal bowel clearance. Laxatives or enemas are administered as needed.
SPECT of the abdomen or occasionally the chest is useful in selected cases.

uptake occurs in the bone and bone marrow, which can be seen prominently throughout the central and proximal peripheral skeleton (Figure 7-1). Other areas of normal uptake include the nasopharynx and lacrimal and salivary glands; uptake in these sites can be quite variable from patient to patient. The kidneys and bladder are seen during the first 24 hours after tracer injection owing to normal renal clearance. By 48 to 72 hours, the kidneys are usually only faintly seen unless there is renal failure.

Lung uptake is often seen at 24 hours but clears by 48 hours. Breast uptake may be variable, depending to some extent on the phase of the woman's hormonal cycle. Breast uptake may be very prominent post partum (Figure 7-2), and Ga-67 is excreted in breast milk. Thymus uptake is common in children, particularly after chemotherapy (Figure 7-3). Other normal areas of low-grade uptake include the scrotum, testes, and the female perineal region. After 24 hours, biological clearance is mainly through the large bowel. Prolonged retention in the cecum or rectosigmoid colon is not uncommon.

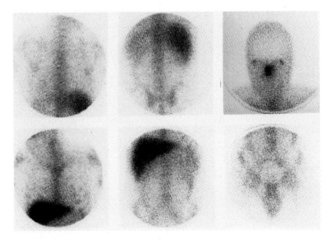

Fig. 7-1   Normal Ga-67 distribution at 48 hours. The highest uptake is seen in the liver. Bone and marrow uptake is quite prominent. Lesser uptake is seen in the spleen and scrotum. Lacrimal gland and nasopharygeal uptake is present. *Left column,* Posterior (*above*) and anterior chest (*below*). *Middle column,* Posterior (*above*) and anterior abdomen. *Right column,* Anterior head (*above*) and pelvis (*below*).

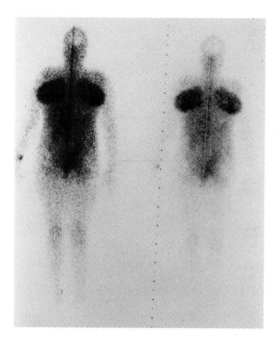

Fig. 7-2 Postpartum breast uptake of Ga-67. Breast uptake of Ga-67 is normal, can be quite variable from patient to patient, and is often quite intense postpartum. Two intensity settings are shown.

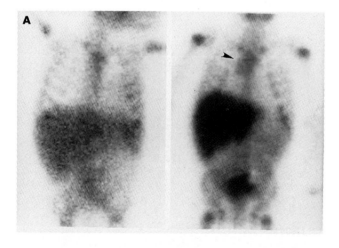

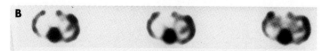

Fig. 7-3 Ga-67 uptake in myocarditis. This 20-month-old child received azothioprine and steroids for treatment of idiopathic myocarditis. **A**, *Left*, Pretherapy planar image of the chest showed no abnormal uptake; *Right*, Posttherapy planar image shows prominent uptake by the thymus (*arrowhead*). **B**, In contrast to the planar study, the pretherapy SPECT study showed definite myocardial uptake (best seen on middle image). Three sequential transverse slices through the myocardium are shown.

In vivo Ga-67 distribution can be altered by whole body irradiation, an excess of carrier gallium or ferric ion (e.g., with multiple transfusions), or gadolinium exposure (e.g., following a recent MR study). The mechanism of the latter two is saturation of protein-binding sites.

Uptake may be seen in surgical wounds for 2 to 3 weeks post operatively and in sterile abscesses associated with frequent intramuscular (IM) injections (e.g., insulin injections in diabetics, depot-injections of iron). Increased salivary gland uptake may be seen following radiation or chemotherapy.

Clinical Applications

In addition to acute localized infections such as abscesses, Ga-67 can reveal infection without pus or well-formed borders, such as cellulitis, peritonitis, and inflammatory and granulomatous processes. Leukocytic infiltration is not necessary to detect foci of infection, a factor that can make Ga-67 useful for studying leukopenic patients.

Pulmonary infectious and inflammatory diseases Although the use of labeled leukocytes has replaced many of the initial indications for Ga-67, the detection of a variety of interstitial and granulomatous pulmonary diseases remains an important role for Ga-67. The radiopharmaceutical accumulates in virtually all pulmonary infections, inflammatory sites, and granulomatous diseases, including pneumonia, lung abscesses, tuberculosis, pneumoconioses, idiopathic pulmonary fibrosis, sarcoidosis (Figure 7-4), *Pneumocystis carinii* infection (Figure 7-5), adult respiratory distress syndrome, and cytomegalovirus infection (Box 7-2).

Sarcoidosis   Sarcoidosis is a chronic granulomatous disease of unknown etiology. Pulmonary manifestations usually predominate, but the disease may involve any organ of the body.

CLINICAL MANIFESTATIONS   The initial presentation varies. Thirty percent of patients with sarcoidosis are initially asymptomatic, and the diagnosis is suggested by findings on an incidental chest x-ray. Another third present with complaints of dysnea and dry cough. Pulmonary involvement occurs in over 90%. Systemic symptoms of weight loss, fatigue, weakness, malaise, and fever are common (40%). Extrathoracic disease can involve any organ, most commonly the liver and spleen, but also the skin, eye, heart, central nervous system (CNS), bones, and muscle.

The clinical course is variable. Spontaneous resolution occurs in about one third of patients. Another 30% to 40% of patients have a smoldering or progressively worsening course, and 20% develop permanent loss of lung function; 5% to 10% die of respiratory failure.

PATHOGENESIS   Intrathoracic manifestations may consist of hilar or mediastinal adenopathy, endobronchial granuloma formation, interstitial or alveolar pulmonary infiltrates, or pulmonary fibrosis. Histologic and

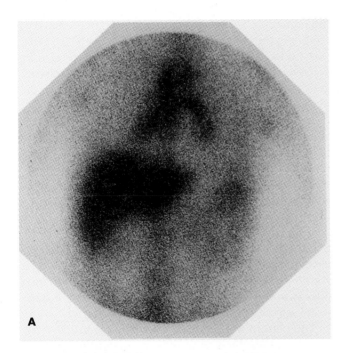

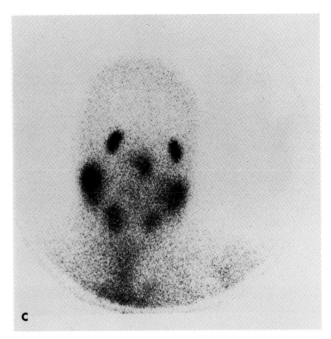

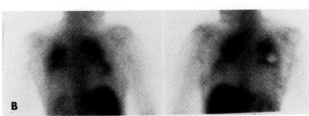

Fig. 7-4   Sarcoidosis. **A**, Paratracheal and hilar nodal uptake seen in early active sarcoidosis (λ sign). **B**, Diffusely increased pulmonary Ga-67 uptake is seen in a patient with active sarcoidosis involving predominantly the upper lobes. The cold defect is due to a pacemaker. **C**, Prominent Ga-67 uptake is seen in the parotids, salivary and lacrimal glands in a patient with active sarcoidosis (panda sign).

bronchopulmonary lavage findings reveal an alveolitis with an increase in both the relative and absolute numbers of lymphocytes (particularly T-cells), monocytes, and macrophages.

Chest radiographic findings can be categorized into four stages (Table 7-5), progressing from nodal to parenchymal involvement. The alveolitis of sarcoidosis can produce an interstitial pattern on the chest radiograph.

DIAGNOSIS AND ASSESSMENT OF DISEASE ACTIVITY   The diagnosis of sarcoidosis is often one of exclusion; however, pathologic evidence of noncaseating granulomas in the absence of vasculitis or fungal or mycobacterial disease is usually diagnostic.

The *Kveim-Siltzbach test* requires intradermal injection of human sarcoid tissue. A nodule develops in 2 to 6 weeks at the injection site, and biopsy reveals a noncaseating granulomatous reaction. Sensitivity is reported to be high in patients with active disease, but false positives occur, and accurate results require meticulous attention to preparation technique and careful selection of splenic tissue.

Bronchoalveolar saline lavage (BAL) with examination for inflammatory cells is an accurate method of making the diagnosis. An increase in the percentage of

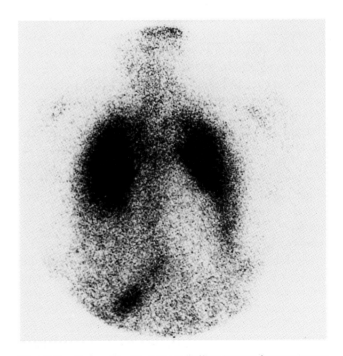

Fig. 7-5   *Pneumocysitis carinii*. Diffuse intense homogeneous or heterogeneous uptake is typical of this infection. The characteristic pattern is different from that of other common pulmonary infections in AIDS patients.

Box 7-2 Interstitial and Granulomatous Pulmonary Diseases Associated With Ga-67 Uptake

Tuberculosis
Histoplasmosis
Sarcoidosis
Idiopathic pulmonary fibrosis
Pneumocystis carinii
Cytomegalovirus
Pneumonconioses
Asbestosis
Silicosis

Table 7-5 A Classification of Chest Radiographic Findings in Sarcoidosis

Stage	Radiographic Findings
0	No demonstrable abnormalities.
1	Hilar and/or mediastinal node enlargement with normal lung parenchma.
2	Hilar and/or mediastinal node enlargement and diffuse interstitial pulmonary disease.
3	Diffuse pulmonary disease without node involvement.
4	Pulmonary fibrosis

T-lymphocytes has been used as indication for therapy. However, the technique is invasive, and controversy exists as to whether this test can be used to predict either the clinical course or response to corticosteroids.

Serum markers such as angiotensin-converting enzyme (ACE) can be used to diagnose active sarcoidosis and predict response to therapy. Serum ACE levels are elevated in up to 80% of patients with active disease. The percentage of patients with elevated ACE levels increases from 33% to 77% as sarcoid progresses from stages 0 and 1 to 2, although ACE levels do not correlate well with the degree of alveolitis. Elevated ACE levels are not specific to sarcoid and may be seen in other pulmonary and nonpulmonary diseases.

SCINTIGRAPHIC DIAGNOSIS   Ga-67 has been used to evaluate the activity of alveolitis with sarcoidosis and can help guide the course of therapy. It can distinguish active granuloma formation and/or alveolitis from fibrotic changes. Increased uptake in the lungs is more than 90% sensitive for clinically active sarcoidosis. Scans are usually negative in dormant cases. Ga-67 can also help localize nonpulmonary sites of disease activity.

Controversy exists as to whether or not increased pulmonary Ga-67 uptake correlates with the degree of inflammation, serum ACE levels, or the percentage of lymphocytes obtained on BAL. Proponents believe that Ga-67 uptake correlates with disease activity and is more sensitive than serum ACE levels for following disease activity. Studies have shown a correlation between the degree of uptake on serial Ga-67 scans and response to therapy with steroids, both early in treatment and later, after 1 year of therapy. However, because of the ease of determining serum ACE levels, some pulmonologists think that the Ga-67 scan should be reserved for cases in which focal involvement must be discriminated from general disease activity.

IMAGE INTERPRETATION   In early sarcoidosis, Ga-67 uptake on scintigraphy may be seen before changes are present on chest radiographs. Up to one third of patients have normal radiographs at this stage of disease. Ga-67 is also more sensitive than radiography for demonstrating hilar lymph node involvement. Patients with a normal Ga-67 scan nearly always have a negative biopsy.

The pattern of uptake in sarcoidosis is usually symmetric and may be that of hilar or mediastinal involvement alone, diffuse parenchymal uptake, or both (Figure 7-4A,B). In contrast, patients with malignant lymphoma typically have asymmetric hilar or mediastinal uptake, often involving the anterior and paratracheal nodes.

The degree of pulmonary uptake is usually judged subjectively relative to uptake in the liver, bone marrow, and soft tissue. Lung uptake greater than liver uptake is highly positive, while lung uptake less than soft tissue uptake is negative. A number of semiquantitative indexes of Ga-67 uptake have been proposed. Although more objective quantitation is desirable, the problem with these methods is that uptake by normal overlying soft tissue, bone, and marrow limits accuracy.

Low-grade pulmonary uptake can sometimes be hard to ascertain, owing to the normal overlying sternum, ribs, scapula, and spine. Because the heart may obscure much of the left lung field in the anterior view, the posterior view is preferred for estimating uptake. Oblique views can be useful for discerning mediastinal and hilar uptake; SPECT may be helpful here.

Characteristic image patterns of Ga-67 uptake seen with sarcoidosis have been described. Increased uptake in the paratracheal and hilar lymph node groups has been referred to as the lambda (λ) sign (Figure 7-4A). A diffuse parenchymal uptake pattern with or without nodal uptake is seen in a later stage of disease (Figure 7-4B). Increased uptake in the nasopharyngeal region, parotids, and salivary glands has been referred to as the panda sign (Figure 7-4C) and is characteristic of sarcoidosis.

The combination of ocular involvement (iritis or iridocyclitis) with accompanying lacrimal gland inflammation and bilateral salivary gland involvement is known as Mikulicz's syndrome or uveoparotid fever. Although para-aortic, mesenteric, and retroperitoneal lymph node involvement may be seen in sarcoidosis, this is much more commonly seen with lymphoma.

Idiopathic interstitial pulmonary fibrosis   In this disease of unknown etiology there is a pathologic progression through progressive stages of alveolitis, with derangement of the alveolar-capillary units, leading to end-stage fibrotic disease. Ga-67 has been used to monitor the course of disease and response to therapy. The amount of Ga-67 uptake correlates with the degree of cellular infiltration; however, unlike the situation with sarcoidosis, it does not predict the results of steroid treatment.

Adverse pulmonary drug reactions   Ga-67 uptake can sometimes be an early indicator of drug-induced lung injury before the chest radiograph is abnormal. This occurs most commonly with cytoxin, nitrofurantoin, bleomycin, and amiodarone toxicity (Box 7-3). Pulmonary uptake may also be seen after lymphangiography as a result of a chemical-induced alveolitis.

Abdominal and pelvic infections   In general, radionuclide whole body scintigraphy is most useful when the site of infection cannot be localized clinically. With localizing symptoms, ultrasonography is usually the imaging modality of choice for examining the right upper quadrant, pelvis, and kidney region, while computed tomography (CT) is used for examining the rest of the abdomen.

When the diagnosis remains uncertain, scintigraphy can be helpful. Although Ga-67 scintigraphy has been successfully used to diagnose intra-abdominal infection, In-111 leukocyte scintigraphy is usually preferable, because the tracer is not cleared through the intestines or kidneys and the study can be completed in 24 hours.

Intrahepatic abscesses may be diagnosed with Ga-67 scintigraphy, although normal hepatic uptake can make interpretation difficult. A concomitant Tc-99m sulfur colloid study to serve as a template can aid in making the diagnosis (Figure 7-6). Ga-67 scans have also proved helpful in confirming the diagnosis of active progressive inflammatory disease of retroperitoneal fibrosis.

Genitourinary infections   Because 10% to 25% of the injected Ga-67 citrate dose will be excreted via the kidneys during the first 24 hours, the diagnosis of renal inflammatory disease should be made from images obtained 48 to 72 hours after tracer injection. Renal

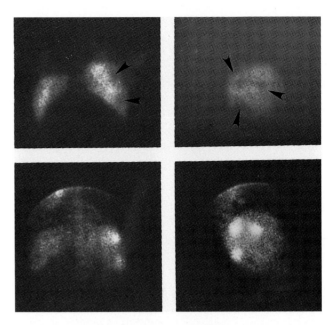

Fig. 7-6   Multiple liver abscesses. The diagnosis was made with Ga-67 in conjunction with a Tc-99m SC liver spleen scan. Posterior (*left*) and right lateral (*right*) views are displayed. *Top,* Tc-99m SC study. *Bottom,* Comparable Ga-67 study. Note increased focal uptake on the Ga-67 scan corresponding to the focal photopenic defects seen on the Tc-99m SC study (*arrowheads*).

parenchymal infection such as pyelonephritis or diffuse interstitial nephritis (Figure 7-7), lobar nephronia (focal interstitial nephritis), and perirenal infections (Figure 7-8) can be diagnosed with Ga-67 scintigraphy. Caution is indicated in the setting of renal or hepatic failure or iron overload, where increased kidney uptake is often seen.

Bone infections   Because Ga-67 is taken up by normal bone and increased uptake may be seen in reactive bone, false positive studies can occur in patients with underlying bone disease, previous surgery, fractures, and prostheses. To improve specificity for the diagnosis of osteomyelitis, Ga-67 has been used in conjunction with a Tc-99m bone scan. Direct comparison studies with In-111 leukocytes have revealed Ga-67 scintigraphy to be generally less accurate. However, Ga-67 scintigraphy can be useful in diagnosing disk space infections, which often have an associated soft tissue component (Figure 7-9).

Ga-67 scintigraphy can be used to differentiate necrotizing external otitis, a life-threatening *Pseudomonas* infection seen in diabetics and associated with a poor prognosis, from other less serious causes of therapy-resistant external otitis. In necrotizing otitis, increased uptake can be seen in the temporal bone on Tc-99m bone scans and Ga-67 studies. The bone scan can be used to establish the intial diagnosis, whereas the Ga-67 scan is useful for evaluating the effectiveness of therapy.

Box 7-3	Ga-67 Lung Uptake Associated With Adverse Drug Reactions
Cytoxin	Amiodarone
Busulfan	Nitrofurantoin
Bleomycin	

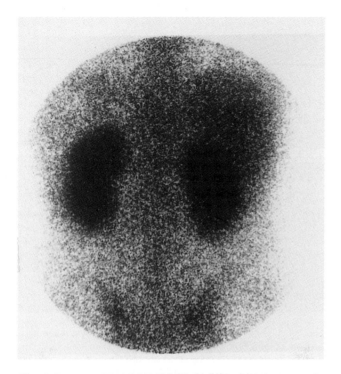

Fig. 7-7   Interstitial nephritis. Bilateral intense renal Ga-67 uptake is seen at 48 hours (posterior view). Normal uptake is seen in the liver, bone, and bone marrow.

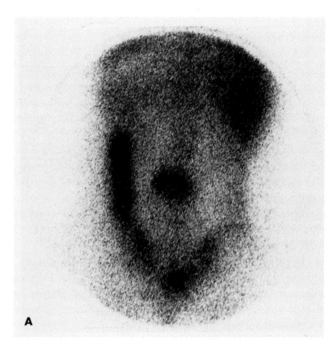

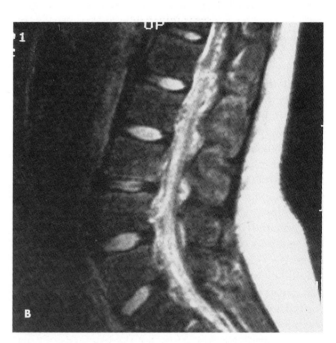

Fig. 7-9   Disk space infection. **A**, Prominent focal Ga-67 uptake is seen at L3–L4 (posterior view). **B**, MRI showed only a narrowed interspace with evidence of degenerative disk disease.

RADIOLABELED LEUKOCYTES FOR INFECTION IMAGING

Scintigraphy using radiolabeled WBCs has long been a physiologically appealing method for detecting infection. In 1976, McAfee and Thakur demonstrated that the In-111 chelate of oxine was well suited for in vitro leuko-

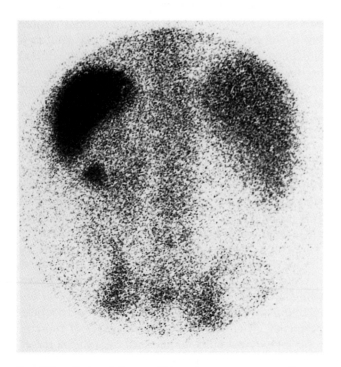

Fig. 7-8   Perirenal abscess. This patient underwent renal stone removal and a nephrostomy. Postoperatively, fever and pain developed. Note the focally increased Ga-67 uptake just inferior to the spleen and adjacent to the left kidney, consistent with an abscess.

cyte labeling. Subsequent studies proved the clinical value of In-111 oxine-labeled leukocytes, and this FDA-approved radiopharmaceutical is now widely available.

Physiology of White Blood Cells

Leukocytes are the major cellular components of inflammatory and immune responses. They protect against infection and neoplasia and assist in the repair of damaged tissue. The nucleated precursor cells differentiate into mature cells within the bone marrow. The normal blood leukocyte count ranges from 4.5 to 11×10^6 cells/mm^3 and includes the granulocyte series of neutrophils (55%-65%), eosinophils (3%), and basophils (0.5%), as well as lymphocytes (25%-35%) and monocytes (3%-7%).

Leukocytes spend a small fraction of their short life span in the peripheral blood (6-7 hours), using it mainly for transportation to sites where they are needed—the spleen, liver, lung, and to a lesser extent the gastrointestinal (GI) tract and oropharynx. Normally about 90% of the neutrophil pool is in the bone marrow, 2% to 3% is in the circulation, and the remainder is in the tissues. Neutrophils exist in two compartments: a "marginated" pool adherent to vascular endothelial cells and a circulating pool. The former can be marshalled into the circulating pool by exercise, epinephrine, or exposure to bacterial endotoxin.

In response to an acute inflammatory stimulus, neutrophils migrate toward an attractant (chemotaxis), increase their adhesiveness, aggregrate, adhere to endothelial surfaces, phagocytize the infectious agent or foreign body, and enzymatically destroy it within cytoplasmic vacuoles. Neutrophilic migration into tissues involves crawling (diapedesis) between postcapillary endothelial cells. Neutrophils survive in tissue for only 2 to 3 days. Both adherence and migration of neutrophils are inhibited by exposure to corticosteroids or ethanol.

Monocytes act as tissue scavengers, phagocytizing damaged cells and bacteria and detoxifying chemicals and toxins; they also have immunologic functions. At sites of inflammation they transform into tissue macrophages. *Eosinophils* mediate allergic reactions and help protect against parasitic infestations.

Lymphocytes play an important role in immune reactions. Although their nonimmunologic role in inflammation is less well understood, they arrive at inflammatory sites during the chronic phases of many inflammatory responses. T-lymphocytes are primarily responsible for cell-mediated immune respones. These cells originate from the marrow and are processed into mature T-lymphocytes in the thymus. They represent 50% to 80% of peripheral lymphocytes and concentrate in the marrow, spleen, tonsils, intestines, thymus, and lymph nodes. They recirculate and have a life span of 100 to 200 days. B-lymphocytes are primarily involved in antibody synthesis, do not usually recirculate, and have a short turnover in the lymph nodes and spleen.

Indium-111-Labeled White Blood Cells

Leukocyte labeling Oxine (8-hydroxyquinolone), a chelating agent, forms a lipophilic complex with In-111 that allows cell membrane penetration. Intracellularly, the In-111-oxine complex dissociates; the In-111 binds to nuclear and cytoplasmic proteins, while the oxine diffuses out of the cell. To label leukocytes efficiently, the cells must be removed from plasma, because In-111 has a higher affinity for serum transferrin than for oxine. Proper labeling does not adversely affect normal physiologic function, and the tag usually remains stable in vivo over 24 hours. Labeling efficiencies of 75% to 95% are obtainable.

In-111, a cyclotron produced radionuclide with a 67-hour (2.8-day) half-life and two gamma photons of 173 keV and 247 keV (Table 7-3), permits imaging at 24 hours with an acceptable estimated radiation dose to the patient (Table 7-4).

In-111 oxine labels blood cells indiscriminately, whether granulocytes, lymphocytes, monocytes, platelets, or erythrocytes. Mixed populations of leukocytes have proved satisfactory for detection of infection. Pure granulocyte preparations have been used, but they require complex separation methods and a clinical advantage has not been shown.

Methodology Cell labeling takes about 2 hours. Careful handling is necessary to avoid damaging the cells. Erythrocytes and platelets must be removed because they are many times more numerous than leukocytes. A technique that simultaneously combines red cell sedimentation with centrifugation (Box 7-4) to reduce platelets and proteins can produce a high yield of leukocytes. Hydroxyethyl starch (Hetastarch), a settling agent, hastens RBC clumping.

Alternatives to oxine have been proposed. Tropolone, unlike oxine, can be labeled with In-111 in plasma. Although clinical studies have not shown improved accuracy with tropolone-labeled leukocytes, earlier diagnosis (at 4 hours versus 24 hours) is possible. In-111 MERC (mercaptopyridine-*N*-oxide) is another chelating agent proposed as an alternative to oxine. It has several potential advantages. Being water soluble, it can label cells efficiently in plasma and is reportedly less cytotoxic than oxine. Less uptake occurs in muscle, liver, and spleen. Neither tropolone nor In-111 MERC is approved for clinical use, and further investigation is needed.

Quality control Viability studies on labeled leukocytes are complex and time-consuming and, therefore, not routinely performed on a clinical basis. The real test of leukocyte viability is the in vivo function as manifested by a normal distribution within the body and ulti-

---

Box 7-4   Labeling Autologous Leukocytes With In-111 Oxine

PREPARATION:

The patient's peripheral WBC count should be greater than 4,000 cells/ μL

PROCEDURE

1. Collect autologous blood
   Draw 30-50 mL into an anticoagulated (heparin or ACD) syringe using a 19-gauge needle.
2. Isolate leukocytes
   Separate RBCs by gravity sedimentation and 6% Hetastarch, a settling agent.
   The leukocyte-rich plasma (LRP) is centrifuged at 300-350 g for 5 min to remove platelets and proteins. A WBC button forms at the bottom of the tube.
   Draw off and save the leukocyte poor plasma (LPP) for later washing and resuspending.
3. Label leukocytes
   Suspend white cells (LRP) in saline (includes granulocytes, lymphs, monocytes, and some RBCs).
   Incubate with In-111 oxine for 30 min at room temperature and gently agitate.
   Remove unbound In-111 by centrifugation. Save wash for later calculation of labeling efficiency.
4. Prepare injectate
   Resuspend 500 uCi In-111 leukocytes in saved plasma (LPP).
   Inject via peripheral vein within 2-4 hr.
5. Quality control
   Microscopic examination of cells.
   Calculate labeling efficiency. Assay the cells and wash in dose calibrator. ($E = C/(C + W)$ x100%, where C is the activity associated with the cells, W is the activity associated with the wash, and E is the labeling efficiency.)

Box 7-5   In-111 Leukocyte Scintigraphy: Protocol Summary

RADIOPHARMACEUTICAL

In-111 oxine in vitro labeled leukocytes, 500 μCi

INSTRUMENTATION

Camera: Large field of view.
Windows: 20%, centered over 173 and 247 keV photopeaks.
Collimator: Medium energy.

PATIENT PREPARATION

A Tc-99m SC liver-spleen scan performed before or after can be helpful in detecting intra- or perihepatic or splenic infection.

PROCEDURE

Inject in vitro labeled cells IV.
Imaging at 4 hour may be helpful to diagnose an acute abscess and is critical in localizing inflammatory bowel disease.
Routine whole body imaging at 24 hr.
Image anterior abdomen for 500k counts and acquire remainder of images for equal time. Images should include anterior and posterior views of the chest, abdomen, and pelvis, and spot images of specific areas of interest (e.g., the feet) for a minimum of 200k counts or 20 min.
SPECT in selected cases.

---

mately its ability to detect infection. Increased lung uptake may be seen with cell damage. Prolonged blood pool uptake can be seen with RBC and platelet labeling.

Routine quality control should include a microscopic examination to look for structural integrity, RBC contamination, and the presence of clumping. Labeling efficiency should be calculated (Box 7-4).

Imaging protocol   Imaging of In-111 WBCs is routinely performed at 18 to 24 hours after tracer injection (Box 7-5). Further delayed images do not add additional information. However, early imaging at 4 hours may occasionally be useful for diagnosis of an abscess that requires prompt intervention. Localizing the site of active inflammatory bowel disease requires imaging at 4 hours, for by 24 hours inflamed mucosal cells will have sloughed, become intraluminal, and moved distally.

Normal distribution and dosimetry   Immediately after injection, radioactivity can be seen in the blood pool, lungs, liver, and spleen. By 4 hours, lung activity and blood pool activity decrease and marrow activity increases. By 24 hours, no blood pool activity should be seen, and bone marrow activity becomes prominent (Figure 7-10); if significant blood pool activity is still noted, it indicates a high percent of erythrocyte or platelet labeling. On images obtained at 18 to 24 hours after tracer injection, the most intense uptake is seen in the spleen, followed by the liver, and then the bone marrow. Each receives about one third of the total activity. Unlike Ga-67, In-111 leukocytes are not cleared through the bowel or kidneys.

The target organ is the spleen, which in an adult receives about 13 to 20 rads, probably somewhat more in children because of the small volume of distribution. The whole body absorbed dose is only 0.37 rads (Table 7-4).

Abnormal uptake   Activity outside the expected normal organs of uptake is evidence of infection or inflammation. Focal uptake equal to or greater than that in the liver or spleen is typical for an abscess; activity equal to that of the liver generally signifies a clinically

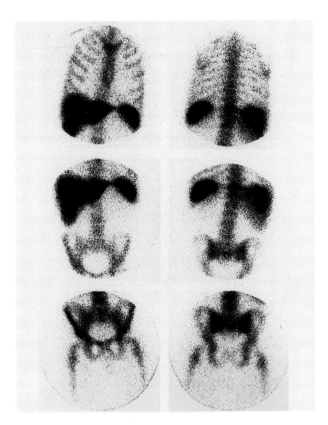

Fig. 7-10 Normal distribution of In-111 leukocytes at 24 hours. Note that the greatest uptake is in the spleen, followed by the liver, then the bone marrow. There is no intestinal or renal activity.

① imp. for inflammatory bowel disease.

important inflammatory site; and activity less than that of the bone marrow usually suggests a low-level inflammatory response.

Clinical applications

Fever of unknown origin Fever of unknown origin has been defined as persistence of fever reaching 38.3° C for at least 3 weeks on more than three occasions and resulting in at least 7 days of hospitalization. In patients who have not had recent surgery, Ga-67 may be the most sensitive test for uncovering a source of the fever, since in addition to acute infection, Ga-67 can detect tumors, as well as chronic, granulomatous, and indolent infections. However, postoperative patients with persistent fever would be better served with In-111 leukocytes, because recently acquired infection is the likely cause and there is no bowel clearance to confound interpretation.

Intra-abdominal abscess Because of the morbidity and mortality associated with intra-abdominal infection, prompt diagnosis is critical. Ga-67 has disadvantages. Although early imaging at 6 to 24 hours can sometimes demonstrate an abscess, imaging delayed as long as 3 to 4 days after tracer injection is often needed to differentiate focal infection from normal bowel clearance. As a result, In-111-labeled leukocytes are preferable (Figure

7-11). Combined data from three large series showed an overall sensitivity of 90% and a specificity of 95% for In-111 leukocytes in detecting intra-abdominal infection.

Abnormal In-111 leukocyte uptake has been described in a variety of inflammatory diseases, including severe pancreatitis, pancreatic abscess, polyarteritis nodosa, rheumatoid vasculitis, and acute cholecystitis. For the routine diagnosis of acute cholecystitis, the Tc-99m HIDA study is preferable: cell labeling is unnecessary, and the study has a high accuracy and lower dose requirements. However, in selected cases In-111 leukocytes may prove useful, such as in settings where a false positive HIDA study may occur (prolonged fasting, hyperalimentation, severe intercurrent illness) or in the case of a suspected false negative HIDA study, eg, for acute *acalculous* cholecystitis.

Inflammatory bowel disease Ulcerative colitis and Crohn's disease (granulomatous or regional enteritis) are characterized by intestinal inflammation. Although barium enema examination and colonoscopy are routinely used to make these diagnoses, the procedures are contraindicated in severely ill patients. Studies have shown good correlation between the site and amount of In-111 leukocyte uptake compared to the endoscopic and radiologic localization.

Imaging should be performed at 4 hours rather than 24 hours because shedding of leukocytes into the bowel lumen from the inflammatory sites and the subsequent peristalsis often result in incorrect assignment of disease

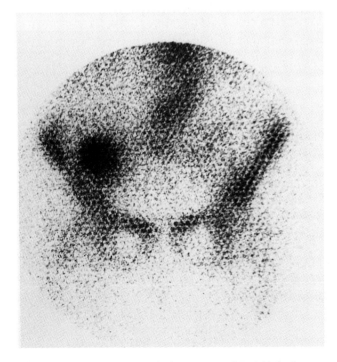

Fig. 7-11 Intra-abdominal abscess. Focal In-111 leukocyte uptake (anterior pelvic view) is seen in the right lower quadrant secondary to a perforated appendix with abscess formation.

to sites distal to the true pathology. The In-111 leukocyte study is useful not only in acute fulminant enteritis or colitis, but also for evaluating areas hard to see with endoscopy and for monitoring the effectiveness of therapy. Inactive colitis is negative on scintigraphy.

In-111-labeled leukocytes can differentiate reactivation of inflammatory bowel disease from abscess formation secondary to bowel perforation. This is a serious clinical problem, with very different therapy required (medical versus surgical). Scintigraphically, In-111 leukocyte uptake within an abscess is usually focal, while uptake in inflamed bowel typically follows the contour of the intestinal wall. Leukocyte uptake may also be seen in ischemic colitis (common in elderly patients), pseudomembranous colitis (antibiotic related), and bowel infarction.

Neutropenic patients Neutropenic patients may have fever and infection without localizing signs. An In-111 labeled WBC study can be suboptimal because of the patient's low granulocyte count. Although a leukocyte count above 5,000/mm^3 is preferred, diagnostic scintigraphy can often be performed in patients with lower cell counts (3,000/mm^3).

Crossmatched donor leukocytes have been successfully used in patients with severe leukopenia. An alternative method that does not require cell labeling or heterologous cells would be preferable, such as the use of Ga-67, or, better, labeled nonspecific polyclonal immunoglobulins (discussed later). This would be particularly advantageous in AIDS cases, where working with blood products exposes medical personel to some risk.

Pediatric patients In-111 leukocyte scintigraphy has been used in children to detect infection; however, the large volume of blood required for labeling, the low recommended administered dose based on weight and size resulting in a low count rate, and the relatively high splenic dosimetry have tended to make this an uncommonly used test in children. Ga-67 scintigraphy, with its limitations, is more frequently used. Tc-99m HMPAO–labeled leukocytes may presently be the preferred tracer in children.

Renal disease In-111 labeled leukocytes can localize and diagnose genitourinary infection. Focal uptake can localize in sites of acute pyelonephritis, focal nephritis (lobar nephronia), and renal or perirenal abscess. However, In-111-labeled WBCs have limited utility for evaluation of renal transplants. For unclear reasons, almost all transplant recipients exhibit uptake, regardless of the presence or absence of clinically significant disease or rejection.

Cardiovascular disease In-111-labeled leukocytes are not useful in making the diagnosis of subacute bacterial endocarditis. The vegetative lesions often contain high concentrations of bacteria, platelets, and fibrin adherent to damaged valvular endothelium but relatively few leukocytes. Uptake can be seen in acute myocardial

infarction and transplant rejection, but the study is not generally used clinically for making these diagnoses.

Labeled leukocytes can be used to diagnose graft infection (Figures 7-12, 7-13). Infection of arterial prosthetic grafts, such as femoropopliteal and aortofemoral grafts, is associated with significant morbidity (amputation) and mortality. Prompt diagnosis of graft infection is critical but often delayed because of the indolent and insidious course of these infections.

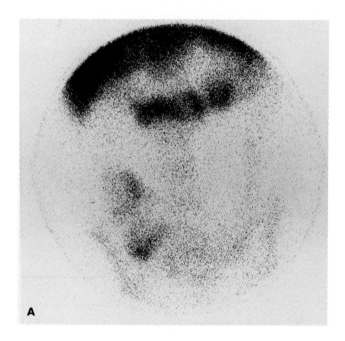

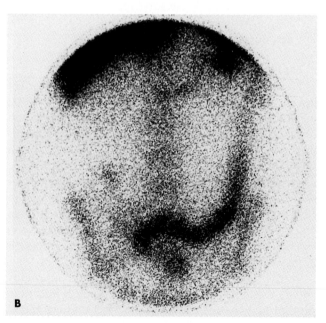

Fig. 7-12 False positive In-111 WBC study due to acute gastrointestinal bleeding. Images obtained at 4 hrs (**A**) and 24 hrs (**B**). Note movement of tracer through the bowel. No intra-abdominal infection was diagnosed. The acute bleeding resolved without specific therapy.

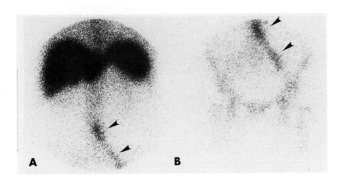

Fig. 7-13 Infected aortofemoral graft. **A**, Abdominal view. **B**, Anterior pelvic view. In-111 leukocyte uptake confirms the clinically suspected graft infection (*arrowheads*).

Pulmonary infection Pulmonary uptake of In-111 leukocytes should be interpreted cautiously. Low-grade diffuse uptake has been associated with a variety of noninfectious causes, including atelectasis, congestive heart failure, and adult respiratory distress syndrome, and therefore should not be considered diagnostic of infection. Focal intense uptake is much more likely to be due to infection (Figure 7-14). Tuberculosis and chronic granulomatous diseases do not take up In-111-labeled leukocytes. Ga-67 is the preferred agent for the scintigraphic evaluation of most pulmonary diseases.

False positive studies Leukocytes often accumulate at sites of inflammation without infection, such as intravenous catheter insertion sites and the placement sites of nasogastric tubes, drainage tubes, tracheostomies, colostomies, and ileostomies. Unless very intense, this uptake should be considered normal. Uninfected postsurgical wounds commonly show faint uptake for up to 10 days. If uptake is intense, persists, or extends beyond the surgical wound site, infection should be suspected.

Intraluminal intestinal activity may be secondary to swallowed or shedding cells as may occur with herpes esophagitis, sinus or pulmonary infection, and nasogastric tubes. Other false positive studies may potentially occur due to GI bleeding, noninfected hematomas, and accessory spleens (Figure 7-15, 7-16, Table 7-6). Rarely, tumors may have increased uptake.

Infection within or adjacent to the liver and spleen may be missed because of normal In-111 leukocyte uptake in these organs. As mentioned earlier, a Tc-99m SC (sulfur colloid) scan can be helpful in confirming or excluding this diagnosis. One study reported that a concomitant Tc-99m SC study was necessary to diagnose an upper abdominal abscess in over half of the patients studied. We routinely perform a Tc-99m SC study prior to reinjecting the labeled cells in patients with suspected intra-abdominal infection.

One study reported a false negative rate approaching 30% for In-111 leukocyte scans for chronic infection; however, a subsequent larger series found no significant

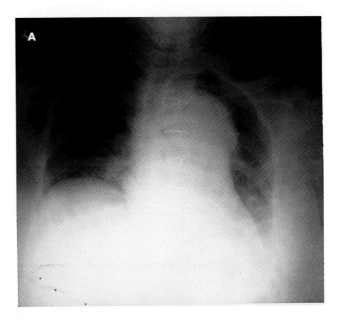

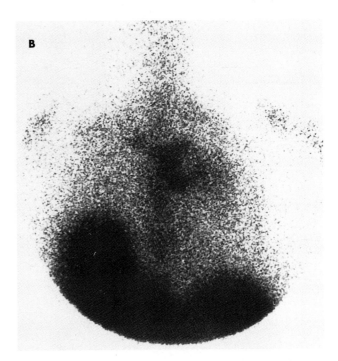

Fig. 7-14 Infected thoracic aortic graft. **A**, Postoperative chest x-ray. **B**, In-111 leukocytes localize in the region of the aortic knob.

difference in sensitivity between acute and chronic infections. Although chronic inflammation consists largely of monocytes, macrophages, lymphocytes and plasma cells, chronic bacterial infections also have significant neutrophilic infiltration and sometimes frank pus.

A lower test sensitivity for In-111 leukocytes has been reported in patients with tuberculosis and fungal infections. Ga-67 is preferable. Conflicting data exist on the

Table 7-6   Optimal Imaging time for Infection-seeking radiopharmaceuticals

Radiopharmaceutical	Time (hr)
Ga-67	48 *(So bone scan on day 1 & Ga on day 2*
In-111 leukocytes	24
Polyclonal IgG antibodies	10, occasionally 24 required
Monoclonal IgG antibodies	4, occasionally later
Tc-99m HMPAO leukocytes	2
Chemotactic peptides	1
Tc-99m albumin colloid	<1
Tc-99m nanocolloids	1

Box 7-6   Causes of False Negative and False Positive In-111 Leukocyte Studies

FALSE NEGATIVE
Encapsulated, nonpyogenic abscess
Vertebral osteomyelitis
Chronic low-grade infection
Parasitic, TB, or fungal infections
Intra- or perihepatic or splenic infection
Hyperglycemia (?)
Steroids (?)

FALSE POSITIVE
Gastrointestinal bleeding
Pseudoaneurysm
Healing fracture
Soft tissue tumor
Swallowed WBCs from disease in the oropharynx, esophagus, or lungs
Surgical wounds, stomas, or catheter sites
Hematomas
Tumors
Accessory spleens

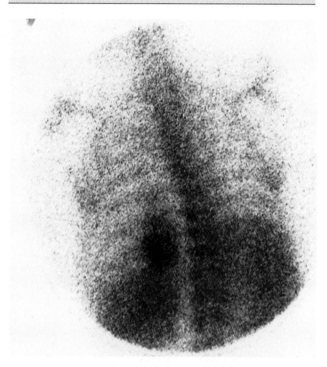

Fig. 7-15   Pneumonia. Focal In-111 leukocyte uptake seen in the left lower lobe (posterior chest). The study was performed to search for a source of postoperative fever. The previous chest radiograph was made 10 days earlier. Pneumonia was not suspected; however, a subsequent radiograph confirmed the diagnosis.

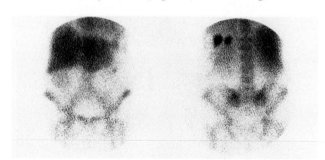

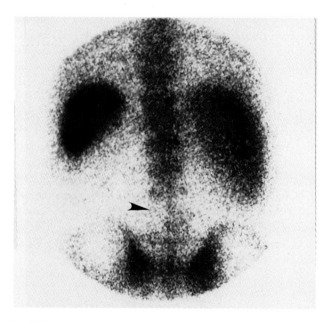

Fig. 7-17   Vertebral osteomyelitis. A cold defect at L5 was seen with In-111 leukocyte scintigraphy. The diagnosis of infection was confirmed by biopsy.

Fig. 7-16   Potentially false positive In-111 leukocyte scan due to accessory spleens in a 78-year-old woman with subacute bacterial endocarditis who had previously undergone splenectomy. The In-111 WBC study was ordered to localize any extracardiac infection. A heat-damaged Tc-99m RBC study confirmed that the focal uptake in the left upper quadrant represented accessory spleens (see also Figure 9-48B).

sensitivity of In-111 leukocyte scintigraphy for detecting infection in patients on antibiotics; however, this is probably not a major determinant.

A low sensitivity for osteomyelitis of the spine has been repeatedly noted. In fact, vertebral osteomyelitis may appear as a cold defect (Figure 7-17). Questions have been raised about the study's sensitivity in patients with diseases or undergoing therapies that alter leukocyte function, such as steroid therapy, hyperglycemia, chemotherapy, hemodialysis, and hyperalimentation. No firm data exist.

Technetium-99m-Labeled Leukocytes

Labeling with Tc-99m rather than In-111 has theoretical advantages. It has lower radiation dosimetry and permits a higher administered activity. The higher photon yield of Tc-99m and its optimal Tc-99m photopeak for modern-day gamma cameras would be expected to produce superior planar and SPECT images. A number of new Tc-99m-labeled radiopharmaceuticals for infection imaging are being investigated, and some are clinically available.

Technetium-99m HMPAO   Tc-99m hexamethylpropyleneamine oxine (HMPAO), used for cerebral perfusion imaging, is lipophilic and readily crosses the white cell membrane. Intracellularly, it changes into a hydrophilic complex and becomes trapped, bound to the mitochondria and the nucleus. Because HMPAO has a predilection for granulocytes, an almost pure labeled granulocyte preparation is obtained without the need for cell separation. With HMPAO, leukocyte labeling can be performed in plasma. The FDA views Tc-99m HMPAO–labeled leukocytes as an alternative use of an approved radiopharmaceutical (Tc-99m HMPAO is approved for cerebral perfusion imaging).

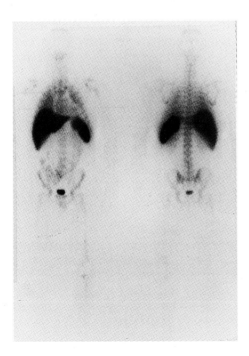

Fig. 7-18   Normal distribution of Tc-99m HMPAO–labeled leukocytes. The study was performed because of suspected left knee prosthesis infection. Imaging at 4 hours shows some normal bowel and bladder clearance. Low-grade normal pulmonary uptake is seen. Marrow is seen, similar to In-111 WBC studies.

Unlike In-111 oxine–labeled leukocytes, the normal biodistribution of Tc-99m HMPAO–labeled leukocytes includes renal and intestinal clearance (Figure 7-18). Kidneys and the bladder may be seen as early as 1 hour after injection. The gallbladder is visualized in 4% of patients at 1 hour, and the percentage increases thereafter. Bowel activity is often seen by 4 hours and increases with time. Abdominal imaging is best performed before significant bowel clearance occurs (Figure 7-19). Gastrointestinal clearance results from excretion of a secondary complex, which can also be seen during Tc-99m HMPAO brain imaging. Early lung uptake similar to that seen with In-111 oxine occurs, but it decreases significantly by 4 hours.

Clinical studies with Tc-99m HMPAO have found the overall accuracy for detection of infection similar to that of In-111-labeled leukocytes (Figure 7-19). An advantage of Tc-99m HMPAO leukocyte imaging is that sensitivity is near maximal by 30 minutes and the study can be com-

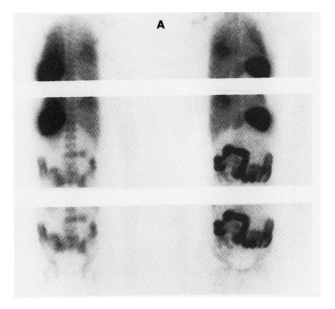
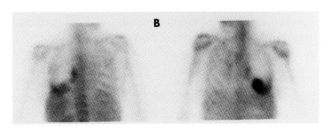

Fig. 7-19   **A**, Abnormal Tc-99m HMPAO study in an HIV-positive patient with fever and diarrhea. *Left column,* Posterior views. *Right column,* Anterior views of chest (*upper*), abdomen (*middle*), and pelvis (*lower*). Imaging was performed at 90 minutes, before bowel clearance would normally be seen. Tc-99m HMPAO uptake is seen in the right lung base and the bowel. Cytomegalovirus was the cause of the colitis. **A**, Pneumonic infiltrate was found on chest x-ray. **B**, Postoperative empyema diagnosed with Tc-99m HMPAO–labeled WBCs. The infection occurred after thoracotomy for lung cancer. *Left,* Posterior view. *Right,* Anterior view.

pleted by 2 hours (Table 7-6). Tc-99m HMPAO may be suboptimal for detecting GI or GU tract infections because of its normal clearance through these organs. In-111-labeled leukocytes may be preferred in chronic infections, where exchange of leukocytes is slower and delayed imaging advantageous.

PROMISING INFECTION-SEEKING RADIOPHARMACEUTICALS

Radiolabeled Antibodies

Nonspecific polyclonal immunoglobulin G   The utility of nonspecific IgG for infection imaging was fortuitously discovered during investigations of monoclonal antibodies for the same purpose. Surprisingly, the nonspecific polyclonal immunoglobulins were found to be equally effective. The mechanism is not well understood, but it seems not to be immunologic. Increased vascular permeability probably plays an important role.

The normal distribution of In-111-labeled IgG includes the liver, spleen, and bone marrow (Table 7-7). The GI and GU systems show varying degrees of uptake. Preliminary results in human studies have been very good, with a sensitivity above 90% and a specificity of 100% in a series of 128 patients. Uptake has been seen with a wide variety of infectious agents, including *Mycoplasma*, *Pneumocystis*, *Candida histoplasma*, and *tuberculosis*. Chronicity of infection, antibiotics, anti-inflammatory drugs, and corticosteroids do not seem to affect the sensitivity.

Radiolabeled nonspecific polyclonal IgG has a number of advantages. It comes in kit form and does not require complicated in vitro cell labeling or handling of blood products. Both In-111 and Tc-99m labels are possible; the most appropriate one could be chosen according to the clinical situtation. Dosimetry, even with the In-111 label, is better than with In-111 leukocytes. Bacterial and nonbacterial infections can be imaged. The disadvantages are that azotemia reduces its sensitivity and tumor uptake occurs more frequently with it than with In-111 labeled leukocytes.

Monoclonal antibodies   Radiolabeled monoclonal antibodies directed against specific leukocyte cell-surface antigens have been investigated. Although hundreds of antibodies have been produced, the most successful one to date, BW 250 183, was originally developed as an antibody against CEA, a tumor glycoprotein; it cross-reacts with a leukocyte cell-surface antigen. Early clinical trials have found most studies to be positive by 3 to 5 hours. The reported sensitivity is greater than 95%. An inherent problem is that murine proteins have the potential for allergic reactions. Fab fragments are being investigated, the advantages being less immunoreactivity and a better target-to-background ratio due to rapid renal clearance.

Chemotactic Peptides

Chemotactic Peptides, produced by bacteria, bind to receptors on the cell membrane of polymorphonuclear leukocytes, stimulating the cells to undergo chemotaxis. Analogues of these peptides have been synthesized and radiolabeled. Localization at sites of infection is rapid, owing to the small size of these compounds; they easily pass through vascular walls and rapidly enter an abscess. The highest target-to-background ratio occurs at 1 hour. Animal studies have been promising; human studies are pending.

Radiolabeled Colloids

Tc-99m albumin colloid   Tc-99m albumin colloid (Microlite, Dupont NEN, North Billerica, Mass.), with a particle size of 0.4 to 2.0 μm, can label leukocytes by taking advantage of the white cell's ability to phagocytize radiolabeled colloid particles. About 50% of the radioactivity is tightly bound to leukocytes. However, the neutrophils tend to lose activity after 2 to 3 hours and in vivo, Tc-99m is easily oxidized to pertechnetate. Because the initial intense uptake fades with time, imaging must performed early. To date, its main application has been in the diagnosis of acute appendicitis. One study reported a sensitivity and specificity of around 90%. Studies were positive between 10 to 60 minutes after injection. However, because there have been a

Table 7-7 Normal Distribution of Radiopharmaceuticals Used for Infection								
Radiopharmaceutical	**Liver**	**Spleen**	**Marrow**	**Bone**	**GI**	**GU**	**Lung**	**Salivary**
Gallium-67	***	*	*	*	***			*
In-111 leukocytes	**	***	**				*	
Tc-99m HMPAO WBCs	**	***	**		**	**	*	
Polyclonal IgG antibodies	***	**	**		*	*	*	

number of indeterminate studies in which the patients had appendicitis, and because of the nonspecificity of Tc-99m albumin colloid for differentiating pelvic inflammatory disease from appendicitis in women, this agent has not found widespread use.

Tc-99m nanocolloids Tc-99m-labeled nanocolloids, most commonly used for bone marrow imaging and lymphoscintigraphy, have also been used for infection imaging. These colloids of human serum albumin are less than 50 nm in size and are preferentially taken up by the reticuloendothelial system of the marrow and to a lesser extent by the liver and spleen. They leave the circulation and localize in the extracellular space at sites of infection, probably due to increased vascular permeability. Nonocolloids have proved useful in the early diagnosis (within 60 minutes) of bone and joint infections; however, the radiotracer has poor sensitivity for infections outside the musculoskeletal system.

SPECIAL CLINICAL PROBLEMS

Osteomyelitis

Pathogenesis In osteomyelitis, bone infection is most commonly bacterial in origin. Organisms reach bone by three mechanisms: (1) hematogenous spread, (2) extension from a contiguous site of infection, and (3) direct introduction of organisms into bone by trauma and surgery.

A) *Acute hematogenous osteomyelitis* involves bone with red marrow. In children, the long bones are most frequently affected because of relatively slow blood flow in metaphyseal sinusoidal veins and the paucity of phagocytes. Infection is often secondary to staphylococcal skin infection.

In adults, acute osteomyelitis rarely involves the long bones because adipose tissue has replaced red marrow. Instead, it most commonly occurs in the vertebral bodies, where the marrow is cellular and has an abundant vascular supply. The initiating event is usually septicemia, often secondary to a urinary tract infection, bacterial endocarditis, or IV drug abuse. Infection usually begins in the vertebral body near the anterior longitudinal ligament and spreads to adjacent vertebrae by direct extension through the disk space or via communicating venous channels. Because the disk in the adult posseses no vascular supply, disk space infection secondary to hematogenous infections is always due to osteomyelitis in an adjacent vertebra.

B) Osteomyelitis due to *extension from a contiguous site of infection* often occurs secondary to soft tissue infection after trauma, radiation therapy, burns, or pressure sores. In patients with vascular insufficiency, organisms may enter the soft tissues through a cutaneous ulcer, often in the foot, causing cellulitis and then osteomyelitis.

C) *Direct introduction of organisms* into bone may occur during open fractures, open surgical reduction of closed fractures, or pentrating trauma by foreign bodies such as bullets. Osteomyelitis may also arise from perioperative contamination of bone during surgery for nontraumatic orthopedic disorders, as in the placement of a joint prosthesis, laminectomy, or diskectomy. Here the causative organism is often normal flora, such *Staphylococcus epidermidis*.

Pathology Pathologic findings during the acute phase of osteomyelitis include neutrophilic inflammation, edema, and vascular congestion. Because of the bone's rigidity, increased intramedullary pressure results, compromising the blood supply and causing ischemia and vascular thrombosis. After several days, the suppurative and ischemic injury may cause bone to fragment into devitalized segments called *sequestra*. Inflammation spreads via Haversian and Volkmann canals to reach the periosteum, where abscesses form. This can lead to soft tissue abscesses or sinus tracts.

With persistent infection, chronic inflammatory cells (lymphocytes, histiocytes, and plasma cells) join the neutrophils. Fibroblastic proliferation and new bone formation occur. Periosteal osteogenesis may surround the inflammation to form a bony envelope or *involucrum*. Occasionally a dense fibrous capsule confines the infection to a localized area of suppuration (Brodie's abscess).

Hematogenous osteomyelitis acquired in childhood or adulthood may present as intermittent or persistent drainage from sinus tracts communicating with the involved bone, usually the femur, tibia, or humerus, or as a soft tissue infection overlying it. Signs of infection may recur after years of quiescence.

Diagnosis Biopsy with culture is the most definitive method for making the diagnosis, but this is invasive and often contraindicated. Contamination of noninfected bone may occur if there is an overlying soft tissue infection and there is the risk of pathological fractures in the small bones of the hands and feet. Noninvasive methods are preferred (Box 7-5).

Plain radiography should be performed in all patients suspected of having osteomyelitis, but the characteristic changes of permeated radiolucencies, destructive changes, and periosteal new bone formation may take 10 to 14 days to develop.

Although not used for diagnosis, CT can be helpful in defining the cortical extent of bone infection and can guide biopsy in suspected vertebral osteomyelitis. However, for the most part, MRI has replaced CT because it can image the marrow as well as demonstrate the extent of cortical infection. It has a reported sensitivity for

> **Box 7-7   Scintigraphic Diagnosis of Osteomyelitis in Different Clinical Situations**
>
> Normal x-ray: 3-phase bone scan.
> Neonates: 3-phase bone scan. If negative; Ga-67.
> Suspected osteomyelitis in non-marrow-containing skeleton (distal extremities); Combined Tc-99m bone scan and In-111 white blood cell study.
> Suspected osteomyelitis in bone marrow-containing skeleton (hips and knees): Combined Tc-99m bone marrow scan and In-111 white blood cell study.
> Suspected vertebral osteomyelitis: Ga-67 or polyclonal IgG studies.

[handwritten annotations: "To confirm osteomyelitis (vs. other pathology)"]

cleared of radiotracer by this time, further delayed images at 18 to 24 hours (fourth phase) can sometimes be helpful when edema slows soft tissue clearance and prevents good bone visualization at 2 to 4 hours. With osteomyelitis, an increased bone-to-soft tissue uptake ratio is seen by 18 to 24 hours. Cellulitis alone will be positive only in the first two phases, with no increased bone uptake on delayed images.

The sensitivity of the three-phase bone scan for osteomyelitis is high, above 95%. A negative three-phase scan (no bony uptake) excludes osteomyelitis with a high degree of certainty. An exception to this is in patients with vascular insufficiency, where flow may actually be decreased.

Table 7-8   Diagnosis of Osteomyelitis: Summed Results From a Literature Review

Type of study	Sensitivity (%)	Specificity (%)
Three-phase bone scan (normal x-ray)	94	95
Three-phase bone scan (underlying bone disease)	95	33
Gallium-67	81	69
In-111 white blood cells	88	85
Tc-99m HmPAO	87	81
MRI	95	88

osteomyelitis of 95% and a specifity of 88%. Typical findings include low signal intensity on T_1-weighted images and high signal intensity on T_2-weighted images. However, any disease that replaces bone marrow and causes increased tissue water, such as healing fractures, tumors, and Charcot joints, may not be distinguishable. Artifacts due to joint implants can degrade images sufficiently to make diagnosis impossible.

Scintigraphic diagnosis

Bone scan   The three-phase bone scan is useful for confirming the diagnosis of osteomyelitis. It will be positive in all three phases (flow, blood pool, and delayed) in osteomyelitis (Figure 7-20). The flow phase shows increased perfusion of the entire vascular region involved secondary to local vasodilation and reactive hyperemia. There is similarly increased uptake on the blood pool images (high count images immediately after the 60-second flow) that represents an expanded extracellular fluid space. Finally, there is increased uptake on the delayed images at 2 to 4 hours which localizes to the bone involved. Although soft tissue has often been

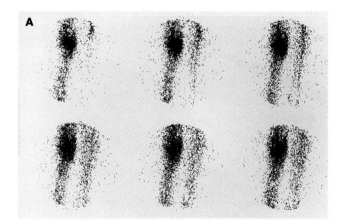

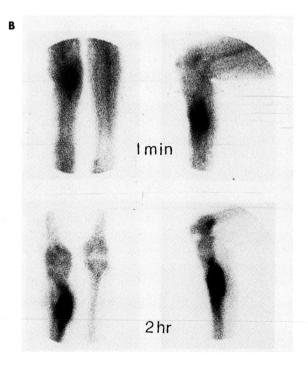

Fig. 7-20   Osteomyelitis of the tibia occurring after compound fracture and multiple operations. The bone scan is positive in three phases. **A**, Increased flow to the right tibia. **B**, Immediate and delayed (2 hour) images are also highly positive at this site.

Specificity depends on the underlying condition of the bone (Table 7-8). In adults with normal radiographs and no reason for increased bone turnover, the specificity of the scan is high (95%) and the diagnosis can be made from the three-phase study alone. When bone remodeling is increased, as may happen with fracture, tumor, an orthopedic device, old, "healed" osteomyelitis, neuropathic joints, or pseudoarthrosis, the specificity of the three-phase scan is reduced and imaging with Ga-67 or In-111 leukocytes may be needed to confirm or exclude the diagnosis (Figures 7-21 to 7-23).

Bone scans in neonates have been reported to have an increased false negative rate for osteomyelitis. Optimal modern instrumentation and methods can minimize this problem. Special attention to the metaphyseal areas is important. The patient and camera must be positioned so that the hot growth plates appear thin and linear; otherwise, apparent "ballooning" of the epiphyseal plates will obscure subtle, asymmetrically increased uptake in a metaphyseal region, often the site of osteomyelitis in children. This requires that both extremities be similarly positioned and the camera head be carefully positioned perpendicular to the growth plate. Cold lesions may occasionally be seen in children; they are due to subperiosteal abscesses that disrupt the predominantly periosteal blood supply.

Gallium-67   Ga-67 has a sensitivity of 81% and a specificity of 69% for the diagnosis of osteomyelitis (Table 7-8). The specificity suffers from the facts that this tracer is normally taken up in cortical bone as well as marrow and that increased uptake occurs whenever there is bone remodeling. To improve specificity, Ga-67 images should be interpreted in conjunction with a bone scan. A positive study is defined as one where Ga-67 uptake is *incongruent* with the bone scan—that is, either there is increased uptake on the Ga-67 study compared to the bone scan, or the uptake occurs in different distributions on the two studies; low-grade uptake (less than bone) on the Ga-67 scan or congruent uptake is interpreted as a negative study (Figure 7-24). However, intense uptake on both is considered equivocal, and infection cannot be ruled out.

Radiolabeled leukocytes   Labeled white cells can be very helpful in making the diagnosis of osteomyelitis. Several studies comparing Ga-67 with In-111-labeled WBCs have favored the latter. The results from numerous studies reported in the medical literature gives a summed mean sensitivity of 88% and a specificity of 85% for In-111-labeled leukocytes. Two prospective studies using In-111 WBCs to evaluate osteomyelitis complicating fracture nonunion had a combined sensitivity of 91% and a specificity of 97%.

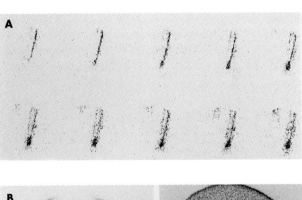

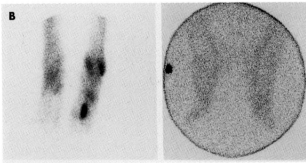

Fig. 7-21   Osteomyelitis; positive on a Tc-99m MDP bone scan and an In-111 leukocyte scan, in a diabetic with peripheral vascular disease, cellulitis, and infection of the first metatarsal. A bone scan was ordered to diagnose osteomyelitis. *Left,* The 2-hour delayed bone scan shows markedly increased uptake in the distal first metatarsal. The first two phases of the study were also positive. *Right,* An In-111 leukocyte study was performed to confirm the diagnosis. Intense uptake is seen in the same distal metatarsal. No uptake is noted in other areas of the foot that were hot on the bone scan (e.g., the distal phalanx of the first toe and the second distal metatarsal), excluding concomitant infection there.

Fig. 7-22   Three-phase positive bone scan compatible with osteomyelitis, but the In-111 WBC scan was negative. **A,** Radionuclide angiogram shows increased flow in the region of the distal left midfoot. **B,** *Left,* A 3-hour delayed image shows increased uptake by the third metatarsal. Ankle uptake is also noted. *Right,* The In-111-leukocyte study is negative for infection. Radiography showed a metatarsal fracture.

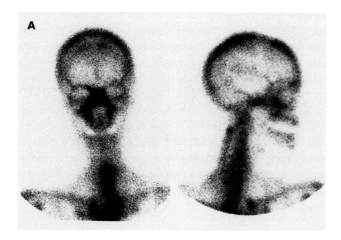

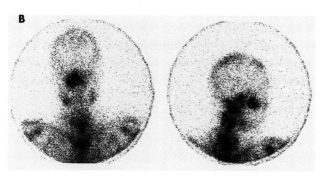

Fig. 7-23   Osteomyelitis of the right maxillary sinus in a patient with previous bilateral sinus surgery. **A**, Bone scan shows bilateral ethmoid and maxillary sinus uptake. **B**, The In-111 WBC study shows uptake just right of midline in a pattern different from the bone scan, consistent with focal maxillary infection—abscess or osteomyelitis.

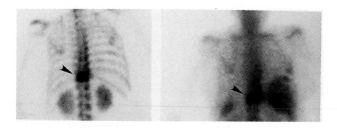

Fig. 7-24   Discordance of Ga-67 and Tc-MDP bone scan. The question of infection arose following a laminectomy. Vertebral Ga-67 uptake was judged to be less than that seen on the Tc-99m MDP bone scan, and the study was interpreted as negative for vertebral osteomyelitis. The low grade Ga-67 uptake was secondary to reactive healing bone.

A lower sensitivity for *vertebral osteomyelitis* using labeled leukocytes has been reported by investigators, with false negatives occurring in 10% to 40% of patients with chronic osteomyelitis of the central skeleton. In this situation, infection cannot be differentiated from metastasis, fracture, Paget's disease, surgical defects, or irradiation. Although Ga-67 will have better sensitivity in the spine, its specificity is poorer, because increased uptake occurs in bone reactive for various reasons, among them fracture, previous infection, and surgery. Radiolabeled IgG may be the best study if preliminary results are confirmed.

Investigations with Tc-99m HMPAO–labeled leukocytes has been encouraging, with results similar to those achieved with In-111 leukocytes. Similar false positive and false negative studies would be anticipated; however, the Tc-99m label has the potential advantage of a higher photon yield that might improve sensitivity and resolution. Like In-111 leukocytes, Tc-99m HMPAO requires about 2 hours of labeling time. Tc-99m nanocolloid has been reported to have a similar sensitivity and specificity for infectious bone and joint disease. In-111 chloride, closely related to Ga-67 citrate, has been reported to have good accuracy for the diagnosis; however, data are limited, and it is not an FDA-approved radiopharmaceutical. Preliminary results with investigational human polyclonal IgG and antigranulocyte antibodies are encouraging, particularly since these agents do not require cell labeling.

Diabetic osteopathy and osteomyelitis   The diagnosis of osteomyelitis in patients with underlying diabetic osteoneuropathy can be difficult. These patients often have overlying soft tissue infection and bone remodeling secondary to neuropathic joints, fractures, or previous surgery.

Although one study in patients with neuropathic foot disease has reported that the combination of a bone scan and In-111 leukocyte study correctly localized infection to bone or soft tissue in 89% of cases, others have not been as successful. One study found rapidly progressing noninfected neuropathic osteoarthropathy of recent on-set to be indistinguishable from osteomyelitis on either scintigraphy or MRI.

Both physical examination of the involved foot to determine the presence or absence of overlying cellulitis, the site of ulcers or drainage, and evidence of previous surgery and correlation with radiographs are extremely important for proper interpretation of the scintigraphic studies. An In-111 or Tc-99m HMPAO leukocyte study in conjunction with a three-phase bone scan is frequently needed to make the diagnosis. Neuropathic joints and recent fractures can have low-grade uptake on white cell imaging.

Bone infarction versus osteomyelitis in sickle cell disease   Neither a bone scan nor a bone marrow scan often makes this differential diagnosis alone. Although decreased uptake on a bone scan might be anticipated with infarction, this early finding is rarely seen, and increased uptake is the rule. With marrow scanning, decreased uptake will be seen with infection and infarction. Infection imaging with In-111 or Tc-99m HMAPO leukocytes is usually necessary for differentiation.

Infected joint prostheses Differentiation of loosening from infection in surgically implanted joint prostheses is often a difficult clinical problem. The symptoms and signs of infection are frequently indolent and often are not associated with systemic signs and symptoms. Joint aspiration has a low sensitivity for the diagnosis of infection (12%-66%). Radiography also has poor sensitivity, while bone scans have poor specificity for this diagnosis.

The use of Ga-67 scintigraphy in conjunction with Tc-99m bone scans and more recently the use of In-111 leukocyte scintigraphy in combination with a Tc-99m SC bone marrow study have proved quite useful for diagnosing infection. Ga-67 scintigraphy is suboptimal because of the increased uptake invariably seen secondary to reactive bone as a result of surgery and the implanted prosthesis. In-111-labeled leukocyte imaging is superior. A good prospective comparison study of Ga-67 and In-111-labeled WBC scintigraphy in patients with prostheses demonstrated an accuracy for In-111 leukocytes of 94%, versus 75% for Ga-67.

Increased uptake at the tip of the prosthesis on In-111 leukocyte scintigraphy can be seen normally after surgery and sometimes persists for years. However, the intensity of uptake is usually low grade and decreases over time. Intense uptake or increasing uptake would suggest infection.

In-111 leukocyte imaging alone may sometimes yield false positive results in areas where there is an altered distribution due to reactive or displaced marrow, as may occur as a result of surgery. The Tc-99m SC marrow scan can serve as a template for comparison. Normal In-111 leukocyte imaging gives a picture of marrow distribution nearly identical to that seen with Tc-99m SC bone marrow imaging. If the In-111 leukocyte study shows increased uptake in an area that is cold or dissimilar to the marrow study, the diagnosis of infection is made (Figure 7-25). No infection is present if the In-111 leukocyte study shows an uptake pattern identical to that seen on the marrow scan. Because of its proven high accuracy, this combination of studies has become the standard approach to diagnosing infection in hip prostheses.

DIAGNOSIS OF INFECTION IN AIDS

This section discusses radionuclide studies useful for establishing the cause of infections in patients with AIDS, arranged by organ systems.

Pulmonary Infections

Ga-67 is very useful for the differentiation of AIDS-related pulmonary disorders. *Pneumocystis carinii* pneumonia is usually the first pulmonary manifestation in AIDS patients, and with time, more than 80% of patients develop the infection. Ga-67 scans are abnormal in 85% to 95% of cases. It is not uncommon for patients with normal chest radiographs to have increased Ga-67 uptake as the earliest finding. With severe pulmonary involvement and an abnormal chest radiograph, the lung uptake of Ga-67 may actually decrease, reflecting a deficient immune response and poor prognosis.

The characteristic pattern of *Pneumocystis* infection is that of *diffuse*, either uniform or nonuniform, bilateral pulmonary Ga-67 uptake with intensity greater than liver (no nodal or parotid uptake) (Figure 7-5). In the proper clinical setting, this pattern has a specificity of greater than 90%. Ga-67 uptake at initial presentation typically is higher than that after the treatment of recurrences. Prophylactic aerosolized pentamidine therapy can result in a very atypical and heterogeneous pattern of uptake.

Cytomegalovirus The characteristic scintigraphic pattern is low-grade lung uptake with perihilar prominence, eye uptake (due to associated retinitis), adrenal and renal uptake, and persistent colon uptake associated with diarrheal symptoms (Figure 7-19A).

Bacterial infections Unusual infections with *Actinomyces* or *nocardia* may be suspected if pulmonary and local bone invasion are noted in AIDS patients. Intense Ga-67 uptake in a lobar configuration in the absence of nodal and parotid uptake suggests bacterial pneumonia. In acute bacterial infections, In-111 leukocyte scintigraphy has an 80% sensitivity. However, it is not useful for most other pulmonary infections.

Mycobacterial infection *M. avium-intracellulare* causes widespread disease in 25% to 50% of AIDS patients and requires more aggressive therapy than

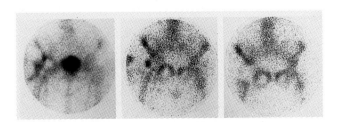

Fig. 7-25 Infected hip prosthesis. *Left,* Tc-99m MDP bone scan shows increased uptake in the region of the right hip prosthesis laterally. *Middle,* In-111 leukocyte study shows focal intense uptake consistent with infection (*arrowhead*). *Right,* Tc-99m SC marrow study shows a normal bone marrow distribution. The mismatch of the bone marrow and In-111 leukocyte study is diagnostic of an infected prosthesis.

that used for tuberculosis. Delays in diagnosis, often due to initial treatment for *Pneumocystis*, contribute to a high morbidity. Patchy lung uptake with hilar and non-hilar nodal (axillary and inguinal) Ga-67 uptake suggests this disease.

Lymphoid interstitial pneumonia   Although the radiographic appearance in this disease may be normal or similar to that seen in *P. carinii* pneumona, viral infections, or miliary tuberculosis, Ga-67 has a diagnostic pattern of low grade diffuse pulmonary uptake *without* nodal uptake and associated symmetrically increased parotid uptake.

Neoplasms   AIDS-related lymphoma is less common than mycobacterial infection and can be differentiated on Ga-67 scintigraphy by its characteristic bulky nodal pattern of uptake. Kaposi's sarcoma is Ga-67 negative, but positive on Tl-201 imaging.

Gastrointestinal Infections

Oral and esophageal candidiasis are common fungal infections in AIDS patients. The diagnosis can usually be made with an upper GI series or endoscopy but may be seen on Ga-67 scintigraphy. Debilitating diarrhea is most commonly caused by the protozoon *Cryptosporidium*. Ga-67 uptake in bowel equal to or greater than liver uptake that intensifies over time often represents infection. Proximal small bowel uptake is usually due to *Cryptosporidium*. In-111 leukocytes may be more specific than Ga-67 for intestinal infection because of the latter's normal bowel clearance.

When stool cultures are negative for *Salmonella* or *Shigella*, diffuse uptake that does not change may be due to cytomegalovirus infection or antibiotic-induced colitis. Concomitant eye, adrenal, esophageal, and low-grade pulmonary uptake is suggestive of cytomegalovirus. Multifocal activity (right paratracheal and bowel) activity is indicative of myocobaterial infection.

COMMENTS ON METHODOLOGY

When more than one study is required to make the diagnosis of infection, attention to the imaging characteristics of the various radionuclides becomes important. Which study should be done first? How much time is required between studies? Can they be performed simultaneously? One needs to consider the various photopeaks of the radiopharmaceuticals, the half-lives, relative administered doses, and the camera's capability for multichannel acquisition.

The simplest method is to perform the Tc-99m scan first. With a 6-hour half-life, most has decayed by 24 hours. If a Tc-99m marrow or bone scan is done in combination with a Ga-67 study, the Ga-67 can be injected immediately after imaging the Tc-99m tracer because the Tc-99m will decay before Ga-67 imaging is performed, usually at 48 hours. If In-111 leukocytes are used, the blood for cell labeling can be drawn immediately before injection of the Tc-99m tracer, and the labeled cells reinjected after the bone scan; In-111 imaging is then performed at 18 to 24 hours. The two radiopharmaceuticals can be imaged simultaneously with dual-isotope acquisition. This approach ensures identically positioned images. With this method, only the upper 247 keV photopeak of In-111 should be used because of overlap of the 140 keV Tc-99m and the 173 In-111 keV 20% windows.

Labeling lymphocytes

Labeled lymphocytes could potentially be used for diagnose more chronic infections as well as to detect rejection of kidney and heart transplants. Only limited investigation has been done in this area, some of it encouraging. Unlike neutrophils, however, lymphocytes are quite radiosensitive. There are concerns about radiation effects on function and the potential for oncogenesis because of the lymphocytes' long life span.

SUGGESTED READINGS

Coleman RE: Radiolabeled leukocytes. In Freeman LM and Weissmann HS, editors: *Nuclear medicine annual 1982*, New York, 1982, Raven Press, Ltd.

Datz FL: The current status of radionuclide infection imaging. In Freeman LM, editor: *Nuclear medicine annual 1993*, New York, 1993, Raven Press, Ltd.

Datz FL and Taylor AT Jr: Cell labeling: Techniques and clinical utility. In *Freeman and Johnson's clinical radionuclide imaging*, ed 3, Update, 1986, Grune & Stratton, Inc.

Ganz WI and Serafini A: The diagnostic role of nuclear medicine in acquired immunodeficiency syndrome, *J Nucl Med* 30:1935-1945, 1989.

McAfee JG and Samin A: In-111 labeled leukocytes: A review of problems in image interpretation, *Radiology* 155:221-229, 1985.

Merkel KD, Brown ML, Dewanjee MK, and Fitzgerald RH Jr: Comparison of Indium-labeled-leukocyte imaging with sequential Technetium-Gallium scanning in the diagnosis of low-grade musculoskeletal sepsis, *J Bone Joint Surg* 67-A:465-476, 1985.

Schauwecker DS: The scintigraphic diagnosis of osteomyelitis, *AJR* 158:9-18, 1992.

CHAPTER 8

Tumors

Oncology has always represented a significant portion of the studies performed in nuclear medicine and continues to be a growing area of application. Many radionuclide studies performed for the detection of primary and metastatic tumors are described in other chapters. Most are organ specific, and not tumor specific; among these are Tc-99m MDP bone scans, I-123 and Tc-99m pertechnetate thyroid scans, Tc-99m sulfur colloid liver-spleen scans, and Tc-99m DTPA or Tc-99m glucoheptonate (Tc-99m GH) brain scans. Although these studies can detect tumor, the hot spot or cold spot abnormalities could also be due to benign nontumorous diseases of these organs (Box 8-1).

Box 8-1 Overview of Tumor Scintigraphy

ORGAN-SPECIFIC TUMOR IMAGING RADIONUCLIDES

Cold spot imaging

Thyroid imaging: I-123 or Tc-99m pertechnetate
Liver imaging: Tc-99m SC

Hot spot imaging

Conventional brain imaging: Tc-99m DTPA or glucoheptonate
Bone imaging: Tc-99m MDP, HDP
Hepatic arterial perfusion imaging: Tc-99m MAA
Lymphoscintigraphy: Tc-99m antimony SC

NONSPECIFIC TUMOR IMAGING RADIONUCLIDES

Gallium-67
Thallium-201
Tc-99m sestamibi
PET (F-18 FDG)

TUMOR-TYPE-SPECIFIC RADIONUCLIDES

Thyroid cancer: I-131
Adrenal tumors: I-131 MIBG or I-131 NP-59
Hepatocyte origin tumors: Tc-99m HIDA
Hemangiomas: Tc-99m RBCs
Radiolabeled monoclonal antibodies against tumor surface antigens
Radiolabeled peptides (e.g., somatostatin receptor imaging)

A few radionuclide studies are tumor-type specific, such as I-131 whole body thyroid cancer scans performed post thyroidectomy, and adrenal tumor imaging with I-131 metaiodobenzylquanidine (MIBG) and I-131-6-β-iodomethyl-19-norcholesterol (I-131 NP-59).

This chapter focuses on radiopharmaceuticals and radionuclide techniques not discussed elsewhere, nonspecific tumor imaging radionuclides, such as gallium-67 (Ga-67), thallium-201 (Tl-201), and Tc-99m sestamibi, and some newer radiopharmaceuticals that are potentially tumor-specific imaging agents, such as radiolabeled monoclonal antibodies and peptides. Lymphoscintigraphy will be briefly reviewed, and the exciting and rapidly growing role for positron emission tomography (PET) in oncology will be discussed.

GALLIUM-67 TUMOR IMAGING

Although initially investigated as a bone imaging agent, Ga-67 citrate was first used clinically in 1969 for tumor localization in Hodgkin's disease. Later its infection and inflammation imaging capability was appreciated. To date, the staging and follow-up of Hodgkin's disease and non-Hodgkin's lymphoma remain a predominant clinical indication for Ga-67 scintigraphy, although Ga-67 is taken up to varying degrees by many other tumors. Clinical studies have found Ga-67 particularly useful for imaging metastatic melanoma and diagnosing hepatocellular carcinoma. Although sometimes used to detect other tumors, among them tumors of the lung, head and neck, and soft tissues, its overall clinical role here is less certain.

An important area of increasing interest is the use of Ga-67 as a marker of tumor viability. It is particularly useful for determining the effectiveness of radiation therapy or chemotherapy.

Chemistry and Physics

Gallium is a group III element (see the periodic table in the Appendix) with biological behavior similar to that of the ferric ion. The radionuclide Ga-67 is cyclotron produced by bombardment of Zn-68. It decays by electron capture and has a physical half-life of 78 hours. Ga-67 emits a complex spectrum of gamma rays ranging from 91 to 394 keV (approximately 100, 200, 300, and 400 keV) (Table 8-1); the lower two or three photopeaks are used for imaging because of their higher percent abundance.

Table 8-1 Physical Characteristics of Tumor Imaging Radiopharmaceuticals

Radiopharmaceutical	Physical Half-life	Principal Mode of Isotopic Decay	Photopeaks keV	(% Abundance)	Usual Dose
Gallium-67	78 hr	Electron capture	93	(41)	10 mCi
			185	(23)	
			300	(18)	
			394	(4)	
Thallium-201	73 hr	Electron capture	69-83	(94)	3 mCi
			167	(10)	
			135	(3)	
Tc-99m (Sestamibi)	6 hr	Isomeric transition	140		25 mCi
F-18 (FDG)	120 min	Positron	511		10 mCi
In-111 (OncoScint)	67.2 hr (2.8 d)	Electron capture	173	(90)	5 mCi
			247	(94)	

Pharmacokinetics and Normal Distribution

After injection, Ga-67 binds to serum transferrin in the blood. Unlike the ferric ion, it cannot be reduced in vivo from its +3 oxidation state, and therefore it does not interact with protoporphyrins to form heme. Within 24 hours, 15% to 25% is excreted by the kidneys. Thereafter clearance is slow (biological $T_{1/2}$ of 25 days), with the colon being the major route of excretion. Ga-67 localizes intracellularly within normal liver, lacrimal and salivary glands, spleen, bone marrow, and bone, primarily by binding to iron-binding proteins of ferritin and lactoferrin. Because iron competes with gallium for binding to transferrin, saturation of transferrin with iron in vivo, as seen clinically with iron overload from repeated transfusions, will result in an altered biodistribution, with less hepatic and greater renal uptake.

Mechanism of Tumor Localization

The mechanism of Ga-67 localization is incompletely understood. After binding to transferrin in the blood, it enters the tumor's extracellular fluid space via the tumor's leaky capillary endothelium. Ga-67 is bound to the tumor cell surface by tranferrin receptors and then transported into the cell, where it binds to iron-binding proteins such as ferritin and lactoferrin. These proteins are found in increased concentration in tumors. The radiopharmaceutical localizes intracellularly in the lysosomes of tumor cells. Importantly, Ga-67 is taken up by actively growing and viable tumor, not by necrotic tumor or fibrosis.

Dosimetry

Larger doses of Ga-67 are administered for tumor imaging than for infection and inflammation imaging. With an adult dose of 10 mCi, the large bowel receives the highest radiation dose, about 9.0 rads (Table 8-2).

Table 8-2	Ga-67 Estimated Radiation Absorbed Dose	
	rads/mCi	rads/10 mCi (cGy/370 MBq)
Large intestine	0.90	9.0
Marrow	0.58	5.8
Spleen	0.53	5.3
Liver	0.46	4.6
Small intestine	0.36	3.6
Skeleton	0.44	4.4
Kidneys	0.41	4.1
Ovaries	0.28	2.8
Testes	0.24	2.4
Total body	**0.26**	**2.6**

From MIRD Dose Estimate Report No. 2. MIRD Primer, Loevinger R, Budinger TF, and Watson EE, Editors, 1988.

The spleen and bone marrow are next receiving 5 to 6 rads; the total body dose is 2.6 rads. Appreciable amounts of Ga-67 are excreted in breast milk.

Methodology

Ga-67 is not an ideal radionuclide for scintigraphic imaging. Neither the low- nor the high-energy photons are well suited for present-day gamma cameras. Slow background clearance, normal uptake by liver, bone, and marrow, and considerable activity in the bowel result in suboptimal images. Nevertheless, Ga-67's tumor avidity makes it a clinically useful radiopharmaceutical.

Much of the medical literature on the utility of Ga-67 was published by the early 1980s, when older camera technology and now outdated techniques were used. These reports often underestimated Ga-67's present-day accuracy with state-of-the-art imaging. Major technical advances in gamma cameras and changes in methodology have greatly improved image quality and tumor detectability.

Technical factors To maximize sensitivity and minimize false negative studies, images must contain an adequate count density to detect small foci of active tumor. Limitations include camera sensitivity, activity administered, and acquisition time. Multiple photopeaks (at least two, and preferably three) should be used to maximize photon detectability. Because imaging time has practical limits, the administered dose is of primary importance. Although 3 to 5 mCi of Ga-67 is typically used for infection imaging in adults, higher doses of 8 to 10 mCi are recommended for tumor imaging. The superior images and improved capability for performing single photon emission computed tomography (SPECT) result in a clear-cut benefit-risk ratio for the higher dose in these cancer patients.

Although 500k counts per view may be adequate for routine whole body imaging, higher count images (1,000k) are needed for evaluating areas of previous disease or regions that are positive on computed tomography (CT) but negative on routine planar imaging. These high count images should be performed with organs of normally high uptake (e.g., liver) mostly out of the field of view.

The larger dose also permits delayed imaging when more background has cleared. This increases detectability, owing to the improved tumor-to-background ratio. The exact protocol varies, depending on the laboratory; some image at 48 and 72 hours and obtain delayed images as needed 7 to 10 days after injection, others prefer to initiate imaging at 72 hours and do delayed imaging 10 to 14 days after tracer injection. Box 8-2 describes a typical tumor imaging protocol.

Improvements in camera technology over the years have also been a major factor in improving image quality and the detectability of Ga-67. Much of the older litera-

---

Box 8-2 Ga-67 Tumor Imaging: Protocol Summary

PATIENT PREPARATION

Bowel preparation optional.

RADIOPHARMACEUTICAL DOSE

Adult dose—10 mCi; pediatric dose—75-100 μCi/kg (minimum 500 μCi)

IMAGING PLAN

Whole body images at 48 and 72 hr and 7 days. SPECT of chest and/or abdomen at 48 and 72 hr.

PLANAR

Camera: Large field of view.
Collimator: Medium energy parallel hole.
Photopeaks: 20% windows around 93, 184, and 296 keV.
Computer acquisition matrix: 128×128 byte mode.

PROCEDURE

1. Inject Ga-67 IV.
2. Acquire 500k spot images for the anterior chest and the other whole body spot images for equal time. Views should include anterior and posterior images of the chest, abdomen, and pelvis, and an anterior head view. Regions of special interest require 1,000k. Axillae should be imaged with the arms elevated; inguinal views are seen in the anterior pelvic view.

SPECT

Camera:	Single-headed	Dual-headed
Collimator:	Medium energy	Two medium energy
Rotation:	360°	360°
Patient:	Supine	Supine
Computer acquisition parameters:	64×64 matrix	128×128 matrix
	128 images/360° arc	120 images/360° 60 stops/head
	20 sec/image	40 sec/stop at 48 hr
PROCESSING		
	Filtered backprojection	Filtered backprojection
	Attenuation correction:	Attenuation correction:
	Chest: no	Chest: no
	Abdomen: yes	Abdomen: yes

---

ture on tumor detectability used what would be now considered outdated instrumentation, such as rectilinear scanners or gamma cameras of older vintage. The modern-day high-resolution gamma cameras with multichannel acquisition and tomographic capability have clearly improved image quality (Figures 8-1 to 8-4).

SPECT has been an exceedingly important advance. Chest and abdominal SPECT should be performed routinely, especially in areas of clinical concern when planar imaging is negative or uncertain. With 8 to 10 mCi Ga-67 doses, high quality SPECT images can be obtained at 48, 72, and often 96 hours. SPECT image acquisition on sequential days has been suggested for the abdomen to ensure that bowel activity is not misinterpreted as tumor. The latter will be unchanged, while bowel activity will normally clear.

Because chemotherapy can affect biodistribution of Ga-67, it is recommended that there be a 3- to 6-week interval from the last complete course of therapy.

False positive Ga-67 studies are not common. Other than in the abdomen, where delayed bowel clearance of the radiotracer may occasionally cause misinterpretation, Ga-67 uptake in hilar lymph nodes can occasionally pose a problem due to concomitant inflammatory dis-

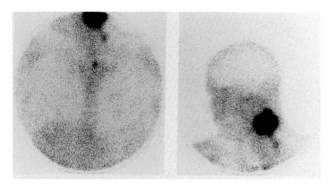

Fig. 8-1   Hodgkin's disease in a 25-year-old man presenting as a left neck mass. *Right*, Prominent Ga-67 uptake is seen in the neck mass. *Left*, Anterior view. Two additional foci of tumor are noted, one just inferior to the large mass on the left and a second one in the mediastinum.

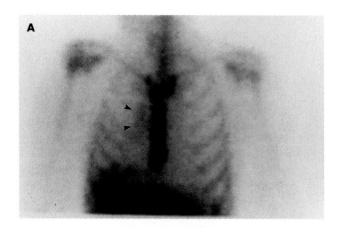

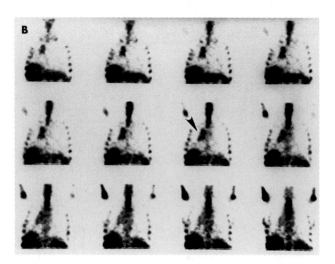

Fig. 8-3   Ga-67 planar and SPECT study in a 35-year-old patient with Hodgkin's disease. **A**, The anterior planar chest image shows low-intensity uptake in the right hilum (*arrowheads*). **B**, SPECT sequential coronal chest slices show clear-cut hilar uptake (*arrowhead*) caused by improved contrast resolution compared to planar imaging.

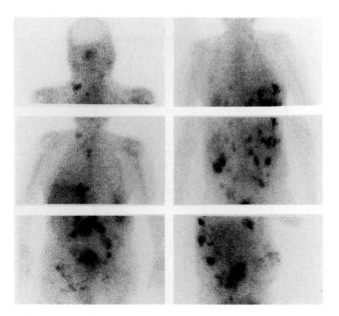

Fig. 8-2   Ga-67 whole body scan in a 67-year-old man with non-Hodgkin's lymphoma. Many sites of tumor uptake are seen. *Left column*, Anterior views of the head, chest, and abdomen/pelvis (*top to bottom*). *Right column*, Posterior views of the chest, abdomen, and a right lateral view of the abdomen/pelvis (*bottom*).

ease; in these uncertain cases, Tl-201 can be used to differentiate benign nodal uptake from tumor. Tl-201 is not usually taken up in inflammatory disease. Benign nodal processes will be gallium avid but thallium negative.

Image Interpretation

Normal Ga-67 distribution   Gallium-67 normally localizes in the liver, spleen, bone, and bone marrow (see Figure 7-1). Splenic uptake is less than liver. Variable uptake is seen in the salivary and lacrimal glands, nasal mucosa, external genitalia, and the female breast.

Breast uptake varies with changes in the hormonal state and may be particularly prominent post-partum (see Figure 7-2).

Salivary gland uptake may become quite prominent following radiation therapy to the head and neck or sometimes after chemotherapy, and this can persist for years. Faint hilar uptake can sometimes be seen. Thymus uptake occurs in children and must be differentiated from mediastinal disease. The kidneys are seen at 24 hours but usually appear faint by 48 to 72 hours.

Large bowel clearance is variable and can pose problems in interpretation. Laxatives and enemas may speed

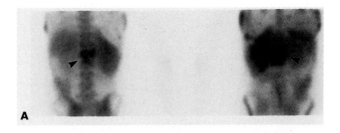

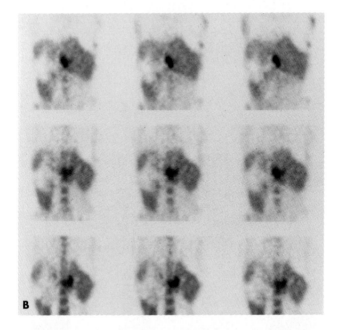

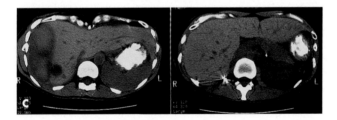

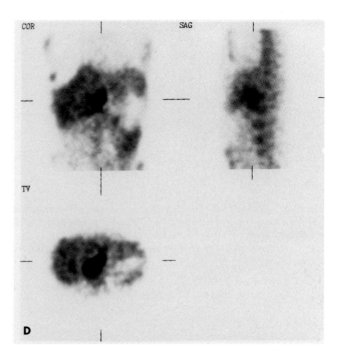

Fig. 8-4 Non-Hodgkins lymphoma in a 26-year-old woman. **A,** The anterior (*left*) and posterior (*right*) planar images suggest uptake in the periaortic or vertebral region (*arrowheads*). **B,** High-contrast SPECT coronal views clearly confirm prevertebral peri-aortic node involvement. Also seen is a subcapsular defect in the right lobe of the liver due to a hematoma caused by liver biopsy. **C,** *Left,* CT shows the large hematoma in a superior cut. *Right,* The tumor mass is anterior to the spine in a lower cut. **D,** Three-view SPECT study of the same patient shows the tumor to be anterior to the spine. This is best seen in the lateral view.

clearance, but more delayed imaging at 3 to 7 days is often necessary to differentiate intra-abdominal tumor from normal bowel clearance.

Faint or absent liver uptake may occur secondary to competition from extensive tumor uptake or, occasionally, from nonmalignant noninflammatory causes of hepatic insufficiency. Chemotherapeutic agents, such as vincristine administered within 24 hours of Ga-67 injection, can depress liver uptake. Iron overload may decrease liver uptake and increase renal clearance. Increased renal uptake is also seen with hepatic failure and has been associated with cytoxan and vincristine therapy.

Pitfalls Pitfalls in interpretation that should be kept in mind include the following: Surgical wounds may have increased uptake for 1 to 2 weeks postoperatively; faint activity may persist for up to a month. Focal bone uptake may occur following marrow biopsy (Figure 8-5). Soft tissue uptake may be seen at injection sites, (e.g., intramuscular iron therapy). Lymphangiography can result in prominent pulmonary uptake. If required, it should be performed after Ga-67 imaging. Axillary node uptake can be missed if imaging is performed with the arms down instead of elevated (Figure 8-6).

Tumor Detectability

The ability of Ga-67 to detect tumors depends on multiple factors. The histology of the tumor is an important

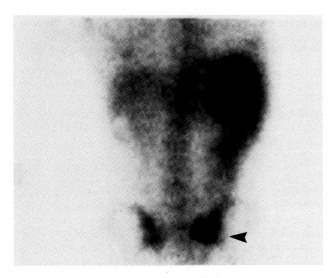

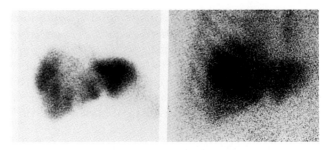

Fig. 8-7   Hepatocellular carcinoma: planar imaging. Tc-99m SC (*left*) and Ga-67 (*right*) anterior planar images in a patient with cirrhosis and suspected hepatoma. The Tc-99m liver scan (*left*) shows an extensive area of decreased uptake in the right and left lobes. The Ga-67 study shows increased uptake in most of these same areas, consistent with hepatoma. Note the separation of the chest wall laterally from the liver due to ascites.

Fig. 8-5   Posterior pelvic view showing Ga-67 uptake in the right superior iliac spine (*arrowhead*) following recent bone marrow biopsy.

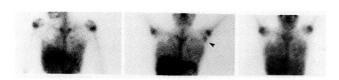

Fig. 8-6   Abnormal axillary node uptake in non-Hodgkin's lymphoma. Initial study (*left and middle*). Left axillary Ga-67 uptake (*arrowhead*) is seen only with the arms elevated. A follow-up study 3 months later (*right*) shows resolution of the nodal involvement.

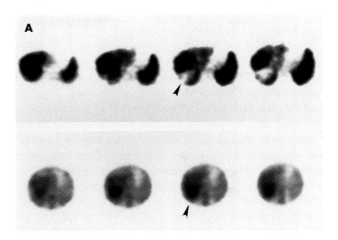

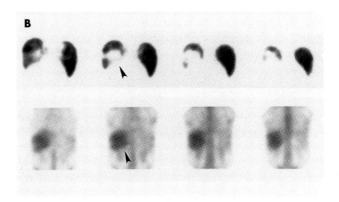

Fig. 8-8   Hepatoma: SPECT imaging (different patient from Figure 8-7), transaxial (**A**) and coronal slices (**B**). SPECT was performed using an aging, single-headed rotating gamma camera. The Tc-99m SC liver spleen sections (*top*) show a large defect (*arrowheads*) in the posterior aspect of the right lobe. In comparable sections, the Ga-67 study (*bottom*) shows increased uptake (*arrowheads*) in the same area, consistent with a hepatoma.

determinant. Lesion size is another. Tumors less than 2 cm in size are not reliably detected with conventional planar imaging. Those 2 to 5 cm in diameter can usually be seen, while tumor masses larger than 5 cm are sometimes poorly visualized, probably due to tumor necrosis. Anatomic location also affects sensitivity for tumor detection. Superfical lesions are easier to detect than deep ones. The improved contrast resolution of SPECT allows detection of smaller and more centrally located lesions.

Detection of tumor in the liver and spleen is complicated by the normal uptake of Ga-67 in these organs. When intrahepatic tumor is suspected, a Tc-99m SC study should be obtained prior to Ga-67 injection and used for comparison. Cold regions (photopenic defects) on the Tc-99m SC study that "fill in" on Ga-67 imaging are positive for tumor or infection. This observation has been particularly useful for diagnosing hepatoma in a cirrhotic liver (Figures 8-7, 8-8).

The detection of mediastinal, hilar, and paratracheal uptake on planar imaging is enhanced by acquiring both anterior oblique views, for normal uptake in the sternum, spine, and ribs can obscure good visualization. SPECT is particularly useful here—in fact, it is mandatory for state-of-the art Ga-67 imaging (Figure 8-2). Breast uptake may occasionally be confused with intrathoracic disease. Lateral or oblique images can clarify the question.

Bowel preparation with laxatives and enemas is used routinely in some laboratories to clear intestinal activity. Others have not found this helpful. Excessive enema use may even induce mucosal inflammation and Ga-67 uptake. Sequential imaging over several days is often necessary to determine if the activity in question remains fixed and represents tumor uptake or moves intraluminally through the bowel.

Clinical Applications

Ga-67 has been used for staging tumors, determining the extent of disease, and following disease course and response to therapy in tumors shown to be Ga-67 avid. However, tumors are highly variable in their ability to take up gallium (Table 8-3). Even though a tumor type may generally be gallium avid and have a high sensitivity for tumor in a particular patient group, any individual patient may have tumor that does not take up Ga-67. In addition, in the same patient, Ga-67 avidity of a primary lesion may be different from that of metastases.

Hodgkin's disease and non-Hodgkin's lymphoma

Cures and long-term complete remissions can be achieved in a large percentage of patients with Hodgkin's disease and in many with high-grade and intermediate-grade non-Hodgkin's lymphomas, using aggressive combination chemotherapy and/or radiation therapy.

Hodgkin's disease and non-Hodgkin's lymphoma differ clinically as well as pathologically (Table 8-4). *Hodgkin's disease* normally presents as an orderly, contiguous spread of lymph node involvement in young patients. It is associated with a high cure rate. *Non-Hodgkin's lymphomas* are characterized by variable histologies, multicentric disease, a highly variable clinical course that may be indolent or rapidly lethal, and a high inci-

Table 8-4 Malignant Lymphomas		
	Hodgkin's Disease	**Non-Hodgkin's Lymphoma**
Cellular derivation	Unresolved	90% B-cell
		10% T-cell
Sites of disease		
Localized	Common	Uncommon
Nodal spread	Contiguous	Discontiguous
Extranodal	Uncommon	Common
Mediastinal	Common	Uncommon
Abdominal	Uncommon	Common
Bone marrow	Uncommon	Common
Systemic symptoms	Uncommon	Common
Curability	>75%	<25%

dence of extranodal tumor involvement. Although mediastinal masses are common with Hodgkin's disease, they are present in only 20% of patients with non-Hodgkin's lymphoma, in whom abdominal presentations involving mesenteric and retroperitoneal nodes are more common. Treatment and prognosis depend on the stage of disease in Hodgkin's disease but on histologic subtype in non-Hodgkin's lymphoma.

Tumor staging and accuracy   Ga-67 can detect both nodal and visceral tumor involvement in Hodgkin's disease and in high- and intermediate-grade non-Hodgkin's lymphomas. It is a highly sensitive method for detecting mediastinal disease, superficial regional lymph nodes, and, to a lesser extent, intra-abdominal and para-aortic nodal involvement.

Detection of Hodgkin's disease   The reported accuracy of Ga-67 in tumor imaging is probably underestimated, for a number of reasons. Many of these studies were performed with what are considered today low doses of Ga-67 and outdated camera technology and techniques. Despite these limitations, however, even the older medical literature noted a high sensitivity for Ga-67 in Hodgkin's disease, approaching 90%. Nodular sclerosing, mixed cellularity, and lymphocyte-depleted tumor types are detected with the highest sensitivity, while lymphocyte-predominant tumors have a lower rate of detection, 79% (Table 8-5).

Detection of non-Hodgkin's lymphoma   Ga-67 imaging also has good sensitivity for high-grade non-Hodgkin's lymphoma, but its sensitivity for low- and intermediate-grade lymphomas is poorer. It is very sensitive for histiocytic lymphoma (89%) and Burkitt's lymphoma (85%) but less sensitive for mixed-cellularity and poorly differentiated lymphocytic subtypes (70%) and well-differentiated lymphocytic lymphomas (59%).

Tumor terminology has now changed to emphasize B-cell and T-cell origin, and studies are needed to reevalu-

Table 8-3 Sensitivity of Ga-67 for Tumor Detection		
Tumor	**Sensitivity (%)**	**Clinical Utility**
Hodgkin's disease	>90	+++
Non-Hodgkin's lymphoma	59-85	+++
Hepatoma	90	+++
Soft tissue sarcomas	93	+++
Melanoma	82-99	++
Lung cancer	85-90	++
Head and neck tumors	56-86	++
Abdominal and pelvic tumors	25-74	+

Table 8-5 Rye Classification of Hodgkin's Disease		
Histologic Subgroup	Incidence (%)	Prognosis
Lymphocyte predominant	2-10	Excellent
Nodular sclerosis	40-80	Very good
Mixed cellularity	20-40	Good
Lymphocyte depleted	2-15	Poor

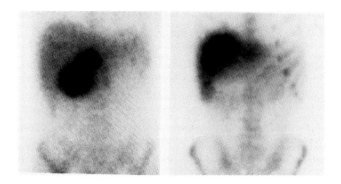

Fig. 8-9 Resolution of Ga-67 uptake with appropriate chemotherapy in a patient with non-Hodgkin's lymphoma. *Left,* A large portal hepatis mass is seen prior to therapy. *Right,* After therapy, no Ga-67 uptake is seen, although there appears to be a photopenic mass effect just below the liver due to residual nonviable tumor.

ate sensitivity with these changes in classification. However, because Ga-67 is less sensitive than CT for detecting disease, it is not commonly used for preoperative staging. Its primary role is in determining tumor viability after therapy.

Tumor viability post therapy Inability to achieve a complete remission is associated with limited survival. Chest radiography and CT often do not reliably distinguish between complete and partial remissions. A common problem after radiation therapy or chemotherapy is the residual mediastinal or abdominal mass detected radiographically without other evidence of active disease. This is particularly common in patients with bulky disease and often does not represent viable tumor post therapy, but rather necrosis and fibrosis. Only complete extraction of the mass can provide definitive proof, and this is usually impossible. Biopsy and needle aspiration are associated with severe sampling errors.

Ga-67 can resolve the dilemma of a residual post-therapy mass by virtue of being an indicator of tumor viability, and as a result it can have signficant impact on the management of patients with lymphoma. A pretherapy study is required to ensure initial Ga-67 uptake at sites involved with disease before scintigraphy is used to evaluate the effectiveness of therapy. Ga-67 uptake within a residual mass is consistent with viable tumor, while a negative scan confirms a complete response to therapy (Figure 8-9). The Ga-67 scan is best interpreted in conjunction with CT, and the highest accuracy is obtained when both studies are interpreted together.

SPECT greatly improves contrast resolution and is often able to demonstrate disease when planar images appear normal. It is particularly valuable in separating superimposed normal Ga-67 activity (e.g., uptake by soft tissue, sternum, liver, and bone) from underlying pathology (Figures 8-2, 8-3). Recent data have shown a sensitivity of 95% and a specificity of 90% for SPECT in demonstrating mediastinal Hodgkin's disease, and a sensitivity of 92% and specificity of 99% for non-Hodgkin's lymphoma, representing a 10% to 15% improvement over planar imaging.

Malignant melanoma Most malignant melanomas and metastases are gallium avid. At some institutions,

Ga-67 has been used to detect and follow metastatic melanoma in patients undergoing chemotherapy or immunotherapy. The overall sensitivity and specificity for detecting metastatic melanoma are reported to be 82% and 99%, respectively, with a tomographic scanner.

Hepatoma Although hepatocellular carcinoma often presents as a single mass lesion in an otherwise normal liver, it is frequently multifocal in patients with cirrhotic livers. Because most hepatomas are gallium avid, Ga-67 can be useful for differentiating hepatoma from regenerating hepatic nodules (pseudotumors) that are seen on CT in patients with cirrhosis (Figures 8-7, 8-8). Approximately 90% of hepatomas are gallium avid, with 63% concentrating more Ga-67 activity than the liver, 25% having uptake equal to that of surrounding liver, and 12% showing less uptake. Although other hepatic lesions besides hepatoma may take up Ga-67, such as abscess or gallium-avid metastatic disease, proper interpretation is aided by knowing the clinical setting. Biopsy will still likely be required.

Lung cancer CT has been the primary imaging modality for staging lung cancer. Cancers of the lung (excluding small cell) are usually treated by resection of the primary lesion with lobectomy. The detection of hilar and mediastinal involvement is critical for determining operability, prognosis, and appropriate treatment. In the absence of hilar or mediastinal node disease, survival approaches 50% at 5 years. However, with hilar or mediastinal involvement, the disease-free survival rate is less than 10% at 5 years, and thoracotomy is not indicated.

The high spatial resolution of CT makes it a sensitive screening modality. However, nodal enlargement is not specific for tumor, and tumor can present in normal-sized nodes. Although mediastinoscopy is diagnostic, it carries some surgical risk and is subject to considerable sampling error. Some investigators have postulated a role here for Ga-67.

The overall sensitivity of Ga-67 for lung cancer is reported to be 85% to 90%, although it is somewhat dependent on tumor type and size (Figure 8-10). There has been controversy as to its value in preoperative staging. The general consensus has been that the accuracy is suboptimal. Recent investigation with SPECT has not changed that perception, although further investigations are underway. Preliminary evidence suggests that Tl-201 is superior to Ga-67 for the detection of lung cancer; however, its clinical utility has yet to be proved. Although useful in individual cases, as yet there is no clearcut routine role for Ga-67 imaging in the detection of metastatic lung cancer.

In patients with pleural-based *mesotheliomas*, Ga-67 can be used to determine the local extent of disease and the presence or absence of distant metastases, although clinical experience with this uncommon tumor is somewhat limited. Ga-67 has been found more sensitive than chest radiography for differentiating malignant mesothelioma from benign pleural thickening.

Head and neck tumors   Varying results have been reported for Ga-67 in head and neck tumors, with the sensitivity ranging from 56% to 86%. Because CT and magnetic resonance imaging (MRI) can demonstrate smaller lesions, Ga-67 is usually reserved for detecting of recurrent tumor following therapy when normal anatomic landmarks have been disrupted. The prognosis is poor in patients who have Ga-67 uptake in recurrent tumor as compared with gallium-negative patients with a residual mass.

Abdominal and pelvic tumors   In general, the sensitivity of Ga-67 in pelvic and abdominal tumors is not particularly good. Ga-67 has been successfully used for detecting metastases from draining nodes in *testicular cancer*. Uptake depends to some extent on histologic type: the sensitivity for metastatic embryonal cell carcinoma is 74%, for metastatic seminoma it is 57%, and for testicular teratomas, 25%.

Results in *gynecologic tumors* have been poor. Similarly, poor accuracy has been found in gastrointestinal tumors (e.g., gastric tumors), 47%; in colon cancer, 25%, and in pancreatic tumors, 16%. The normal bowel excretion of Ga-67 complicates interpretation.

Soft tissue sarcomas   Most soft tissue sarcomas are quite Ga-67 avid, with a 93% overall sensitivity for disease detection and good sensitivity for primary lesions, local recurrences, and metastatic disease. Tumor grade predicts Ga-67 avidity, explaining why liposarcomas, typically a low-grade tumor, are associated with a higher false negative rate. Intra-abdominal detection of tumor sites is high (88%), except for the liver (56% sensitivity), where CT is superior. Although older reports suggest poor sensitivity in bone, recent studies with modern imaging techniques have found a high sensitivity for bone lesions (94%). A Ga-67-positive site that becomes negative after therapy is indicative of a favorable clinical response.

THALLIUM-201 TUMOR IMAGING

Thallium-201 has been used since the 1970s to evaluate myocardial perfusion. There is now a growing and convincing amount of data to show that it can also play an important clinical role in tumor imaging. Much of the initial tumor work was done for the evaluation of thyroid nodules in an effort to differentiate benign and malignant causes. Tl-201 was subsequently used to diagnose parathyroid adenomas in conjunction with Tc-99m pertechnetate. Recent investigations have demonstrated Tl-201 uptake in a wide variety of tumor types.

Mechanism of Uptake

A number of factors seem to influence the uptake of Tl-201 by tumors (Box 8-3). Tumor blood flow is critical for

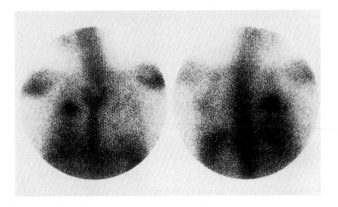

Fig. 8-10   Ga-67 scans of the chest anterior (left) and posterior (right) views in a patient with primary lung cancer showing focal uptake in the right upper lung field.

Box 8-3   Factors Affecting Tl-201 Uptake by Tumor Cells
Blood flow
Viability
Tumor type
Sodium-potassium ATPase system
Cotransport system
Calcium ion channel system
Vascular immaturity with "leakage"
Increased cell membrane permeability

delivery of the radiotracer. Biologically, Tl-201 behaves similar to potassium, and an important mechanism for Tl-201 entry into tumor cells is the action of the ATPase system in the cell membrane, which actively extrudes sodium from the cell in exchange for potassium. A high gradient of intracellular to extracellular potassium and Tl-201 is maintained. This transport system is inhibited by ouabain. A second cotransport system for Tl-201 has been described that is inhibited by furosemide. Tl-201 is accumulated by viable tumor tissue, to a much lesser degree by connective tissue, and not at all by necrotic tissue. It is reported to reside in free form in tumor fluids. Only a small amount localizes in the nuclear, mitochondral, and microsomal fractions of the cell.

Physical Properties and Pharmacokinetics

Tl-201 is a metallic element in group IIIA of the periodic table (See Appendix). It decays by electron capture with a half-life of 73 hours and emits a cluster of x-rays between 69 and 83 keV (94% abundant) and gamma rays of 167 keV (10% abundant) and 135 keV (3% abundant) (Table 8-1).

After intravenous (IV) injection, it is distributed to all parts of the body in proportion to regional blood flow. The heart receives only 3% to 5% of the dose, with the majority going to the liver, spleen, skeletal muscles, brain, and kidneys. It is excreted primarily through the kidneys (Figure 8-11). As with Ga-67, there is considerable background activity and some, but less, bowel clearance.

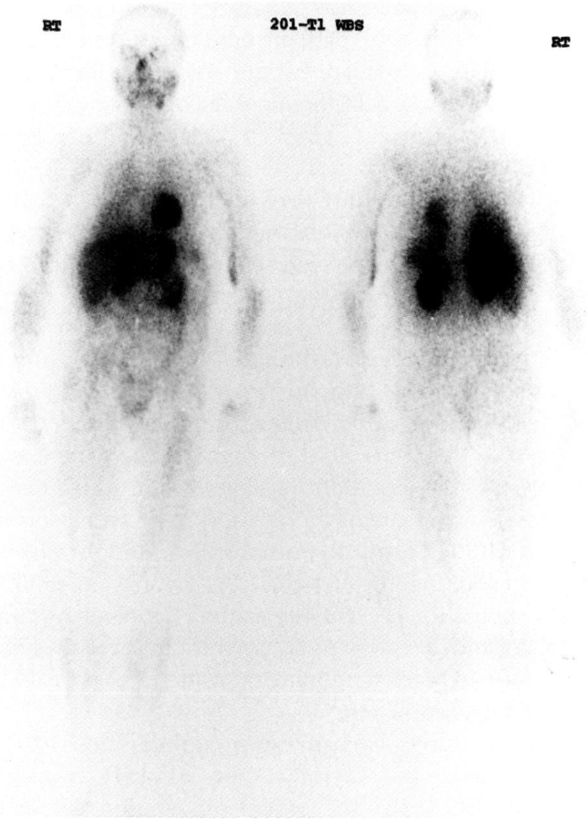

Dosimetry

The kidney is the target organ, receiving 3.6 rads/mCi (Table 8-6). The testicle receives about 1.5 rads/mCi. The whole body dose is 0.63 rads/mCi.

Methodology

Optimal imaging time is 10 to 30 minutes after injection. Because the maximum approved dose is 3 mCi, limiting photon yield, an imaging time similar to that for I-131 or Ga-67 is required. A typical protocol is described in Box 8-4.

Fig. 8-11   Normal resting Tl-201 distribution. Note prominent distribution to the kidneys, heart, liver, and to a lesser extent the bowel. Normally the thyroid would be prominently seen. This patient has undergone total thyroidectomy for thyroid cancer.

Table 8-6   Tl-201 Radiation Absorbed Dose

Organ	rads/mCi
Kidneys	1.7
Thyroid	2.3
Heart wall	1.0
Liver	0.37
Testes	3.0
Ovaries	0.37
Large bowel	1.2

Modified from package insert, Mallinkrodt Medical Inc., St. Louis, Mo.

Box 8-4   Tl-201 Tumor Imaging: Protocol Summary

PATIENT PREPARATION

Fasting if abdominal imaging is required.

DOSE

3 mCi

INSTRUMENTATION

Camera: Large field of view with LEAP collimator; 20% photopeak over 80 keV and 167 keV

IMAGING PROTOCOL

Inject Tl-201 IV.
Begin imaging 10 min after injection.
Whole body imaging: 1,000k.
Large field of views spot imaging: 500k or 5 min.
SPECT: May be useful for intracranial or chest disease.

Image Interpretation

Normal uptake is seen in the heart, kidneys, muscles, and soft tissue. Myocardial uptake can be a problem in evaluating lung and breast cancer, and variable GI clearance poses a similar problem in the abdomen. Lesions as small as 1 cm can usually be detected.

Clinical Applications

Brain tumors Multiple studies have shown the clinical utility of Tl-201 for evaluation of cerebral tumors (See Figure 11-23). The uptake in gliomas has been correlated with the tumor grade; the higher the tumor grade, the more uptake. Perhaps more important, Tl-201 can accurately determine viability when CT and MRI cannot differentiate residual tumor from postoperative or post-radiation changes. Tl-201 has been extremely valuable for evaluating the effectiveness of therapy. The results are similar to those achieved with F-18 FDG PET imaging.

Tl-201 has also been used to determine the cause of intracerebral masses in HIV-positive patients. It is taken up by lymphomas but not in infectious etiologies (e.g., toxoplasmosis).

Primary tumors of bone Tl-201 is more accurate than Tc-99m MDP or Ga-67 in determining the extent of involvement of primary bone tumors and is valuable for following tumor response to chemotherapy. It is particularly sensitive and accurate for demonstrating osteosarcoma (Figure 8-12), and there is a high correlation between Tl-201 uptake and response to chemotherapy, superior to both Tc-99m MDP and Ga-67. Unlike what is seen with Tl-201, uptake of the latter two radiopharmaceuticals is determined by factors other than healing response.

Lung cancers Tl-201 has been successfully used to detect primary carcinoma of the lung in lesions as small as 1.5 cm. Hilar and mediastinal metastases can be detected as well. One study has reported good accuracy for Tl-201 in differentiating malignant lung tumors from tumors of benign causes. Tl-201 uptake is usually greater than that seen with Ga-67. Although Ga-67 is taken up in both inflammatory disease (e.g., sarcoidosis) and tumor, Tl-201 is, with few exceptions, taken up only by tumor. No study has yet compared Tl-201 scintigraphy with the results of CT and biopsy to determine how well Tl-201 is able to predict operability of lung cancer patients.

Lymphoma Tl-201 has a high degree of affinity for low-grade, non-Hodgkin's lymphoma. In contrast, Ga-67 is more useful than Tl-201 for evaluating intermediate- and high-grade lymphomas. Tl-201 appears to be valuable in determining the efficacy of chemotherapy in these lower-grade tumors.

Breast cancer Tl-201 is taken up with a good sensitivity in adenocarcinoma of the breast. The highest tar-

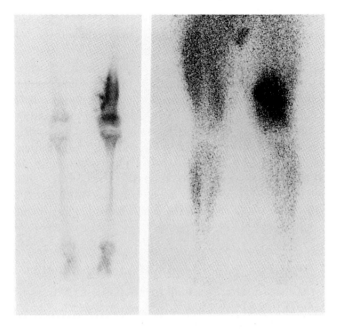

Fig. 8-12 Osteosarcoma. *Left*, Tc-99m HDP bone scan shows uptake in the distal left femur extending into soft tissue medially in a young patient with an osteosarcoma. *Right*, Tl-201 study shows a similar pattern of uptake as Tc-99m HDP, but more clearly shows soft tissue involvement superiomedially.

get-to-background ratio occurs 15 minutes post injection. In a study of 45 patients with breast lesions greater than 1.5 cm, Tl-201 had a sensitivity of 97% for detecting breast cancer and 38% for adenoma of the breast, whereas fibrocystic disease showed no thallium uptake (0% sensitivity). The smallest detectable primary lesion is about 1 cm. This study may be very useful in patients with indeterminate lesions on mammography. A positive Tl-201 study would suggest an aggressive approach (biopsy). The sensitivity of Tl-201 for the detection of axillary nodes is lower.

Thyroid cancer Although I-131 scintigraphy has been used successfully for years in the post-thyroidectomy evaluation of patients with differentiated thyroid cancer, it has some disadvantages. A major one is the necessity for the patient to have discontinued thyroid hormone replacement therapy for 4 to 6 weeks prior to the study to ensure hypothyroidism and an elevated TSH. In addition, the 364 keV I-131 gamma emissions are not optimal for present-day gamma cameras. Adequate imaging and detection of disease require a relatively high dose of I-131 and long imaging times. There is about a 10% false negative rate.

Several studies have investigated the use of Tl-201 for thyroid cancer post-thyroidectomy whole body imaging. An advantage is that the patient can continue taking thyroid hormone therapy. These studies have found Tl-201 to be more sensitive than I-131 in the detection of tumor. The downside is that Tl-201 is not specific for thyroid cancer and does not give predictive information on the therapeutic potential of I-131. In clinical practice, the clearest role for Tl-201 is in localizing the site of tumor when the I-131 whole body scan is negative but the serum thyroglobulin level is elevated. Some of these tumors will then respond to high-dose radioactive iodine I-131 therapy, as evidenced by a fall in the serum thyroglobulin level. A 5- to 7-day post-therapy I-131 scan may show tumor uptake even though it was not seen on the routine 5 mCi I-131 diagnostic scan. Tl-201 can then be used in follow-up of these patients.

AIDS

While all AIDS opportunistic infections are Ga-67 ⊕.

Kaposi's sarcoma is Ga-67 negative but Tl-201 positive. This can be helpful in the differential diagnosis of chest disease in patients with AIDS, in whom many of the infectious conditions take up Ga-67 (e.g., Pneumocystis, atypical Mycobacterium). Tl-201 scintigraphy is usually negative in infectious and inflammatory diseases.

TECHNETIUM-99M SESTAMIBI

Tc-99m sestamibi is a new myocardial perfusion agent that, like Tl-201, has tumor imaging capability. Its Tc-99m label would suggest that it may have some imaging advantages over Tl-201. However, it has disadvantages similar to those associated with Tl-201 scintigraphy for lung and breast imaging, such as uptake by the heart and other soft tissues. The large amount of hepatobiliary clearance poses a problem for intra-abdominal imaging. Tc-99m sestamibi has been found clinical utility for localizing parathyroid adenomas. Interestingly, there seems to be a differential washout from parathyroid tumor compared to normal thyroid—that is, a slower clearance from tumor than from the thyroid (Figure 8-13). Only

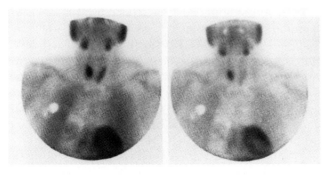

Fig. 8-13 Parathyroid adenoma diagnosed on Tc-99m sestamibi scintigraphy. *Left*, Imaging at 15 minutes shows bilateral thyroid uptake with somewhat more *prominent* focal uptake on the right. *Right*, Imaging at 2 hours shows that focal uptake remains in the region of the right lobe of the thyroid. There has been washout bilaterally of normal thyroid activity between 15 minutes and 2 hours. This is consistent with the diagnosis of a parathyroid adenoma, which was subsequently proved correct at surgery.

preliminary studies have been done for other tumors. This agent shows considerable promise in breast cancer imaging similar to Tl-201. Further work is needed to better define the role of this agent in tumor imaging.

MONOCLONAL ANTIBODIES

Most tumor imaging in nuclear medicine has not been specific for tumor type, whether "cold spot" or "hot spot" imaging (Box 8-1). There have been a few exceptions, most notably I-131 whole body thyroid cancer scanning post thyroidectomy, which is tumor specific for differentiated papillary-follicular thyroid cancer. Likewise, I-131 6ß-iodomethyl-19-norcholesterol (NP-59) and I-131 metaiodobenzylguanidine (MIBG) are radiopharmaceuticals with specificity for cortical adrenal tumors and medullary adrenal tumors and neuroblastomas, respectively. This section will deal with a new, potentially specific form of whole body tumor imaging, radiolabeled monoclonal antibodies (MoAbs).

Mechanism of uptake

Antibodies are glycoproteins produced in the bone marrow, lymph nodes, and spleen by plasma cells following exposure to a foreign antigen. These immunoglobulins may be of various types (IgA, IgD, IgE, IgG, and IgM). In the past, most available antibodies were produced in rabbits or other animals, were of limited purity, were polyclonal (derived from different lymphocyte clones), and were bound to multiple sites on an antigen.

In 1975, Kohler and Milstein described a method that produced unlimited quantities of a single monoclonal type of antibody that bound to only one antigenic site. The technique involved fusing mouse myeloma cells with lymphocytes from the spleen of mice immunized with a particular antigen (Figure 8-14). These "hybridoma" cells retain both the specific antibody production of the lymphocytes and the immortality of the myeloma cells. Immunoassays screen the hybrid cells to identify specific cell lines that produce an MoAb with the desired features, such as high affinity and specificity. The individual hybdridoma cells can then be maintained in culture to produce large quantities of antibody directed against a single antigenic determinant.

Unique cell-surface antigens are preferentially expressed in many disease states, thus allowing antibody targeting for a variety of diseases (Table 8-7). Importantly, many tumors have antigens preferentially expressed on their surfaces.

Antibodies consist of two identical heavy (H) and light (L) chains linked by a disulfide bridge (Figure 8-15). Each chain is made up of a *variable* region, responsible for antigenic binding, and a *constant* region, responsible

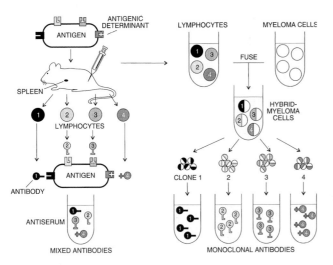

Fig. 8-14 Monoclonal antibody production. The process starts with injection of an antigen into a mouse, causing proliferation of B-lymphocytes that can make antibody to the antigen. The mouse spleen is removed and the B-cells harvested, many of which are capable of making antibody to the specific antigen, others that can make other specific antibodies. If they were cultured at this point (*left*), they would make a mix of antibodies (antiserum) and would soon die off. If instead the B-cells are mixed with mouse myeloma cells in polyethylene glycol, some of the normal B-cells will fuse with the myeloma cells, producing a population of *hybridomas* that can be cultured indefinitely. When this population is selectively cloned for those that make the desired antibody, a pure culture of target antibody-producing cells can be grown in great quantities. Its product is the desired monoclonal antibody. More recently, efforts have succeeded in making human-human hybridomas, those derived by using human rather than mouse myeloma cells and human spleen lymphocytes obtained at laparotomy.

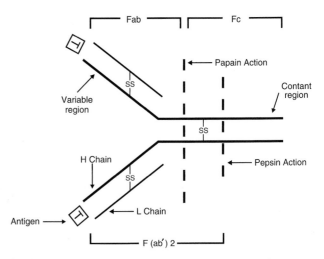

Fig. 8-15 IgG antibody. The molecule can be digested enzymatically by papain, resulting in three parts, two Fab fragments and one Fc fragment, or by pepsin to produce F(ab')₂ fragments and subfragments of Fc. Fab' may be produced by splitting the disulfide bond of F(ab')₂.

for effector functions such as complement fixation and antibody-dependent cell cytoxicity.

The biodistribution of MoAbs is affected by multiple factors. Specificity is determined by the variable regions of the molecule's heavy and light chains (Fab region). The antibody's effector functions are determined by the structure of the constant region, which lies mostly within the molecule's Fc portion. Antibody fragments can have biological properties more desirable than those of the intact molecule, such as less antigenicity and less background due to more rapid blood clearance.

Different radionuclides have been used as labels for immunoscintigraphy, including I-131, I-123, In-111, and Tc-99m (Table 8-8). Various methods have been developed by chemists for attaching these isotopes to a particular MoAb. It must be done without changing the antibody's immunoreactivity or biological properites. Early antibody imaging studies were performed with polyclonal antibodies, often labeled with I-131, which showed promising results in a variety of tumors.

Most studies in the past decade have used MoAbs labeled with shorter-lived isotopes that have better imaging characteristics, such as In-111. Recently, Tc-99-labeled antibodies have also been investigated. Most studies using Tc-99m, with a short half-life of 6 hours, have used antibody fragments because of their more rapid clearance. Studies with In-111 (2.8-day $T_{1/2}$) have usually used intact antibodies, which allows more time for accumulation and background clearance.

Table 8-7	Diseases With Antigenic Sites That Can Be Targeted With Radiolabeled Antibodies
Disease	**Antigens**
NONTUMOR	
Cardiac disease (infarction, myocarditis, graft rejection)	Cardiac myosin
Venous thrombosis	Fibrin, platelet glycoproteins
Infection	Granulocyte
Bone marrow disease	Granulocyte
TUMOR	
Colon and ovarian cancer	CEA, TAG-72
Melanoma	Transferrin receptor, gangliosides
Lymphoma	Differentiation antigens, transferrin
Hepatoma	α-Fetoprotein
Head and neck cancer	CEA, epidermal growth factor
Breast cancer	Human milk fat globule/mucin
Prostate cancer	Normal prostate, prostate-specific antigen
Neuroblastoma	Gangliosides

Table 8-8   Radionuclides Used for Immunoscintigraphy

Radionuclide	Energy (keV)	Half-life	Advantages	Disadvantages
Tc-99m	140	6 hr	Pure gamma Inexpensive high photon flux	Complex chemistry Short half-life High counts in kidney, bladder
In-111	173 247	2.8 d	Gamma emitter Delayed imaging possible	Affinity for liver and RES
I-123	159	13 hr	Gamma emitter Ease of labeling	Dehalogenates Cyclotron produced Expensive due to short half-life
I-131	364	8 d	Ease of labeling	Dehalogenates Low count rate High radiation dose

Clinical Applications

MoAbs have been used for a variety of applications in both benign and malignant disorders. They are used clinically for in vitro testing (radioimmunoassay), in vivo for the early detection and staging of disease and for assessing the effectiveness of intervention (radioimmunoscintigraphy), and investigationally as vehicles for the delivery of radioimmunotherapy.

Although a number of radiolabeled MoAbs have been extensively investigated as tumor imaging agents, only one to date, Oncoscint CR/OV (Cytogen Corp., Princeton, NJ) has been approved by the Food and Drug Administration (FDA) for clinical use. Approvals are pending for a number of other immunoscintigraphic agents for cancers of the colon, prostate, and lung, and lymphoma.

Colorectal cancer   Colorectal cancer is the third most common noncutaneous malignancy. The 5-year survival is 85% with localized disease, 50% with regional spread, and less than 7% with distant spread. The first recurrence occurs at a single site in 75% of cases. These sites include the liver (33%), local-regional sites (21%), intra-abdominal sites (18%), and retroperitoneal lymph nodes (10%).

Serum carcinoembryonic antigen (CEA) levels are used to follow the course of disease and to predict recurrence; however, one third of patients with recurrence do not have elevated CEA levels. Colonoscopy and barium studies are of low yield in determining the site of recurrence because they can detect only intraluminal disease. CT and MRI have limited sensitivity for evaluating the extrahepatic abdomen, tumors in normal-sized lymph nodes, and in distinguishing postoperative and postradiation changes from tumor.

Oncoscint CR/OV is a B72.3 murine IgG MoAb directed against a high molecular weight glycoprotein, TAG-72, which is expressed in the majority of colorectal and ovarian carcinomas. This radiopharmaceutical has been approved for immunoscintigraphy to locate extrahepatic recurrences of colorectal and ovarian cancer (Figure 8-16). Box 8-5 describes its pharmacokinetics.

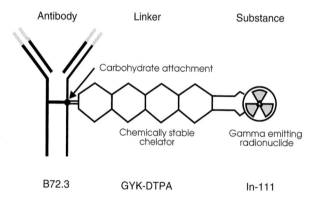

Fig. 8-16   OncoScint CR/OV formulation. The site of attachment of the linker does not interfere with the effector or binding functions of the antibody. (From Cytogen Corp., Princeton, New Jersey, Distributed by Knoll Pharmaceutical Co., Whippany,

Box 8-5   Pharmacokinetics of OncoScint CR/OV (In-111 B72.3)

Biological half-life:	56 ± 14 hr.
Clearance pattern:	Mono- or biexponential, mean 56 ± 14 hr.
Plasma clearance:	Slow, mean 50 ± 15 mL/hr.
Volume of distribution:	Small, mean 71 ± 32 ml/kg.
Urine exretion at 72 hr:	10%.

Most recurrences and metastases of these two tumors occur in the abdomen and pelvis (Figures 8-17 to 8-18). In a large multicenter trial of 192 patients with colorectal carcinoma, the overall sensitivity per patient was 69%, the specificity was 76%, the positive predictive value was 97%, and negative predictive value was 19%. It detected occult disease in 10% and changed patient management in 25%. Although CT was more sensitive than antibody imaging in the liver, OncoScint was superior in the pelvis and extrahepatic abdomen (Table 8-9). The combined sensitivity of CT and OncoScint CR/OV immunoscintigraphy was higher than the sensitivity of either study alone (88%).

Table 8-9 Imaging Sensitivity of OncoScint by Antatomic Site

| | Per-patient sensitivity, % | |
Anatomic site	OncoScint	CT
Pelvis	74	57
Extrahepatic abdomen	66	34
Liver	41	84

Methodology OncoScint CR/OV, 1 mg, and In-111 chloride, 5 mCi, are incubated at room temperature for 3 minutes. After aseptic filtration (0.22 μ) and instant thin-layer chromatography (ITLC) to determine radiochemical purity, the combination can be used for up to 8 hours after labeling. An imaging protocol is described in Box 8-6.

Dosimetry The estimated radiation absorbed dose for OncoScint CR/OV is shown in Table 8-10. The liver and spleen receive the highest dose, followed by the bone marrow.

In *primary* colorectal cancer, OncoScint can be used to detect synchronous lesions, to determine the extent of regional disease, and to find occult metastases. Its main role is likely to be in *recurrent disease*, where it can be used to detect occult disease, such as rising CEA levels but an otherwise negative workup, and in *potentially resectable disease*, such as single metastases, to exclude evidence of other tumor. Fifty percent of first recurrences occur in the extrahepatic abdomen and

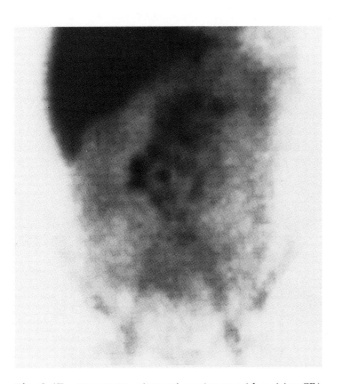

Fig. 8-17 Metastatic colorectal carcinoma with a rising CEA level. Midabdominal area of Oncoscint uptake proved to be metastatic tumor. CT of the abdomen was abnormal, with post-therapy changes, but was interpreted as negative for residual tumor.

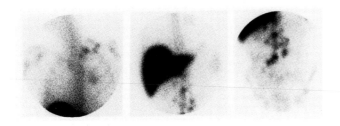

Fig. 8-18 Recurrent colon cancer in a 55-year-old man. OncoScint uptake is seen in the left supraclavicular nodes and left hilum (*left*), the periaortic nodes, and more diffusely throughout the abdomen (*middle and right*). Retrosternal uptake was detected with SPECT.

Box 8-6 OncoScint CR/OV imaging: Protocol Summary

RADIOPHARMACEUTICAL

Dose: 5 mCi In-111 OncoScint.

INSTRUMENTATION

Camera: Large field of view gamma camera.
Collimator: Medium energy.
Photopeaks: 20% symmetric windows around 173 and 247 keV.
Computer: 128 × 128 matrix size.

IMAGING PROCEDURE

Infuse Oncoscint CR/OV IV over 5 min.
Image: 48-72 hr post injection and 72-120 hr post-injection.
Planar images: Anterior and posterior views of the chest, abdomen, and pelvis at 1,000k or for 10 min per view.
SPECT: Use protocol similar to Ga-67.

Table 8-10 Radiation Dosimetry for OncoScint CR/OV

Organ	rads/5 mCi (cGy/185 MBq)
Liver	15
Spleen	16
Red marrow	12
Kidney	9.7
Stomach wall	3.2
Large intestine	3.1
Ovaries	2.9
Bladder	2.8
Testes	1.4
Total body	2.7

Modified from package insert, Cytogen Corp., Princeton, NJ.

pelvis. It can also be used to clarify equivocal CT and MRI findings.

Human antimouse antibodies (HAMA) occur in 40% of patients, although 50% become negative over time. This has implications for using this MoAb in a serial manner to evaluate the effectiveness of therapy or as a prelude to a therapeutic dose of the MoAb. At present, only single administrations have been approved.

No correlation has been found between the development of HAMA and adverse reactions, and HAMA is not related to any change in hematology, blood chemistry, or urine values. HAMA can interfere with murine-based immunoassays of CEA and CA-125, producing falsely high values. Alternative assay methods are available that are not adversely affected.

HAMA can also alter the biodistribution and pharmacokinetics of MoAbs and may interfere with the quality or sensitivity of the imaging study. Investigations using antibodies from a human rather than murine source, *chimeric antibodies* ("humanized" murine antibodies designed using recombinant DNA technology), and antibody fragments are being investigated to minimize this problem.

Adverse effects with OncoScint have been seen in less than 4% of patients, were not serious, and were readily reversible, generally without intervention. They included fever, chills, hypotension, hypertension, rash, and pruritus. In a study of patients receiving repeat infusions, the adverse reaction rate was similar, less than 4%. OncoScint is not presently approved for repeat use.

Image interpretation NORMAL DISTRIBUTION The highest normal uptake of In-111 B72.3 (OncoScint CR/OV) is in the liver, followed by the spleen, then the bone marrow. The kidneys may occasionally be seen faintly, bladder activity is not uncommon, and male genitalia can also be seen. Large bowel activity is variable. Localization may occur at colostomy sites, sites of degenerative joint disease, abdominal aneurysms, postoperative bowel adhesions, and local inflammatory lesions,

such as inflammatory bowel disease or inflammation secondary to surgery or radiation.

ABNORMAL UPTAKE (Figures 8-17, 8-18) The probability that uptake represents a site of tumor is increased if it is located over the expected distribution of lymph nodes or an organ under investigation.

Certain image patterns are unlikely to represent tumor. For example, long linear zones of uptake are more likely to be a vessel or a loop of bowel, rather than a site of tumor.

Extrahepatic uptake not associated with normal structures and equal to or greater than hepatic uptake has a high probability of being tumor. Activity less intense than that of liver, but which meets all or most of the above criteria, is highly probable for tumor.

Uptake in tumor will either remain stable or become more intense over sequential imaging days. Potential false positive sites of uptake, such as the large bowel and blood pool structures, may show a rapid drop-off in activity in subsequent images, or activity may remain static in the bowel for the duration of the study. Bladder activity may or may not clear during the study duration.

Hepatic metastases will generally appear as photopenic defects due to the normal intense uptake of OncoScint in the liver. Hepatomegaly and heterogeneous distribution should be classified as possible tumor. Occasionally, hot liver lesions may also be present.

Other colorectal MoAbs are still under investigation. In-111 and Tc-99m labeled CEA antibodies have shown encouraging results. Approval is pending.

Ovarian cancer Ovarian cancer is the fourth most frequent cause of cancer deaths in women. The average age at diagnosis is 53 and the overall 5-year survival rate is 39%. Accurate surgical staging and the amount of residual disease influence the selection of therapy and its success. The diagnosis of recurrent disease requires a variety of blood tests (CA-125, liver function), x-rays (chest x-ray, IVP, BE, CT, US), and surgery (laparotomy or laparoscopy). However, serum CA-125 assay has a high false negative rate and does not predict the extent of disease or location; CT is limited in the detection of small tumor deposits, tumor in normal-sized lymph nodes, and diffuse miliary disease, and in distinguishing adhesions or scar from tumor. No reliable method has been available to detect disease in the clinically relevant size range (≤2 cm).

Ovarian cancer is difficult to diagnose and stage with current imaging methods because it presents as small peritoneal implants not detectable on CT. Exploratory laparotomy is the best approach to surgical staging in ovarian cancer. However, it does not detect extra-abdominal tumors, is expensive, has a 20% complication rate, and is inaccurate in 20% to 50% of patients, with negative results on second-look surgery.

OncoScint CR/OV (In-111 B-72.3) can also be used to

locate and define the extent of extrahepatic ovarian cancer, to detect occult disease, including miliary spread, and can help direct the surgical approach for ovarian cancer. In a multicenter trial of patients with primary or recurrent diease, OncoScint had a sensitivity of 60% to 70% and a specificity of 55% to 60% (Table 8-11). The positive predictive value was 83% and the study was able to detect occult disease in 35% (some of whom had normal CA-125 levels). Of occult lesions detected, 43% were less than 2 cm in size, including some miliary and microscopic lesions. The antibody scan changed patient management in 25% of cases. It was superior to CT in patients with recurrent disease and carcinomatosis (60% vs. 30%).

Other MoAbs under investigation

Lung cancer Antibody scanning with a Tc-99m-labeled antibody fragment has a sensitivity of 77% and 88% respectively, for non-small cell and small cell lung cancers.

Melanoma Several trials have shown good results. One multicenter imaging trial found a greater than 80% sensitivity and specificity.

Prostate cancer Correctly staging a newly diagnosed prostate carcinoma is critical in ascertaining prognosis and therapy. However, due to inadequacies of current noninvasive diagnostic studies, including CT and MRI, many patients must undergo surgical staging to determine the presence or absence of lymph nodes. MoAb imaging has the potential for demonstrating involved nodes, as well as skeletal and visceral metastases. MoAbs against prostate cancer are under investigation.

TUMOR RECEPTOR IMAGING

Tumor growth may be affected by hormones and growth factors that interact with tumor-associated receptors which could potentially be imaged with radionuclide scintigraphy.

Somatostatin is a peptide hormone produced in the hypothalamus, pituitary, brain stem, GI tract, and pancreas that has an inhibitory effect on the secretion of many gastric hormones. Many endocrine-related tumors, among them carcinoid, meningiomas, gastrinomas, pancreatic endocrine tumors, and paragangliomas, have high-affinity receptors for somatostatin.

A somatostatin analogue (octreotide) has been radiolabeled with I-123 and now In-111. A variety of receptor-positive tumors have been imaged. Most neuroedocrine tumors (derived from cells belonging to the amine precursor uptake and decarboxylation [APUD] system) have been successfully imaged, including pituitary tumors, pancreatic islet cell tumors, carcinoids, medullary carcinoma of the thyroid, paragangliomas, neuroblastomas, and pheochromocytomas.

Other tumors with somatostatic receptors have been imaged, including central nervous system tumors (meningiomas, astrocytromas), breast cancer, small cell cancer of the lung, and lymphoma. Other tumor receptors, such as estrogen receptors, epidermal growth factor, dopamine, and bombesin, have been radiolabeled and are being investigated.

PET IMAGING OF TUMORS

PET imaging of tumors with F-18 fluorodeoxyglucose (FDG) is an exciting new avenue of investigation with considerable potential clinical importance. Preliminary studies demonstrate uptake of F-18 FDG in a wide variety of tumors.

A characteristic of malignant cells is an enhanced rate of glycolysis. Unlike glucose, F-18 FDG-6-phosphate cannot enter most metabolic pathways and as a result accumulates within cells. The metabolic trapping of F-18 FDG in tisssue following phosphorylation by hexokinase facilitates imaging and quantitation.

The high target-to-background ratio of F-18 FDG combined with the high sensitivity and good resolution obtainable with PET results in excellent functional images, far superior to what has been available with radiolabeled MoAbs to date. Many studies are now under way investigating its clinical utility in a wide range of malignancies. PET's quantitative potential is an additional advantage. Tc-99m SC is suboptimal since a large percent remains at the site of injection.

Clinical Studies

Astrocytomas Considerable experience has been gained in the imaging and quantitation of F-18 FDG uptake with PET in astrocytomas. The glucose metabolic rate has been linearly correlated with histologic grade, providing noninvasive tumor grading and prognostic information. PET F-18 FDG studies have been used to detect tumor recurrences and for differentiating post operative and post radiation changes from tumor recurrence.

Head and neck tumors A good correlation has also been found between the histologic grade of head and

Table 8-11 OncoScint CR/OV for Ovarian Cancer		
	Primary Disease (%)	Recurrent Disease (%)
Sensitivity	68	58
Specificity	55	60
Positive predictive value	83	
Negative predictive value	29	
Occult disease	35	

neck tumors and F-18 FDG uptake. In a study of 16 patients with primary squamous cell carcinoma, PET identified all primary tumors, whereas MRI and CT did not demonstrate one superficial tumor of the anterior tongue. PET demonstrated 71% of all pathologically positive nodes, whereas CT and MRI showed only 59%.

Breast cancer   This is an area of considerable promise for determining the etiology of palpable breast masses as well as lesions first detected on mammography. It may aid in deciding which patients require biopsy or surgery (Figure 8-19A). It may also be useful in determining the presence or absence of axillary adenopathy in patients with breast cancer, thereby affecting therapeutic decisions. Preliminary studies in this area are encouraging.

Miscellaneous tumors   Lung carcinomas, lymphomas, colorectal carcinomas (Figure 8-19B-D), and thy-

roid cancer have all consistently demonstrated increased glycolytic rates in primary and metastatic lesions. Quantitative measurements of glucose metabolism in tumors with PET F-18 FDG are proving useful in monitoring the effects of radiation therapy and chemotherapy.

Imaging cancers with PET F-18 FDG offers considerable clinical promise. The images have a high target-to-background ratio, much better than any MoAbs studied to date. This may be an important area where PET can have a definite clinical impact.

Although most oncologic studies to date have utilized F-18 FDG, future investigation will include other radiolabeled compounds, such as those that measure blood flow, oxygen metabolism, amino acid incorporation (protein synthesis), and cell division rates by analysis of C-11 thymidine incorporation.

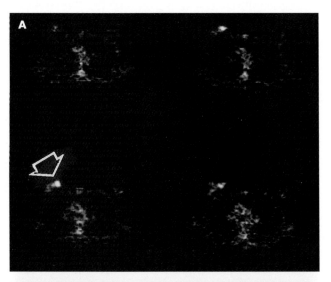

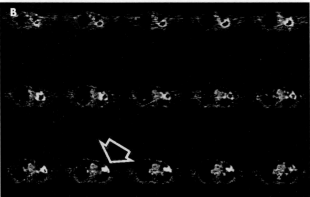

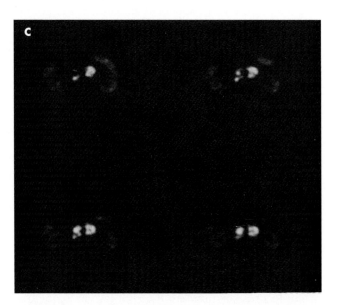

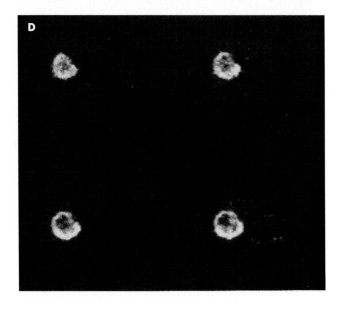

Fig. 8-19   Transverse cross-sectional F-18 FDG PET scan sections. **A**, Breast cancer. Focal increased uptake (*open arrowhead*) is seen in the right breast in four sequential transverse sections. **B**, Bronchogenic lung cancer. Sequential transverse sections show uptake in the left lung (*open arrowhead*). **C**, Abdominal lymphoma involving mesenteric nodes as seen in four sequential transverse sections. **D**, Colon cancer metastatic to the liver. The high target-to-background ratio makes the normal liver uptake fade into background.

LYMPHOSCINTIGRAPHY

Radionuclide lymphoscintigraphy can help define the nodal drainage patterns of tumors that are not routinely accessible to evaluation by routine diagnostic methods. Lymphoscintigraphy has been most commonly used in patients with truncal melanomas, breast cancer, and prostate cancer to help determine the most effective surgical or radiation therapy.

Radiopharmaceuticals

A number of radiopharmaceuticals have been used for lymphoscintigraphy, including Tc-99m SC, Tc-99m HSA, Tc-99m antimony sulfur colloid, and Tc-99m dextran. The last two are not commercially available. Colloidal clearance rate is very dependent on particle size. Tc-99m HSA has a much more rapid clearance than Tc-99m SC. Tc-99m SC is suboptimal since a large percent remains at the site of injection.

Clinical Studies

Malignant melanoma   The major use of lymphoscintigraphy has been in the pretherapeutic evaluation of patients with malignant melanoma. This tumor spreads via lymphatics to regional lymph node groups. In midline truncal tumors, the route of drainage is difficult to predict. Lymphoscintigraphy can demonstrate the drainage pattern and potential site of spread. Surgical resection of the nodes at risk has been recommended as a means of improving prognosis for patients with Stage I disease, although there is some controversy about this.

A small volume of tracer is injected intradermally at multiple sites surrounding the skin lesion. Sequential imaging is performed to determine the flow pattern. The exact timing depends on the radiopharmaceutical used.

Breast cancer   Investigators have found internal mammary lymphoscintigraphy useful for defining the routes of lymphatic dissemination of breast cancer. The internal mammary nodes are a primary site of tumor dissemination.

The radiopharmaceutical is injected into the subxiphoid rectus sheath ipsilateral to the midline, followed by contralateral injection once the ipsilateral pattern is established. Nodal metastases usually appear as areas of diminished or absent uptake. Obstuction appears as intense focal activity without distal nodal uptake. Nodal chains should be seen bilaterally. Although there is some variability, approximately seven nodes can be imaged with internal mammary scintigraphy. Cross-drainage may be seen. For interpretation, bilateral studies must be done. Abnormal patterns include faint or absent uptake, collateral channels, and crossover with poor filling of the contralateral side.

Genitourinary tumors   A number of genitourinary malignancies, among them prostate and testicular cancer, spread primarily via lymphatics and often involve the iliopelvic lymphatics. Lymphoscintigraphy can aid in the evaluation of this relatively inaccessible group of lymphatics.

Injection into the ischiorectal fossa is performed for ileopelvic scintigraphy. Imaging is typically performed immediately and at 3 hours.

Normal iliopelvic lymphoscintigraphy will display the internal, common iliac, and the para-aortic nodes. Decreased or asymmetric uptake or obstructed flow is abnormal.

Accuracy

None of these studies has achieved widespread clinical use. Good correlation has been shown between the findings on melanoma scans and surgery. Limited results have been good with internal mammary scintigraphy, but this study has been used only at a few investigational centers. Abnormal results are associated with a twofold increase in recurrent breast cancer and a threefold increase in distant metastases. Encouraging preliminary results have also been reported with iliopelvic lymphoscintigraphy. Occasional false positive studies occur with the latter two techniques. The clinical role of lymphoscintigraphy is yet to be defined.

SUGGESTED READINGS

Collier BD, Abdel-Nabi H, Doerr RJ, et al: Immuno-scintigraphy performed with In-111-labeled CYT-103 in the management of colorectal cancer: comparison with CT, *Radiology* 185:179-186, 1992.

Front D, Israel O, and Ben-Haim S: The dilemma of a residual mass in treated lymphoma: the role of Gallium-67 scintigraphy. In Freeman LM, editor: *Nuclear medicine annual 1991*, New York, 1991, Raven Press.

Kaplan WD, Jochelson MS, and Herman TS: Gallium-67 imaging: a predictor of residual tumor viability and clinical outcome in patients with diffuse large-cell lymphoma, *J Clin Oncology* 8:1966-1970, 1990.

Monoclonal antibody-based imaging agents in nuclear medicine: a supplement to the *J Nucl Med* 34:531-566, 1993.

Sullivan DC, Croker BP, Harris CC, et al: Lymphoscintigraphy in malignant melanoma: Tc-99m antimony sulfur colloid, *AJR* 137:847-851, 1981.

Wahl RL, Cody RL, Hutchins GD, et al: Primary and metastatic breast carcinoma: initial clinical evaluation with PET with the radiolabeled glucose analogue 2-(F-18)-fluoro-2-deoxy-D-glucose, *Radiology* 179:765-770, 1991.

Waxman AD: Thallum-201 in nuclear oncology. In Freeman LM, editor: *Nuclear medicine annual 1991*, New York, 1991, Raven Press.

Waxman AD, Ramanna L, Memsic LD, et al: Thallium scintigraphy in the evaluation of mass abnormalities of the breast, *J Nucl Med* 34:18-23, 1993.

Nuclear medicine has played an important role in imaging of the liver and spleen for over 20 years, but that role has changed considerably in recent years with the availability of alternative high-resolution imaging modalities and the approval of new nuclear medicine radiopharmaceuticals. Until the advent of computed tomography (CT), the Tc-99m sulfur colloid (Tc-99m SC) liver-spleen scan was the primary imaging method used to diagnose and evaluate diseases of the liver and spleen. Tc-99m SC imaging now plays a much more limited role, owing to the availability of alternative superb anatomic abdominal imaging methods such as CT, magnetic resonance imaging (MRI), and ultrasonography (US).

However, other clinically important nuclear medicine liver studies have been developed that provide unique functional and pathophysiologic information not available from anatomic imaging methods. These include *cholescintigraphy* (Tc-99m IDA), commonly used to diagnose acute cholecystitis as well as an increasing number of other hepatobiliary diseases; Tc-99m-labeled *red blood cell liver imaging*, used to diagnose cavernous hemangiomas of the liver; and Tc-99m macroaggregated albumin (Tc-99m MAA) *hepatic arterial perfusion imaging*, used to evaluate intra-arterially administered chemotherapy of liver neoplasms.

Each of these studies uses a radiopharmaceutical with a different physiologic mechanism of uptake and localization that illustrates a different aspect of hepatic

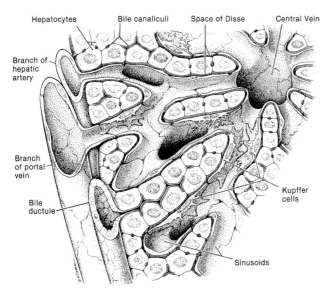

Fig. 9-1 Anatomy of a liver lobule. The plates of hepatic cells (hepatocytes and Kupffer cells) are distributed radially around the central vein. Branches of the portal vein and hepatic artery located at the periphery of the lobule deliver blood to the sinusoids. Blood leaves via the central vein (proximal branch of hepatic veins). The peripherally located bile ducts drain bile canaliculi that run between hepatocytes.

anatomy, physiology, and function: blood flow (Tc-99m MAA), intravascular blood pool distribution (Tc-99m-labeled RBCs), hepatocyte function and biliary patency (Tc-99m IDA), and Kupffer cell extraction (Tc-99m SC) (Figure 9-1).

The emphasis of this discussion will be on the current clinical role for each of these studies. For example, although considerable experience has been gained with Tc-99m SC liver-spleen imaging in a wide variety of diseases, the discussion will emphasize current indications and uses for the study. Because cholescintigraphy is increasingly used to diagnose a large number of hepatobiliary diseases, it will be discussed first, and in more detail. Hepatic arterial perfusion imaging will be discussed briefly. Finally, splenic imaging is reviewed.

CHOLESCINTIGRAPHY

Radiopharmaceuticals

I-131-labeled rose bengal, introduced in 1955, was for 20 years the only available liver radiopharmaceutical that was extracted and cleared by hepatocytes. However, it had a limited clinical role, owing to its poor imaging characteristics and high radiation dosimetry. Labeling rose bengal with I-123 was superior in both regards, but it never gained widespread use because of its limited availability and, more important, the introduction of Tc-99m-labeled hepatobiliary imaging radiopharmaceuticals in

Box 9-1   Clinical Indications for Cholescintigraphy

Acute cholecystitis
Acute acalculous cholecystitis
Biliary diversion procedures
Postoperative leaks
Common duct obstruction
Postcholecystectomy syndrome
  Cystic duct remnant
  Recurrent or retained common duct stone
  Sphincter of Oddi dysfunction
Chronic acalculous cholecystitis
Focal nodular hyperplasia
Hepatoma
Biliary stent follow-up
Sclerosing cholangitis
Enterogastric biliary reflux

the mid-1970s. The Tc-99m-labeled iminodiacetic acid analogues (IDAs) have found a clinically important role in the diagnosis of a variety of hepatobiliary disorders (Box 9-1), and imaging with these agents is now the most commonly performed liver study in nuclear medicine.

Chemistry

The technetium-labeled IDA radiopharmaceuticals were initially synthesized to develop a heart imaging agent, based on the structural similarities between IDA and lidocaine molecules (Figure 9-2). The high liver

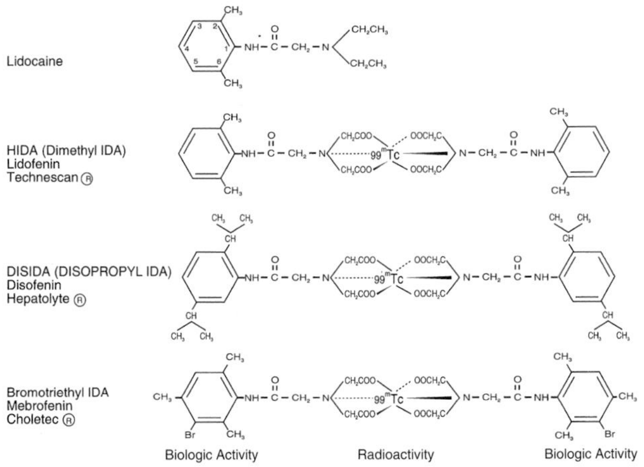

Lidocaine

HIDA (Dimethyl IDA)
Lidofenin
Technescan ®

DISIDA (DISOPROPYL IDA)
Disofenin
Hepatolyte ®

Bromotriethyl IDA
Mebrofenin
Choletec ®

Biologic Activity   Radioactivity   Biologic Activity

Fig. 9-2 Chemical structure of HIDA radiopharmaceuticals. Note the similarity of the Tc-99m IDAs to lidocaine. The radioactivity is located centrally (Tc-99m) bridging two ligand molecules; iminodiacetate (NCH_2COO) attaches to the Tc-99m, while the acetanilide (IDA) analogue of lidocaine at the periphery carries the biological activity. Substitutions on the aromatic rings differentiate the various Tc-99m IDA analogues and determine their pharmacokinetics.

extraction of one early IDA compound (dimethyl IDA) tested prompted the acronym HIDA, for hepatobiliary IDA. Tc-99m HIDA was cleared from blood more rapidly than radioiodinated rose bengal but with a similar hepatobiliary clearance rate. A variety of analogues followed, with different chemical substitutions around the aromatic ring. The newer analogues offered improvements in hepatocellular uptake and more rapid blood clearance. These IDA analogues go by many acronyms—BIDA, DIDA, EIDA, PIPIDA, and so forth. The Food and Drug Administration (FDA) has approved three: Tc-99m lidofenin (HIDA), Tc-99m disofenin (DISIDA), and Tc-99m mebrofenin (BrIDA). Only the latter two are currently used clinically in the United States.

The IDA radiopharmaceuticals are organic anions that act as bifunctional chelates. The iminodiacetate (NCH$_2$ COO) attaches at one end to the radioactivity (Tc-99m) and at the other end to an acetanilide analogue of lidocaine, which carries the biological function (Figure 9-2). Relatively minor structural changes in the phenyl ring (N-substitutions) result in significant alterations in the IDA biokinetics (e.g., uptake, retention, and excretion times). The final Tc-99m IDA complex exists as a dimer, with two molecules of the chelating agent (IDA) reacting with one atom of Tc-99m. This dimeric configuration, with Tc-99m serving as a bridging atom between the two ligand molecules, confers stability to the technetium complex and determines hepatobiliary excretion.

Mechanism of Uptake and Clearance

Tc-99m IDA radiopharmaceuticals share the same hepatocyte uptake, transport, and excretion pathways as bilirubin. After intravenous (IV) injection, the Tc-99m IDA is bound to protein in the blood, minimizing renal clearance. The radiotracer is transported into the hepatocyte by a high-capacity carrier-mediated anionic clearance mechanism. Following hepatocellular uptake, these substances are transported into the bile canaliculi (Figure 9-3) by an active membrane transport system. The Tc-99m IDA compounds are stable in vivo and, in contrast to bilirubin, are excreted in their original radiochemical form without being conjugated or undergoing significant metabolism. Because these compounds have the same hepatocyte uptake, transport, and excretion pathways as bilirubin, the Tc-99m IDA compounds are subject to competitive inhibition by high serum bilirubin levels.

Pharmacokinetics and Preparation

Once Tc-99m IDA reaches the bile canaliculi, the radiopharmaceutical follows the flow of bilirubin into the gallbladder via the cystic duct and into the duodenum via the common duct (Figure 9-3). The differential flow is

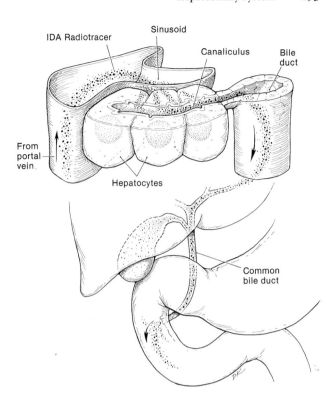

Fig. 9-3   Pharmacokinetics of Tc-99m IDA. The hepatic uptake and clearance of Tc-99m IDA are similar to that of bilirubin except that these radiopharmaceuticals are not conjugated or metabolized. Bilirubin is transported in the blood bound to albumin. It is then extracted by the hepatocyte, secreted into the bile canaliculi, and then cleared through the biliary tract into the bowel.

determined primarily by the patency of the bile ducts, intraluminal pressure, and tone at the sphincter of Oddi. Within the gallbladder, bile is concentrated and stored for later discharge into the bowel. The gallbladder contracts and empties in response to rising serum levels of cholecystokinin (CCK), a hormone produced and secreted into the blood by duodenal mucosa in response to ingested fat and protein passing through the proximal small bowel. CCK simultaneously relaxes the sphincter of Oddi.

Tc-99m disofenin and Tc-99m mebrofenin are considerably more effective than Tc-99m HIDA in competing with bilirubin for uptake (Table 9-1). Although bilirubin levels greater than 5 mg/dL result in poor image quality with Tc-99m HIDA, Tc-99m disofenin and Tc-99m mebrofenin can be effectively used with serum bilirubin levels as high as 20 to 30 mg/dL. Tc-99m mebrofenin has an edge over Tc-99m disofenin at very high serum bilirubin levels because of its greater resistance to displacement by bilirubin. Renal excretion serves as the alternative route of clearance for all IDA radiopharmaceuticals, is greater in those with less hepatic extraction, and increases with worsening hepatic insufficiency.

Table 9-1   Normal Pharmacokinetics of Tc-99m IDAs

Agent	Hepatic uptake (%)	Clearance $T_{1/2}$ (min)	Renal Excretion (2 hr) (%)
Tc-99m lidofenin (HIDA)	84	42	>14
Tc-99m disofenin (DISIDA)	88	19	< 9
Tc-99m mebrofenin (BrIDA)	98	17	< 1

The Tc-99m IDA radiopharmaceuticals are available as radiopharmaceutical kits that contain the IDA analogue and stannous chloride in lyophilized form. The Tc-99m IDA complex is formed by the simple addition of pertechnetate to the vial. The product is stable for at least 6 hours after reconstitution.

Dosimetry

Both Tc-99m disofenin and Tc-99m mebrofenin have similar dosimetry. The highest estimated radiation dose (target organ) is to the large bowel, about 2 rads (Table 9-2). Gallbladder dosimetry is variable, depending on whether the gallbladder fills, its ability to contract, and when it is stimulated to contract after the study.

Patient Preparation

The clinical history should be carefully reviewed prior to starting cholescintigraphy. The following questions are critical to optimally performing and interpreting a Tc-99m IDA study: What is the clinical question being asked? Are the symptoms acute or chronic? When and what did the patient last eat? Has the patient had biliary surgery? If the patient has had a biliary diversion procedure, what is the anatomy? Are there intra-abdominal tubes or drains? If so, where are they placed, and which

Table 9-2   Dosimetry for Tc-99m IDA

Organ	Tc-99m Disofenin (Hepatolite)*	
	rads/5mCi	mGy/185 MBq
Liver	0.19	1.9
Gallbladder	0.60	6.0
Large Intestine	1.90	19.0
Bladder	0.46	4.6
Ovaries	0.41	4.1
Testes	0.03	0.3
Marrow	0.14	1.4
Total body	0.08	0.8

*From package insert, E.I. duPont, Billerica, MA.

tubing drains each? Has US been performed? What did it show? Has the patient received any drugs (e.g., morphine or Demerol) that could affect normal biliary physiology and affect interpretation of the results? The answers to these questions will help determine the proper study protocol and correct interpretation of the study.

The patient should be fasting for at least 4 hours before the study is initiated. A recently ingested meal containing fat and protein stimulates production of endogenous CCK from the duodenal mucosa which continues until the food has emptied from the stomach and upper small bowel. The rising serum CCK level causes gallbladder contraction. This prevents radiotracer entry and may result in a false positive study for acute cholecystitis (nonvisualization of the gallbladder). On the other hand, fasting for longer than 24 hours without any stimulus to contraction results in concentrated, viscous bile within the gallbladder that may also prevent radiotracer entry. Clear liquids are not an adequate stimulus to gallbladder contraction.

In patients fasting greater than 24 hours, administration of IV CCK to stimulate contraction prior to beginning the study may prevent a false positive study for acute cholecystitis (gallbladder non-visualization). Of course, CCK can only be successful if the gallbladder is able to contract. For example, chronic cholecystitis is often associated with a nonfunctioning gallbladder. In this case, CCK administration prior to the study may not produce the desired result. (See below for further discussion.)

Box 9-2 summarizes the protocol for cholescintigraphy.

Image Interpretation

Because hepatic blood flow, Tc-99m IDA extraction, and biliary clearance are ongoing dynamic processes, image acquisition must be rapid enough to visualize each phase (Figure 9-4). The liver will not normally be seen on a blood flow study until 6 to 8 seconds after the spleen and kidneys became visible, since liver blood flow is predominantly portal in orgin (75% portal vein and 25% hepatic artery). Early diffusely increased blood flow may be seen if the liver is arterialized, as in cirrhosis or generalized tumor involvement, or focally due to a tumor mass or abscess, or in the region of the gallblad-

Box 9-2 Cholescintigraphy: Protocol Summary

PATIENT PREPARATION

1. NPO for 4 hr prior to the study.
2. If NPO >24 hr: infuse sincalid, 0.02 μg/kg in 30 mL normal saline over 30 min using a constant infusion pump.

RADIOPHARMACEUTICAL

Tc-99m mebrofenin or Tc-99m disofenin, injected IV.
Dosages: Adults: bilirubin <2mg/dL 5.0 mCi (185 MBq)
                    2 mg/dL   7.5 mCi (278 mCi)
                    10 mg/dL 10.0 mCi (370 MBq)
         Children: 200 μCi/kg (no less than 1 mCi or 35 MBq)

INSTRUMENTATION

Camera: Large field of view gamma camera.
Collimator: Low-energy all-purpose parallel hole.
Window: 15% over a 140-keV photopeak.
Computer acquisition: 1-sec frames for 60 sec (optional), then 1-min frames for 60 min.
Static film images: 500-1,000k count immediate anterior image, then images for equal time every 5 min × 60 min.

PATIENT POSITIONING

Supine, with upper abdomen in field of view.

IMAGING PROTOCOL

1. Inject Tc-99m IDA as a bolus and start computer.
2. If acute cholecystitis is suspected and there is biliary-to-bowel transit but the gallbladder has not filled by 30-60 min, inject morphine sulfate (MS) IV, 0.04 mg/kg over 1 min.
3. At end of routine study (30 min after MS or at 60 min if MS is not given), acquire a right lateral and LAO view.
4. Perform delayed imaging at 2-4 hr if:
   a. Neither CCK nor MS was administered and the gallbladder did not fill. Shielding of bowel activity and a longer acquisition time may be necessary to visualize the gallbladder fossa if most tracer has cleared from the liver. Occasionally Tc-99m IDA reinjection will be necessary.
   b. Where otherwise clinically indicated (e.g., hepatic insufficiency, partial common duct obstruction, suspected biliary leak).

CCK ADMINISTRATION

1. Computer set for 30 1-min frames; acquire high-count images on film every 5 min.
2. Start the computer 1 min before injection. Infuse 0.02 ug/kg sincalide diluted in 30-mL volume slowly over 15-30 min, using a constant infusion pump.
3. Calculate the percent gallbladder emptying (maximum counts minus minimum counts divided by maximum counts, all corrected for background).

der fossa due to the inflammation associated with acute cholecystitis (Figure 9-5).

Hepatic extraction can best be evaluated by comparing the immediate high count image after injection with one obtained at 5 minutes. The initial image will predominantly represent blood pool activity because extraction of the Tc-99m IDA is just beginning. By 5 minutes, most of the blood pool seen in the heart should normally have been cleared of radiotracer, owing to its rapid hepatic extraction. Delayed blood pool clearance is a sign of hepatic insufficiency (Figure 9-6).

During the early hepatic phase, before biliary clearance, an assessment can be made of liver size, shape, and the presence of intrahepatic lesions. A small amount of early renal clearance may be seen normally; relatively more occurs with increasing severity of hepatic insufficiency. With good hepatic function, biliary excretion usually begins by 10 minutes after injection. Although the smaller peripheral biliary structures usually cannot be visualized unless enlarged, the left and right hepatic bile ducts, common hepatic, and common bile duct are usually seen with frequent image acquisition or on computer cinematic display (Figures 9-4, 9-5, 9-7). The left hepatic ducts are often more prominent than the right. Although evidence of dilation can be seen on cholescintigraphy, the study should not be used to anatomically size ducts, but rather to determine their functional patency.

About two thirds of biliary flow travels directly through the common duct and the sphincter of Oddi into the second portion of the duodenum. The remaining third enters the gallbladder via the cystic duct. The normal gallbladder is usually seen by 30 minutes, al-

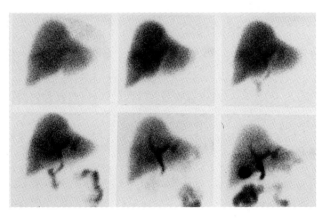

Fig. 9-4 Normal Tc-99m IDA study: analog immediate and sequential images acquired every 5 minutes (*left to right*). Note rapid heart blood pool clearance between the immediate and 5-minute image. Right and left and common hepatic ducts can be seen by 10 minutes; the common bile duct begins to be visualized by 10 minutes and is well seen by 15 minutes concomitant with duodenal clearance. Normal gallbladder visualization is subsequently noted. In this case the study was completed in 30 minutes.

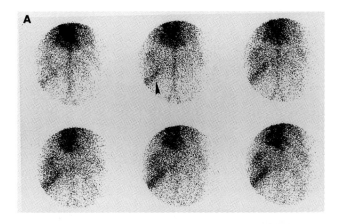

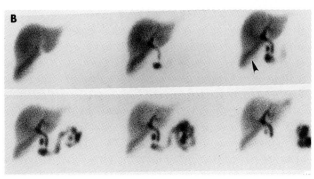

Fig. 9-5 Acute cholecystitis. **A**, Increased flow to the inferior aspect of the right lobe of the liver adjacent to the gallbladder fossa (*arrowhead*). **B**, Rim sign. Increased uptake in the liver adjacent to the gallbladder fossa is seen on all sequential images through 60 minutes (*arrowhead*). There is normal biliary-to-bowel transit, but no gallbladder visualization. Transient duodenal activity is seen inferior and medial to the common duct.

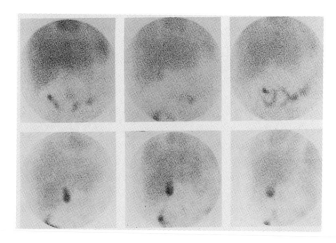

Fig. 9-6 Severe hepatic insufficiency. *Top*, Images acquired at 10 minutes, 2 hours, and 4 hours (*left to right*) show a low liver-to-background ratio consistent with poor liver function. Note persistent heart blood pool. The gallbladder is not visualized. *Bottom*, Delayed images acquired at 12 hours (*left to right*, RAO, Anterior, LAO) show delayed gallbladder visualization.

though visualization by 60 minutes is defined as normal. Biliary-to-bowel transit should also occur by 60 minutes. However, about 10% to 20% of normal subjects will have common duct visualization but delayed biliary-to-bowel transit as a result of a physiologic "hypertonic" sphincter of Oddi. Although delayed imaging at 1 to 2 hours can confirm common duct patency, CCK administration can promptly differentiate this normal variation from partial common duct obstruction (see below) (Figures 9-7, 9-8).

Cholecystokinin

There are various diagnostic indications for the interventional use of CCK before, during, or after routine cholescintigraphy (Box 9-3). Sincalide (Kinevac; E.R. Squibb & Sons, Princeton, NJ) is the synthetic C-terminal

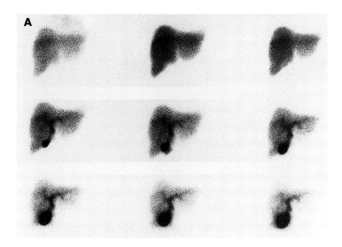

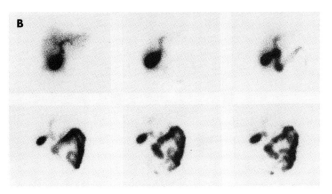

Fig. 9-7 Normal HIDA variation with delayed biliary-to-bowel transit. Sequential 5 minute images were acquired for 40 minutes. **A**, The gallbladder begins to fill at 15 minutes and the common hepatic and proximal common bile duct are fully seen by 30 minutes, but there is no biliary-to-bowel clearance. **B**, *Upper left* image was acquired at 70 minutes just before CCK infusion. After sincalide infusion, the gallbladder contracts (EF = 41%) and there is rapid transit into the bowel due to concomitant sphincter of Oddi relaxation. This is a normal study.

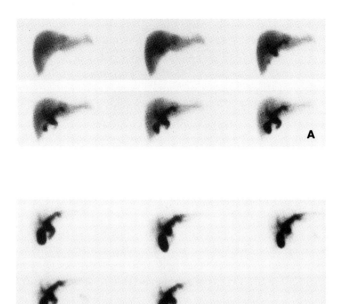

A

B

Fig. 9-8   Partial common duct obstruction. **A,** The gallbladder visualizes early. The common bile duct appears prominent and probably dilated. Retained or refluxed bile is seen in the left hepatic duct. No biliary-to-bowel transit occurs by 60 minutes. **B,** Thirty-minute CCK infusion with immediate, 5, 10, 20, and 30-minute images. No gallbladder contraction or further biliary-to-bowel transit occurs. This pattern is diagnostic of partial common duct obstruction.

octapeptide of CCK. It is the only form of CCK available for clinical use in the United States. Its pharmacokinetic effect is dependent on the total administered dose, the dose rate, and the length of infusion. Bolus infusions of less than 60 seconds' duration can cause biliary spasm; short infusions of 2 to 3 minutes have been recommended and are often used clinically but are nonphysiologic and may give unpredictable and variable results. Continuous slow infusions over 15 to 30 minutes are preferable and give more reproducible and complete gallbladder emptying. Tc-99m IDA should not be injected until 30 minutes after sincalide infusion to allow time for gallbladder relaxation.

The clinical use of sincalide is discussed below under the appropriate clinical sections. Sincalide can be infused IV more than once in a study because its serum half-life is only 2.5 minutes. For example, in a patient who has fasted longer than 24 hours, sincalide can be given before the study and again at the end of the study to calculate a gallbladder ejection fraction. Sincalide administered prior to cholescintigraphy can change the normal pharmacokinetics of Tc-99m IDA and result in delayed biliary-to-bowel transit time. CCK should not be used after morphine sulfate because of the latter's rela-

tively long and variable serum half-life of 3 to 6 hours, which can counteract the effect of CCK.

Clinical Applications

Acute cholecystitis   Clinically suspected acute cholecystitis is the most common indication for cholescintigraphy. The usual presenting symptoms include acute colicky right upper quadrant pain and nausea and vomiting, accompanied by leukocytosis. Acute cholecystitis is initiated by cystic duct obstruction, usually due to an impacted stone. A progression of histopathologic changes in the gallbladder wall then ensues: edema, white cell infiltration, hemorrhage, necrosis, and finally gangrene and perforation. Cholecystectomy is the standard treatment.

Cholescintigraphy is generally considered to be the study of choice to make the diagnosis of acute cholecystitis. It defines the underlying pathophysiology, obstruction of the cystic duct, as manifested by nonfilling of the gallbladder (Figure 9-5).

Although US is sometimes reflexively ordered for the diagnosis of symptomatic biliary disease, the results usually are not specific enough to make the diagnosis of acute cholecystitis. A stone impacted in the cystic duct can confirm the diagnosis; however, this is uncommonly seen (<5%) with US. Although patients with acute cholecystitis frequently have cholelithiasis, gallstones are also common in the asymptomatic general population. Their presence is not an indication of *acute* cholecystitis but rather of *chronic* cholecystitis.

Other typical findings on US in acute cholecystitis include thickening of the gallbladder wall and pericholecystic fluid, both of which are nonspecific findings and can occur with other disease processes. The diagnostic utility of the "ultrasonographic Murphy's sign" (localized tenderness on examination in the region of the gallbladder on US examination) is controversial; in some hands it has been found quite accurate, but it is subjective and highly technician dependent.

Scintigraphic diagnosis In the proper clinical setting (as described in the previous section), nonfilling of the gallbladder by 60 minutes after Tc-99m IDA injection is diagnostic of acute cholecystitis. The accuracy of cholescintigraphy is very high. However, causes of false positive studies should be noted (Box 9-4). If the patient has eaten within 2 to 4 hours of the start of the study, the gallbladder will likely be contracted due to the meal-induced endogenous production of CCK, thus preventing radiotracer entry into the gallbladder. Prolonged fasting of greater than 24 hours often results in a gallbladder filled with viscous bile due to the lack of CCK-stimulated gallbladder contraction.

Hepatic insufficiency may result in either nonvisualization or very delayed visualization of the gallbladder (Figure 9-6). Some controversy exists as to whether pancreatitis and alcoholism are associated with an increased incidence of false positive studies. Clearly, an increased incidence of false positive studies is seen in hospitalized patients with intercurrent serious illness and in patients who have been fasting or who are receiving hyperalimentation.

Although most patients with chronic cholecystitis have gallbladder filling by 60 minutes, some (<5%) will not; in most of the latter the gallbladder will fill by 2 to 4 hours after injection, ruling out acute cholecystitis. The reason for delayed visualization is partial cystic duct obstruction as a result of recurrent inflammation and cellular debris. Administration of CCK prior to injecting Tc-99m IDA reduces gallbladder filling time in these patients to the first hour; however, this is not routinely done, for two reasons. First, it would require administering CCK to all patients, and second, it would prevent differentiation of patients without gallbladder disease from those with

chronic cholecystis. Therefore, delayed imaging up to 4 hours has been recommended and routinely performed in patients without gallbladder visualization at 1 hour.

Certain scintigraphic findings can increase the certainty of the diagnosis of acute cholecystitis in patients with nonfilling of the gallbladder who are in a clinical setting associated with potential false positive studies. These are (1) increased blood flow to the region of the gallbladder fossa and (2) increased hepatic uptake in the gallbladder fossa (Rim sign) (Figure 9-5).

The Rim sign is a very specific sign of acute cholecystitis and is seen in about 25% of patients. It is seen in patients presenting at a later stage in the pathologic spectrum of acute cholecystitis and has been associated with an increased risk for the serious complications of perforation and gangrene. The pathophysiologic mechanism producing the Rim sign is believed due to a combination of increased blood flow delivered to inflamed liver adjacent to the gallbladder, resulting in increased extraction as well as delayed clearance due to the edematous and inflamed biliary canaliculi.

Morphine augmentation The 2- to 4-hour time delay required to ensure the diagnosis of acute cholecystitis when the gallbladder does not visualize in the first hour is not optimal in sick patients. The interventional use of morphine sulfate as an alternative to delayed imaging has gained wide popularity and is now often routinely used to shorten the duration of this test. Morphine sulfate increases intraluminal pressure at the sphincter of Oddi. This results in preferential biliary flow via the cystic duct, if it is patent. Once biliary-into-bowel clearance is seen, but there has been no gallbladder filling, morphine sulphate can be given IV (0.04 mg/kg). With cystic duct patency, the gallbladder begins to fill within 5 to 10 minutes and the study is complete by 30 minutes. The entire Tc-IDA study takes a total of 60 to 90 minutes (Figures 9-9A,B).

Sometimes it may be difficult to differentiate gallbladder filling from radioactivity in adjacent or overlapping common duct and duodenum. Right lateral and left anterior oblique (LAO) views can help make this distinction (Figure 9-10). In the right lateral projection, the gallbladder is usually anterior. In the LAO projection, the gallbladder will move to the right and the common duct and duodenum will move to the left, the latter being more posterior structures. Upright imaging or a drink of water to clear duodenal activity can also be helpful. Morphine sulfate may also be helpful, for contraction of the sphincter of Oddi prevents further biliary-to-bowel clearance and the duodenal activity usually moves on (Figure 9-9A).

Acute acalculous cholecystitis Acute acalculous cholecystitis is a serious life-threatening disease that typically occurs in predisposed patients, such as sick, hospitalized patients with severe burns, sepsis, massive trauma, or

---

Box 9-4   Causes of False Positive Cholescintigraphy for Acute Cholecystitis

Fasting < 4 hr
Fasting > 24 hr
Intercurrent severe illness
Hepatic insufficiency
Chronic cholecystitis
Hyperalimentation
Alcoholism (?)
Pancreatitis (?)

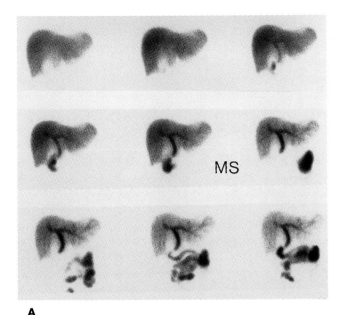

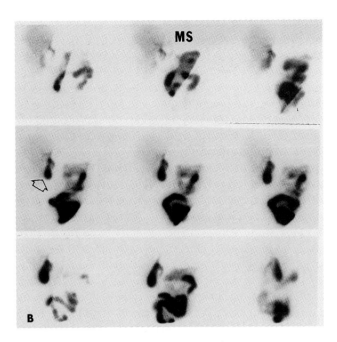

Fig. 9-9   Morphine-augmentation cholescintigraphy. **A**, Tc-IDA study performed to confirm the clinical diagnosis of acute cholecystitis. Images shown were acquired at 1, 5, 10, 20, 30, 40, 50, 60, and 70 minutes. At 30 minutes there was good visualization of the common hepatic and common bile duct, biliary clearance into the duodenum, but no gallbladder visualization. Morphine sulfate (MS) was given intravenously. The gallbladder did not visualize, making the diagnosis of acute cholecystitis within 1 hour. **B**, In another patient, there was no gallbladder filling at 60 minutes *(upper left)*, so morphine sulfate was given. Gallbladder filling began within 5 minutes and was definite by 10 minutes *(arrowhead)*. Acute cholecystitis has thus been ruled out.

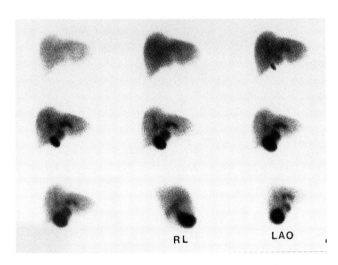

Fig. 9-10   Use of the right lateral (RL) and left anterior oblique (LAO) view to differentiate gallbladder from common duct and duodenal overlap. In this study, separating the gallbladder from the common bile duct and duodenum is problematic *(middle row)*. The RL view confirms gallbladder filling since it is anterior. The LAO view nicely demonstrates the common bile duct, but there has been no biliary-to-bowel clearance and therefore no duodenal activity. In the LAO view the gallbladder moves to the right (anteriorly) and the common bile duct and duodenum move to the left (posteriorly).

recent surgery. Because of its high mortality, early diagnosis is imperative. The etiology is cystic duct obstruction caused by inflammatory debris and inspissated bile or sometimes infection or ischemia of the gallbladder wall without duct obstruction.

Although cholescintigraphy can usually be used to make the diagnosis (nonfilling of the gallbladder), cystic duct obstruction in acute acalculous cholecystitis may be incomplete or not present, allowing tracer to enter the gallbladder, resulting in a false negative study. If the diagnosis is suspected but the gallbladder has filled, infusion of CCK to evaluate gallbladder function may be helpful. An inflamed gallbladder does not contract normally, and an ejection fraction of less than 35% suggests the diagnosis. This finding is not specific because it does not differentiate acute from unrelated chronic gallbladder disease. A radiolabeled white blood cell study can confirm the diagnosis.

Common duct obstruction   Common duct obstruction may be caused by choledocholithiasis, neoplasm or stricture. The diagnosis of obstruction is usually made by observing common duct dilation on US. Although high-grade common duct obstruction has a classic appearance on cholescintigraphy (good uptake, but no biliary clearance) (Figure 9-11), it is not usually needed to make the diagnosis. There are two exceptions: (1) In the first

24 hours of obstruction before ductal dilation has occurred, US may be normal, but the HIDA study will be abnormal, showing the physiologic abnormality. (2) In patients who have had previous common duct obstruction or surgery, dilated ducts usually do not return to normal size. Cholescintigraphy can differentiate obstructive from nonobstructive dilation by demonstrating biliary dynamics, that is, the presence or absence of normal biliary-to-bowel transit.

Biliary atresia   In pediatric patients, cholescintigraphy has been found to be quite accurate in the diagnosis of biliary atresia and in differentiating it from other causes of neonatal jaundice. Early diagnosis is critical, because surgery must be performed before irreversible liver failure ensues. The congenitally atretic bile ducts produce a picture of high-grade obstruction (Figures 9-12A,B). However, severe hepatic insufficiency of any cause may result in very delayed biliary-to-bowel transit. Pretreatment with phenobarbital (5 mg/kg/day for 5 days) prior to Tc-99m IDA imaging maximizes the sensitivity of this test by revving up the liver excretory enzymes. Nonobstructive causes of neonatal jaudice will show biliary-to-bowel transit by 24 hours. Biliary atresia will not. The serum phenobarbital level should be checked prior to initiating the study to ensure a therapeutic blood level.

Partial common duct obstruction   Tc-99m IDA studies can be useful for detecting partial common duct obstruction (Figures 9-8, 9-13). Common duct stones causing partial obstruction are infrequently seen with US or intravenous cholangiography (<10%), and dilation may not be present. Cholescintigraphy can be diagnostic or at least suggestive of the diagnosis, thereby determining the need for more invasive workup. Delayed biliary-to-bowel transit (>60 minutes) is the least specific finding. It may be normal in up to 50% of patients with partial common duct obstruction. In addition, delayed

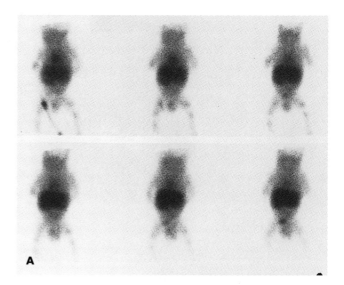

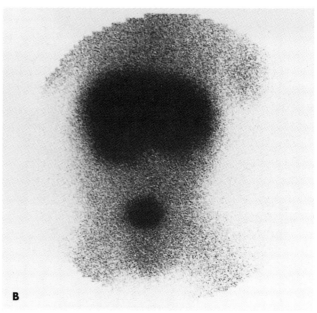

Fig. 9-12   Biliary atresia. Serum phenobarbital level was in the therapeutic range. **A**, Imaging every 10 minutes for the first hour after injection of Tc-99m mebrofenin showed no biliary-to- bowel transit. Note very delayed heart blood pool clearance due to some hepatic insufficiency. **B**, Images acquired at 24 hours show no bowel activity, only renal clearance into the bladder. Surgery confirmed the diagnosis of biliary atresia.

transit occurs in up to 20% of normal subjects, so this finding alone is neither sensitive nor specific.

A number of other scintigraphic findings are more specific (Box 9-5). Intraluminal filling defects are uncommonly seen. Segmental narrowing with ductal prominence proximally is characteristic. There may be an abrupt or a gradual cutoff. Abnormal biliary dynamics may be demonstrated with delayed imaging; for example, no decrease or an increase in ductal radioactivity

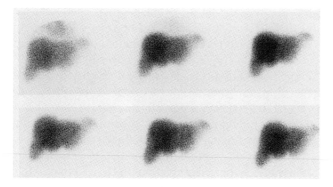

Fig. 9-11   Common bile duct obstruction. Good hepatic uptake is seen, but no secretion into the biliary ducts. This is the classic picture of high-grade common duct obstruction. The high back pressure prevents tracer from entering the biliary system.

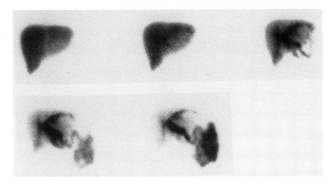

Fig. 9-13   Postoperative stricture causing partial common duct obstruction. Images were acquired at 5, 10, 20, 40, and 60 minutes. Note the dilated common hepatic and common bile duct with an abrupt distal cutoff. However, biliary-to-bowel transit is normal.

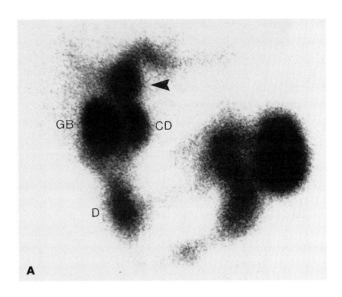

may be seen between 1 and 2 hours, or persistent pooling may be seen after CCK infusion.

Other causes of partial common duct obstruction may produce characteristic findings on cholescintigraphy. A *choledochal cyst* often presents clinically as obstruction, although many remain asymptomatic. Pathologically, it is not really a cyst but merely a dilation that can occur anywhere within the biliary system. Although a complete obstruction would result in nonvisualization of the biliary tract, a partial obstruction can often be confirmed on cholescintigraphy (Figures 9-14A,B). US will often show a cystic structure but many times does not show for certain whether it is part of the biliary tract. Tc-99m IDA tracer will fill the choledochal cyst, although delayed images are frequently needed; there will be prolonged retention within the cystic structure.

The *postcholecystectomy pain syndrome* is a common and clinically perplexing entity that has a variety of causes. Partial common duct obstruction may be caused by a retained stone, postoperative stricture, or *sphincter of Oddi dysfunction*. The latter syndrome is manifested by elevated sphincter pressure, usually without anatomic obstruction. However, pressure measurements are technically difficult to perform and not always success-

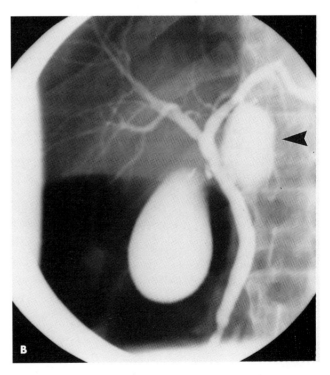

Fig. 9-14   Choledochal cyst in a 25-year-old patient who presented with abdominal pain. US defined a cystic structure, possibly a choledochal cyst, adjacent to the common hepatic duct; however, a definite connection to the biliary system could not be ascertained. **A**, The Tc-99m IDA study showed evidence for a choledochal cyst in the region of the common hepatic duct (*arrowhead*). This image was acquired at 90 minutes after the liver had cleared of most tracer. The common duct (CD), gallbladder (GB), and duodenum (D) are labeled. **B**, A subsequent cholangiogram confirmed the diagnosis.

Box 9-5   Scintigraphic Findings of Partial Common Duct Obstruction
Segmental narrowing
Abrupt or gradual cutoff
Intraluminal filling defect
Ductal prominence above narrowing
Abnormal biliary dynamics
Delayed biliary-to-bowel transit

ful. In the setting of a normal ERCP that excludes anatomic obstruction, evidence of partial obstruction on cholescintigraphy would suggest the diagnosis and therefore select out patients for sphincter pressure measurement. Recent data suggest that CCK infusion during cholescintigraphy may increase detectability.

Tc-99m IDA studies are also useful for follow-up of patients treated for obstruction with *papillotomy* or *biliary stents* (Figure 9-15) and can be used to confirm patency or diagnose restenosis.

Evaluation of a suspected *postoperative biliary leak* is an important use of cholescintigraphy. The study can be used to confirm the diagnosis when CT or US demonstrates a fluid phase of uncertain cause, such as ascites, abscess, or bile leak (Figure 9-16). The rate of leakage can be estimated. Rapid leaks often require surgery, while slow ones may resolve with time. Follow-up studies can confirm resolution.

Primary benign and malignant hepatic tumors Tc-99m IDA studies can play a role in the differential diagnosis of primary benign and malignant hepatic tumors, among them *focal nodular hyperplasia, hepatic adenoma*, and *hepatoma* (Table 9-3). These tumors all con-

Table 9-3   Differential Diagnosis of Primary Hepatic Tumors With Cholescintigraphy

	Flow	Uptake	Clearance
Focal nodular hyperplasia	Increased	Immediate	Delayed
Hepatic adenoma	Normal	None	—
Hepatocellular carcinoma	Increased	Delayed	Delayed

tain hepatocytes and therefore might be expected to take up Tc-99m IDA.

Focal nodular hyperplasia and adenoma Focal nodular hyperplasia (FNH) and hepatic adenoma have quite different natural histories and require different therapy. FNH is usually asymptomatic, found incidentally, and requires no specific therapy, whereas hepatic adenomas are often symptomatic, may hemorrhage, and can be life-threatening. Adenomas have a strong association with oral contraceptive use. They must be discontinued.

FNH is a benign tumor containing heptocytes, Kupffer cells, and bile canaliculi. The characteristic findings on cholescintigraphy are increased blood flow, prompt hepatic uptake, and very delayed clearance (Figure 9-17); the latter finding is probably due to abnormal biliary canaliculi. One might expect similar findings with hepatic adenoma, a benign tumor made up only of hepatocytes, but this seems not to be the usual case; adenomas do not usually exhibit uptake on cholescintigraphy.

Hepatocellular carcinoma   Hepatocellular carcinoma (hepatoma) also has diagnostic findings on Tc-99m

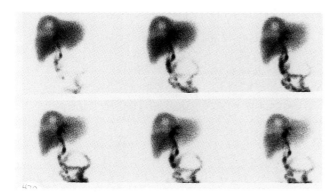

Fig. 9-15   Patent biliary stent. A common duct stent was placed to relieve obstruction from tumor. This 60-minute HIDA study confirms its patency. Note the hepatic mass in the dome of the liver.

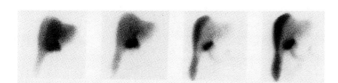

Fig. 9-16   Postoperative biliary leak. CT performed 4 days after cholecystectomy showed intra-abdominal fluid. A HIDA study was ordered to determine if the fluid collection was of biliary origin. Scintigraphic evidence of biliary leakage is seen on sequential images acquired 60 minutes (*left*) to 6 hours (*right*) after tracer injection. The bile localized between the liver and chest wall, over the liver dome, and in the portal area.

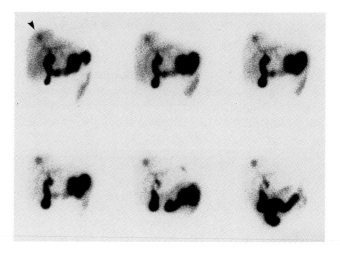

Fig. 9-17   Focal nodular hyperplasia. Sequential images acquired every 5 minutes show early uptake in a tumor in the dome of the liver that persists through the 60-minute study, while the normal liver has cleared of tracer. This focal uptake persisted on delayed images acquired at 3 hours.

IDA imaging. The malignant hepatocytes usually retain function but are hypofunctional compared to normal liver. On cholescintigraphy, images made during the first hour usually show no uptake within the lesion (cold defect). However, delayed imaging at 2 to 4 hours often shows "filling in," or continuing uptake within the tumor and concomitant clearing of adjacent normal liver (Figure 9-18). This pattern is specific for hepatoma. Some poorly differentiated tumors will not fill in on delayed imaging. Tc-99m IDA uptake can sometimes indicate sites of metastases.

Chronic cholecystitis Chronic cholecystitis, unlike acute cholecystitis, is appropriately diagnosed with US. Routine cholescintigraphy is usually normal in patients with chronic cholecystitis, although occasionally gall-bladder filling defects (uncommon), delayed gallbladder filling (<5%), or delayed biliary-to-bowel-transit (nonspecific) can be seen.

Symptomatic chronic cholecystitis is often associated with poor gallbladder contraction as demonstrated by a decreased ejection fraction when stimulated with a fatty meal or CCK. Although it has been suggested that CCK cholescintigraphy may help differentiate patients with symptomatic cholelithiasis from those with stones but chronic abdominal pain from other causes, cholescintigraphy more clearly plays a well-established clinical role in making the diagnosis of chronic *acalculous* cholecystitis.

Chronic acalculous cholecystitis is relatively uncommon compared to chronic *calculous* cholecystitis, but it is a perplexing clinical problem because the diagnosis is difficult to make preoperatively. These patients' pain often goes undiagnosed. They have recurrent biliary colic-like pain, but extensive clinical workups, including US, oral cholecystography, and routine cholescintigraphy, are usually normal. A low gallbladder ejection fraction (<35%) after sincalide infusion can preoperatively predict histopathologic evidence of chronic cholecystitis and symptomatic relief with cholecystectomy (Figure 9-19). Although a fatty meal can effectively produce contraction of the gallbladder, sincalide infusion is more predictable, faster, and not dependent on gastric function.

Enterogastric bile reflux Enterogastric bile reflux can sometimes cause an alkaline gastritis resulting in symptoms similar to those of acid-related disease. This is most commonly seen after gastric resection operations. Cholescintigraphy can be used to make this diagnosis noninvasively (Figure 9-20). Although some reflux is normal, particularly if morphine sulfate or CCK has been given, the larger the quantity of reflux and the more persistent it is, the more likely that it is related to the patient's symptoms.

Accuracy The sensitivity and specificity of cho-

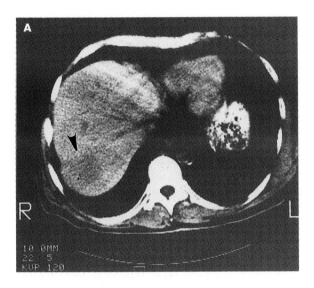

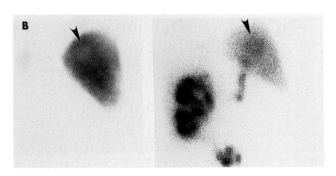

Fig. 9-18 Hepatocellular carcinoma. **A**, CT scan shows large lesion in posterior aspect of the right lobe (*arrowhead*). **B**, *Left*, Tc-99m HIDA posterior image acquired at 5 minutes shows a cold defect in the same region as seen on CT (*arrowhead*). *Right*, Posterior view. HIDA at 2 hours shows increased uptake within the lesion (*arrowhead*) and considerable washout of the remainder of the liver. Surgery confirmed a hepatoma.

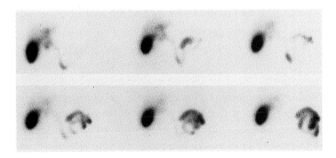

Fig. 9-19 Chronic acalculous cholecystitis. There was extremely poor contraction of the gallbladder after sincalide infusion (ejection fraction <5%). Biliary-to-bowel transit occurs due to relaxation of the sphincter of Oddi.

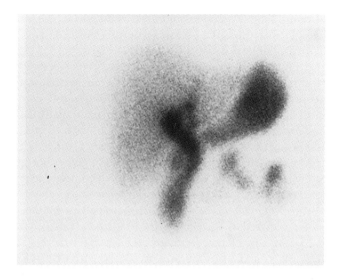

Fig. 9-20   Enterogastric reflux. At 60 minutes after injection of Tc-99m IDA, considerable enterogastric reflux of labeled bile into the stomach is seen. Bile gastritis was confirmed at endoscopy.

lescintigraphy for making the diagnosis of acute cholecystitis are very high in the proper clinical setting (sensitivity >95%, specificity >98%). However, patients with intercurrent illness, who are fasting, who are on hyperalimentation, who have hepatic insufficiency, or who have chronic cholecystitis have an increased incidence of a false positive studies. Alcoholism and pancreatitis have also been associated with false positive studies, although this is more controversial. Morphine-augmented cholescintigraphy is as accurate as 2-4-hour delayed imaging for making the diagnosis. The sensitivity for *acute* acalculous cholecystitis is slightly less, (85%-90%). A low gallbladder ejection fraction in a patient referred with suspected *chronic* acalculous cholecystis is more than 90% accurate for making the diagnosis.

TC-99M RED BLOOD CELL LIVER SCINTIGRAPHY

Cavernous hemangiomas are the most common benign tumor of the liver and the second most common hepatic tumor, exceeded in incidence only by hepatic metastases. They are usually asymptomatic and discovered incidentally on CT or US during the clinical workup or staging of a patient with a known primary malignancy, or during evaluation of unrelated abdominal symptoms or disease. They almost never require specific therapy. However, they must be differentiated from other, more serious hepatic tumors.

Tc-99m-labeled red blood cell (Tc-99m RBC) scintigraphy is highly accurate for making the diagnosis and can obviate the need for biopsy, which, on occasion, may

result in hemorrhage-associated morbidity and even mortality. The radionuclide imaging technique has an exceedingly low false positive rate.

Pathology

Cavernous hemangiomas of the liver are made up of abnormally dilated endothelial-lined vascular channels of varying sizes separated by fibrous septa; they are essentially large varix-filled spaces. Cavernous hemangiomas are not pathologically related to capillary hemangiomas, angiodysplasia, or infantile hemangioendotheliomas. Ten percent of these benign liver tumors are multiple. Lesions larger than 4 cm are often referred to as giant cavernous hemangiomas.

Radiopharmaceutical

Red blood cell labeling with Tc-99m pertechnetate is performed in much the same way as discussed in Chapters 4 and 10 under Radionuclide Ventriculography and Gastrointestinal Bleeding Scintigraphy. The in vitro kit method is now the preferred method because of its high labeling efficiency and ease of preparation.

Mechanism of Localization and Pharmacokinetics

After injection, the Tc-99m-labeled RBCs distribute within the blood pool of the liver. Time is required for the labeled cells to exchange and equilibrate within the large, relatively stagnant, nonlabeled blood pool of the hemangioma (Figure 9-21). This equilibration time

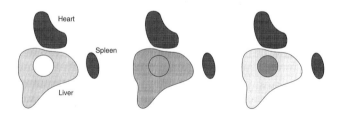

Fig. 9-21   Schematic diagram illustrating the classic pharmacokinetics of Tc-99m RBCs used for the diagnosis of cavernous hemangioma of the liver. *Left*, Immediately after injection the hemangioma is "cold." The blood pool activity within the liver is considerably greater than activity within the large hemangioma. It requires time for the injected Tc-99m labeled RBCs to equilibrate with the large number of unlabeled RBCs in the enlarged blood pool volume of the hemangioma. *Middle*, As the Tc-99m-labeled cells increasingly enter the hemangioma and mix with the unlabeled cells, the relative uptake in the hemangioma equalizes with normal liver. *Right*, When the RBCs have fully equilibrated (60-120 minutes), uptake within the lesion exceeds uptake in surrounding liver and is often equal to activity in the heart and spleen.

varies, depending to some extent on the size of the hemangioma, between 30 and 120 minutes. When the RBCs are fully equilibrated, the radioactivity per pixel within the hemangioma will typically be greater than in adjacent normal liver and usually equal to heart blood pool radioactivity.

Dosimetry

The total body radiation absorbed dose is about 0.4 rads. The the target organ is the heart wall, which receives 1.2 rads; the bladder and spleen radiation dose are slightly less (Table 9-3).

Box 9-6   Tc-99m RBC Scintigraphy: Protocol Summary

PATIENT PREPARATION

None.

RADIOPHARMACEUTICAL

Tc-99m pertechnetate, 25 mCi, labeled to RBCs (in vitro kit method).
Inject IV. Bolus injection for flow images.

INSTRUMENTATION

Camera: Large field of view gamma camera with SPECT capability.
Energy window: 15% centered over 140-keV photopeak.
Collimator: Low-energy, high-resolution parallel-hole collimator.

IMAGE ACQUISITION

Planar imaging

1. Blood flow: 1-sec frames X 60 on computer and 2-sec film images.
2. Immediate images: Acquire a 750-1,000k count planar image in the same projection and other views as necessary to best visualize the lesion(s).
3. Delayed images: Acquire 750-1,000k count planar static images 1-2 hr after injection in multiple projections (anterior, posterior, lateral, and oblique views).

SPECT

1. Position the patient supine on the imaging table. Raise the patient's arms above the head.
2. Center the liver in the field of view.
3. Rotate the camera head around the patient to ensure that the camera does not come in contact with the patient. Observe the liver on the camera monitor or computer display. It should remain completely in the field of view during a test rotation.

SINGLE- VERSUS MULTIHEADED SPECT IMAGING PARAMETERS

	Single-Headed SPECT	**Triple-Headed SPECT**
CAMERA SETUP		
Window:	15% window centered over 140-keV Tc-99m photopeak	15% window centered over 140-keV Tc-99m photopeak
Setup:	Step and shoot	Step and shoot
Collimator(s):	High resolution	Ultra-high resolution
COMPUTER SETUP		
Aquisition parameters		
Patient orientation:	Supine	Supine
Rotation:	Clockwise	Clockwise as viewed from feet
Matrix:	64 × 64 word mode	128 × 128 word mode
Image/arc combination:	128 images/360°	40 images/120° for each detector (120 images/360°)
Time/frame:	10 sec/stop	40 sec/stop
Reconstruction parameters		
Filters:	Dependent on manufacturer and personal preference	Dependent on manufacturer and personal preference
Attenuation correction:	Chang	Chang
Reformatting:	Sagittal/coronal	Sagittal/coronal

Methodology

A combined three-phase planar and SPECT technique is described in Box 9-6. If SPECT instrumentation is available, it is the preferred method and provides diagnostic information. The planar flow and immediate images are not really necessary for diagnosis if SPECT is performed; however, many investigators still routinely obtain all three phases because of the characteristic findings.

Proper performance of the study as well as correct interpretation requires using the patient's prior imaging study (CT, MRI, US, or Tc-99m SC liver-spleen scan) to determine in which projection the flow study and immediate images should be acquired to give optimum visibility to the lesion and for correlative image interpretation, which is particularly important with SPECT and small lesions.

The exact methodology used for image acquisition and processing will depend on the particular instrumentation available—whether it is a single-, dual-, or triple-headed camera, the manufacturer, computer, software, and personal preferences. The protocols described in Box 9-6 serve as a general guideline for both a single-headed and triple-headed system.

Image Interpretation

Normal hepatic vascular anatomy   The liver has a complex vascular system (Figures 9-1, 9-22, 9-50). It receives only about one third of its blood supply from the hepatic artery; the remaining two thirds comes from the portal vein. The sinusoids act as the capillary bed for the liver cells. Blood leaves the liver via the hepatic veins, which then empty into the inferior vena cava. The caudate lobe is an exception in that it also has a direct connection with the vena cava. Much of this normal vascular anatomy of the liver is seen with Tc-99m-labeled RBCs (Figures 9-23 to 9-27).

The organs with the highest activity per pixel are the heart and spleen, followed by the kidney; the normal liver has much less blood pool activity. The aorta and inferior vena cava and sometimes the portal vein can be seen with planar imaging; portal branching vessels and hepatic veins can be seen with SPECT.

Diagnostic criteria   The diagnostic scintigraphic pattern of cavernous hemangioma is that of increased activity of Tc-99m-labeled RBCs within the lesion compared to adjacent liver on 1- to 2-hour delayed imaging. The uptake is usually equal to that of blood pool of the heart and spleen (Figures 9-24 to 9-27). With rare exceptions, benign and malignant liver tumors, abscesses, cirrhotic nodules, and cysts have decreased activity (Figure 9-28).

The arterial blood flow to a hemangioma is usually normal, although increased or decreased flow has occasionally been described. Immediate blood pool images usually have decreased uptake within the hemangioma

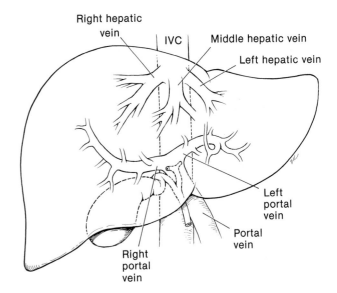

Fig. 9-22   Normal vascular anatomy of the liver. The blood supply to the liver is predominantly from the portal vein (75%) and to a lesser extent from the hepatic artery (25%). Both enter the liver in the portal area. The hepatic artery and its branches are not shown here. The portal vein divides into a right and a left branch and then further subdivides. The smaller branches in conjunction with the hepatic artery branches and canaliculi define the periphery of lobules (see Figure 9-1). The hepatic veins originate at the lobule center (central veins), feeding into the right, middle, and left hepatic veins, which drain into the inferior vena cava.

compared to adjacent liver (Figures 9-23 to 9-25), although early increased uptake may sometimes be seen. Very large giant cavernous hemangiomas often show heterogeneity of uptake with areas of decreased as well as increased uptake (Figure 9-23). These cold regions, which are often located centrally, are due to thrombosis, necrosis, and fibrosis.

Other Imaging Methods: US, CT, and MRI

The classic sonographic pattern of a homogeneous, hyperechoic mass with well-defined margins and posterior acoustical enhancement is neither sensitive nor specific for the diagnosis of cavernous hemangioma.

Strict criteria for the classic CT appearance include relative hypoattenuation prior to IV contrast agent injection, early peripheral enhancement during the rapid bolus dynamic phase of contrast agent administration, progressive opacification toward the center of the lesion, and complete isodense fill-in, usually by 30 minutes after contrast agent administration. Frequently not all criteria are satisfied. When these criteria are used to maximize specificity, the sensitivity of CT is only 55%; less strict criteria result in a high false positive rate. Accuracy is even poorer with multiple hemangiomas.

Cavernous hemangiomas have a characteristic appear-

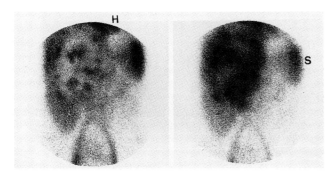

Fig. 9-23   Giant cavernous hemangioma. *Left,* Immediate postinjection image shows a large relatively photopenic area involving most of the left lobe and a large portion of the right lobe. Some focal areas of increased uptake are seen. *Right,* Delayed image acquired at 1 hour shows filling in of the initial cold area and now increased uptake throughout this large hemangioma that is equal to heart *(H)* and spleen *(S).*

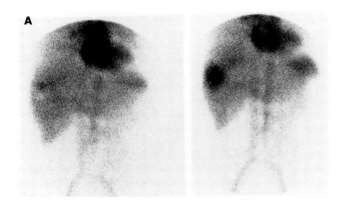

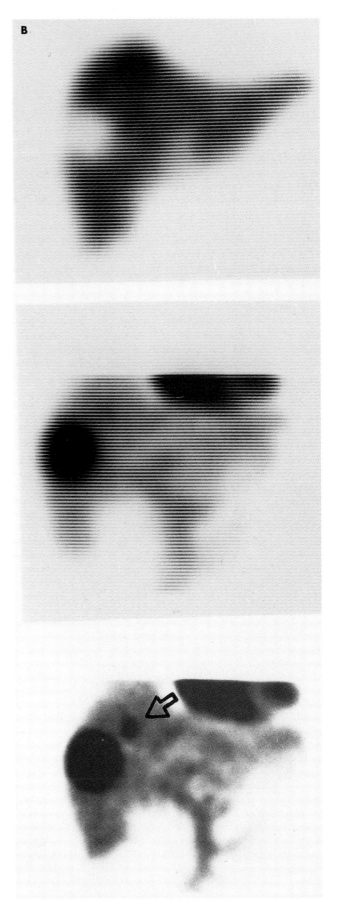

Fig. 9-24   Comparison of planar, single-headed, and triple-headed SPECT. **A,** Planar study. *Left,* Immediate postinjection image shows a cold defect in the superior lateral portion of the right lobe. A small portion of the cold lesion has increased uptake superiorly. *Right,* Delayed image acquired at 60 minutes shows complete filling in, diagnostic of a hemangioma. **B,** SPECT coronal section views. *Top,* The single-headed Tc-99m SC SPECT section shows a well-defined cold defect. *Middle,* The comparable Tc-99m RBC coronal section, obtained with the same single-headed camera, shows increased uptake in that lesion, consistent with a hemangioma. This illustrates the improved contrast resolution of SPECT, but there is no diagnostic advantage over planar imaging. *Bottom,* Triple-headed SPECT study in the same patient shows the hemangioma, but also resolves an additional small hemangioma immediately adjacent *(open arrow)* that was not diagnosed on single-headed SPECT. The small lesion measured 0.9 cm on CT but did not meet all diagnostic criteria for a hemangioma.

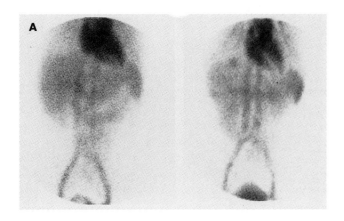

Fig. 9-25 Improved visualization of small lesion with SPECT **A**, *Left*: immediate postinjection image shows neither decreased nor increased uptake, probably due to the small size of the lesion. *Right:* the 1.5-hour delayed planar study shows mildly increased focal uptake in the superior anterior aspect of the liver. If this lesion had been more central it likely would not have been seen, due to overlying activity. **B**, The SPECT coronal (*above*) and transverse (*below*) sections are strongly positive for a hemangioma with a high target-to-background ratio. Note the heart (H) and aorta (A).

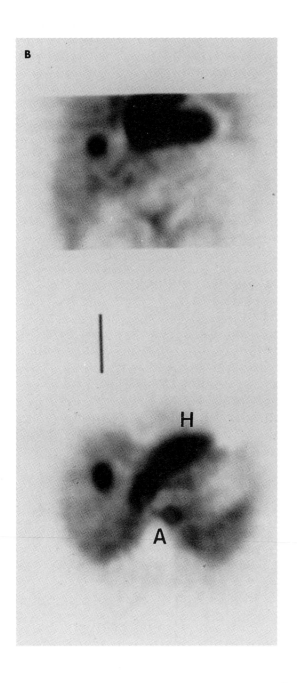

ance on MRI with high signal intensity on T2-weighted spin-echo images (lightbulb sign). Although MRI is much more accurate than CT or US, numerous other benign and malignant tumors have been reported to give false positive results, including metastatic adenocarcinoma of the lung, metastatic carcinoid, pheochromocytoma, islet cell carcinoma, pancreatic and uterine adenocarcinomas, and various sarcomas. MRI is most helpful in the diagnosis of very small lesions, particularly those adjacent to major vessels.

Accuracy

Tc-99m RBC scintigraphy has a very high positive predictive value (approaching 100%). In other words, a positive test is likely to be true positive for cavernous hemangioma of the liver. In over a decade of clinical use, few false positive studies have been reported, including four hepatomas and one angiosarcoma. However, the vast majority of hepatomas are negative on Tc-99m RBC imaging; angiosarcomas are extremely rare.

Although extensive fibrosis or thrombosis may result in a false negative study, this is extremely rare, and some areas of increased uptake are usually seen. The diagnostic sensitivity of Tc-99m RBC imaging is dependent on the instrumentation used and the lesion size. SPECT is clearly superior to planar imaging due to its improved contrast resolution (Figures 9-24 to 9-28). It is especially useful for the detection of small lesions, those located centrally within the liver, multiple hemangiomas, and those adjacent to the heart, kidney, and spleen (Figure 9-26). In seven comparison studies performed between 1987 and 1991, the mean overall sensitivity (all studies combined) for planar imaging was 55%, and for SPECT it was 88%.

Detection of individual hemangiomas is dependent on lesion size and location (Table 9-4). As a general rule, planar imaging can demonstrate hemangiomas down to a size of about 3 cm; single-headed SPECT has good sensitivity for hemangiomas 2 cm and larger, while three-headed SPECT can routinely demonstrate almost all

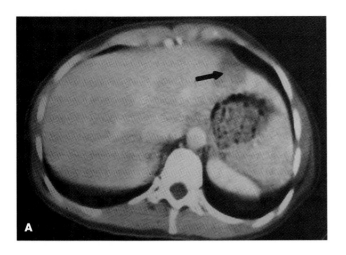

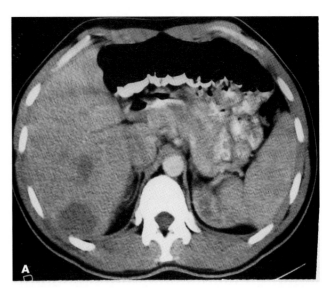

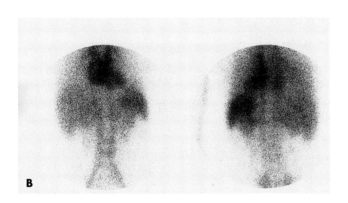

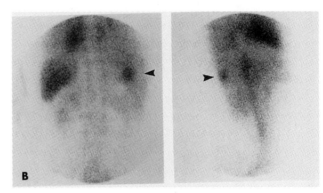

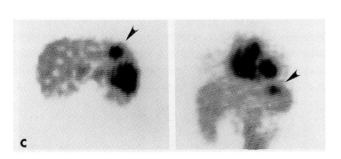

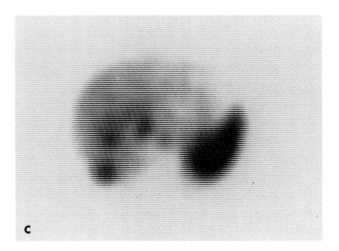

Fig. 9-26   Negative planar and positive SPECT study. **A**, Liver CT shows a lesion in the left lobe of uncertain etiology. **B**, Planar anterior (*left*) and posterior (*right*) Tc-99m RBC study is negative, probably due to the proximity of the lesion to the hot spleen. **C**, The SPECT study performed using a single-headed camera clearly defines the increased uptake of the hemangioma (*arrowheads*) adjacent to the spleen and left ventricle of the heart in the coronal (*right*) and transverse (*left*) slices.

Fig. 9-27   Detection of more lesions with SPECT than with planar imaging. **A**, CT shows two lesions in the posterior aspect of the right lobe. **B**, Only the larger and more posterior one is positive on planar imaging (*arrowheads*). **C**, Both are clearly positive with SPECT. The inferior vena cava and aorta are seen medial to the hemangiomas.

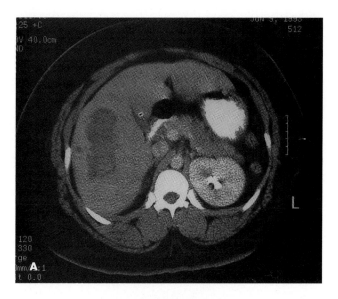

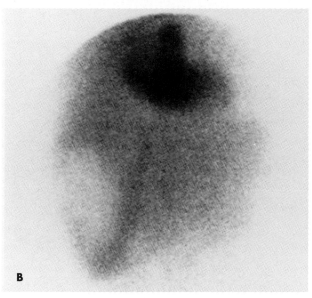

Fig. 9-28 Tc-99m RBC study negative for hemangioma. **A**, CT scan shows a large lesion in the right lobe of the liver. **B**, The planar Tc-99m RBC scan is cold in the same region and therefore negative for hemangioma. Metastatic colon cancer was ultimately diagnosed.

Table 9-4 Dosimetry for In Vitro Tc-99m RBC Scintigraphy

Target	rads/25 mCi (cGy/925 MBq)	rads/mCi
Heart wall	1.350	0.054
Bladder wall	1.275	0.051
Spleen	1.025	0.041
Blood	0.875	0.035
Liver	0.650	0.026
Kidneys	0.625	0.025
Ovaries	0.425	0.017
Testes	0.175	0.007
Total body	0.375	0.015

Modified from Atkins, et al.: *J Nucl Med* 31:378-380, 1990.

TC-99M SULFUR COLLOID LIVER-SPLEEN IMAGING

Radiopharmaceutical

Radiocolloids such as gold-198 colloid have been used for liver imaging since the mid-1950s. Tc-99m SC was introduced in 1963 and became the preeminent method of liver-spleen imaging until the advent of CT. It continues to be used today, but on a more limited basis. The only other radiocolloid preparation commercially available for liver imaging in the United States is Tc-99m microaggregrated albumin colloid.

Mechanism of Localization and Pharmacokinetics

After IV injection, the small colloid particles of Tc-99m SC (0.1 - 0.5 μm) are removed from the blood by cells of the reticuloendothelial system (RES) with a single-pass extraction efficiency of 95% and a blood clearance half-time of 2 to 3 minutes. Tc-99m SC localizes predominantly within the Kupffer cells of the liver (85%) and the macrophages of the spleen (10%) and bone marrow (5%). Hepatic uptake is normally complete by 15 minutes. The SC particles are fixed intracellularly for an indefinite period after phagocytosis. Tc-99m albumin microcolloid (0.4 - 2.0 μm) is metabolized and cleared.

Factors that influence the distribution of colloid particles besides extraction efficiency include blood flow, particle size, and disease states. For example, increased blood flow to a region of the liver (e.g., in FNH) increases the relative regional delivery of colloid, resulting in focally increased uptake on imaging.

The larger the colloid particle size, the greater the proportion taken up by the liver, whereas smaller parti-

hemangiomas less than 1.5 cm in size and may show lesions as small as 0.5 cm in size, although with lower sensitivity. The reason for the improved resolution of multiple-headed SPECT is that the increased sensitivity of the three detector heads is traded for improved resolution by using ultra-high-resolution collimators (Figure 9-24).

cles distribute more to the bone marrow. For example, Tc-99m antimony SC, with a particle size considerably smaller (<0.2 μm) than Tc-99m SC, has been found useful for bone marrow scanning and lymphoscintigraphy. Very large colloid particles—those that may be produced during preparation of Tc-99m SC if high levels of aluminium ions are present in the generator eluate—may result in increased lung uptake. Some RE cells normally reside there.

Kupffer cells are distributed uniformly throughout the liver (Figure 9-1), but make up less than 10% of liver cell mass. Most diseases of the liver affect both hepatocytes and adjacent Kupffer cells similarly, with only occasional exceptions. Focal disease (benign or malignant tumors, abscess, etc.) results in locally decreased uptake due to destruction or displacement of normal liver. Diffuse liver disease produces a generalized reduction in extraction and, therefore, relatively increased distribution to the spleen and bone marrow (colloid shift).

Colloid shift (displacement to the spleen and marrow) may result from portal hypertension with or even without direct cellular damage if less colloid is presented to the Kupffer cells for extraction. An enlarged functioning spleen will have increased uptake of Tc-99m SC because of the increased number and an increased activity of macrophages. Certain immunologically active states, such as systemic tumor without liver involvement, may result in relatively increased uptake, as is commonly seen with melanoma.

Preparation

Tc-99m SC is available commercially in kit form and requires about 15 minutes of preparation. Acid is added to a mixture of Tc-99m pertechnetate and sodium thiosulfate, which is heated in a water bath (95°-100°F) for 5 to 10 minutes. The pH is adjusted with a buffer, gelatin is added to control particle size and stabilize the colloid, and EDTA is added to remove by chelation any aluminum ion present. Labeling yield is greater than 99%. Tc-99m albumin microcolloid is rapidly prepared without any heating using a simple commercial kit formulation.

Toxicity and dosimetry No toxic reactions have been seen experimentally with Tc-99m SC given at 1,000 times the usual adult dose. Pyrogenic or allergic reactions have been very rarely reported and usually are attributed to stabilizers used in the formulations. Tc-99m microcolloid is contraindicated in patients with hypersensitivity to products containing human serum albumin.

The estimated radiation dose from Tc-99m SC is about 1.7 rads to the liver and 1.1 rads to the spleen. The ratio is reversed with diffuse parenchymal disease (Table 9-5).

Table 9-5   Sensitivity for Hemangioma Detection With Triple-Headed SPECT, by Lesion Size

Lesion Size (cm)	Sensitivity (%)
1.4	100
1.3	91
1.0-2.0	65
0.9-1.3	33
0.5-0.9	20

Clinical Applications

Although still occcasionally ordered for liver-spleen imaging, the role of Tc-99m SC today is usually limited to situations where it can add functional information not available with the usual anatomic imaging methods of CT, US, and MRI, or situations in which it provides correlative imaging findings to another radionuclide study (Box 9-7).

Box 9-7   Clinical Indications for Tc-99m SC Liver-Spleen Scintigraphy

1. Modern day indications
   A. CT cannot be performed (e.g., claustrophobia)
   B. Diagnostic correlation with other nuclear medicine studies:
      Tc-99m RBC liver scintigraphy for hemangioma
      In-111 white blood cell imaging for infection
      I-131 MIBG for pheochromocytoma or carcinoid
      Tc-99m MAA hepatic arterial perfusion study
      Ga-67 imaging for hepatoma or other tumors
      Monoclonal antibody studies for tumor localization
      Xe-133 for focal fatty metamorphosis
   C. Aid in differential diagnosis of liver mass, specifically, focal nodular hyperplasia and hepatic adenoma.
   D. Diagnosis of Budd-Chiari syndrome
2. General indications (CT, US, and MRI are more commonly used today) Evaluation for:
      Size, shape and position of liver
      Abdominal masses
      Focal hepatic disease, (e.g., tumors, abscess)
      Follow-up of liver metastases
      Liver trauma
      Abnormal liver function studies
      Spleen

Box 9-8   Tc-99m SC Liver-Spleen Sintigraphy: Protocol Summary

PATIENT PREPARATION AND CONTRAINDICATIONS

None. The study should not be performed immediately after a barium contrast study since attenuation artifacts may result.

RADIOPHARMACEUTICAL DOSE

Planar imaging: 4 mCi (148 MBq)
SPECT: 6 mCi (296 MBq)
Pediatric patients: 30-50 μg/kg (minimal dose, 300 μCi)

INSTRUMENTATION

Camera: Large field of view gamma camera.
Window: 15% window over 140-keV photopeak.
Collimator: Parallel-hole, low-energy, high-resolution collimator.

IMAGING PROTOCOL

1. Inject Tc-99m SC IV.
2. Commence imaging 20 min after injection.

Planar Imaging:

500-1,000k count images in multiple projections (anterior, upright and supine, supine with costal marker, posterior, right and left laterals, anterior and posterior oblique. Upright imaging is preferable when possible to minimize respiratory excursion, a cause of image degradation.

SPECT

Imaging acquisition protocol similar to that used for Tc-99m labeled RBC liver scintigraphy (Box 9-6).

Box 9-9   Normal Liver Variants and Artifacts

Normal variation
  Anatomic variability in liver size, shape, and position
  Prominent porta hepatis
  Prominent gallbladder fossa
  Intrahepatic gallbladder
  Prominent hepatic veins in heart failure
  Costal margin imprint
  Kidney imprint
  Cardiac impression
  Riedel's lobe
Artifacts
  Breast shadow
  Skin and soft tissue folds
  Barium in colon
  Contrast media in gallbladder
  Postsurgical drain
  Foreign objects (metallic)
  Devices for patient immobilization
Extrahepatic compression
  Renal tumors
  Subdiaphragmatic fluid
  Extrahepatic obstructive jaundice (hilar defect)
  Pancreatic mass
  Depression of right diaphragm due to COPD, effusion, tumor

Methodology

No patient preparation is required. SPECT has replaced planar imaging in some laboratories. Box 9-8 describes a typical protocol.

Image Interpretation

Liver imaging   Correct interpretation of Tc-99m SC liver-spleen scans requires an appreciation of *normal* liver anatomy and its variability, the effect of extrinsic liver compression by normal and abnormal structures, and common artifacts (Box 9-9) (Figures 9-29 to 9-36). Additional views and positioning can sometimes be helpful in differentiating normal from pathologic structures. Combined supine and upright anterior views as well as a right anterior oblique (RAO) view can often help determine whether a defect, for example in the portal region, represents normal variation or pathology

(Figures 9- 34, 9-36). SPECT can improve lesion detection because of improved contrast resolution (Figure 9-37) but necessitates a SPECT-capable camera and additional technical expertise. Correct interpretation requires a good knowledge of normal cross-sectional hepatic anatomy (Figures 9-38A,B) and awareness of potential artifacts due to field nonuniformities, center of rotation errors, and movement.

Abnormal scintigraphic findings include hepatomegaly, inhomogeneity, splenomegaly, colloid shift, and focal defects (single and multiple). *Heterogeneity* or inhomogeneity of uptake suggests hepatic dysfunction or an infiltrating process (Box 9-10). Hepatomegaly is a nonspecific finding and may be caused by a variety of disease processes (Box 9-11). Hepatomegaly and inhomogeneity may be the only findings in early tumor involvement. This is more typical of breast and lung cancer than colon cancer, for liver metastases from the latter are usually larger and focal at the time of clinical presentation, while the former may be small, diffuse, and infiltrating.

Liver size is often overestimated on physical examination, particularly in patients with chronic obstructive pulmonary disease, in whom the liver may be more easily palpated due to a depressed diaphragm. A variety of scin-

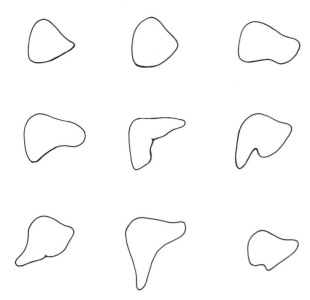

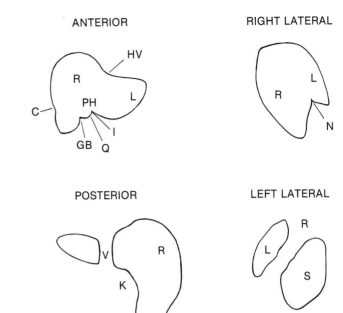

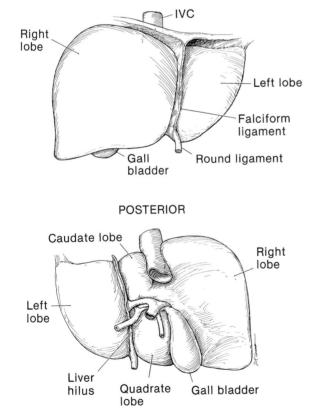

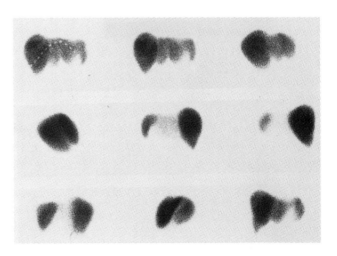

Fig. 9-29 Normal variability of liver contour. Livers come in many shapes—triangular, round, even square. The inferior border may be convex or concave. The inferior lateral aspect of the right lobe may be indented due to rib compression, elongated (Riedel's), notched, or absent. The dome of the liver may be flattened due to depressed diaphragms from COPD or elevated due to phrenic nerve paralysis or congenital weakness (eventration).

Fig. 9-31 Schematic diagram of normal anatomic landmarks and potential interpretative pitfalls for Tc-99m SC liver scintigraphy. *C,* costal indentation of ribs; *GB,* gallbladder fossa; *HV,* notch due to hepatic veins; *I,* incisura umbilicus (ligamentum teres); *K,* kidney impression; *L,* left lobe; *N,* notch between right and left lobes; *PH,* porta hepatis; *Q,* quadrate lobe; *R,* right lobe; *V,* vertebral spine attenuation; *S,* spleen.

Fig. 9-30 Normal anatomic landmarks of the liver are important for proper interpretation of Tc-99m SC liver sections.

Fig. 9-32 Normal Tc-99m SC liver-spleen scan in multiple projections. Two anterior views are displayed: one made with a marker in a supine patient (*upper left*), the other made without a marker in an upright patient (*upper middle*). In sequence the remaining images are right anterior oblique, right lateral, posterior, right posterior oblique (shallow), left posterior oblique, left lateral, and left anterior oblique. Note the normal landmarks as shown in Figure 9-31.

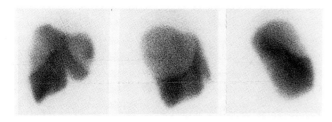

Fig. 9-33 Prominent breast artifact seen in the anterior, right anterior oblique, and right lateral views. A curvilinear line of increased activity at the breast border is attributed to soft tissue short angle scatter.

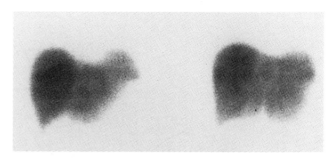

Fig. 9-36 Upright (*left*) and supine (*right*) anterior Tc-99m SC images. Note change in liver contour with position. The gallbladder fossa is better seen in the upright position, whereas the quadrate lobe and ligamentum teres are best seen on the supine image.

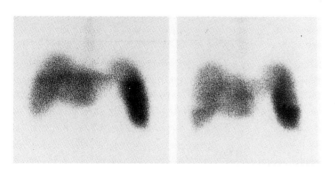

Fig. 9-34 Artifacts due to soft tissue folds and costal indentation in a large man with hepatic insufficiency and splenomegaly. *Left*, decreased activity is seen in the superior portion of the right and left lobe and upper spleen in a linear pattern (arms to the side). *Right*, Soft tissue fold artifact resolves and is replaced with indentations at the inferior lateral border of the liver and spleen due to costal compression (arms elevated).

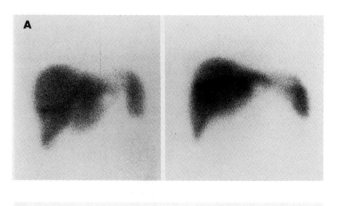

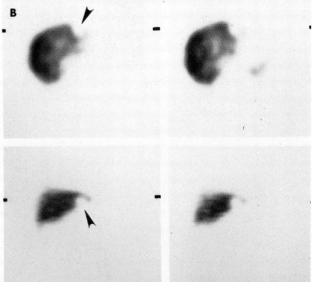

Fig. 9-37 Improved lesion detectability with SPECT. A patient with primary malignant melanoma was referred for a Tc-99m SC study to rule out hepatic metastases. **A**, Anterior planar images in upright (*left*) and supine (*right*) views. A questionable defect is noted at the medial inferior aspect of the left lobe. This was though likely to be normal variation. **B**, Selected SPECT short-axis (*two above*) and coronal (*two below*) sections demonstrate a well-defined lesion in the anterior aspect of the left lobe (*arrowheads*).

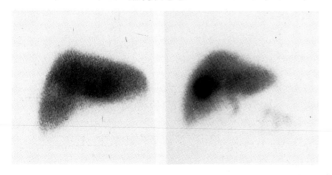

Fig. 9-35 Liver "lesion" due to intrahepatic gallbladder. *Left*, anterior Tc-99m SC liver image with photopenic defect in lateral mid-right lobe. *Right*, a Tc-99m IDA study performed immediately after showed gallbladder filling of the Tc-99m SC defect.

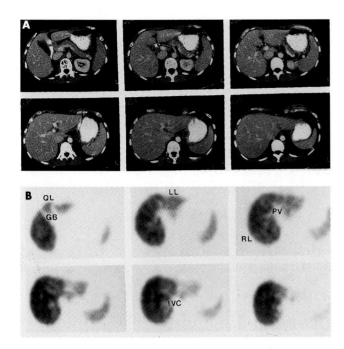

Fig. 9-38 Normal SPECT anatomy and correlation with CT. **A,** Selected CT sections. **B,** Corresponding SPECT sections in the same patient. The most inferior images are at the upper left and the most superior images at the lower right. GB, gallbladder fossa; QL, quadrate lobe; PV, portal vein bifurcation; IVC, inferior vena cava; RL, right lobe; LL left lobe.

tigraphic methods have been used to estimate liver and spleen size. Simple linear measurements with a costal margin marker (e.g., cobalt hot marker with 1-cm intervals or lead cold markers) are often used. Typically the normal liver's longest vertical and midclavicular line dimensions are 17 cm and 15 cm, respectively. Spleen size greater than 14 cm in its longest axis or greater than 110 cm^3 using two perpendicular dimensions is generally considered enlarged. Volume measurements can be made using SPECT, although limited data are available on normal values.

In properly exposed images, no perceptible bone marrow uptake is usually seen. The intensity of the spleen on the posterior view is usually equal to or less than that of the liver (Figure 9-32). Colloid shift is seen with a variety of hepatic diseases, as discussed earlier. Quantitative spleen-to-liver count ratios greater than 1.5 are abnormal.

Lung radiocolloid uptake is uncommon. It may be due to improper labeling (excessive aluminum causing large particle clumping) but more commonly has been associated with a variety of pathophysiologic processes (Box 9-12). The postulated mechanisms include activation of normal lung macrophages and stimulation of RES cell migration from other parts of the body to the lung. This is most commonly seen in patients with irreversible liver disease, and the finding of increased lung uptake has been associated with a poor prognosis. However, it may be completely reversible in patients with treatable or self-limited diseases such as malaria, postpartum fatty metamorphosis of the liver, toxoplasmosis, and so forth (Figure 9-39A,B).

Renal transplants may exhibit uptake in rejection episodes.

Decreased uptake Decreased liver activity on a Tc-99m SC study is the result of displacement or destruction of Kupffer cells, or of alterations in blood flow or function, which may be caused by a large number of different disease processes. Most benign and malignant lesions of the liver produce "cold" or "photopenic" defects on Tc-99m SC liver imaging (Box 9-13; Figures

---

Box 9-10 Causes of Liver Inhomogeneity

Metastases, infiltrative, early
Lymphoma, leukemia
Hepatitis
Fatty infiltration
Chronic passive congestion
Parenchymal liver diseases
Cirrhosis

Box 9-11 Causes of Hepatomegaly

Infiltrative:	Fatty metamorphosis, alcoholic liver disease, amyloidosis, Gaucher's disease, Wilson's disease, granulomas
Congestive:	Heart failure, hepatic vein thrombosis
Neoplastic:	Primary and secondary tumors
Infectious:	Hepatitis, sepsis, malaria
Inflammatory:	Drugs (methyldopa, isoniazid)
Miscellaneous:	Cystic disease

Box 9-12 Causes of Pulmonary Uptake

Incorrect radiopharmaceutical preparation
Severe liver disease, acute or chronic
Pulmonary trauma
Bacterial endotoxin
High serum aluminum level (antacids)
Bone marrow transplantation
Disseminated intravascular coagulation
Histiocytosis X
Various malignancies

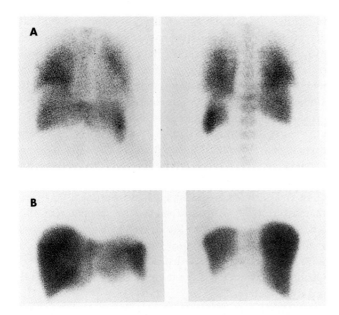

Fig. 9-39 Increased Tc-99m SC lung uptake in a patient with fatty metamorphosis of the liver during pregnancy. **A,** During the acute illness the liver-spleen scan showed increased lung uptake, colloid shift to the marrow and spleen, and inhomogeneous liver uptake. **B,** Follow-up study after the patient clinically recovered. The Tc-99m SC liver spleen-scan has returned to normal.

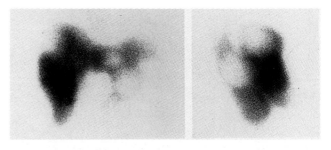

Fig. 9-40 Tc-99m SC study in a patient with colon cancer, anterior and right lateral views. Note large metastases in the right and left lobes.

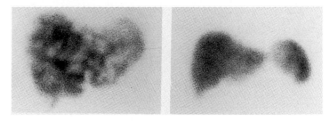

Fig. 9-41 Good response to chemotherapy. Extensive liver metastases on the initial Tc-99m SC study (*left*) and a definite response to therapy seen on follow-up 4 months later (*right*).

Box 9-13   Causes of Focal Liver Defects

Cyst(s)
Benign and malignant tumors
Dilated bile ducts
Abscess(es)
Hematoma
Laceration
Localized hepatitis
Radiation therapy
Infarction
Cirrhosis (pseudotumors)
Fatty infiltration

9-24B, 9-40, 9-41). Ancillary radionuclide tests can sometimes be helpful in making a more specific diagnoses, such as Ind-111 WBC study for infection, Ga-67 citrate for hepatoma, and Tc-99m RBC study for hemangioma (Box 9-7). Xenon-133, an inert gas and fat-soluble radiopharmaceutical, exhibits increased uptake in focal fatty tumors and generalized fatty metamorphosis of the liver.

Radiation therapy can result in characteristic rectangular port-shaped hepatic defects. Diffusely decreased uptake is usually due to hepatocellular disease (Figure 9-42A-C), although early infiltrating tumor involvement may be difficult to differentiate.

Increased uptake   Increased hepatic uptake on Tc-99m SC imaging is uncommon and the causes are few (Box 9-14). Focal areas of increased uptake can result from (1) increased blood flow to an area, resulting in more radiocolloid delivered to normally functioning Kupffer cells, or (2) normal flow to an area of increased density of Kupffer cells. It cannot be due to increased Kupffer cell activity per se because the extraction efficiency is quite high to begin with.

In *superior vena cava obstruction,* collateral thoracic and abdominal wall vessels communicate with the recanalized umbilical vein delivering radiocolloid via the left portal vein to a small volume of tissue usually in the region of the quadrate lobe, producing a "hot spot" (Figure 9-43). This collateral blood flow has a relatively increased concentration of colloid compared to blood delivered to the rest of the liver after systemic mixing. Injection in the lower extremity rather than the upper extremity, not surprisingly, results in a normal scan (Figure 9-43).

Focal nodular hyperplasia may have increased uptake due to both the vascular nature of this benign tumor and an increased density of functioning Kupffer cells (Figure 9-44). The *Budd-Chiari syndrome* (hepatic vein thrombosis) is usually listed as a cause of increased Tc-99m SC uptake (Box 9-14). More correctly, the caudate lobe will have relatively more uptake than the remainder of the liver (Figure 9-45). The impaired venous drainage

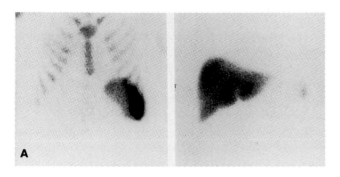

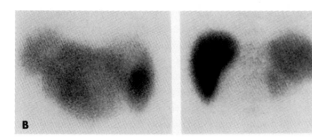

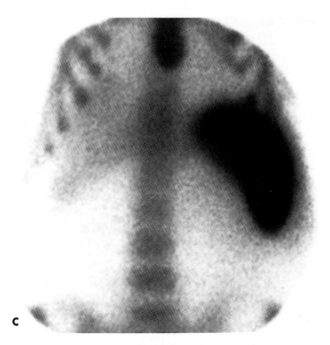

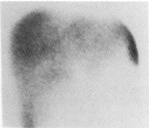

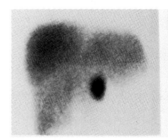

Fig. 9-43 Superior vena cava syndrome. *Left,* Hot spot in the region of the quadrate lobe on Tc-99m SC liver spleen scan in a patient with lung cancer and superior vena cava obstruction. The radiotracer was injected in the arm. *Right,* Repeat study in the same patient with the radiotracer injected in the lower extremity. No hot spot is seen.

Fig. 9-42 Hepatic parenchymal disease imaged with Tc-99m SC. **A,** Acute alcoholic hepatitis. *Left,* Nonvisualization of the liver, splenomegaly, and colloid shift with Tc-99m SC during acute alcoholic hepatitis. *Right,* After recovery and abstinence from alcohol, the liver-spleen scan returned to normal. **B,** Hemochromatosis in a 52-year-old man with hyperpigmentation and biopsy-proved hemochromatosis; anterior (*left*) and posterior (*right*) views. Note the small right lobe, hypertrophied left lobe, large spleen, and colloid shift. **C,** Severe cirrhosis. The anterior image shows a very small liver with poor uptake, enlarged spleen, and a prominent colloid shift to the marrow and spleen.

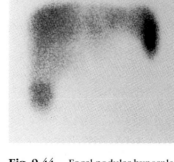

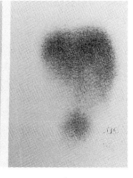

Fig. 9-44 Focal nodular hyperplasia. Anterior (*left*) and right lateral (*right*) views show increased uptake in a lesion at the inferior tip of the right lobe of the liver. Angiography confirmed the diagnosis of focal nodular hyperplasia.

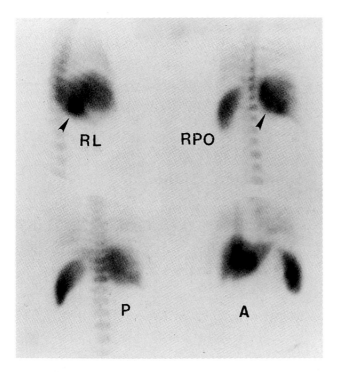

Fig. 9-45   Budd-Chiari syndrome. Good Tc-99m SC uptake in the region of the caudate lobe *(arrowheads)* in a patient with hepatic vein thrombosis. Images were aquired in the right lateral (RL), right posterior oblique (RPO), posterior (P), and anterior (A) projections. Note increased marrow uptake.

of the majority of the liver results in poor hepatic function. The caudate lobe retains good function as a result of its direct venous drainage into the inferior vena cava. This finding is seen in about 50% of patients with the Budd-Chiari syndrome.

Many diseases affect the liver diffusely (Box 9-10, 9-11). In the Western world, *alcoholic liver disease* is the most common cause. It may present with fatty infiltration, acute alchoholic hepatitis, or cirrhosis. With only mild *fatty infiltration,* the liver scan may be normal or may show mild inhomogeneity. As the severity increases, hepatomegaly and colloid shift result (Figure 9-42B,C). *Alcoholic hepatitis* results in hepatic necrosis and widespread inflammation, particularly around the central efferent veins. This regional variation may partly explain the irregular distribution of colloid on scans.

Cirrhosis may be micronodular, macronodular, or mixed; the scan pattern is related to the degree of pathology and the presence or absence of portal hypertension. With increasing severity, the liver, particularly the right lobe, shrinks; the left lobe compensates with hypertrophy, and colloid redistribution becomes more marked (Figure 9-42B,C). With portal hypertension, splenomegaly and marked splenic uptake are common. The very inhomogeneous appearance seen in severe cirrhosis may give the impression of focal defects (pseudo-

tumors). This is due to inhomogeneous blood flow, shunting, and an irregular distribution of the functioning Kupffer cells. This can be a diagnostic dilemma because the incidence of hepatoma is increased in patients with cirrhosis. Ga-67 citrate can aid in this differential diagnosis because it is taken up by tumor but not by regenerating nodules (see Figures 8-7, 8-8).

Tc-99m SC can aid in the differential diagnosis of *focal nodular hyperplasia* and *hepatic adenoma.* Although these two distinct pathologic entities were sometimes confused both pathologically and clinically in the past, they have very different natural histories (see earlier discussion under Cholescintigraphy). Hepatic adenoma, made up almost exclusively of hepatocytes, is typically seen as a cold defect on Tc-SC liver-spleen scans. However, FNH has hepatocytes, bile ducts, and Kupffer cells and has either normal or increased colloid uptake (Figure 9-44) in two thirds of patients.

Nonvisualization   Nonvisualization of the *liver* may occur in the setting of severe hepatocyte-phagocyte damage and diminished blood flow, for example in severe acute hepatitis (Figure 9-42A) or cirrhosis. Nonvisualization of the *spleen* may be due to congenital absence or acquired *functional asplenia.* The latter can result from interruption of blood supply (splenic artery occlusion) or may be secondary to RES dysfunction (sickle cell crisis) (Figure 9-46). This may be irreversible (e.g., thorotrast irradiation, chemotherapy, amyloid) or reversible (e.g., sickle cell crisis). A discordance may be seen between RES phagocytic function and other splenic functions.

Lesion detectability, sensitivity and specificity   Cold focal liver lesions can usually be detected if they are larger than 2 to 3 cm in diameter on planar imaging or 1.5 to 2.0 cm on SPECT. Superficial lesions are more easily detected than deep ones. SPECT is now routinely performed in many laboratories and can aid in detecting smaller and more central lesions because of its improved contrast resolution. Modern multiheaded SPECT cameras using ultra-high-resolution collimators can give resolution in the range of 1.0 to 1.2 cm. Based on the combined data from a large number of studies, the average

Fig. 9-46   Functional asplenia in an 11-year-old African-American girl with sickle cell crisis. Splenic uptake of Tc-99m SC is very decreased. This is reversible with proper therapy and transfusion.

sensitivity for detecting metastatic liver disease with planar Tc-99m SC imaging is 81% and the specificity is 90%. SPECT improves the sensitivity by about 10%.

Several studies have tried to compare the accuracy of Tc-99m SC liver-spleen scintigraphy with the accuracy of CT and US. However, the studies often did not use comparable state-of-the-art instrumentation. Although there seems to be somewhat better detectablility of lesions with CT, the advantage does not reach statistical significance in studies reported to date. Very large series would be needed to prove a small difference in accuracy. Practically, CT offers better image resolution and simultaneous imaging of the entire abdomen, and is usually the study of choice by clinicians, making the question moot.

Spleen imaging The spleen has multiple functions. It serves as a reservoir for formed blood elements, as a site for particle trapping, as a potential site of hematopoiesis during bone marrow failure, and as a source of splenic hormones; it plays a role in white blood cell production, contributes to platelet processing, and has immunologic functions. As a result, the spleen can visualized by various radiopharmaceuticals with different mechanisms of uptake, among them Tc-99m SC (RES function), In-111 WBC imaging (WBC migration), Tc-99m RBC imaging (RBC distribution), damaged RBC imaging (sequestration), and so on.

Radionuclide splenic imaging is most often requested to detect splenic infarcts (Figure 9-47), postoperative splenic remnants, accessory spleens, or splenosis (Figure 9-48A,B). Although Tc-99m SC scintigraphy can often be used to make these diagnoses, liver uptake may sometimes obscure adjacent splenic uptake. In addition, the tip of the left lobe often migrates into the splenic bed after splenectomy and must not be confused with residual splenic tissue on a Tc-99m SC study. Imaging with heat or chemically damaged Tc-99m RBCs will give excellent splenic images without significant liver uptake (Figure 9-48B).

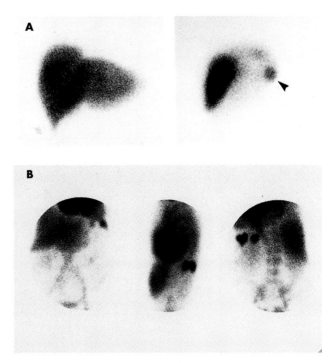

Fig. 9-48 **A,** Splenic remnant detected with Tc-99m SC study, seen in the left lateral view (*arrowhead*). The patient had previously undergone splenectomy. **B,** Splenosis (autotransplantation of splenic tissue following splenic trauma). Damaged Tc-99m-labeled RBC study (*left to right*: anterior, left lateral, and posterior views) shows definite splenic tissue in the left upper quadrant.

TC-99M HEPATIC ARTERIAL PERFUSION SCINTIGRAPHY

Intra-arterial chemotherapy for the treatment of primary and metastatic cancer has been employed by oncologists since the 1960s. Enthusiasm for this form of chemotherapy, which has waxed and waned over the years, seems to peak with the introduction of new technology making administration of the chemotherapy easier, safer, and potentially more effective, and wanes following disenchantment with the overall results in light of the technical difficulties and expense.

Colorectal carcinoma is the third most common cancer in the United States, accounting for 15% of malignancies, and the liver is the most common site for metastatic involvement. Survival in untreated patients with liver metastases varies from 1 to 22 months. Complete surgical resection is curative, but feasible for few patients with solitary or unilobar metastases. Conventional IV chemotherapy yields response rates of only 10% to 30%. Response rates of 34% to 72% have been reported in a number of randomized trials using hepatic arterial chemotherapy for the

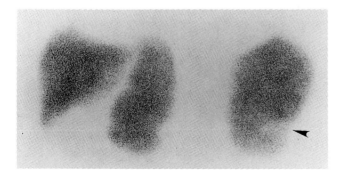

Fig. 9-47 Splenic infarct. *Right*, Large wedge-shaped defect (*arrowhead*) of the spleen in a patient with massive splenomegaly and myeloid metaplasia on a Tc-99m SC study. *Left*, Smaller defects can also be seen on the anterior view.

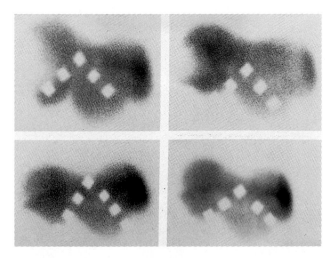

Fig. 9-49 Good response to intra-arterial chemotherapy. The Tc-99m SC studies performed sequentially every 3 months show continuing improvement in a patient with primary hepatocellular carcinoma.

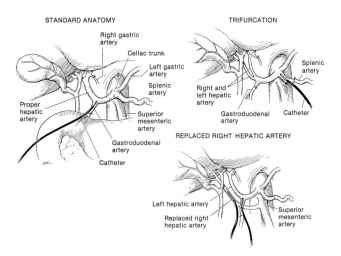

Fig. 9-50 Surgical placement of intra-arterial catheters. *Left,* Patient with standard anatomy. The gastroduodenal artery is ligated and catheter is placed at the junction of the gastroduodenal and common hepatic arteries. The right gastric is ligated. *Upper right,* Surgical placement in a patient with a trifurcation, where the right and left hepatic arteries originate too close to the gastroduodenal artery to allow equal distribution to all areas of the liver. In this normal variation, the gastroduodenal and right gastric arteries are ligated. The splenic artery is ligated and the catheter is positioned at the junction of the splenic artery and celiac axis. *Lower right,* The presence of a replaced right hepatic artery originating from the superior mesenteric artery requires use of two catheters. Similarly, a patient with the left hepatic artery arising from the left gastric would require two catheters.

treatment of metastases. Other primary and metastatic hepatic tumors have also been effectively treated with this regional form of therapy (Figure 9-49).

The attractiveness of this selective intra-arterial approach to chemotherapy is based on the differential blood flow to tumor and normal liver. As tumor in the liver grows, it derives most of its blood supply from the hepatic artery, whereas normal liver cells are supplied predominantly by the portal circulation. Intra-arterial chemotherapy delivers the drug preferentially to the tumor, minimizing exposure to normal liver and to drug-sensitive, dose-limiting tissues such as gastrointestinal epithelium and bone marrow, often the source of side effects common with conventional IV chemotherapy.

Successful application of intra-arterial chemotherapy requires that the drug be reliably and safely delivered to the tumor. After initial arteriographic assessment of the vascular supply of the tumor and liver, a therapeutic catheter is inserted either (1) percutaneously via the transfemoral and transaxillary approach and attached to an external infusion pump, or (2) surgically, and connected to a subcutaneously implanted constant infusion pump (Figure 9-50). Confirmation is needed that the perfusion distribution from the catheter truly encompasses the entire tumor without perfusion of other visceral organs (Figures 9-51 to 9-57).

Although angiography is required for initial catheter placement, it is not a good indicator of blood flow at the capillary level. The high flow rates needed for good contrast angiography often do not reflect the actual perfusion pattern that occurs with the slower infusion rates used with chemotherapy delivery systems. A high-pressure contrast bolus may result in streaming, reflux, or retrograde flow. In addition, contrast angiography can-

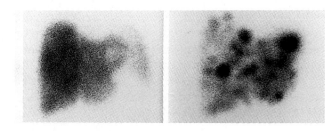

Fig. 9-51 Comparison of Tc-99m SC and Tc-99m MAA studies in a patient with colon cancer and liver metastases. *Left,* Tc-99m SC study shows multiple lesions involving right and left lobes. *Right,* Tc-99m MAA study shows solid tumor nodules involving both lobes of the liver in a pattern similar to the defects seen on Tc-99m SC. Perfusion to the liver is good, and there is no extrahepatic perfusion.

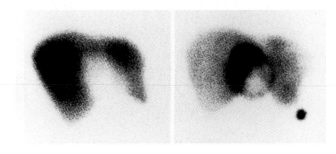

Fig. 9-52 Large tumor mass in the midportion of the liver on Tc-99m SC imaging (*left*). The Tc-99m MAA study (*right*) shows hyperperfusion of the periphery of the large tumor mass with a large, cold, necrotic center.

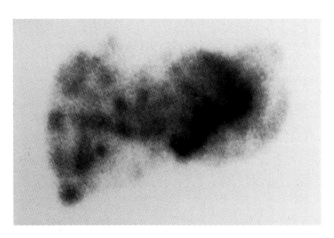

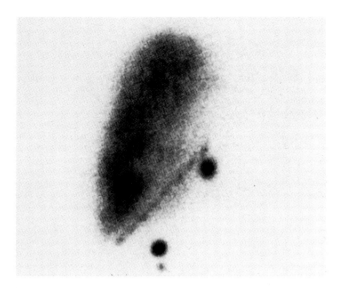

Fig. 9-53 Incomplete hepatic perfusion. Only the right lobe is perfused on the Tc-99m MAA intra-arterial study. The superior hot spot is a clot in the catheter. The lower hot spot is radiotracer in the infusion pump. A hot marker is placed along the costal margin.

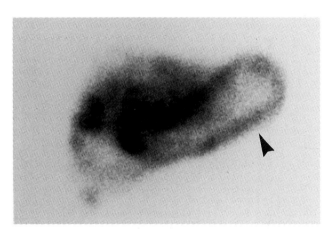

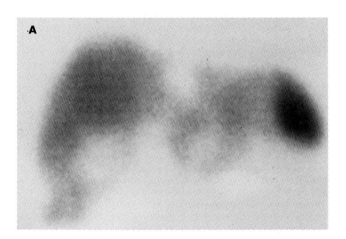

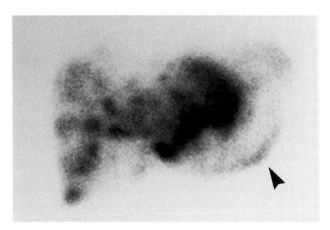

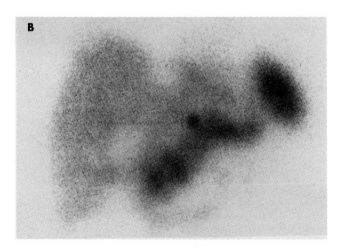

Fig. 9-54 Extrahepatic perfusion to the stomach and spleen. **A,** Tc-99m SC shows multiple large defects in the right and left lobes and colloid shift to the spleen. **B,** Tc-99m MAA study shows extrahepatic perfusion of the stomach, proximal bowel, and spleen.

Fig. 9-55 Extrahepatic perfusion. Images show the value of the left lateral view and the use of effervescent sodium bicarbonate granules in confirming the diagnosis. *Top,* The Tc-99m MAA study is suspicous for gastric perfusion but inconclusive. *Middle,* The left lateral view nicely shows perfusion of the gastric mucosa (*arrowhead*). *Bottom,* After ingestion of sodium bicarbonate effervescent granules, the greater curvature of the stomach moves inferiorly (*arrowhead*), confirming gastric perfusion.

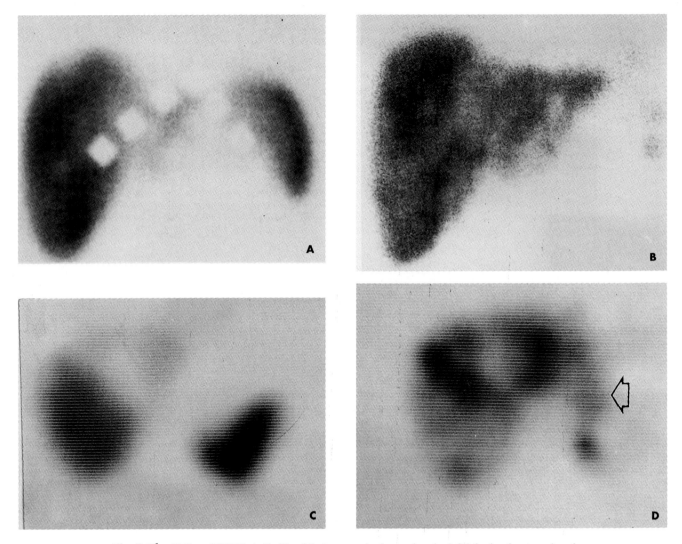

Fig. 9-56   Utility of SPECT. **A**, Tc-99m SC planar study shows that the left lobe has been replaced by tumor. Cold markers overlie the left lobe. **B**, Tc-99m MAA study shows apparent perfusion of the left lobe without definite gastric perfusion. However, there is a suggestion of splenic perfusion, and the perfusion adjacent to the left lobe could represent some gastric perfusion. **C**, Tc-99m SC SPECT study showing a large tumor defect in the left lobe. **D**, Tc-99m MAA SPECT study showing hyperperfusion of the periphery of the tumor nodule which is cold centrally and definite gastric perfusion, clearly seen on the transverse SPECT section. Splenic perfusion was seen on other sections not shown here.

not be performed through the small-bore surgically placed catheters, which deliver chemotherapy at a rate of only 1 to 5 mL/day.

Improper positioning of the intra-arterial catheter will result in inadequate perfusion of the tumor-involved liver and can result in extrahepatic perfusion to the stomach, pancreas, spleen, and bowel (Figures 9-54 to 9-57). Sub-optimal perfusion may occur as a result of difficulties in placement due to normal vascular anatomic variation (Figure 9-50). Even when the catheter is properly placed initially, movement of the catheter, catheter occlusion, or hepatic artery thrombosis may produce a change from

the inital perfusion pattern. Tc-99m MAA hepatic arterial scintigraphy can give a reliable estimate of the adequacy of blood flow to the tumor and can determine the presence or absence of extrahepatic perfusion, a frequent cause of gastrointestinal and systemic toxicity.

Chemistry and Radiopharmaceutical Preparation

The chemistry and radiopharmaceutic preparation are discussed under Lung Scanning in Chapter 6; the information will not be repeated here.

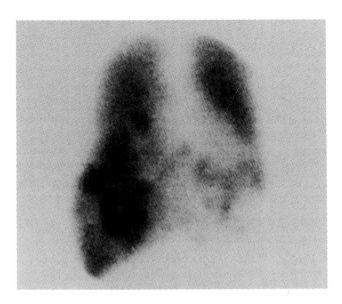

Fig. 9-57   Increased lung uptake of Tc-99m MAA consistent with considerable arteriovenous shunting (40% in this case).

Mechanism of Localization and Pharmacokinetics

Tc-99m Tc-MAA particles are larger than capillary size (range, 10-90 μ; mean, 30-50 μ). When injected into the hepatic artery, they distribute according to blood flow and will be trapped on first pass in the arteriolar-capillary bed of the liver. The irregularly shaped and malleable particles occlude only a small percentage of the liver capillary bed, break down into smaller particles over a relatively short period of time (effective half-life in the liver of approximately 4 hours), and are eventually taken up by macrophages of the RES or cleared through the kidney.

Extrahepatic perfusion is manifested on Tc-99m MAA perfusion imaging as uptake within abdominal visceral organs, usually the stomach, spleen, and bowel (Figures 9-54 to 9-56). Although a small amount of *arteriovenous* (AV) *shunting* is not uncommon (1%-7%), shunting of 10% to 40% can occur (Figure 9-57). AV shunting results in less perfusion of the tumor, increased systemic exposure, and increased potential for side effects.

The typical pattern of tumor perfusion on Tc-99m MAA studies is greater uptake in the tumors compared to normal liver (mean tumor-nontumor ratio of 3:1). Small tumor nodules usually show uniform uptake (Figure 9-51), whereas larger tumors often have increased uptake at the periphery of the tumor and relatively decreased uptake centrally, due to central necrosis (Figure 9-52). Selective hepatic angiography has demon-

strated that most cancers, including colon cancer, are hypervascular, particularly at the periphery of the tumor where active growth occurs (neovascularity). This increased tumor-to-nontumor flow ratio is a major advantage of the intra-arterial technique.

Dosimetry   The estimated radiation dose to the liver is similar to that seen with Tc-99m SC liver spleen imaging. Estimates of doses to other abdominal organs are based on assumptions of the percent extrahaptic perfusion and AV shunting (Table 9-6).

Methodology

The method of Tc-99m MAA administration depends to some extent on the type of intra-arterial catheter and whether it is placed percutaneously or surgically. These methods are described in Box 9-15.

Clinical Applications

Tc-99m MAA hepatic arterial perfusion studies should be performed after initial catheter placement and ideally before each course of chemotherapy, particularly if the patient experiences symptoms suggestive of gastrointestinal toxicity. The effectiveness of intra-arterial chemotherapy will be maximized if there is perfusion of the entire tumor-involved liver, and side effects will be minimized when there is no extrahepatic perfusion to the stomach, spleen, or bowel and no significant AV shunting to the lung. It is often clinically impossible to distinguish the symptoms of tumor progression from those due to extrahepatic perfusion of the stomach and bowel. Extrahepatic perfusion to the stomach is associated with a high incidence of adverse symptoms (70%, vs. 20% in patients without extrahepatic perfusion), including nausea, vomiting, gastritis, ulceration, and hemorrhage.

Image Interpretation

The important diagnostic information to be obtained from this study is (1) the adequacy of perfusion of the tumor and liver, (2) the presence or absence of extrahepatic perfusion, and (3) the amount of AV shunting to the lung.

Hepatic uptake is often somewhat inhomogeneous. Tumor nodules typically have increased uptake compared to surrounding normal liver. Muliple views (right lateral, anterior, posterior, left lateral) are often helpful for establishing the distribution of perfusion. Comparison with a recent Tc-SC liver scan can be quite helpful (Figure 9-54, 9-56).

AV shunting manifests on Tc-99m MAA studies as lung uptake (Figure 9-57). The particles shunted through the tumor bypass the capillary bed and are trapped within the lung. This gives an indication of the percentage of drug administered that would not be delivered to the

Box 9-15 Tc-99m MAA Hepatic Arterial Scintigraphy: Protocol Summary

PATIENT PREPARATION

None. A Tc-99m SC study performed within 24-48 hr is helpful for comparison when interpretating the Tc-99m MAA study.

CLINICAL CONTRAINDICATIONS AND PRECAUTIONS

None.

INSTRUMENTATION

Large field of view gamma camera with low-energy, all-purpose, parallel-hole collimator.

Energy window: 15% centered over 140 keV photopeak.

RADIOPHARMACEUTICAL

Tc-99m MAA, 1-4 mCi (37-148 MBq) for planar imaging and 5-6 mCi (185-222 MBq) for SPECT.

Infuse in a small volume (0.5-1.0 cc) through an intra-arterial catheter.

METHOD OF ADMINISTRATION

Depends on whether catheter was placed percutaneously or surgically.

Surgically implanted infusion pump and catheter

Insert a 22-gauge 1-inch Huber needle into the infusion pump side port. After ascertaining free flow, infuse the Tc-99m MAA slowly over 1-2 min and slowly flush with 10 mL saline. Before removing the needle, inject 5 mL of heparin (10 units/mL).

Percutaneously placed catheter and external infusion pump

1. Place a three-way stopcock as close as possible to the site of catheter entry.
2. With the patient positioned under the camera so that entering flow can be monitored, gently flush catheter with 10-20 mL of normal saline.
3. Infuse Tc-99m MAA in 0.2-mL volume via the three-way stockcock.
4. Advance the external pump flow rate to 200 mL/hr.
5. Monitor the progress of the radioactive injectate on the persistence scope. As the bolus approaches the liver, decrease the flow rate of the pump to the rate at which the chemotherapy is to be delivered, generally 10-20 mL/hr.

IMAGING PROTOCOL

1. Acquire images with the patient lying supine on the table.
2. Acquire 500k count anterior image, then posterior, right and left lateral, and anterior chest views for equal time.
3. If extrahepatic gastric perfusion is suspected, 4 g of sodium bicarbonate-citric acid-simethicone effervescent granules (EZ-gas, Sparkles) should be administered in 100 mL of water by mouth. The patient must be encouraged not to eruct. Repeat anterior and left lateral images.
4. SPECT option. Technique similar to Tc-99m SC SPECT.

Table 9-6 Tc-99m SC Dosimetry

Organ	Normal liver (rads/5 mCi)	Diffuse Parenchymal Disease
Liver	1.7	0.8
Spleen	1.1	2.1
Bone marrow	0.14	0.4
Testes	0.006	0.016
Ovaries	0.028	0.06
Total body	0.095	0.09

Table 9-7 Dosimetry of Intra-arterially Administered Tc-99m MAA

	Good Perfusion No Extrahepatic Perfusion (rads/mCi)	Poor Perfusion: Extrahepatic Perfusion and AV shunting (rads/mCi)
Hepatic perfusion	96%	40%
Extrahepatic perfusion	0%	40%
AV shunting to lungs:	4%	10%
Liver	0.26	0.11
Lungs	0.01	0.06
Intestines		
10 g	0.0	0.10
40 g	0.0	0.03
100 g	0.0	0.01
Total body	0.02	
Gonads	0.02	

Modified from Croft, Schlafke-Stelson AT and Watson EE, editors: *Proceedings of the 4th International Radiopharmaceutical Dosimetry Symposium*, 1986, U.S. Dept. of Energy and Oak Ridge Associated Universities.

tumor and would result in systemic exposure and potential toxicity.

Extrahepatic perfusion, such as perfusion of the stomach and bowel, is often obvious on imaging; at other times, however, it can be hard to differentiate gastric perfusion from perfusion of liver and tumor in the adjacent left lobe. A left lateral view may be helpful in making this important differentiation. The ingestion of sodium bicarbonate effervescent granules (e.g., E-Z Gas) can be quite useful in confirming gastric perfusion (Figure 9-55). SPECT can also be useful in determining the three-dimensional distribution of hepatic and tumor perfusion and the presence or absence of extrahepatic perfusion (Figure 9-56).

Tc-99m MAA has also been used preoperatively to evaluate patients prior to surgical resection. The Tc-99m MAA intra-arterial perfusion studies can detect more intrahepatic tumor nodules than Tc-99m SC scans or CT. The Tc-99m MAA particles are infused at the time of angiography.

SUGGESTED READINGS

Birnbaum BA, Weingreb JC, Megibow AJ et al: Definitive diagnosis of hepatic hemangiomas: MR imaging versus Tc-99m labeled red blood cell SPECT, *Radiology* 176:95-101, 1990.

Choy D, Shi EC, McLean RG et al: Cholescintigraphy in acute cholecystitis: use of intravenous morphine. *Radiology* 151:203-207, 1984.

Fig LM, Stewart RE, and Wahl RL: Morphine-augmented hepatobiliary scintigraphy in the severely ill: caution is in order, *Radiology* 175:473-476, 1990.

Fink-Bennett D, DeRidder P, Kolozsi WZ et al: Cholecystokinin cholescintigraphy: Detection of abnormal gallbladder motor function in patients with chronic acalculous gallbladder disease, *J Nucl Med* 32:1695-1699, 1991.

Freitas JE, Coleman RE, Nagle CE et al: Influence of scan and pathologic criteria on the specificity of cholescintigraphy, *J Nucl Med* 24:876-879, 1983.

Kaplan WD, D'Orsi CJ, Ensminger WD et al: Intra-arterial radionuclide infusion: a new technique to assess chemotheraphy perfusion patterns, *Cancer Treat Rep,* 62:699-703, 1978.

Krishnamurthy GT and Turner FE: Pharmacokinetics and clinical applications of technetium-99m labeled hepatobiliary agents, *Sem Nucl Med* 20:130-149, 1990.

Weissman HS and Freeman LM: The biliary tract. In Freeman LM, editor: Freeman and Johnson's Clinical Radionuclide Imaging, 1984, Grune & Stratton, Inc.

Yap L, Wycherley AG, Morphett AD, and Toouli J: Acalculous biliary pain: cholecystectomy alleviates symptoms in patients with abnormal cholescintigraphy, *Gastroenterology* 101:786-793, 1991.

Ziessman HA: Atlas of cholescintigraphy: Selected update, atlas of Tc-99m labeled red blood cell liver scintigraphy, and atlas of heptic arterial perfusion scintigraphy. In selected atlases of gastrointestinal scintigraphy, New York, 1992, Springer-Verlag.

Ziessman HA, Fahey FN, and Hixson DJ: Calculation of a gallbladder ejection fraction: Advantage of continuous sincalide infusion over the 3-minute method, *J Nucl Med* 33:537-541, 1992.

Ziessman HA, Silverman PM, Patterson J et al: Improved detection of small cavernous hamangiomas of the liver with high-resolution three-headed *SPECT, J Nucl Med* 32:2086-2091, 1991.

Ziessman HA, Thrall JH, Yang PJ et al: Hepatic Arterial Perfusion scintigraphy with Tc-99m MAA. *Radiology* 152:167-172, 1984.

CHAPTER 10

Gastrointestinal System

Gastrointestinal (GI) scintigraphy uses nuclear medicine methods to obtain physiologic information about esophageal and GI function. Computer techniques can quantitate various physiologic parameters, aid in the detection of disordered function, and be used to follow a patient's clinical course and response to therapy.

ESOPHAGEAL TRANSIT

Esophageal transit scintigraphy has theoretical advantages over other methods for the evaluation of esophageal motility. It is noninvasive, relatively simple to perform, and quantitative. Barium radiography can demonstrate structural lesions and mucosal changes and afford a qualitative assessment of motility, but it is not quantitative. Manometry is the reference standard for the diagnosis of motility disorders. It provides quantitative information on peristaltic contraction, sphincter presssure, and the

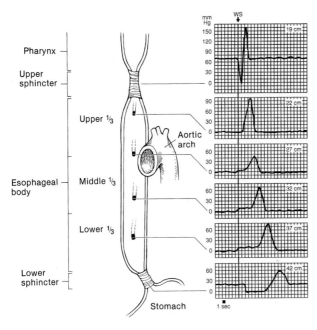

Fig. 10-1 Esophageal anatomy and function. Swallowing initiates a coordinated peristaltic contraction that propagates down the esophagus. The esophagus is a posterior mediastinal structure with three distinct regions: the upper esophageal sphincter (UES), which allows food to pass from the mouth to the esophagus and prevents tracheobronchial aspiration, the esophageal body with striated muscle proximally and smooth muscle distally, and the lower esophageal sphincter (LES), a high pressure smooth muscle region that prevents gastric reflux but relaxes during swallowing to allow passage of food into the stomach. *Right*, manometric pressure changes with a water swallow (WS) of an 8-mL bolus. Immediately after swallowing, UES pressure falls transiently. Shortly thereafter, LES pressure falls and remains low until the peristaltic contraction passes aborally through the UES and the esophageal body, which closes the LES.

Box 10-1 Classification of Esophageal Motility Disorders

PRIMARY/SECONDARY

Primary
  Achalasia
  Esophageal spasm
  Nutcracker esophagus
Secondary
  Scleroderma
  Diabetic enteropathy

DEGREE OF MOTILITY

Amotility
  Achalasia
  Scleroderma
Hypomotility
  Presbyesophagus
Hypermotility
  Diffuse spasm
  Nutcracker esophagus

---

ability of the upper and lower esophageal spincter (LES) to relax. However, manometry is invasive and technically demanding. Although the exact role of radionuclide esophageal transit studies has yet to be clearly defined, these studies can be used as a noninvasive screening test in symptomatic patients and are particularly useful for evaluating the effectiveness of therapy.

The esophagus transports liquids and solids from the mouth to the stomach, clears regurgitated substances, and prevents tracheobronchial aspiration and acid reflux (Fig. 10-1).

Dysphagia is the most common complaint of patients with abnormal esophageal motility. Esophageal motor disorders have been classified as primary or secondary, or, alternatively, by the type of dysfunction (Box 10-1).

Esophageal Motor Disorders

Achalasia Achalasia is a disease of unknown etiology characterized by the absence of peristalsis in the distal two thirds of the esophagus, increased LES pressure, and incomplete sphincter relaxation with swallowing. Esophageal dilation and retention of food result. Common symptoms include dysphagia, weight loss, nocturnal regurgitation, cough, and occasionally aspiration. The diagnosis can be confirmed by esophageal manometry. Radionuclide esophageal transit studies have a high sensitivity for making this diagnosis and are of proven value for determining the effectiveness of therapy.

Diffuse esophageal spasm Diffuse esophageal spasm is characterized by intermittent chest pain or dysphagia without a demonstrable organic lesion. The symptoms are produced by abnormal nonperistaltic contractions of the esophageal body, which can be demonstrated by manometry or radiologic studies. The *nutcracker esophagus* is a somewhat controversial classification defined by its manometric manifestations. These patients have noncardiac chest pain and normal radiographic studies. Manometry reveals high-amplitude persistaltic contractions, sometimes of prolonged duration.

Scleroderma   Scleroderma is a systemic disease involving esophageal smooth muscle. The esophagus is dilated, aperistaltic, and shows barium retention and gastroesophageal reflux (GER) on contrast radiography. Manometry demonstrates decreased or absent LES pressure and decreased amplitude of contractions of the smooth muscle portion of the esophagus. Radionuclide studies show delayed transit.

Other   Esophageal smooth muscle disease is also seen in *systemic lupus erythematosus* (SLE) and *polymyositis*. Striated muscle abnormalities may occur in *muscular dystrophy*, *myasthenia gravis*, and *myotonia*

dystrophica. *Diabetes* and *alcoholism* can be associated with abnormalities of esophogeal motor function. Esophagitis itself, particularly when severe, may result in a motility disorder.

Radiopharmaceutical

Esophageal transit scintigraphy is usually performed with Tc-99m SC, 300 μCi, dispersed in a liquid bolus, usually water. Semisolid food boluses are thought by some investigators to be more sensitive for detecting dysmotility, but further data are needed. Transit is faster for less viscous materials, for smaller volumes than for larger volumes, and in the upright position than in the supine position.

Dosimetry

Tc-99m SC is used for studies of esophageal transit, GER, and gastric emptying. The following dosimetry applies to all three (Tables 10-1, 10-2). The large intestine receives the highest absorbed dose.

Table 10-1   Dosimetry for Tc-99m SC Gastroesophageal Scintigraphy for Children

| | rads/100 μCi : (Usual Dose = 200-500 μCi), by Age | | | | |
Organ	Newborn	1 yr	5 yr	10 yr	15 yr
Stomach	0.383	0.093	0.050	0.031	0.022
Small intestine	0.372	0.164	0.090	0.058	0.036
Large intestine	0.927	0.380	0.194	0.120	0.072
Ovaries	0.099	0.042	0.033	0.072	0.010
Testes	0.018	0.007	0.003	0.011	0.001
Whole body	0.020	0.011	0.006	0.004	0.003

Modified from Castranovo FP: Gastroesophageal scintiscanning in a pediatric population: dosimetry, *J Nucl Med* 27:1212-1214, 1986.

Table 10-2   Dosimetry for Esophageal and Gastric Scintigraphy in Adults

| | mrads/Study Meal, by Organ | | | | | |
	Stomach	Small Intestine	Large Intestine	Ovaries	Testes	Total Body
Liquid						
300 μCi Tc-99m SC	28	83	160	29	2	5
1 mCi Tc-99m DTPA	93	280	520	98	5	20
250 μCi In-111 DTPA	110	490	2000	420	27	60
Solid						
500 μCi Tc-99m SC ovalbumin	120	120	230	42	2	9
250 μCi In-111 chicken liver	240	480	1900	400	28	58
500 μCi Tc-99m chicken liver	120	120	230	42	2	9

Modified from Siegel JA, Wu RK, Knight LC et al: Radiation dose estimates for oral agents used in upper gastrointestinal diseases, *J Nucl Med* 24:835-837, 1983.

Methodology

Many variations of the protocol described in Box 10-2 have been used, including the type of bolus, patient positioning, method of acquisition, and analysis. The supine position is preferable because it eliminates the effect of gravity on esophageal emptying. However, the upright position may be useful for serial quantitative studies in patients with achalasia because gravity is the only mechanism of emptying in this disease. In contrast, emptying occurs in both the supine and upright positions in systemic sclerosis, a differential point. Both anterior and posterior imaging have been used. Multiple swallows are often necessary for complete emptying even in normal subjects because there is a high incidence (25%) of "aberrant" swallows, defined as extra swallows occurring between the two prescribed swallows and resulting in inhibition of the initial swallow with a delay in transit.

Box 10-2   Tc-99m SC Esophageal Transit Imaging: Protocol Summary

RADIOPHARMACEUTICAL

Tc-99m SC, 300 µCi in 10 mL water.

PATIENT PREPARATION

Overnight fast.
Place a radioactive marker on the cricoid cartilage.
Position the patient supine.
Practice swallows with nonradioactive bolus.

INSTRUMENTATION

Camera setup: Tc-99m with 20% photopeak.
Computer setup: 0.8 sec frame × 240;
    byte mode, 64 × 64.

PROCEDURE

Practice swallows with nonradioactive bolus.
Swallow Tc-99m SC as a bolus.
Dry swallow at 30 sec, then radiolabeled bolus
    every 30 sec × 4.
No swallowing between boluses.

PROCESSING

Time-activity curves, condensed dynamic images.

QUANTITATION

Time of 90% emptying
Transit time

Analysis and Quantitation

Although analog film images or cine review on computer is often adequate to diagnose severe abnormalities of motility (Figures 10-2, 10-3), quantitative analysis can be useful for diagnosing less severe abnormalities and for serial studies to evaluate the effectiveness of a particular therapy.

Esophageal transit can be quantitated by calculating either (1) the residual activity in the esophagus or (2) the transit time through it (Figure10-3B). Any normal residual remaining after an initital swallow usually clears when followed by a dry swallow.

$$\text{Percent residual esophageal activity} = \frac{(E_{max} - E_t)}{E_{max}} \times 100,$$

where E_{max} is the maximum counting rate in the esophagus (15-second intervals), E_t is the counting rate after dry swallow number t, and transit time is the time from initial entry of the bolus into the esophagus until all but 10% of peak activity is cleared (abnormal, < 15 seconds).

Pattern analysis and functional images have been used as an aid to diagnosis. Time–activity curves can be derived for the entire esophagus and for the proximal, middle, and distal thirds. Normally, peak activity is seen in sequence from proximal to distal, but this pattern is often lost in disease states (Figure10-4). Functional images can aid in viewing the many images acquired in a single transit study. Because the interpreter is interested only in the craniocaudal transit, not in lateral motion, the dynamic data can be condensed into a single image with one spatial (vertical) and one temporal dimension (Figure10-5). Characteristic disease patterns have been described (Figure10-6A,B).

Fig. 10-2 Normal supine esophageal transit study. Images are obtained at 2-second intervals. The swallowed bolus travels rapidly through the upper esophagus. The transit time is 11 seconds (normal < 15 seconds).

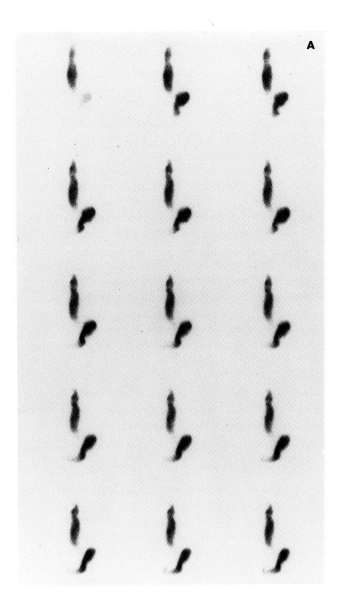

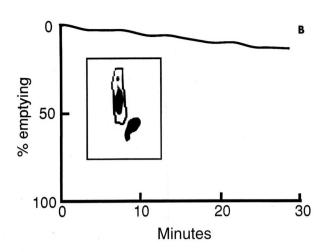

Fig. 10-3 **A**, Abnormal esophageal emptying in achalasia. One-minute images are acquired for 30 minutes. There is considerable stasis within the esophagus. **B**, Quantitative analysis. An ROI was drawn on computer for the entire esophagus and a time-activity curve generated. The percent esophageal emptying over 30 minutes was calculated to be only 12%.

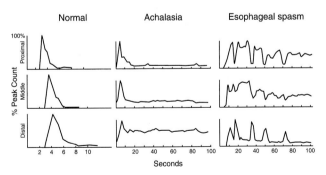

Fig. 10-4 Radionuclide time-activity profiles in a normal control subject (*left*), a patient with achalasia (*middle*), and a patient with diffuse esophageal spasm (*right*) for three esophageal regions of interest: proximal, middle, and distal esophagus. In the normal state the bolus proceeds sequentially from proximal to distal esophagus. In achalasia, retention is seen predominantly in the lower esophagus. With diffuse spasm, uncoordinated contraction shows very poor bolus progression through the esophagus.

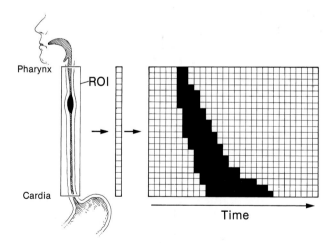

Fig. 10-5 Schematic diagram illustrating the generation of condensed dynamic images. In each consecutive frame, the data in an esophageal ROI are compressed into a single column, displaying the distribution of the tracer from the pharynx to the proximal stomach for each 0.8-second time interval. The columns are arranged consecutively, thus generating a space and time matrix whose vertical and horizontal dimensions represent spatial and temporal activity changes.

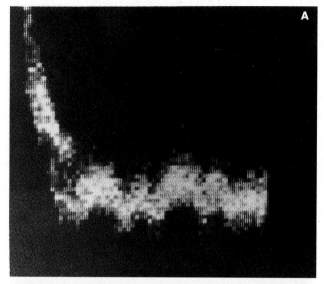

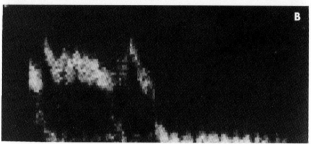

Fig. 10-6   Condensed dynamic images (CDI). **A**, Normal swallow sequence, showing smooth uninterrupted transit of the bolus down the esophagus. **B**, Diffuse esophageal spasm. After the inital swallow, part of the bolus remains in the midesophagus as the remainder is transported to the stomach. A subsequent dry swallow propels the rest of the bolus into the stomach.

Accuracy

Esophageal transit studies can demonstrate achalasia with a high sensitivity; however, a lower or more variable detection rate has been reported in other conditions, limiting its use as a routine screening test. The clearest indication is for monitoring a disease process over time and evaluating its response to therapy, whether pharmacologic, medical, or surgical.

GASTROESOPHAGEAL REFLUX

Symptomatic reflux of gastric contents into the esophagus is a very common GI disorder and heartburn is its most common clinical symptom. Complications include esophagitis, bleeding, perforation, and stricture. The clinical presentation in infants and children differs considerably from that in adults. Besides regurgitation, common symptoms are respiratory problems, iron deficiency anemia, and failure to thrive.

A small amount of reflux occurs in infants as a normal physiologic event and resolves spontaneously by 7 to 8 months of age. Clinically important reflux often is evident by 2 months of age. The majority have a benign course and are symptom free by 18 months of age. However, approximately one third will have persistent symptoms until age 4 and sometimes develop significant sequelae, including strictures and even death due to inanition or recurrent pneumonia (5%–10%).

Esophageal clearance is a critical factor in determining whether reflux becomes clinically evident since this determines the duration of mucosal exposure to refluxate. Other contributing factors include the efficacy of the antireflux mechanism, the volume of gastric contents, the potency of refluxed material (acid, pepsin), mucosal resistance to injury, and mucosal reparative ability.

Although LES pressure is reduced in many patients with reflux, considerable overlap exists between healthy and ill subjects. Reflux events result from either (1) a transient LES relaxation not associated with swallowing, (2) stress reflux due to transient increases in intra-abdominal pressure, or (3) free reflux across an atonic sphincter. Although most patients with moderate to severe esophagitis have a sliding hiatus hernia, the majority of individuals with a hiatus hernia do not have reflux disease.

Diagnostic Tests

A variety of tests have been used to diagnose GER. *Barium esophagography* can detect severe grades of reflux, mucosal damage, stricture, and tumor; however, it has a low overall sensitivity for reflux. *Endoscopy* provides a direct view of the esophageal mucosa and allows biopsy, although histologic evidence of esophagitis is not particularly sensitive for diagnosing reflux disease.

The *Bernstein acid infusion test* attempts to reproduce the patient's symptoms and confirm their esophageal origin with infusion of 0.1N hydrochloric acid into the distal esophagus. The *Tuttle acid reflux test* is generally considered the reference standard but is techically demanding. Reflux events are detected by positioning a pH electode in the distal esophagus; an abrupt drop in esophageal pH (<4.0) is diagnostic of a reflux event. Detection of recurrent events requires clearance of the previous reflux event. Although reflux volume clears within seconds, acid clearance takes several minutes even in normal subjects, because neutralization by swallowed saliva is necessary.

The radionuclide method has a number of potential advantages. It is physiologic, easily performed, well tolerated by the patient, quantitative, involves a low radiation dose to the patient, and is a relatively sensitive method for detecting GER.

The radionuclide study and pH monitoring measure different components of refluxate—volume versus acid

Box 10-3 Gastroesophageal Reflux: Protocol Summaries

ADULT

Patient preparation

Overnight fast.

Procedure

Have patient drink a solution containing 150 mL orange juice, 150 mL of 0.1N HCl, and 300 µCi Tc-99m SC.

Obtain a 30-sec acquisition on computer to ascertain that the bolus has transited the esophagus. If not, give 30 mL of water to clear residual esophageal activity.

Position patient supine over a wide field of view gamma camera.

Have the patient perform a Valsalva maneuver, and acquire a 30-sec image on computer.

Place an abdominal binder below the rib cage and attach a sphygmomanometer to increase the pressure in 20 mm Hg increments from 0 to 100 mm Hg.

Obtain 30 sec images at each pressure gradient.

Calculate GER at each pressure step using the formula:

$$R = (E_t - E_b) \times 100/G_0,$$

where R is % GER, E_t is esophageal counts at time t, E_b is esophageal background counts, and G_0 is gastric counts at the start of the study. A value >4% is considered abnormal.

CHILDREN

Patient preparation

Overnight fast.

Computer setup

Framing rate of 5-10 sec/frame for 60 min.

Test Meal

Tc-99m SC, 0.1-1.0 mCi (5 µCi/mCi).

Procedure

Optional: An *esophageal transit study* may be performed initially or at end of the study.

Give 250 µCi Tc-99m SC in 10 mL sterile water as a bolus via a feeding tube placed in the posterior pharynx. Once the transit study is completed, the remaining meal volume can be fed.

Feed the infant a meal that approximates its normal feeding (formula or milk).

After being burped, place the patient supine, with the gamma camera positioned posteriorly and the chest and upper abdomen in the field of view. *Abdominal compression is not used because it is considered nonphysiological, is poorly tolerated in infants, and does not increase the detection rate.*

Acquire 2-4-hr delayed images of the chest. Review with computer enhancement for aspiration.

Quantitate reflux.

---

concentration—and are influenced by different physiologic events, such as meal ingestion, gastric emptying, and esophageal acid clearance. Whereas the pH probe cannot detect a second reflux event until acid has cleared the pH probe, the radionuclide study can detect reflux only while the radiolabeled meal remains in the stomach.

Methodology

The radionuclide study has been performed differently in adults and children (Box 10-3), although this may not be completely rational or necessary.

Image Interpretation and Analysis

Adults All 30-second frames at each level of abdominal pressure should be reviewed for evidence of reflux, using computer enhancement. Greater than 4% reflux of stomach contents into the esophagus is considered abnormal.

Children All frames should be reviewed with contrast enhancement. GER is seen as distinct spikes of activity into the esophagus (Figure 10-7). Reflux events are graded as low or high level (less or greater than midesophagus), by duration (e.g., less or more than 10 seconds), and by their temporal relationship to meal ingestion. Reflux events of longer duration increase the risk of esophagitis; events that occur with small gastric volumes have more clinical significance because reflux is occurring without the effect of the increased pressure of a full meal volume and acid buffering.

Time-activity curves can be generated and regions of interest (ROI) drawn for the oropharynx, esophagus, and stomach. A variety of quantitative indices have been

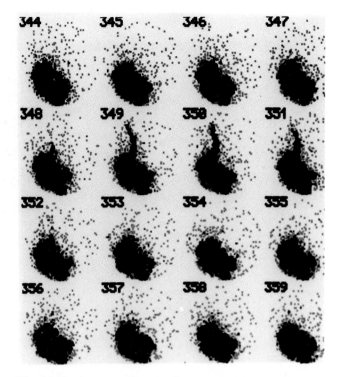

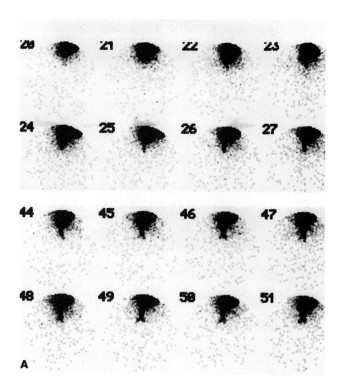

Fig. 10-7   Gastroesophageal reflux. Sequential 5-second frames demonstrate an episode of high-grade reflux of slightly greater than 15 seconds' duration.

used in both adult and pediatric populations (Box 10-4). Peaks greater than 5% generally correspond to reflux. The gastric emptying portion of the study can be quantitiated by drawing a stomach ROI on computer for the initial, 1-hour and 2-hour images. The results must be corrected for physical decay and are usually expressed as the percent emptying. Normal values are not available for children because truly normal infants are not studied; however, 40% to 50% emptying of milk at 1 hour and 60% to 75% at 2 hours is generally considered normal. The 2-hour emptying is more reliable than the 1-hour time period.

Pulmonary aspiration should be looked for carefully and computer enhancement is essential. However, aspiration is infrequently detected. The "salivagram," essentially an esophageal transit study performed by placing a labeled bolus of radiotracer in the infant's posterior pharynx, also acquired in a rapid framing mode, is a more sensitive method of detecting aspiration (Figure 10-8A,B)

Accuracy

Adults   Although the sensitivity of GER scintigraphy has been reported to be as high as 90%, other studies have found a lower sensitivity, in the 60% to 70% range. Because of gastroenterologists' perception that this test is not very sensitive, and because competing modalities

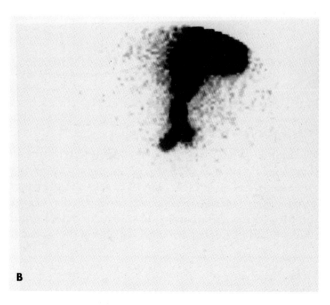

Fig. 10-8   Aspiration diagnosed from a salivagram. A neonate with neurologic deficits and swallowing difficulties had suspected GER with aspiration. A GER (milk) study performed after feeding by nasogastric tube showed numerous reflux events, but no evidence of aspiration. **A,** On another day, a salivagram was performed. After radiotracer was placed in the posterior pharynx, sequential 5-second frames showed slow transit into the tracheal bifurcation with no evidence of esophageal activity. **B,** High-count image at the end of 60 minutes in the same patient. Activity remains at the tracheal bifurcation.

Box 10-4   Methods Used for Quantitifying of Gastroesophageal Reflux in Children

1. The mean value of the esophageal time-activity curve as a percent of the inital gastric activity.
2. Reflux index derived by integrating the esophageal time-activity curve over 60 min and dividing by the initial gastric activity.
3. Percent activity in a specified episode relative to gastric activity at that time, multiplied by duration of the episode.
4. Number of episodes of high-level and low-level reflux, and their duration.

exist, the study is not commonly used in adults. One reason for the reported poor sensitivity in some studies may be the difference in methodology for adults and children, such as the longer framing rate and the nonphysiologic method of relying on external pressure.

Children In contrast, pediatricians generally feel that scintigraphy is very useful for evaluation of GER in children. The reported sensitivity is reasonably good (75%-88%). Children are less likely to be subjected to more invasive tests.

The detection of aspiration with reflux studies is low, variously reported to be 0 to 25%. However, the salivagram can often demonstrate aspiration when the GER study is negative.

GASTRIC EMPTYING

In the past, a variety of nonisotopic techniques were used for evaluating of gastric function, all with serious limitations. Gastric intubation methods require serial aspiration, and marker-dilution techniques with duodenal recovery are cumbersome, disliked by patients, and the tubing itself may alter emptying. Radiographic methods can define anatomy and show mechanical obstructions but are insensitive to motor disturbances of the stomach and cannot provide quantitative information on emptying. Radionuclide gastric emptying studies have become the standard method for evaluating gastric function because the technique is accurate, sensitive, quantitative, and relatively easy to perform.

Gastric Physiology

The stomach is composed of two functionally distinct regions (Figure10-9). The proximal stomach or *fundus* serves as a reservoir and can accept a large fluid volume with only minimal increases in pressure (receptive relaxation). Regular slow tonic muscular contractions produce a pressure gradient between the stomach and duodenum, moving the stomach contents toward the distal stomach. Liquid emptying is largely due to this fundal mechanism; it is volume dependent and therefore exponential in character: the larger the volume the more

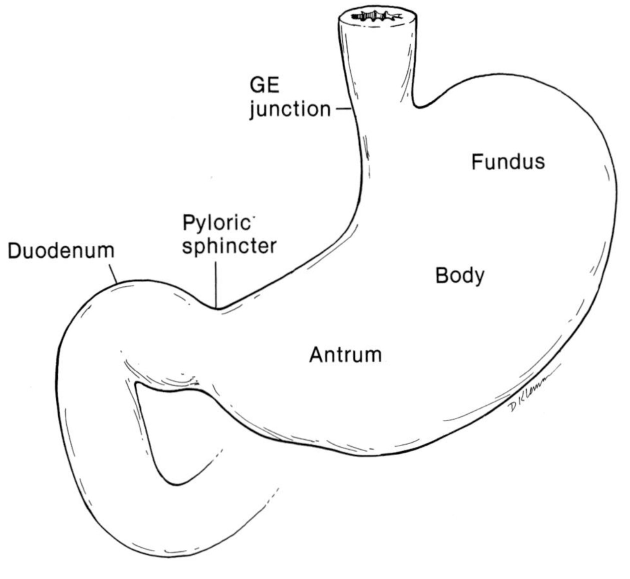

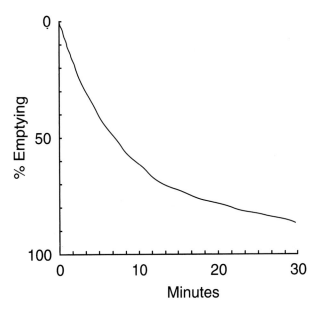

Fig. 10-9 Gastric anatomy and function. The proximal stomach (fundus) accommodates and stores food. The distal stomach (antrum) acts as a preparatory chamber where mixing and grinding of food occurs.

Fig. 10-10 Liquid-only emptying study. The patient ingested 300 mL of water with Tc-99m SC and 1-minute frames were acquired for 30 minutes. A time-activity curve was generated by drawing a whole-stomach ROI on computer. Emptying began immediately and the clearance curve pattern was exponential. Normal half-emptying time is less than 20 minutes.

rapid the emptying (Figure10-10). Nutrients, salts, and acidity all slow liquid emptying.

The distal stomach or *antrum* is responsible for the "grinding and sieving" of food and controls the emptying of solid food. After solid food ingestion, muscular contractions sweep down the antrum in a ringlike pattern, squeezing the food toward the pylorus. Large food particles are not allowed to pass and are retropelled toward the antrum, becoming progressively ground up until this chyme mixture is able to pass through the pyloric sphincter. After this delay before emptying begins (lag phase), solids begin to empty in a linear pattern (Figures 10-11A,B), with the rate of emptying dependent on the size and contents of the meal. Fat, acid, protein, and high osmolality foods all act to slow solid emptying.

In the fasting state between meals, phase III interdigestive contractions empty nondigestible debris from the stomach. These forceful, lumen-obliterating peristaltic waves sweep the gastric contents through the pylorus. Motilin, a peptide hormone secreted by the upper small bowel mucosa, is responsible for this motility pattern.

Gastric function is controlled by sympathetic and parasympathetic neural innervation as well as by a variety of hormones whose interactions are complex and incompletely understood.

Gastric Stasis Syndromes

Symptoms of gastric stasis include early satiety, bloating, nausea, and occasionally vomiting. Although gastric stasis may occur acutely (e.g., in viral gastroenteritis and metabolic derangements), chronic gastric paresis is a more important clinical problem with serious long-term consequences. It can be caused by a variety of disease processes (Box 10-5). Mechanical causes of stasis, such as obstruction by tumor or pyloric channel ulcer, must be excluded by endoscopy or contrast barium radiography.

Chronic gastric stasis may initially be asymptomatic, but it usually becomes clinically manifest with time. Rapid gastric emptying may also produce symptoms, sometimes severe, including palpitations, diaphoresis, weakness, and diarrhea (dumping syndrome) (Box 10-6).

Diabetic gastroparesis   Diabetic gastroparesis is the most common cause of chronic gastroparesis. It usually occurs in the long-standing insulin-dependent diabetic. Although it has been thought to reflect vagal damage as part of a generalized autonomic neuropathy, no morpho-

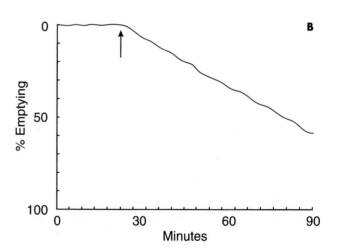

Fig. 10-11 Solid gastric emptying study. **A**, Normal progression of stomach contents during a solid radionuclide gastric emptying study. These are 5-minute sequential images acquired for 60 minutes. The meal moves from the gastric fundus to the antrum in a normal emptying pattern. A radioactive marker has been placed in the right chest as a check for movement. **B**, Solid meal (egg sandwich) computer-generated time-activity curve in a different patient. An initial delay of about 25 minutes is seen before emptying begins. The length of this lag phase (*arrow*) is at the upper end of normal limits (5-25 minutes). A linear pattern of emptying follows. Greater than 50% emptying occurred by 90 minutes (normal, >40%).

Box 10-5   Causes of Functional Gastric Stasis Syndromes

ACUTE STATES OR DISEASES

Trauma
Postoperative ileus
Gastroenteritis
Hyperalimentation
Metabolic disorders: hyperglycemia, acidosis,
    hypokalemia, hypercalcemia, hepatic coma,
    myxedema
Physiologic effects: labyrinth stimulation, physical and
    mental stress, gastric distention, increased intragastric
    pressure
Drugs: anticholinergics, antidepressants, nicotine,
    opiates levodopa, progresterone, contraceptive pills,
    β-andrenergic agonists, alcohol
Hormones: gastrin, scretin, glucagon, cholecystokinin,
    somatostatin, estrogen, progesterone

CHRONIC DISEASES

Diabetes mellitus
Hypothyroidism
Progressive systemic sclerosis
Systemic lupus, dermatomyositis
Myotonic dystrophy
Familial dysautonomia
Fabry's disease
Amyloidosis
Pernicious anemia
Anorexia nervosa
Bulbar poliomyelitis
Gastric ulcer
Post vagotomy for obstruction with or without pylorplasty
Tumor-associated gastroparesis
Idiopathic

---

logic abnormality in the gastric wall or abdominal vagus has been identified. In addition to producing disturbing symptoms, poor gastric emptying may make diabetes control more difficult, since timing of the insulin dose, food ingestion, and absorption is critical. Delayed emptying in the diabetic may be caused by hyperglycemia alone. Because symptoms suggestive of gastric stasis in the diabetic are nonspecific and may be due by other causes, such as infection, metabolic derangements, and so forth, study of gastric function when the patient is under optimal diabetic control is critical to making the correct diagnosis.

Drug therapy for gastroparesis   A number of drugs have been used to treat chronic gastroparesis. The gastrokinetic properties of these drugs are mediated by different mechanisms. *Metoclopramide* has both central and peripheral antidopaminergic properties; it also releases acetylcholine from the myenteric plexus. Neurologic side effects such as drowsiness and lassitude are seen in up to 20% of patients. *Domperidone* is a peripheral dopamine antagonist that penetrates the blood-brain barrier poorly and therefore rarely produces neurologic side effects. *Cisapride* releases acetylcholine from the myenteric plexus. *Erythromycin* acts as an agonist of motilin. All of these drugs improve gastric emptying by increasing the amplitude of antral contractions. Metoclopramide can improve symptoms via a central antinausea effect without improving emptying in some patients. A repeat study on therapy is necessary to determine if gastric emptying has indeed improved.

Radiopharmaceutical

For accurate quantitation of solid gastric emptying, the radioactive marker must be tightly bound to the meal. Elution of the radiolabel in vivo will result in a partially solid, partially liquid labeled mixture that will produce an erroneously shortened solid emptying time, as liquids empty faster than solids.

A physiologically superb method for labeling chicken liver in vivo has been described and used clinically. It involves injecting Tc-99m SC into the wing vein of a chicken; the chicken is killed and the liver removed and cooked. The Tc-99m SC is taken up by the Kupffer cells. This intracellular localization is highly stable and does not dissociate after ingestion. The chicken liver is usually mixed with beef or chicken stew for palatability and volume. Although this method is of proven utility, it is not generally used, for obvious practical reasons.

Alternative acceptable in vitro methods of labeling liver have been developed and are now more commonly used clinically. Cooking injected or surface-labeled liver

---

Box 10-6   Causes of Rapid Gastric Emptying

Postoperative
  Pyloroplasty
  Hemigastrectomy (Billroth I, II)
Diseases
  Duodenal ulcer
  Gastrinoma (Zollinger-Ellison syndrome)
  Hyperthyroidism
Hormones
  Thyroxine
  Motilin
  Enterogastrone
Drugs
  Erythromycin

cubes or liver paté traps the radionuclide within the meat. Another convenient, palatable, and easy to prepare method that is frequently used is to fry eggs with Tc-99m SC and serve it as a sandwich. The Tc-99m SC binds tightly to the egg albumin.

Liquid phase markers must equilibrate rapidly and be nonabsorbable. Tc-99m SC in water is most commonly used to measure liquid-only emptying. In dual isotope combined solid-liquid studies, In-111 DPTA is often used as the liquid marker because of its higher photopeaks (171 and 247 keV) compared to the Tc-99m-labeled solid (Figure 10-12).

Methodology

There is no generally accepted standard protocol for performing gastric emptying studies. Meal composition, patient positioning, instrumentation, data acquisition, and quantitative methods vary from laboratory to laboratory. Therefore, there are also no generally applicable normal values.

Despite the variable methodologies, the radionuclide study is relatively straightforward. The patient ingests a radiolabeled meal and is placed under a gamma camera, and the study is acquired on a computer. Gastric emptying over a specified period of time is then quantitated. Each laboratory must decide for itself how best to perform the study using the instrumentation available and in the circumstances of the facility. A number of factors must be considered (Box 10-7).

Meal   The content of the ingested meal is a primary factor in determining the rate of emptying. Clear liquids

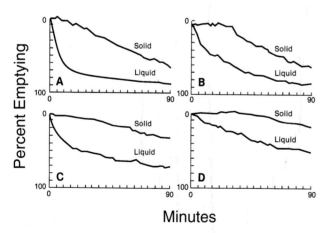

Fig. 10-12 Dual-phase solid-liquid gastric emptying study in three diabetics and a normal volunteer. **A,** Normal subject. Linear solid emptying after a short lag phase and rapid exponential liquid emptying. **B,** Diabetic subject. Normal solid and liquid emptying. **C,** Diabetic subject with delayed solid emptying but normal liquid emptying. **D,** Diabetic subject with delay in solid and liquid emptying. This figure demonstrates the spectrum of gastric emptying in the diabetic population.

Box 10-7	Factors That Affect the Rate of Gastric Emptying

Meal content
Amount of fat, protein, acid, osmolality
   Volume
   Weight
   Caloric density
   Particle size
Time of day
Sex
Postion (standing, sitting, supine)
Stress
Drugs

empty faster than liquids with nutrients; liquids empty faster than soft foods, which empty faster than solids; large meals empty faster than small meals. Therefore, normal values for a laboratory that uses labeled paté mixed with stew do not apply to a laboratory that uses a Tc-99m-labeled egg sandwich or even to a laboratory that uses the same meal but a larger volume or different calorie total. One must either *closely* follow the protocol of a laboratory that has established normal values or establish one's own normal values.

Single- versus dual-isotope studies   A dual-isotope study allows simultaneous evaluation of liquid and solid gastric emptying. Although dual-phase studies are important for the investigation of gastric physiology and pharmacology, they add complexity, cost, and increased radiation exposure to the patient. Solid emptying is all that is needed for most clinical purposes. The liquid phase is less sensitive than the solid phase for detection of delayed gastric emptying. Liquid emptying is always normal when solid emptying is normal. When solid emptying is delayed, liquid emptying may be normal or delayed, depending on the severity of the gastroparesis. A liquid-only study should be reserved for patients who cannot tolerate solids.

Study length   Although ideally one should continue to acquire a gastric emptying study until half-emptying occurs, a practical guideline for the busy clinic would be to use a routine study length equal to the normal mean half-emptying time of the method being used. Large, hard to digest meals (stew) empty slowly and may require a 2.5 to 3.0-hour acquisition time, while smaller and more easily digestible meals (egg sandwich) require a shorter study length of 1.5 to 2.0 hours.

Frequency of image acquisition   Although a gross estimate of gastric emptying could be estimated from a computer-acquired image immediately after ingestion of the meal and another one at the end of the study time, much of the qualitative and quantitative potential of radionuclide gastric emptying studies would be lost. For example, because solid emptying is normally biphasic, delayed emptying may be the result of a prolonged lag phase, a decreased rate of emptying, or both. With multiple data points, a time-activity curve can be generated and a more accurate half-time of emptying or rate of emptying can be determined. If one acquires a study every 30 minutes for 2 hours, only five data points result. A lag phase of 15 minutes would be missed completely, and the slope of the resulting emptying curve would be in error whether one used either the first or the second data point as the start of emptying. More frequent image acquisition would improve accuracy.

Attenuation correction   The ingested meal moves from the gastric fundus, which is relatively posterior and lateral, to the gastric antrum, which is anterior and medial. This posterior to anterior movement of the gastric contents results in a variable detection efficiency of the radiolabel by the gamma camera. A radiolabeled meal will be detected with greatest efficiency when the stomach contents are close to the camera, that is, with the least amount of attenuating material between the camera and stomach. Therefore, if only a single-headed gamma camera is placed in the anterior view, the detected radioactive counts will rise as the meal moves from the fundus to the antrum (Figure 10-13). This can result in underestimation of gastric emptying. The amount of error will vary from patient to patient, depending on the size and configuration of the patient and his or her stomach. This is especially a problem in obese patients. The average error due to attenuation is in the range of 10% to 15%, but it can be considerably greater (30%-50%) in some individuals, and is to a large extent unpredictable.

With dual-isotope meals, such as In-111 with Tc-99m, correction for downscatter and perhaps even upscatter may be necessary. Whether correction is needed and how much can be determined from a simple phantom study. Error is minimal when the dose ratio of Tc-99m/In-111 is 4-5:1.

The standard method for attenuation correction is the *geometric mean* method (Figure 10-13). This method requires acquisition of opposed images, typically the anterior and posterior views, and then mathmatical correction by calculating the geometric mean (square root of the product of the counts in the anterior and posterior views) at each data point. Ideally, both images should be obtained simultaneously, but to do this, a dual-headed gamma camera is required. With a single-headed camera, the two opposing views must be obtained sequentially, commonly every 15 to 30 minutes.

An alternative method of attenuation compensation that requires only a single-headed gamma camera and allows frequent image acquisition is the LAO method. When the study is acquired in the left anterior oblique projection, the stomach contents move roughly parallel to the head of the gamma camera, thus minimizing the effect of attenuation. An advantage of this method is the simplicity of acquisition, with no mathmatical correction required (Figure 10-12). Because of normal anatomic variation, this method is not as accurate in all patients as the geometric mean method, but it is very adequate for clinical purposes and clearly superior to anterior view-only acquisition.

Analysis of Gastric Emptying

To some extent, the method of processing depends on how the study is acquired. Generally, a gastric ROI is drawn on computer for individual or summed images. After correction for decay and attenuation, a time-activity curve is generated and a selected parameter of gastric emptying is calculated, such as a half-time of emptying, percent emptying, or emptying rate (%/min).

Liquid emptying   Emptying of clear liquids only begins immediately after ingestion into the stomach, typically without a lag phase; the computer-generated clearance curve is monoexponential, with a $T_{1/2}$ of 10 to 20 minutes being normal (Figure 10-10).

Liquids in a dual-phase meal also empty exponentially but considerably slower than a liquid-only meal. The emptying rate is very dependent on the type of solid phase meal (Figure 10-12).

Solid emptying   After the initial lag phase, solid gastric emptying has a linear pattern of emptying. The length of the lag phase is affected by the same factors that affect the rate of emptying (Box 10-7). Certain dis-

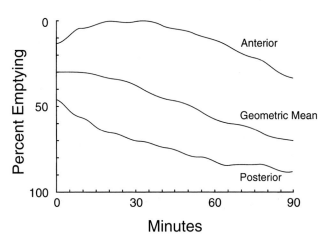

Fig. 10-13   Geometric mean attenuation correction. Anterior and posterior acquisition with GM correction. Both the anterior and posterior view time-activity curves show the effect of attenuation. The anterior acquired data have a rising time-activity curve before it begins to empty. The posterior view shows decreasing counts from time zero. The geometric mean corrects for this attenuation affect. Two phase emptying is seen. The nearly flat, early portion of the GM curve confirms good attenuation correction.

Table 10-3   Gastric Emptying Protocols

	Single-Headed Camera, LAO Method	Dual-Headed Camera, Geometric Mean	Single-Headed Camera, Geometric Mean
Preparation	Overnight fast	Overnight fast	8-hr fast
Marker	Anterior Tc-99m point source on right lower chest		50-100 μCi Tc-99m taped to right anterior rib margin away from stomach; posterior rib marker similarly placed
Meal	Tc-99m SC egg white sandwich, 200 mL water	Tc-99m SC whole, whole egg sandwich, 300 mL water	Tc-99m SC in vitro labeled fried liver paté mixed with beef stew, orange juice
Dose	Tc-99m SC, 1 mCi In-111, 200 μCi	Tc-99m SC, 500 μCi In-111 DTPA, 125 μCi	Tc-99m SC, 600 μCi In-111 DTPA, 100 μCi
Window	15% 140 keV 15% 247 keV 10% 172 keV	10% 140 keV 20% 247 keV	20% 140 keV 20% 247 keV
Patient position	Semiupright (60°) on gurney	Seated	Upright
Projections	Left anterior oblique	Anterior and posterior simultaneously	Anterior and posterior sequentially
Framing rate	90 sec/frame for 90 min	60 sec/frame X 2 hr	40 sec/frame *q* 15 min X 1 hr, then *q* 30 min until 50% emptying
Bkgd correct	No	Yes	No
Decay correct	Yes	Yes	Yes
Scatter correct	No	Yes	Yes
Attenuation correction	LAO view	Geometric mean	Geometric mean
Computer processing	ROI around summed gastric image	ROI around summed gastric image	ROI around each image and counts obtained
Data presentation	Time-activity curve of % emptying vs. time	Time-activity curve of geometric mean counts	Percent of counts remaining at each time interval
Quantitation	Solid: % emptying at 90 min Liquid: half-emptying time	Curve fit to a modified power exponential with estimation of lag phase and emptying rate	Half-emptying time for solids and liquids

ease states have been associated with a prolonged lag phase (e.g., diabetes) and the prokinetic effect of certain drugs (e.g., metoclopramide) improve emptying by shortening the lag phase. Although the half-time of emptying has been used to characterize solid emptying, it infers exponential emptying; the rate of emptying is preferable (e.g., %/min), or, more simply, the amount of emptying at selected time intervals and at the end of the study.

The specific protocol used, therefore, will be determined by factors unique to each laboratory. Three typical protocols used at different institutions are described in Table 10-3.

Evaluation of Therapy and Pharmacologic Interventions

Pharmacologic intervention can help predict the effectiveness of a potential therapy. For example, if poor emptying is noted, metoclopramide can be given IV dur-

ing the study. A change to a steeper emptying slope would confirm a positive response to the drug (Figure 10-14). Alternatively, the study can be repeated after oral ingestion of the drug, either after a single dose or, preferably, after several days or weeks of therapy. The effectiveness of various interventional therapies (e.g., gastroplasty, surgical relief of obstruction) can also be effectively evaluated (Figure 10-15).

HELICOBACTER PYLORI INFECTION

Helicobacter pylori, formerly called *Campylobacter pylori*, a gram-negative bacterium, infects the gastric mucosa of most patients with duodenal ulcer disease, gastric ulcer disease, and antral gastritis. There is increasing evidence that *H. pylori* is the causal agent in most cases. Bacterial eradication markedly decreases duodenal ulcer recurrence rates, reverses histologic gastritis, and hastens healing of active duodenal ulcers.

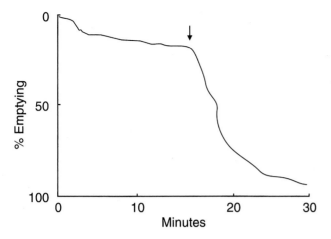

Fig. 10-14   Metoclopramide intervention. Very delayed liquid-only emptying is seen in a diabetic subject. Metoclopramide was infused IV at 17 minutes (*arrow*). Prompt, rapid emptying ensued. This study predicted the potential clinical effectiveness of this drug in this patient.

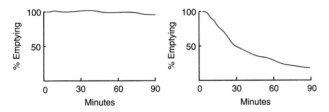

Fig. 10-15   Pre- and postoperative study of a patient diagnosed with pyloric obstruction secondary to peptic ulcer disease. *Left,* preoperative study shows no emptying. A partial gastrectomy was performed. *Right,* postoperative study shows a short lag phase and relatively rapid emptying.

The Urea Breath Test

Utility in duodenal and gastric ulcer disease and antral gastritis   The principle of the urea breath test is that, in the presence of the bacterial enzyme urease, orally administered urea is hydrolyzed to CO_2 and ammonia. If the urea carbon is labeled with either the stable isotope C-13 or radioactive C-14, it can be detected in the breath as labeled CO_2. *H. pylori* is the most common urease-containing gastric pathogen, and therefore a positive urea breath test can be equated with *H. pylori* infection.

Methodology   The urea breath test is easy to perform in a laboratory that has the appropriate breath analyzer equipment. It is inexpensive, noninvasive, and accurate. False negative results may occur due to the use of antibiotics or bismuth-containing medications. False positive results occur in patients with achlorhydria, contamination with oral urease-containing bacteria, colonization with another *Helicobacter,* such as *H. felis,* and so on.

Clinical utility   The clinical role of this test remains to be determined. Whether stable (nonradioactive) C-13 or radioactive C-14 is used will probably depend on the capabilities and facilities of the intitution and the interests of the clinicians and investigators. Serologic tests are being developed, and in the future, a positive test may be sufficient to diagnose infection. The breath test is ideal for following the results of therapy because the antibody titer falls too slowly to be of diagnostic utility. The breath test also will be useful for evaluating new therapies.

GASTROINTESTINAL BLEEDING

Effective and prompt therapy of acute GI bleeding depends on accurate localization of the site of hemorrhage. The history and clinical examination often can distinguish upper from lower GI bleeding. Upper tract hemorrhage can be confirmed with *gastric intubation* and localized with flexible *fiber-optic endoscopy*; however, lower GI bleeding is more problematic. During active hemorrhage, *endoscopy* and *barium radiography* are of limited value in the small bowel and colon.

Nonradionuclide Diagnostic Methods

Angiography is diagnostic but will only demonstrate the bleeding site if the contrast agent is injected during active hemorrhage. Bleeding is typically intermittent, however, and the clinical determination of whether the patient is actively bleeding is very difficult. The clinical signs of active bleeding often present after the hemorrhage has ceased. Because repeated angiographic studies are not practical, it is often the angiographers who request that radionuclide GI bleeding studies be performed prior to angiography, both to ensure that the patient is indeed actively bleeding and to localize the approximate bleeding site so that the length of the angiographic study and the amount of contrast agent used can be minimized.

Radionuclide Studies

In 1977, Alavi et al. first described scintigraphic imaging of active GI bleeding using Tc-99m SC. In 1979, Winzelberg et al. described the use of Tc-99m labeled red blood cells (Tc-99 RBCs) for the same purpose.

Tc-99m SC scintigraphy   After injection of Tc-99m SC, it is rapidly extracted by the reticuloendothelial cells of the liver, spleen, and bone marrow (serum $T_{1/2}$ of 3 minutes); by 15 minutes after injection, most activity has cleared from the vascular system. During active GI bleeding, radiotracer will extravasate at the bleeding site into the bowel lumen with each recirculation of blood. Continued extravasation with simultaneous background clearance results in a high target-to-background ratio, permitting visualization of the intra-abdominal active bleeding site (Figure 10-16).

Methodology Details of Alavi's method, the Tc-99m SC method, are given in Box 10-8. In summary, the protocol requires the IV injection of 10 mCi of freshly prepared Tc-99m SC and acquisition of serial 500k to 750k count images of the abdomen and pelvis every 1 to 2 minutes for 20 to 30 minutes. In experimental animal studies, bleeding rates as low as 0.05 to 0.1 mL/min have been detected.

Image interpretation Rapid bleeding may be detected on the 1 sec/frame blood flow images. Vascular blushes of tumors, angiodysplasia, and arteriovenous malformations may be seen in the absence of active bleeding. Active hemorrhage is most commonly detected in the first 5 to 10 minutes of imaging on the static

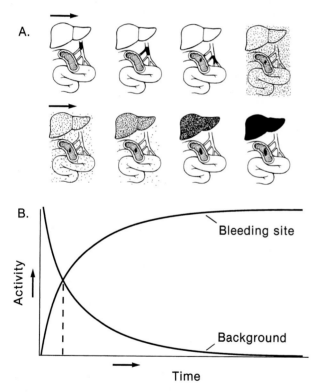

Fig. 10-16 Schematic diagram illustrating the mechanism by which Tc-99m SC scintigraphy can demonstrate an acute GI bleed. **A,** After IV injection, Tc-99m SC is cleared by the RES with a short serum half-life of 3 minutes so that by 15 minutes, most is cleared from the vascular system. With active bleeding, a fraction of the injected radiotracer will extravasate at the site of bleeding; this occurs with each recirculation. Due to rapid background clearance, a high-contrast image of acute bleeding can be produced. **B,** The time-activity curve demonstrates rapid exponential clearance of background and inversely increasing activity at the bleeding site. Contrast improves as the target-to-background ratio increases with time.

high-count images. The site of bleeding is seen as a focal area of radiotracer accumulation that increases in intensity and moves through the intestinal tract during the course of the study (Figure 10-17).

Because blood acts as an intestinal irritant, movement can often be rapid and bidirectional. A fixed region of radiotracer accumulation that does not move is not likely to represent intraluminal hemorrhage. An ectopic spleen is a common cause of this finding, and renal transplants may also accumulate Tc-99m SC. Asymmetric bone marrow activity can be misleading, for marrow replacement by tumor, infarction, or fibrosis may make the adjacent marrow appear as focal uptake and suggest a bleeding site. The critical diagnostic point is that the region of tracer accumulation is fixed and does not move. When the initial study is negative but recurrent active bleeding is suspected clinically, a repeat injection is indicated.

Detection of bleeding in the splenic flexure and the transverse colon can sometimes be difficult, although flow images, frequent repeated static images, and the rapid movement of intraluminal contents may allow identification of the bleeding site. The main disadvantage of the Tc-99m SC method, like angiography, is that bleeding must be active at the time of injection.

Tc-99m-labeled RBC scintigraphy Because GI bleeding is intermittent, the use of Tc-99m labeled RBCs to diagnose GI bleeding has a major theoretical advantage over Tc-99m SC: A hemorrhagic site can be detected over a much longer period of time, dependent only on the physical half-life of Tc-99m and the stability of the radiolabel.

Red blood cell labeling techniques A high labeling efficiency is very important for proper interpretation of the Tc-99m RBC bleeding study. Free unbound Tc-99m pertechnetate is taken up by the salivary glands and gastric mucosa and then secreted into the GI tract, potentially complicating interpretation of the study. Various labeling techniques (in vivo, modified in vivo or in vivtro, and in vitro) with varying labeling efficiencies have been used (Box 10-9). Although the Brookhaven in vitro method has the highest labeling efficiency (>98%), it is not an FDA-approved method, is technically demanding, requires centrifugation (which is potentially damaging to RBCs), and contamination is possible when transferring RBCs into sterile containers.

A simple kit technique for labeling RBCs in vitro is now FDA approved and commercially available. This method uses whole blood and does not require centrifugation or transferring of red cells (Figure 10-18). Although the in vivo and modified in vivo method depend on biological clearance of undesirable extracellular reduced stannous ion and the Brookhaven in vitro method removes it by centrifugation, the in vitro kit method prevents extracellular reduction of stannous ion by the addition of an oxidizing agent (sodium hypochlorite) which

Box 10-8   Tc-99m SC Scintigraphy for Gastrointestinal Bleeding: Protocol Summary

PATIENT PREPARATION

None.

INSTRUMENTATION

Camera setup: Large field of view gamma camera with a high-resolution, low-energy parallel hole collimator interfaced with a nuclear medicine computer. Intensity: Set so that bone marrow can be seen.
Computer setup: 1 sec/frame anterior flow images obtained for 1 min, then acquire 500-750k images of the abdomen every 1-2 min for 20 min.

PATIENT POSITION

Supine. The field of view should include the entire abdomen and pelvis.

IMAGING PROCEDURE

Inject 10 mCi Tc-99m SC as a bolus after starting computer and beginning camera acquisition.
In addition to anterior views, oblique, lateral, and posterior views may be obtained as needed to confirm the site of bleeding.
If no bleeding site is detected, obtain a 1,000k count image of the upper abdomen with oblique views to evaluate the hepatic and splenic flexures. If negative, repeat views of the lower abdomen are taken 15 min later to check for activity that may have been obscured in the hepatic and splenic flexures.
If the scan is negative and recurrent active bleeding is suspected, a repeat dose of Tc-99m SC is given and the same protocol is repeated.

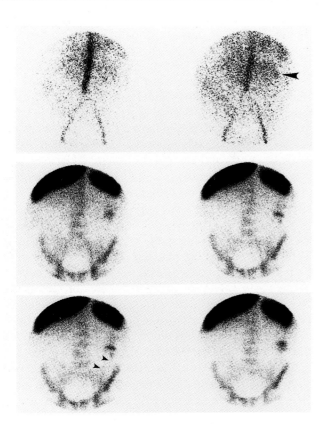

Fig. 10-17   Tc-99m SC GI bleeding study positive in the descending colon. *Top,* two sequential 3-second flow images; the second flow image indicates the site of bleeding (*large arrowhead*). *Bottom,* four sequential 5-minute images showing the site of bleeding. The lower images show some movement to the more distal left colon (*small arrowheads*).

cannot enter the red cell (labeling efficiency of >98%).

Methodology   A Tc-99m labeled RBC study protocol is outlined in Box 10-10. Sequential images are initially acquired for 90 minutes. If the study is negative, repeat 30-minute acquisitions are performed at 2 to 4 hours and whenever recurrent active bleeding is suspected.

Image interpretation   In addition to detecting active bleeding sites, the flow phase may show vascular bleeding sources that are not actively bleeding at the moment (e.g., angiodysplasia or tumors), define vascular structures such as the kidneys, ectatic vessels, and uterus that help interpret later images, and occasionally be helpful for detecting bleeding sites difficult to see on later high-count dynamic imaging, such as those adjacent to the bladder.

Active bleeding can often be diagnosed from frequent intermittent static images during the first 60 minutes of acquisition (Figures 10-19, 10-20). However, in order to diagnose the site of active GI bleeding, the extravascular activity must be judged to be intraluminal, to be increasing over time, and to be moving through the GI tract (Box 10-11). Activity that is not moving with time should not be diagnosed as an active bleeding site and is usually due to a fixed vascular structure such as a hemangioma, accessory spleen, or ectopic kidney.

Some pitfalls in diagnosis that may lead to misinterpretation are listed in Box 10-12. Pitfalls are normal, pathologic, or technical findings that can usually be distinguished from active hemorrhage if one is aware of the potential problems. For example, a poor label can result

Box 10-9 Methods of Tc-99m Red Blood Cell Labeling

In vivo method (labeling efficiency, 75%-80%)
1. Inject stannous pyrophosphate.
2. Wait 10-20 min.
3. Inject Tc-99m sodium pertechnetate.

Modified in vivo (in vivtro) method (labeling efficiency, 85%-90%)
1. Inject stannous pyrophosphate.
2. Wait 10-20 min.
3. Withdraw 5-8 mL whole blood into shielded syringe containing Tc-99m sodium pertechnetate.
4. Gently mix syringe contents for 10 min at room temperature.

In vitro (Brookhaven) method (labeling efficiency, 98%)
1. Add 4 mL heparinized whole blood to reagent vial containing 2.0 mg Sn^{+2}, 3.67 mg Na citrate, 5.5 mg dextrose, 0.11 mg NaCl.
2. Incubate at room temperature for 5 min.
3. Add 2.0 mL 4.4% EDTA.
4. Centrifuge tube for 5 min at 1,300 g.
5. Withdraw 1.25 mL of packed red cells, transfer to sterile vial containing 1-3 mL Tc-99m sodium pertechnetate.
6. Incubate at room temperature for 10 min.

In-vitro commercial kit (labeling efficiency, 98%)
1. Add 1.0-3.0 mL of whole blood (heparin or ACD as anticoagulant) to reagent vial (50-100 µg stannous chloride, 3.67 sodium citrate) and mix. Allow to react for 5 min.
2. Add syringe 1 contents (0.6 mg sodium hypochlorite) and mix by gently inverting 4-5 times.
3. Add contents of syringe 2 (citric acid 8.7 mg, sodium citrate 32.5 mg, dextrose) and mix.
4. Add 370-3,700 MBq (10-100 mCi) Na pertechnetate Tc99m to reaction vial.
5. Mix and allow to react for 20 min, with occasional mixing.

Modified from Swanson, Chilton, and Thrall: Pharmaceuticals in Medical Imaging, New York, 1990, Macmillan.

in bladder activity; and lateral images may be needed to differentiate rectosigmoidal bleeding from radioactivity in the bladder, uterus, or penis (Figure 10-21). Free Tc-99m pertechnetate can be a particularly troublesome problem due to gastric uptake simulating a gastric bleed or bleeding more distally (Figure 10-22), particularly on delayed images.

If the inital study is negative, delayed acquisitions can be performed 2 to 4 hours later or for up to 24 hours if there is clinical suspicion of recurrent bleeding. Dynamic computer acquisition is also suggested at these times.

The radionuclide study is a very sensitive test for locating the site of lower GI bleeding, for example in the hepatic flexure, transerse colon, splenic flexture, rectosigmoid, and so forth. Frequent image acquisition is important for localizing the site of bleeding because hemorrhage may be rapid and may move retrograde as well as antegrade. Although the bleeding site can often be identified by viewing static images acquired every 5 to 10 minutes, review of the 1-minute frames acquired on computer in a cinematic display is often helpful in confirming and better defining the site of bleeding. For example, it can aid in differentiating ureteral clearance from GI bleeding.

Small bowel bleeding can be particularly trouble-

some to diagnose. The cecum is often the site for pooling of a more proximal small bowel bleed, but the original source (duodenum, jejunum, ileum) is not always certain. Glucagon has been advocated as a method to aid in the diagnosis of small bowel bleeding. After injection, bowel peristalsis is inhibited, often resulting in pooling of the radiotracer in the small bowel at the site of active bleeding.

Note should always be made of any evidence of bleeding from the stomach and duodenum. Although upper GI bleeding should be detected clinically by aspiration from a nasogastric tube placed in the stomach prior to scintigraphy, this is not always the case. Images of the thyroid and salivary glands may be helpful in excluding free Tc-99m pertechnetate as a source of gastric activity (Figure 10-22, 10-23). This is now a less common problem with the availability of the in vitro kit for labeling RBCs.

Intraluminal radioactivity first detected on delayed images can be a diagnostic dilemma. Blood first seen in the sigmoid colon or rectum on a single delayed image obtained at 18 to 24 hours may have originated from anywhere in the GI tract or could be due to the transit of free Tc-99m pertechnetate from the stomach. This isolated finding should not be misinterpreted.

Bleeding rates as low as 0.1 mL/min can be clinically detected. Only 2 to 3 mL of extravasated blood is neces-

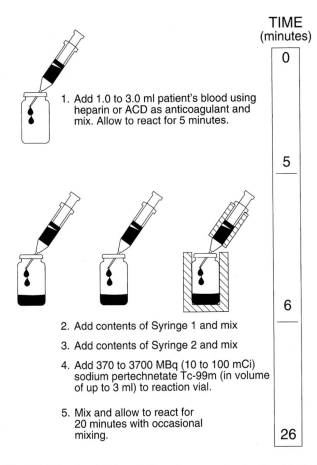

TIME
(minutes)

0

1. Add 1.0 to 3.0 ml patient's blood using heparin or ACD as anticoagulant and mix. Allow to react for 5 minutes.

5

2. Add contents of Syringe 1 and mix

3. Add contents of Syringe 2 and mix

4. Add 370 to 3700 MBq (10 to 100 mCi) sodium pertechnetate Tc-99m (in volume of up to 3 ml) to reaction vial.

6

5. Mix and allow to react for 20 minutes with occasional mixing.

26

Fig. 10-18 Simple kit technique for preparing in vitro labeled Tc-99m RBCs (UltraTag RBC, Mallinkrodt Medical, Inc., St. Louis, MO). Each kit consists of three nonradioactive components: a 10-mL vial containing stannous chloride; syringe I, containing sodium hypochlorite; and syringe II, containing citric acid, sodium citrate, and dextrose. The typical percent labeling efficiency is 98%.

sary for detection. This compares favorably with the ability of contrast angiography to detect bleeding rates of about 1.0 mL/min or greater.

Dosimetry The radiation absorbed dose to the patient using the Tc-99m SC technique and the Tc-99m-labeled RBC method is relatively low, particularly when compared with contrast angiography (Tables 10-4, 10-5). The target organ for Tc-99m SC is the liver, and for Tc-99m labeled RBCs the myocardial wall. The whole body dose for the latter is about 0.4 rads/25 mCi.

Tc-99m RBCs versus Tc-99m SC There has been considerable controversy over which radiopharmaceutical, Tc-99m SC or Tc-99m-labeled RBCs, is best for detection of acute GI bleeding. A comparison of the two methods and the theoretical advantages and disadvantages of both are listed in Table 10-6. Although the controversy has not completely abated, a general consensus has evolved in favor of Tc-99m-labeled RBCs in light of the results of several comparison studies.

A large multicenter study compared the results of these two approaches in 100 patients referred with clinical evidence of acute GI bleeding. A 20-minute Tc-99m SC study was performed first, followed by an in vitro labeled Tc-99m RBC study. Tc-99m SC showed only five sites of hemorrhage, while Tc-99m RBC imaging accurately disclosed the source of bleeding in 38 cases. The sensitivity of the Tc-99m RBC study was 93% and the specificity was 95%. Continuous imaging for 90 minutes revealed 83% of all active hemorrhages. Delayed imaging revealed the remainder. Other smaller studies have found similar results.

It has been argued that the comparative studies were biased against Tc-99m SC because the protocols allowed no repeat injections of this radiotracer. This may be true,

---

Box 10-10   Tc-99m RBC Scintigraphy: Protocol Summary

RADIOPHARMACEUTICAL

Tc-99m labeled RBCs.

INSTRUMENTATION

Camera: Large field of view gamma camera interfaced with computer parallel hole high resolution collimator.
Computer setup: 1-sec frames × 60; 1-min frames × 60-90 min.
Aquire 2-4 hr delayed images as 1-min frames × 20-30 min.
Static images: acquire 2-sec flow images and 1,000k count images every 5 min. Set intensity so that aorta, IVC, and
  iliac vessels are well visualized.
Patient position
  Supine; image anteriorly. Field of view to include entire abdomen and pelvis.

IMAGING PROCEDURE

Inject Tc-99m-labeled RBCs as a bolus.
Acquire flow images, followed by static images for 60-90 min.
If study is negative, repeat 30-min acquisition at 2-4 hr and if recurrent active bleeding is suspected.

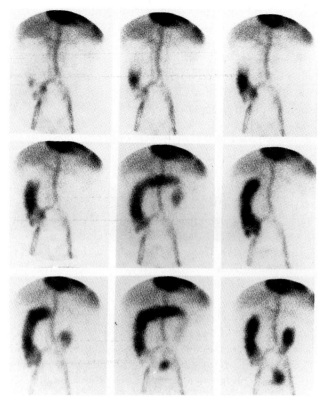

Fig. 10-19 Hepatic flexure bleeding in an elderly man. The blood can be seen moving along the low-lying transverse colon and into the left colon by the end of the 60-minute study. A tortuous aorta is noted. The source of bleeding in this patient was cancer of the colon.

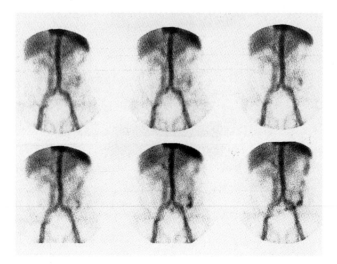

Fig. 10-20 Left colonic bleeding. Dynamic images acquired over 60 minutes show increasing activity in the region of the sigmoid colon that moves distally.

Box 10-11 Criteria for Positive Tc-RBC Scintigraphy

1. Abnormal radiotracer "hot spot" appears and conforms to bowel anatomy.
2. Persistence or increase in abnormal activity over time.
3. Essential: Movement of activity by peristalsis, retrograde or antegrade.

Box 10-12 Pitfalls in Interpretation of Tc-99m RBC Scintigraphy

Common
  Physiologic
    Gastrointestinal (due to free Tc-99m pertechnetate)
    Stomach, small and large intestine
    Genitourinary
    Pelvic kidney
    Ectopic kidney
    Renal pelvic activity
    Ureter
    Bladder
    Uterine blush
    Penis
Uncommon
  Accessory spleen
  Hepatic hemangioma
  Varices, esophageal and gastric
Rare
  Vascular
    Abdominal aortic aneurysm
    Gastroduodenal artery aneurysm
    Abdominal varices
    Caput medusae and dilated mesenteric veins
    Gallbladder varices
    Pseudoaneurysm
    Hemobilia from false hepatic artery aneurysm
    Arterial grafts
    Cutaneous hemangioma
    Duodenal telangectasia
    Angiodysplasia
  Miscellaneous
    Gallbladder (heme products)
    Gluteal hematoma
    Nonhemorrhagic gastritis
    Factitious gastrointestinal bleeding

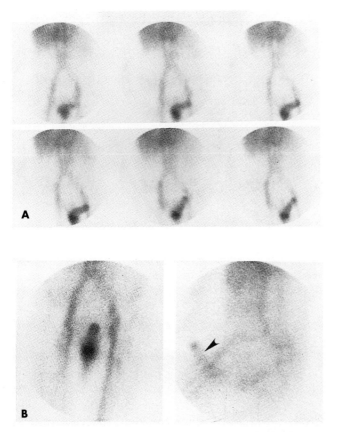

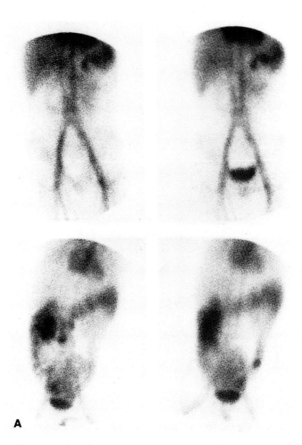

Fig. 10-21 False positive GI bleeding study. **A,** Images acquired every 10 minutes over about 1 hour show changing, increasing activity in the lower left and middle pelvis. **B,** Anterior (*left*) and left lateral (*right*) images acquired 90 minutes after tracer injection show the activity to be the penile blood pool. Not recognizing a potentially false positive study can be an embarrassing and serious error. Left lateral views should be obtained whenever pelvic activity is seen to separate out rectal, bladder, and penile activity.

but the results still seem convincing: the major advantage of Tc-99m RBC scintigraphy is the ability to image over a prolonged period of time. However, Tc-99m-labeled RBCs studies have the potential for false positive results because of (1) misinterpretation of normal variations, or pitfalls (Box 10-12), (2) free Tc-99m pertechnetate, or (3) misinterpretation of delayed images. Tc-99m SC still has a role to play. For example, in a patient who is actively bleeding and clinically unstable, the Tc-99m SC study will likely be positive and the 20-minute study can be promptly performed and completed prior to angiography. A labeled RBC study requires that much time just to label the patient's blood, and 60 additional minutes for imaging.

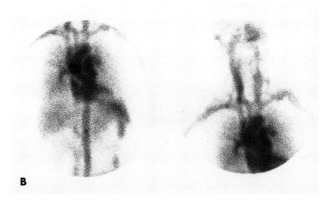

Fig. 10-22 Hemorrhagic gastritis vs. free Tc-99m pertechnetate. Hemorrhagic gastritis may occasionally be diagnosed with a labeled RBC study; however, evidence of free pertechnetate should be vigorously sought. **A,** Images obtained at 10, 20, 60, and 90 minutes show prominent gastric uptake at 10 and 20 minutes; however, on the later images, there is no longer gastric activity and the activity has passed to the colon. **B,** Images of the neck show no thyroid or salivary activity, which rules against free pertechnetate. Endoscopy confirmed hemorrhagic gastritis.

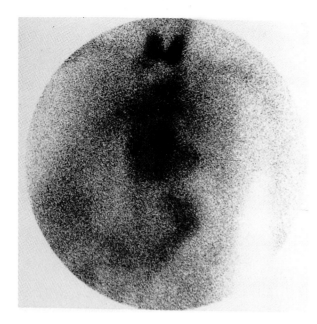

Fig. 10-23 Free Tc-99m pertechnetate. In contrast to Figure 10-22 there is gastric and thyroid uptake and a poor target-to-background ratio.

Table 10-5   Dosimetry for In-vitro Tc-99m-Labeled RBCs

Target	rads/mCi	rads/25 mCi (cGy/925 MBq)
Heart wall	0.054	1.4
Bladder wall	0.051	1.3
Spleen	0.041	1.0
Lungs	0.041	1.0
Blood	0.035	0.9
Liver	0.026	0.7
Kidneys	0.025	0.7
Red marrow	0.019	0.5
Ovaries	0.017	0.5
Testes	0.007	0.2

The calculations are based on a 2.4-hour voiding schedule.

Modified from Atkins HL, Thomas SR, Buddemeyer U, and Chervu LR: MIRD dose estimate report no. 14: Radiation absorbed dose from technetium-99m labeled RBCs, *J Nucl Med* 31:378-380, 1990.

ECTOPIC GASTRIC MUCOSA

Ectopic gastric mucosa is found most commonly in a *Meckel's diverticulum* but may be associated with a *duplication of the GI tract* and *Barrett's esophagus.* After partial gastrectomy for peptic ulcer disease, a *retained gastric antrum* with gastric mucosa may inadvertently be left behind. In all these clinical situations, acid and pepsin secretion from the gastric mucosa may produce ulceration of adjacent tissue and result in serious complications. Tc-99m pertecthnetate scintigraphy has been sucessfully used to help make these diagnoses.

Mechanism of Uptake

Normal mucosa of the gastric fundus contains *parietal cells,* which secrete hydrochloric acid and intrinsic

Table 10-4   Dosimetry for Tc-99m Sulfur Colloid

Target	rads/mCi	rads/10 mCi (cGy/370 MBq)
Spleen	0.210	2.100
Liver	0.340	3.400
Red marrow	0.027	0.270
Ovaries	0.006	0.060
Testes	0.001	0.010
Whole body	0.019	0.190

Modified from Atkins HL, Cloutier RJ, Lathrop KA et al: Report No. 3, Technetium-99m-SC in various liver conditions. In MIRD primer for absorbed dose calculations, New York, 1988, Society of Nuclear Medicine.

Table 10-6   Comparison of Tc-99m SC and Tc-99m RBC Scintigraphy for Gastrointestinal Bleeding

	Tc-99m SC	Tc-99m RBCs
Administered dose	10 mCi (may be repeated)	25 mCi
Dosimetry		
Whole body	0.2 rads	0.3 rads
Target organ	3.6 rads (liver)	1.2 rads (heart)
Minimal bleeding detectable	0.1 mL/min	0.05 - 0.4 mL/min
Labeling	Commercial kit	Commercial kit
Imaging duration	20-30 min; repeat study if needed	60-90 min, then 30-min acquisition 2 and 4 hr later and up to 24 hr later, as needed
Advantages	Short imaging time; high target-to-background ratio	Repeat imaging up to 24 hr
Disadvantages	Difficulty detecting hepatic and splenic flexure bleeding: only detects bleeding over short time period	False positive studies due to excretion of free Tc-99m

factor, and *chief cells,* which secrete pepsinogen. The antrum and pylorus contain *G-cells,* which secrete the hormone gastrin. Columnar *mucin-secreting epithelials cells* are found throughout the stomach. Gastric secretions in both normal and ectopic gastric mucosa are stimulated by neural and hormonal mechanisms in response to the ingestion of food, which increase the volume and acidity of gastric secretions over the basal fasting state. The presence or absence of symptoms, the clinical presentation (e.g., bleeding vs. obstruction), and the ability of Tc-99m pertechnetate to image ectopic gastric mucosa are all dependent on gastric mucosal cell types present.

It has been assumed that the parietal cells are responsible for gastric mucosal uptake and secretion. The technetium ion, in the same periodic table group as chloride (see Appendix), might be expected to compete with chloride in the formation of acid by the parietal cell. Although there is some experimental evidence to support this hypothesis, the predominance of evidence lies with the mucin-secreting cells. These cells excrete an alkaline juice that protects the mucosa from the highly acidic gastric fluid. Tc-99m pertechnetate uptake has been found in gastric tissue with no parietal cells, such as pernicious anemia, retained gastric antrum, and some cases of Barrett's esophagus. Animal studies confirm this, and several autoradiographic studies localize Tc-99m pertechnetate uptake to the mucin cell rather than the parietal cell.

A hypothesis explaining the conflicting data suggests that the predominant mechanism is specific mucin cell uptake and secretion which is suppressible by perchlorate in a manner similar to iodide, while parietal cell uptake is a minor factor, non-specific, secondary, and, like chloride uptake, not suppressed by perchlorate.

Box 10-13 Epidemiology of Meckel's Diverticulum

1%-3% incidence in the general population.
50% or more occur by age 2 yr.
10%-30% have ectopic gastric mucosa.
25%-40% are symptomatic; 50%-67% of these have ectopic gastric mucosa.
>95% of those that bleed have gastric mucosa.

Dosimetry

The target organ for Tc-99m pertechnetate is the stomach, followed by the thyroid (Table 10-7).

Clinical Indications

Meckel's diverticulum Meckel's diverticulum is the most common congenital anomaly of the GI tract, occurring in 1% to 3% of of the population. It results from failure of closure of the omphalomesenteric duct of the embryo. (The omphalomesenteric duct connects the yolk sac to the primitive foregut via the umbilical cord.) This true diverticulum arises on the antimesenteric side of the small bowel, usually 80 to 90 cm proximal to the ileocecal valve. It is usually only 2 to 3 cm in size but may be considerably larger. Gastric mucosa is present in 10% to 30% of all cases, in approximately 60% of symptomatic patients, and, importantly, in 98% of those with bleeding (Box 10-13).

Clinical manifestations Gastric mucosa is responsible for most symptoms of Meckel's diverticulum. Gastric secretions may cause peptic ulceraton of the diverticulum itself or adjacent ileum, resulting in pain, bleeding, or perforation. Sixty percent of all patients seen with complications of Meckel's diverticulum are under the age of 2, and bleeding accounts for the majority of cases.

Other manifestations of Meckel's diverticulum seen most commonly in adults include intussusception, obstruction, infection, and abnormal fixation of the diverticulum. Bleeding from Meckel's diverticulum after age 40 is unusual.

Diagnosis The preoperative diagnosis of Meckel's diverticulum was quite difficult prior to scintigraphy. It is often not identified on small bowel follow-through films because the diverticulum may have a narrow or stenotic ostium; they are often not well filled and have rapid emptying. Small bowel enteroclysis is a better method for detection because the higher pressure of the barium column more reliably fills the diverticulum. Angiography is useful only if there is brisk active bleeding, and is rarely used. Tc-99m pertechnetate scintigra-

---

Table 10-7 Radiation Absorbed Dose for Tc-99m pertechnetate

Target Organ	Absorbed Dose	
	rads/mCi	rads/5 mCi
Bladder wall	0.053	0.265
Stomach wall	0.250	1.250
Large intestine wall	0.068	0.340
Ovaries	0.022	0.110
Red marrow	0.019	0.095
Testes	0.009	0.045
Thyroid	0.130	0.650
Total body	0.014	0.070

From MIRD dose estimate report no. 8. Summary of current radiation dose estimates to normal humans from 99mTc as sodium pertechnetate, *J Nucl Med* 17:74-77, 1976.

Box 10-14   Radionuclide Scintigraphy for Meckel's Diverticulum: Protocol Summary

PATIENT PREPARATION

4-6 hr fasting prior to study to reduce size of stomach.
No pretreatment with perchlorate, but it may be given after completion of the study.
No barium studies should be performed within 3-4 days of scintigraphy.
Void prior to study, during if possible, and after.

PREMEDICATION

None, or:
Pentagastrin: 6 µg/kg SC 5-15 min before study
Cimetidine: 20 mg/kg PO for 2 days prior to study
Glucagon: 50 µg/kg IV 10 min before study

RADIOPHARMACEUTICAL

Tc-99m pertechnetate
   Children: 30-100 µCi/kg
   Adults: 5-10 mCi IV

IMAGING PROCEDURE

Large field of view gamma camera with low-energy all-purpose or high-resolution collimator interfaced with computer.
Place patient supine under camera with xiphoid to symphysis pubis in field of view.
For flow images, acquire 60 1-sec frames. For static images, acquire 500k counts for first image, others for same
   time every 5-10 min for 1 hr.
Erect, right lateral, posterior, or oblique views may be helpful at 30-60 min.
Obtain Postvoid image.

---

phy (Meckel's scan) is considered the standard method for making the initial diagnosis of Meckel's diverticulum.

Methodology Attention to patient preparation is important. A full stomach or urinary bladder may obscure an adjacent Meckel's diverticulum. Therefore, fasting for 3 to 4 hours prior to the study or continuous nasogastric aspiration to decrease the size of the stomach is recommended. Voiding prior, during, and at the end of the study is also important. Perchlorate is not used prior to scintigraphy because it may block uptake of Tc-99m pertechnetate by the gastric mucosa; however, it may be administered after the study to wash out the radiotracer from the thyroid, minimizing radiation exposure.

Barium studies should not be performed for several days before scintigraphy because attenuation by the contrast material may prevent lesion detection. Procedures (proctoscopy) or drugs (laxatives) that irritate the intestinal mucosa and result in nonspecific Tc-99m pertechnetate uptake should be avoided. Certain drugs (e.g., ethosuximide [Zarontin]) may also cause unpredictable uptake. A typical imaging protocol is described in Box 10-14.

Pharmacologic augmentation Various pharmacologic maneuvers have been reported to improve the detection of Meckel's diverticulum, including the use of *pentagastrin, glucagon,* and *cimetidine.* Although some

authors recommend routine premedication with one or a combination of these drugs, we reserve their use for situations in which an initial false negative study is suspected. No large series has evaluated their relative effectiveness.

Pretreatment with *pentagastrin* experimentally increases the rapidity, duration, and intensity of Tc-99m pertechnetate uptake; in one case, an initially false negative scan was converted to positive with use of the drug. The mechanism is uncertain but may be the result of increased acid production, leading to increased activity of the mucin-producing cells and increased tracer uptake. However, pentagastrin also increases intestinal motility, leading to rapid movement into the small bowel. The antiperistaltic effect of *glucagon* has been used to prevent washout of the tracer from the stomach and from Meckel's diverticulum. One study reported optimal visualization of Meckel's diverticulum with the use of a combination of pentagastrin and glucagon.

The use of *cimetidine*, a histamine antagonist, has also been reported to improve the detection of ectopic gastric mucosa. The more intense and prolonged uptake of Tc-99m pertechnetate by gastric mucosa is thought to be due to inhibition of its release from the gastric mucosa. Although no controlled studies have been performed, some investigators recommend its routine use because it does not have significant risks or side effects.

Image interpretation   Meckel's diverticulum appears scintigraphically as a focal area of increased intraperitoneal activity, usually in the right lower quadrant, although it may be seen anywhere within the abdomen (Figure 10-24). Increased activity is usually first seen 5 to 10 minutes after tracer injection, and activity increases over time as gastric uptake increases.

Lateral or oblique views are sometimes helpful in confirming the anterior position of the diverticulum. Lateral and posterior images can help confirm renal or ureteral origin of activity. Upright views can help distinguish fixed activity (e.g., duodenum) from ectopic gastric mucosa, which moves inferiorly in response to the altered position; it also serves to empty renal pelvis activity. The intensity of activity within the lesion may sometimes fluctuate due to intestinal secretions, hemorrhage, or increased intestinal motility that carries the radiotracer away. Postvoiding images are suggested to help empty collecting system activity and better see uptake adjacent to the bladder.

Diagnostic accuracy   False negative studies may occur due to poor technique, washout of the secreted Tc-99m pertechnetate, or the lack of sufficient gastric mucosa. Experimentally, an area smaller than 2 cm^2 cannot be detected scintigraphically. Meckel's diverticulum with impaired blood supply due to intussusception, volvulus, or infaction may also result in a false negative study.

A variety of causes of false positive studies have been reported (Box 10-15). Normal structures can be confused with ectopic gastric mucosa if careful technique is not followed. False positives are often the result of inflammatory or obstructive lesions. Lesions with increased blood pool, such as arteriovenous malformations and tumors, may be seen on flow and blood pool imaging but do not take up Tc-99m pertechnetate; therefore, they are seen early and then fade.

The reported accuracy of scintigraphy in the detection of Meckel's diverticulum has varied considerably and seems to depend in part on the referral population studied (children or adults), the presenting symptom (rectal bleeding or abdominal pain), and the technology used (rectilinear scanners or modern-day gamma cameras). One report, summarizing the results in 954 patients—mostly children—who had undergone scintigraphy for suspected Meckel's diverticulum performed using mod-

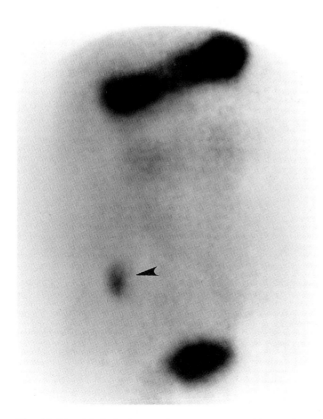

Fig. 10-24   Meckel's diverticulum in an 8-year-old boy with rectal bleeding. Focal uptake in right lower quadrant is Meckel's diverticulum (*arrowhead*). Above is the stomach and below, bladder activity. Over the first 30 minutes the gastric activity and RLQ activity increased simultaneously. The diagnosis was confirmed at surgery.

Box 10-15   Causes of False Positive Scintigraphy in Meckel's Diverticulum and Their Mechanism

Urinary tract	Hyperemia and inflammatory
Ectopic kidney	Peptic ulcer
Extrarenal pelvis	Crohn's disease
Hydronephrosis	Ulcerative colitis
Vesicoureteral reflux	Abscess
Horseshoe kidney	Appendicitis
Bladder diverticulum	Colitis
Vascular	Neoplasm
Arteriovenous	Carcinoma of sigmoid colon
malformation	Carcinoid
Hemangioma	Lymphoma
Aneurysm of intra-	Leiomyosarcoma
abdominal vessel	Small bowel obstruction
Angiodysplasia	Intussusception
Other areas of ectopic	Volvulus
gastric mucosa	
Gastrogenic cyst	
Enteric duplication	
Duplication cysts	
Barrett's esophagus	
Retained gastric antrum	
Pancreas	
Duodenum	
Colon	

ern imaging methods, found an overall sensitivity of 85% and a specificity of 95%.

Experience in differentiating nonspecific accumulation of pertechnetate from true ectopic gastric mucosa makes this high specificity possible. Earlier studies, often using rectilinear scanners, noted sensitivities and specificities in the range of 78%. Scintigraphy for Meckel's diverticulum in adults appears to have a poorer sensitivity than in children; one series reported a sensitivity of only 63%. There were ten false positive studies, although seven of the subjects had surgically treatable disease. The lower sensitivity may be related to the lack of gastric mucosa in the adult diverticula.

Gastrointestinal duplications Duplications are cystic or tubular lesions of congenital origin that are composed of GI muscular walls with mucosal linings. Fifty percent occur in the small bowel, most in the ileum and 20% in the mediastinum. Although most are symptomatic by the age of 2 years, some remain asymptomatic into adulthood. The presenting symptoms are similar to those of Meckel's diverticulum because 30% to 50% have gastric mucosa.

The diagnosis is usually made at surgery. Occasionally a preoperative diagnosis may be made following barium radiography or US. Scintigraphy has occasionally been reported to be helpful—for example, mediastinal GI cysts have been diagnosed with Tc-99m pertechnetate scintigraphy. Duplications often appear as large, sometimes multilobulated areas of increased activity.

Retained gastric antrum The gastric antrum may occasionally be left behind in the afferent loop after a Billroth II gastrojejunostomy for peptic ulcer disease. The antrum continues to produce gastrin, which is no longer inhibited by acid in the stomach because it has been diverted through the gastrojejunostomy. The resulting high acid production often leads to marginal ulcers. Other causes of recurrent ulcers after a partial gastrectomy include an incomplete vagotomy and the Zollinger-Ellison syndrome. In the latter, a pancreatic tumor causes continued production of gastrin. The clinical diagnosis is usually based on the response of serum gastrin to IV calcium or secretin infusions.

Endoscopy or barium radiography can often demonstrate the retained gastric antrum. However, Tc-99m pertechnetate scintigraphy can be confirmatory. The protocol used is similar to that for imaging Meckel's diverticulum. Uptake in the gastric remnant occurs simultaneously with gastric uptake and is seen as a collar of radioactivity in the area of the duodenal stump of the afferent loop. The retained antrum usually lies to the right of the gastric remnant. In one reported series, Tc-99m pertechnetate uptake was demonstrated in 16 of 22 patients with a retained antrum .

Barrett's esophagus Barrett's esophagus is a condition in which the distal esophagus becomes lined by columnar epithelium rather than the usual esophageal squamous epithelium. It is generally thought to be secondary to chronic GER and is associated with ulcers, high strictures, and an 8.5% incidence of esophageal adenocarcinoma.

Although Tc-99m pertechnetate scanning first demonstrated Barrett's esophagus in 1973, the diagnosis is now usually made with endoscopy and mucosal biopsy. Scintigraphy should be performed with the patient erect to minimize GER. LAO views may be helpful. Although the normal esophagus ends at the esophagogastric junction, a positive scan shows intrathoracic uptake contiguous with the stomach but conforming to the shape and posterior location of the esophagus. A potential problem is differentiating Barrett's esophagus from a simple hiatal hernia. To avoid problems, the scan should be interpreted in conjunction with an upper GI series. False negative results have been reported, and the scan does not replace endoscopic biopsy. At best it is a complementary or confirmatory procedure.

MALABSORPTION AND INTESTINAL TRANSIT

Protein-Losing Enteropathy

Excessive protein loss through the GI tract has been assocated with a variety of GI and non-GI diseases, including intestinal lymphangectasia, Crohn's disease, Menetrier's disease, amyloidosis, and intestinal fistula. The resulting hypoproteinemia can be a serious clinical problem.

α_1-Antitrypsin α_1-Antitrypsin is an endogenously produced macromolecule that has been used as a fecal marker of malabsorption. It has been found to be as accurate and reproducible as Cr-51-labeled albumin, the generally accepted reference standard. However, because daily stool collection for 48 to 72 hours and fecal quantitation are required for both, they have not been well accepted by the patient or laboratory personnel.

Radionuclide imaging Two radiopharmaceuticals have been used to make this diagnosis scintigraphically, Tc-99m human serum albumin (Tc-99m HSA) and In-111 transferrin. Tc-99m-labeled HSA was first used for qualitative assessment of protein loss. Serial abdominal images acquired for 30 minutes after IV injection reveal radiotracer collection in the small bowel that increases in amount over 24 hours (Figure 10-25). When injected IV, In-111 chloride binds in vivo to serum proteins, most notably transferrin, and abdominal imaging can be used to visualize the protein leak. However, better binding and imaging may be obtained with in vitro labeling.

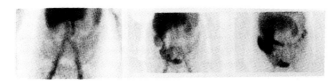

Fig. 10-25 Protein-losing enteropathy. The patient received Tc-99m HSA IV. Immediate, 1-hour and 2-hour images (*left to right*). Note the increasing activity seen in the small bowel initially (*middle*) and subsequent transit to the colon (*right*). The cause of this patient's GI protein loss was uncertain.

Table 10-8	Clinical Breath Analysis Tests	
Clinical Application	**Substrate**	**Metabolic End Product Measured**
Bacterial overgrowth	^{14}C-glycocholate	$^{14}CO_2$
	^{14}C-xylose	$^{14}CO_2$
	glycose	H_2
Ileal dysfunction	^{14}C-glycocholate	$^{14}CO_2$
Steatorrhea	^{14}C-triolein	$^{14}CO_2$
Lactase deficiency	^{14}C-lactose	$^{14}CO_2$
	lactose	H_2
Small Bowel Transit Time	^{14}C-lactulose	$^{14}CO_2$
	lactulose	H_2

Malabsorption of Fat and Carbohydrates

Radioactive breath analysis tests A variety of radiolabeled breath analysis techniques have been used over the years to diagnose malabsorption of fat and carbohydrates. Because the terminal step of oxidative metabolism of carboydrates, lipids, and other organic substrates always results in the production of CO_2 and H_2O, the rate-limiting step in the production of these metabolic end products after oral administration is intestinal absorption. Thus, breath $^{14}CO_2$ analysis after oral administration of a ^{14}C-labeled compound provides information about the amount and rate of absorption of that compound. For example, if a labeled fat is administered and less than normal amount of $^{14}CO_2$ is collected, then some defect in intestinal fat absorption must be present. If, on the other hand, the compound is not absorbed but metabolized by intestinal bacteria, the measurement of $^{14}CO_2$ output after oral administration of the compound may provide information to suggest that the compound is exposed to excessive numbers of intestinal bacteria.

This same scheme is the basis for the use of ^{14}C-bile acid and ^{14}C-xylose administration. Increased amounts of $^{14}CO_2$ are produced when metabolism of these compounds occurs in the small bowel because of the presence of bacterial overgrowth, because small bowel dysfunction results in malabsorption of the bile acids or xylose, allowing these compounds to appear in the colon where metabolism by normal colonic bacteria occurs. Most of the clinically validated breath analysis tests are listed in Table 10-8.

Intestinal Transit

Small and large intestinal transit scintigraphy is relatively new and optimal methods are still being developed. Unique technical problems exist. The radiolabeled meal must be able to withstand the acid environment of the stomach and the alkaline milieu of the small bowel. Quantitation is more problematic than for gastric emptying since the input into the intestine is not a single food bolus, but rather a protracted infusion from the stomach, with no single time zero. In quantitation of gastric emptying, all the radiolabled meal resides in the stomach at the beginning of the study; quantitation depends only on the rate of clearance. Although this is an area of increasing interest, most of the work to date is investigational, and its clinical role is yet to be defined. Therefore, only a brief overview will be presented.

Nonscintigraphic diagnostic methods The transit of barium through the *small bowel* during a routine barium follow-through study is qualitative, not quantitative. Mixing barium with food and plotting its movement on a monitor using image intensification provides an index of the transit rate through the small bowel into the colon, but radiation dosimetry is relatively high and the meal is nonphysiologic.

The hydrogen breath analysis test measures hydrogen produced when a carbohydrate (^{14}C lactose) is fermented by colonic bacteria. It measures the transit time of the leading edge of the meal from the mouth to the cecum and is not an index of the transit of the bulk of the meal. It has other limitations: the lactose itself alters transit, the transit time is affected by the gastric emptying rate, and the test requires fermentative bacterial in the colon, which may be absent in one fourth of the population. Various radiographic methods have been used for studing *large bowel transit,* including cineradiography, fluoroscopy to estimate transit times, and the use of radiopaque plastic cuttings. All give relatively large radiation doses to the patient and are not physiologic.

Radionuclide scintigraphy: radiopharmaceuticals and meals *Small bowel* Radiomarkers such as Tc-99m SC or Tc-99m DTPA in water or mixed with a semisolid meal have been used because of their simplicity; however, study of the semisolid phase of the intestinal contents is more complex. Accurate measurement requires a stable, nondigestible meal. Fiber is the only normal dietary constituent that is unaffected by gastric antral grinding and progresses along the small intestine in solid form without hydrolytic ingestion. Labeled with I-131, it is stable in acid and alkaline environments, but synthesis is laborious and the dosimetry relatively high. Other radiopharmaceuticals include Tc-99m-labeled cellulose fiber, In-111-labeled plastic paricles, and In-111-labeled resin pellets. Various quantitative methods have been used.

Large intestine   For most accurate results and to minimize the length of the study, direct placement of the radiotracer via intubation at the site of interest (proximal small bowel for small bowel transit studies or distal small bowel or cecum for colonic studies) is optimal. Tc-99m DTPA has been used. I-131 fiber cellulose and In-111 DTPA encapsulated in nondigestible capsules have also been used. Cecal or jejunal instillation ensures a clear starting time. Oral ingestion would require a prolonged imaging time. However, intubation methods are not practical for routine clinical performance because they are invasive, technically demanding, and unpleasant for the patient.

An interesting alternative approach is the use of In-111 polystyrene cation exchange resin pellets. They are placed in a gelatin capsule coated with a pH-sensitive polymer that is resistant to disruption at the levels of pH found in the stomach and proximal small bowel but will disrupt at the ileocecal valve due to the increasing pH. A large field of view camera is used for imaging. The frequency and the duration of image acquisition depend on the methodology, the length of the study, and the information needed. Different quantitative methods have been used.

Clinical results   Considerable normal variation in small bowel transit times exists. Generally groups with diarrhea tend to have rapid mean transit times whereas patients with constipation have longer transit times, although there is considerable overlap with normal values. More data are needed.

SUGGESTED READINGS

Datz FL: Considerations for accurately measuring gastric emptying, *J Nucl Med* 32:881–884, 1991.

Fahey FH, Ziessman HA, Collin MJ, and Eggli DF: Left anterior oblique projection and peak-to-scatter ratio for attenuation compensation of gastric emptying studies, *J Nucl Med* 30:233–239, 1989.

Heyman S: Pediatric Nuclear Gastroenterology: Evaluation of gastroesophageal reflux and gastrointestinal bleeding. In Freeman LM and Weissman HS, editors: *Nuclear Medicine Annual 1985*, New York, 1985, Raven Press.

Klein HA and Wald A: Esophageal Transit Scintigraphy. In *Nuclear Medicine Annual 1988*, pp 79–124, New York, 1985, Raven Press.

Malmud LS, Vitti RA, and Fisher RS: Gastroesophageal Reflux. In Freeman LM, editor: *Freeman and Johnson's Clinical Radionuclide Imaging*, Vol III, pp 1669–1693, 1986, Grune & Stratton, Inc.

Sfakianakis GN and Haase GM: Abdominal scintigraphy for ectopic gastric mucosa: a retrospective analysis of 143 studies, *AJR* 138:7–12, 1982.

Vitti RA, Malmud LS, and Fisher RS: Gastric emptying. In Freeman LM, editor: *Freeman and Johnson's Clinical Radionuclide Imaging*, Vol III, pp 1694–1728, 1986, Grune & Stratton, Inc.

Winzelberg GG: Radionuclide evaluation of gastrointestinal bleeding. In Freeman LM, editor: *Freeman and Johnson's Clinical Radionuclide Imaging*, Vol III, pp 1729–1775, 1986, Grune & Stratton, Inc.

Ziessman HA: Gastrointestinal Scintigraphy: Esophagus and Stomach. In Neumann R, Harbert J, and Eckelman W, editors: *National Institutes of Health Series in Nuclear Medicine*, New York, 1995, Thieme Medical Publishers, Inc.

CHAPTER 11

Central Nervous System

Brain scintigraphy has always played an important part in the practice of nuclear medicine. Until the advent of computed tomography (CT) in the 1970s radionuclide brain scintigraphy was the only noninvasive brain imaging method available and represented a large portion of the practice of clinical nuclear medicine. In current practice, magnetic resonance imaging (MRI) and CT play preeminent roles in clinical brain imaging, producing superb anatomic images of the central nervous system (CNS). The role of nuclear medicine imaging has been redefined as *functional* brain imaging. Positron emission tomography (PET), using both blood flow and metabolic agents (F-18 FDG), produces images of physiologic and biochemical processes in the brain that have both important research and clinical impact. The success of PET in this area led to the development of new single photon radiopharmaceuticals (Box 11-1) that, together with vastly improved dedicated SPECT instrumentation, have resulted in a revival of nuclear medicine brain scintigraphy.

Box 11-1   Radiopharmaceuticals for Single Photon Brain Scintigraphy

CONVENTIONAL BRAIN SCINTIGRAPHY

Tc-99m Pertechnetate
Tc-99m Glucoheptonate
Tc-99m DTPA

BRAIN PERFUSION SCINTIGRAPHY

I-123 Iodoamphetamine
Tc-99m HMPAO
Tc-99m ECD

BRAIN TUMOR IMAGING

Thallium-201
Tc-99m Sestamibi

CISTERNOGRAPHY

Yterbium-169
In-111 DTPA

BLOOD POOL IMAGING

Tc-99m RBCs

CONVENTIONAL BRAIN SCINTIGRAPHY WITH BLOOD-BRAIN BARRIER AGENTS

Brain imaging using radiopharmaceuticals that distribute within the extracellular space and do not enter brain tissue unless there is a break in the blood-brain barrier was successfully used in the late 1960s and early 1970s to noninvasively diagnose intracerebral diseases of cerebrovascular, traumatic, inflammatory, infectious, and neoplastic origin. Because the role for this technique today is substantially more limited, it will be discussed briefly, with an emphasis on current indications.

Radiopharmaceuticals

The blood-brain barrier is both an anatomic and a physiologic barrier that prevents most substances in the blood from entering the CNS. Selective movement of substances across this barrier for the most part occurs by active transport. Diseases of the brain cause a breakdown in the blood-brain barrier, allowing uptake of conventional brain imaging agents.

Three Tc-99m-labeled radiopharmaceuticals have been used for conventional brain scintigraphy. Tc-99m pertechnetate was the first. Although inexpensive and readily available, it results in prolonged blood pool activity and is concentrated in the salivary glands and choroid plexus. Although this uptake can be prevented by prior ingestion of sodium or potassium perchlorate, the technetium chelates of DTPA and glucoheptonate (GH) are associated with faster clearance from the blood, no salivary or choroid plexus uptake, a higher target-to-background ratio, better lesion detection, and a lower radiation dose to the patient.

Both Tc-99m DTPA and Tc-99m GH distribute throughout the extracellular space. Because of their hydrophilic character they penetrate the blood-brain barrier only when it is disrupted, then diffuse into the altered tissue and bind by uncertain mechanisms. Tc-99m GH has been preferred by some because of its better uptake in tumors, which may be due to the fact that it is a glucose analogue and serves as a substrate for tumor metabolism. Prior administration of corticosteroids may diminish uptake on brain scintigraphy owing to the effect of corticosteroids on blood-brain barrier permeability.

Dosimetry

For dosimetry of Tc-99m DTPA and Tc-99m glucoheptonate, see Chapter 12 on the Genitourinary System.

Methodology

Box 11-2 describes a typical protocol. Dynamic flow images are routinely acquired. Certain vascular lesions, such as early stroke, carotid occlusion, and arteriovenous malformations, may be better seen on the flow phase, and the findings on dynamic imaging can help in the differential diagnosis of lesions seen on later static images. Immediate high count blood pool images can sometimes be helpful for the diagnosis of vascular malformations or venous sinus occclusions or for confirming a hypervascular abnormality noted on an initial dynamic flow study. Normally the anterior view is used for the flow phase, although the posterior projection may be preferable in children and in patients with cerebellar, occipital, or posterior parietal symptoms and signs. Delayed static planar images are acquired in multiple views 1.5 to 2.0 hours after tracer injection. SPECT can be helpful in selected cases and is routinely performed in some laboratories.

Image Interpretation

The conventional nuclear medicine brain scan does not really image the brain, because the radiotracer enters the brain only where there is a pathologic break in the blood-brain barrier. In the normal scan (Figure 11-1), the peripheral activity corresponds to the outer scalp and inner meninges. The normal cerebral cortex is devoid of activity.

Venous structures define most of the anatomic re-

Box 11-2   Conventional Blood-Brain Barrier Scintigraphy: Protocol Summary

PATIENT PREPARATION

None.

RADIOPHARMACEUTICAL

Tc-99m GH or Tc-99m DTPA, 20 mCi.

INSTRUMENTATION

Camera setup: Large field of view gamma camera. High-resolution, low-energy collimator. 140 keV photopeak
    with 15% window.
Camera formatter setup: 2-3 sec flow images × 30, then immediate and delayed static images in multiple views.
Computer setup: 1-sec flow images x 60 (64 × 64 byte mode), then static images (128 × 128 frame mode).

IMAGING PROCEDURE

1. Inject radiopharmaceutical as an IV bolus.
2. Acquire dynamic flow study.
3. (Optional) *Immediate* 750k static images in the anterior, posterior, right and left lateral views.
4. Two hr after injection, acquire *delayed* 750k static images in same views.
    Vertex view if needed
SPECT (optional): Acquire similar to cerebral perfusion study (Table 11-4).

gions seen on the conventional brain scan. The cerebral veins include an external group of veins that course over the surface of the calvarium, and an internal group of veins from which the great vein of Galen drains the deep structures of the brain (Figure 11-2). All drain into the

sinuses of the dura mater and carry blood to the internal jugular vein.

An understanding of the normal arterial vascular distribution of the brain and associated perfusion patterns is needed for the accurate diagnosis of cerebrovascular

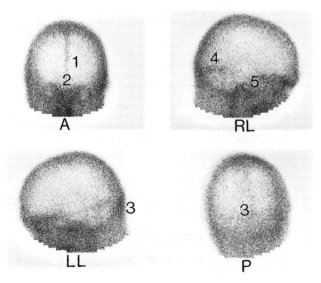

Fig. 11-1   Normal conventional brain scan in anterior (A), right lateral (*RL*), left lateral (*LL*), and posterior (*P*) projections. The cerebral hemispheres are surrounded by the peripheral activity of the scalp, bone, and the superficial cerebral vessels. The superior sagittal sinus (*1*) is seen in the anterior and posterior views. The floor of the frontal sinus (*2*) is the inferior border in the anterior view. The confluence of the sinuses, the torcular Herophili (*3*), is seen on the left lateral and posterior views. The transverse sinuses (*4*) are seen on the lateral views as well as the sphenoid sinus (*5*). Compare these images with the schematic diagram in Figure 11-2.

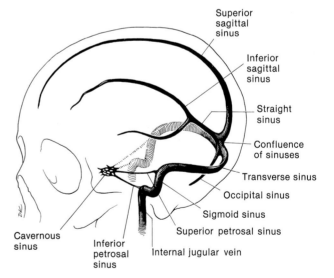

Fig. 11-2   Schematic diagram of normal cerebral venous anatomy. The superior sagittal sinus runs along the falx within the superior margin of the interhemispheric fissure. The inferior sagittal sinus is smaller and courses over the corpus callosum, joins with the great vein of Galen to form the straight sinus that drains into the superior sagittal sinus at the confluence of sinuses (torcular Herophili) at the occipital protuberance. The transverse sinuses drain the sagittal and occipital sinuses into the internal jugular vein.

A

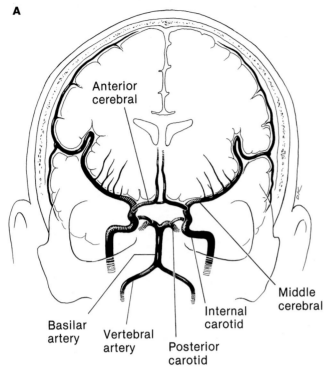

C

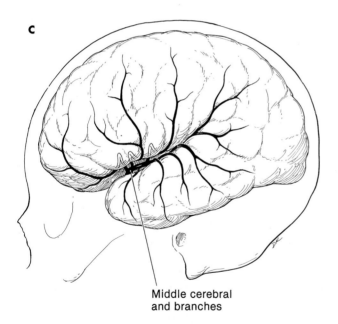

Middle cerebral
and branches

B

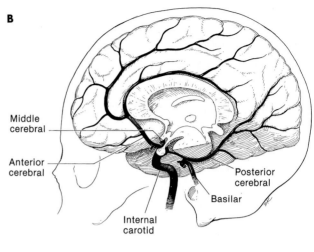

Fig. 11-3   Arterial anatomy. **A,** Coronal section showing circle of Willis and course of the middle and anterior cerebral arteries. The internal carotids divide at the base of the brain (circle of Willis) into the anterior and middle cerebral arteries. The middle cerebral artery runs laterally in the Sylvian fissure and then backward and upward on the surface of the insula, where it divides into branches distributed to the *lateral* surface of the cerebral hemisphere as well as to portions of the basal ganglia. **B,** Midline saggital view showing distribution of anterior, middle, and posterior cerebral arteries. The anterior cerebral artery supplies the cerebrum along its *medial* margin above the corpus callosum and extending posteriorly to the parietal fissure as well as to the anterior portion of the basal ganglia. The vertebral arteries fuse into the basilar artery, which branches at the circle of Willis into the two posterior cerebral arteries supplying the occipital lobe and the inferior half of the temporal lobe. **C,** Left lateral view showing distribution of the middle cerebral artery over the cerebral cortex.

disease (Figures 11-3A-C, 11-4). The brain is perfused by two internal carotid arteries and two vertebral arteries. The internal carotid arteries deliver blood to the majority of the cerebral cortex while the vertebral arteries supply the inferior portion of the cerebrum, cerebellum, and brain stem.

Clinical Applications

Trauma   The major application of neuroscintigraphy in trauma has been in cases of suspected subacute or chronic subdural hematomas. The radionuclide study has been found particularly helpful when CT is negative or equivocal during the isodense phase.

Dynamic flow images typically show peripherally decreased activity due to the hematoma's mass effect (Figure 11-5A). Delayed images show increased activity in the same distribution (crescent sign) (Figure 11-5B). Although characteristic, this finding is not specific and can be seen in peripherally located lesions of other causes, such as infarction, or scalp trauma. Radioactivity in the hematoma continues to increase with time; there-

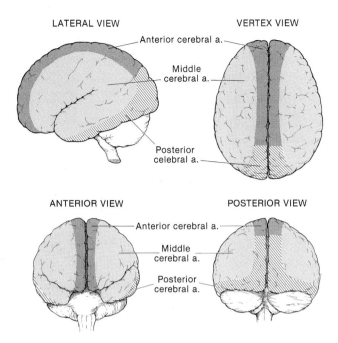

LATERAL VIEW   VERTEX VIEW

Anterior cerebral a.

Middle cerebral a.

Posterior celebral a.

ANTERIOR VIEW   POSTERIOR VIEW

Anterior cerebral a.

Middle cerebral a.

Posterior cerebral a.

Fig. 11-4 Regional cerebral cortex perfusion patterns of the anterior, middle, and posterior cerebral arteries.

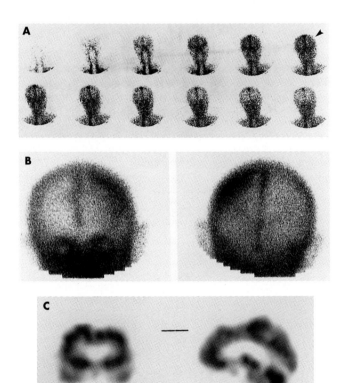

Fig. 11-5 Subdural hematoma. **A**, Radionuclide angiogram shows decreased perfusion of the left cerebral cortex peripherally (*arrowhead*). **B**, The 2-hour postinjection Tc-99m GH scan shows increased uptake at the periphery of the left cerebral cortex. **C**, In another patient, a Tc-99m HMPAO brain perfusion scan shows a peripheral perfusion defect due to a subdural hematoma.

fore, further delayed images can be helpful. The study is most sensitive for subacute or chronic subdural hematomas, since accumulation of tracer is related to the presence of a well-developed subdural membrane, which can take 10 days or more to form.

Inflammation and infection Radionuclide brain imaging is quite sensitive for demonstrating inflammatory lesions of the brain such as viral cerebritis and ventriculitis. Increased blood flow is characteristic. Ventriculitis typically shows a pattern of bilaterally increased lateral ventricle activity.

Intracerebral *abscess* appears as a focal area of increased radionuclide accumulation on delayed imaging. With disease progression, a "doughnut" pattern (hot lesion with cold center) may result. Although these findings may be seen with other benign and malignant CNS lesions, in the proper clinical setting the findings are strongly suggestive of infection.

The early diagnosis of *herpes encephalitis* is essential for effective treatment. Because brain biopsy is usually required to confirm the diagnosis, imaging localization is extremely important. Radionuclide imaging is more sensitive than CT for demonstrating encephalitis in its early phase. The combination of brain scintigraphy and CT has a higher sensitivity than either study alone. Increased flow and increased uptake within the temporal lobe are the usual findings in herpes encephalitis. The diagnosis can be made with Tc-99m DTPA or Tc-99m GH, or Tc-99m HMPAO (see discussion under Cerebral Perfusion Imaging) (Figure 11-6A-C). This is still an important modern-day indication.

Brain tumors The detectability of brain tumors depends on their size and location. Tumors less than 2 cm in size and those that are deep-seated, centrally located, or adjacent to areas of normally high activity (e.g., base of skull and vascular structures) may be missed. Tumor type also influences detectability. Meningioma and malignant gliomas are detected with high sensitivity, while pituitary and parasellar tumors, low-grade gliomas, and brain stem tumors are detected with relatively low sensitivity. Intermediate results are reported with posterior fossa tumors and acoustic neuromas.

The appearance on conventional brain scintigraphy is often not specific for malignancy; however, suggestive features include a spherical configuration, extension across vascular distributions, and a doughnut appearance (Figure 11-7). Blood flow is often increased. Increased uptake in the tumor is usually seen on immediate images and is definitely seen on 1- to 2-hour delayed imaging. Benign tumors may also be associated with increased flow and uptake. Although meningiomas have prominently increased arterial flow, this often fades during the venous phase. Interpretation following surgery may occasionally be complicated by uptake at the craniotomy site.

Although the pattern for *metastatic* brain tumor is

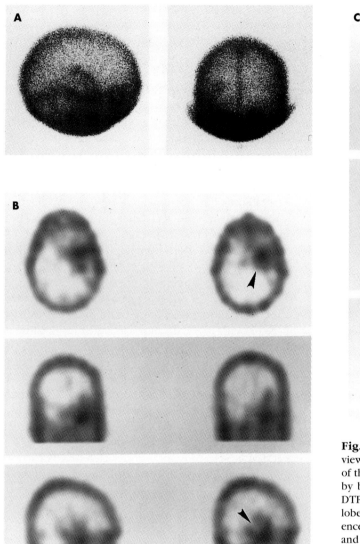

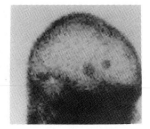

Fig. 11-6   Herpes encephalitis. **A**, Right lateral and anterior views of Tc-99m GH scan showing increased uptake in the region of the temporal parietal cortex. The abnormal uptake was proven by biopsy to be due to herpes encephalitis. **B**, SPECT Tc-99m DTPA brain scan showing increased uptake in the left temporal lobe (*arrowheads*) in another patient with biopsy-proven herpes encephalitis. Paired consecutive transverse (*top*), coronal (*middle*), and sagittal (*bottom*) sections. **C**, Similar cross-sectional SPECT slices using Tc-99m HMPAO (same patient as in **B**). Increased uptake is seen in the left temporal lobe (*arrowheads*).

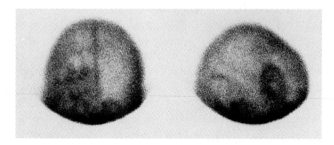

Fig. 11-7   Primary brain tumor—glioblastoma. Increased uptake on a Tc-99m GH brain scan is seen in the right frontal parietal region on both the anterior and right lateral views.

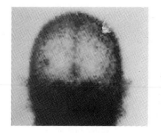

Fig. 11-8   Metastatic brain tumor. Several focal areas of increased uptake are seen on the anterior and right lateral views of this Tc-99m DTPA brain scan in a patient with lung cancer metastatic to the brain.

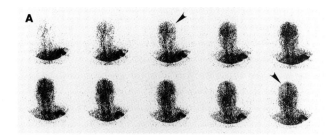

not specific, multiple lesions are typical (Figure 11-8). Infection and infarcts may be difficult to differentiate from tumor. Discrete rounded lesions that cross vascular boundaries are more likely to be tumor. Increased perfusion may be seen with vascular metastatic tumors (e.g., kidney or thyroid tumors or melanoma). CT and MRI are superior to brain scintigraphy for the demonstration of most intracranial tumors because of their superior anatomic resolution.

Cerebrovascular disease The radionuclide angiogram phase can be quite helpful in making the diagnosis of cerebrovascular disease, increasing the yield over static imaging alone. The characteristic "flip-flop" phenomenon consists of delayed cerebral blood flow and clearance compared to the opposite normal side (Figure 11-9A). This may be seen with a high-grade carotid artery stenosis with or without cerebral infarction. Flow abnormalities alone may be seen without uptake on delayed images acquired during the first days after a stroke.

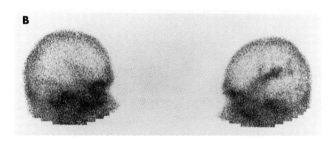

Occasionally, increased perfusion or "luxury perfusion," may be seen after a recent stroke. Luxury perfusion represents an uncoupling of blood flow from metabolism and oxygen demand (blood flow without metabolism) and may be seen by 5 days after an acute event.

Carotid and middle cerebral artery flow abnormalities are more easily detected than those of the vertebral-basilar or anterior cerebral arteries. Visual interpretation can be aided by the use of time-activity curves derived from computer-drawn regions of interest (ROIs) for both carotid arteries and the associated cerebral cortex.

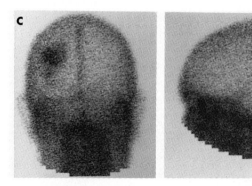

Following cerebral infarction, static images may be normal during the first week, become positive by 2 to 3 weeks, and return to normal by 2 to 3 months. Characteristic wedge-shaped patterns of increased uptake in the vascular distribution involved are typical of strokes (Figure 11-9B-D).

The sensitivity for stroke detection is in the 75% to 80% range. The spectrum of patterns seen on static images overlaps with that of tumor and infection, limiting the specificity of the study. Variations in the typical stroke pattern include central necrosis resulting in a doughnut appearance, associated hemorrhage producing a spherical abnormality crossing vascular distributions, occlusion of multiple branches, and watershed

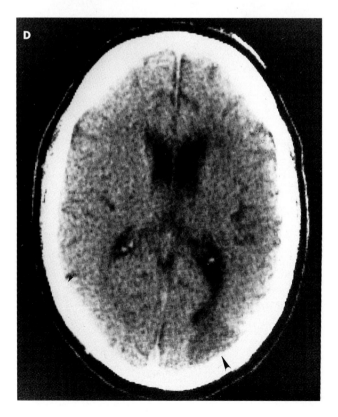

Fig. 11-9 Stroke. **A,** The radionuclide angiogram (ant. view) shows a "flip-flop" pattern. Decreased cerebral perfusion is noted on the left (*arrowhead*) compared to the right in the early arterial parenchymal phase (*arrowhead*); this pattern then reverses on later images showing delayed perfusion on the left, while the right has cleared (*arrowhead*). **B,** In a different patient presenting with right hemiparesis and stroke, there is uptake in the left parietal area in a vascular pattern is strongly suggestive of a left middle cerebral artery infarct. **C,** Tc-99m DTPA brain scan (posterior and left lateral views) showing uptake in the posterior parietal region in a patient with a recent CVA. **D,** The CT scan of the patient in C confirmed a stroke in that cortical region (*arrow*).

infarctions (cortical regions at the edge of two different vascular sources).

CT can demonstrate acute cerebral infarctions during the first week with better sensitivity and more specificity for distinguishing ischemic from hemorrhagic infarction. It is also better able to demonstrate intracerebral hematomas, tumors, and brain herniation and to estimate ventricular size. However, there is a 2- to 4-week period after an acute ischemic infarction when CT may be negative as the infarction evolves through an isodense phase. The radionuclide brain scan may be helpful at that time.

Bone radiotracers such as Tc-99m MDP may be taken up in cerebral infarctions, and this radiotracer may occasionally be helpful in the differential diagnosis of tumor versus infarct when the CT or MRI diagnosis is uncertain (Figure 11-10A-D).

Venous sinus thrombosis Although rapid dynamic flow and immediate static imaging with conventional brain scanning agents can be used to make this diagnosis, the use of Tc-99m-labeled RBCs is a superior method. The target-to-lesion ratio is higher, and static imaging alone is diagnostic. Imaging should be performed in mul-

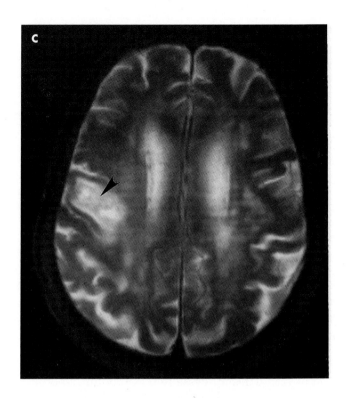

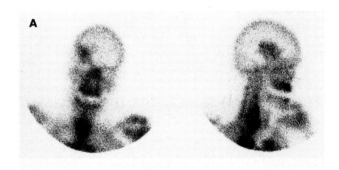

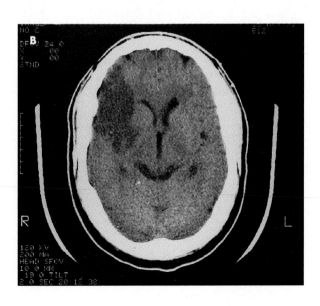

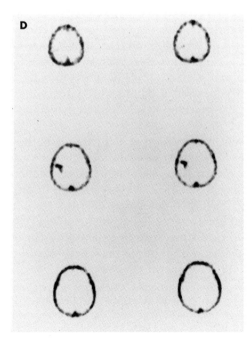

Fig. 11-10 Tc-99m MDP SPECT of brain tumor. **A**, The planar Tc-99m MDP bone scan shows intense uptake in the right parietal cortex. **B**, CT confirmed a CVA. **C**, In another patient, clinical evaluation and CT were uncertain as to the cause (stroke vs. tumor) of this patient's neurologic symptoms, hemiparesis, and right parietal lesion (*arrowhead*). **D**, Tc-99m MDP SPECT bone scan showing prominent uptake within the lesion, making the diagnosis of stroke likely.

tiple views for suspected sinus thrombosis. Good visualization of these sinuses excludes thrombosis. Normal asymmetry of the lateral sinuses occurs; however, an abrupt termination of the midportion (stump sign) is pathognomonic for thrombosis (Figure 11-11A,B).

Vascular malformations The diagnosis of arteriovenous malformation (AVM) can best be made during the dynamic flow phase. It is seen as a focal area of intense blush and rapid washout. The sensitivity for detection is high. Although the pattern is characteristic, hypervascular tumors occasionally look similar. Large AVMs may sometimes show persistence of peak activity throughout the venous phase. Because the blood-brain barrier is intact in uncomplicated AVM, static brain imaging will often be negative and therefore less sensitive than flow imaging. Immediate static images are more likely to be positive than delayed ones.

The diagnosis of cerebral venous angiomas may be confirmed with Tc-99m-labeled RBC imaging. Increased

uptake on delayed imaging is diagnostic. Post-therapy follow-up scintigraphy can be done to evaluate the effectiveness of treatment (Figure 11-12A, B).

Brain death The diagnosis of brain death is a clinical determination. The accuracy and promptness of this diagnosis are critical whenever organ donation transplantion is considered and for the efficacious use of expensive life support systems.

Specific criteria for brain death have been defined. The patient must be in deep coma with total absence of brain stem reflexes or spontaneous respiration. Potentially reversible causes must be excluded, such as drug intoxication, metabolic derangements, or hypothermia. The cause of the brain dysfunction must be diagnosed (trauma, stroke, etc.) and the clinical findings of brain death must be present for a defined period of observation (6-24 hours).

Confirmatory tests may be used to increase certainty, but the diagnosis is still primarily clinical. Electroencephalography (EEG) and radionuclide angiography evaluate cortical activity and function, not the brain stem. An isoelectric EEG by itself does not establish brain death and at least one repeat study is required. In the setting of intoxication with barbiturates and other depressive drugs, or hypothermia, the EEG may be flat even though there is still cerebral perfusion and recovery is possible.

Edema, softening, necrosis, and autolysis of brain tissue lead to increased intracranial pressure sufficient to overcome arterial pressure and prevent cerebral blood flow. Lack of blood flow to the brain is diagnostic of brain death. No filling on four-vessel arteriography is

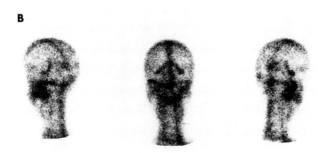

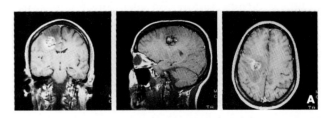

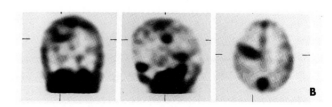

Fig. 11-11 Cerebral venous thrombosis. **A,** Normal Tc-99m-labeled RBC brain blood pool study. Compare the clearly defined venous anatomy with the schematic diagram in Figure 11-2. *Top,* posterior, LPO, and RPO views. *Bottom,* left lateral, right lateral, and anterior views. **B,** Abnormal study in a patient with a frontal lobe brain abscess, cerebritis, and increased intracerebral pressure. CT was suggestive of a superior sagittal sinus thrombosis. The Tc-99m-labeled RBC study demonstrated reduced activity in the posterior aspect of the superior sagittal sinus and abrupt cutoffs in the transverse sinuses bilaterally, diagnostic of thrombosis.

Fig. 11-12 Venous hemangioma. **A,** MRI shows a lesion in the right parietal cortex on coronal, sagittal, and transverse sections (*right to left*). **B,** The Tc-99m RBC study confirms the diagnosis of hemangioma (corresponding SPECT and MRI sections). This study can be used to confirm the effectiveness of ablative therapy.

diagnostic; however, it is invasive, usually impractical, and unnecessary.

The radionuclide brain death study can serve as an important ancillary test in confirming brain death. It is simple to perform, rapid, and can be done at the bedside. Scintigraphy is not affected by drug intoxication or hypothermia. An abnormal radionuclide angiogram showing no cerebral perfusion is more specific for brain death than an isoelectric EEG. This study is usually performed when the patient meets clinical criteria for brain death but the EEG is equivocal.

Radiopharmaceuticals   A number of radiopharmaceuticals have been used to diagnose brain death. The brain scintigraphic agents Tc-99m pertechnetate, Tc-99m DTPA, or Tc-99m GH can be used. Because only perfusion is being evaluated, they are equally useful.

Recently cerebral perfusion agents such as Tc-99m HMPAO (see discussion under Cerebral Perfusion Imaging) have been used, because cerebral perfusion can be evaluated on delayed static images as well as with flow images (Figure 11-13A-C). Therefore, one is not solely dependent on a good bolus. SPECT is not practical in these patients, nor is it necessary; planar delayed imaging with Tc-99m HMPAO can give the needed information.

Methods   The radionuclide angiogram protocol for cerebral perfusion has already been described (Box 11-2). A scalp tourniquet is utilized by some to minimize flow through the external carotid arteries, thereby making image interpretation of brain perfusion easier. However, it is regarded as contraindicated in children because it could increase intracranial pressure. Many believe it is also not really necessary for adults, since peripheral scalp activity can usually be easily differentiated from cerebral perfusion.

Image interpretation   An adequate radiopharmaceutical dose and good bolus infusion are required to ensure a diagnostic flow study. When the study is performed properly, flow to both common carotid arteries will be seen to the level of the base of the skull. Diagnostic findings of brain death include the lack of intracranial arterial flow and no visualization of major venous sinuses on subsequent static images.

Often the "hot nose" sign is seen (Figure 11-13). Diversion of flow from the intracranial to extracranial circulation results in relatively increased flow to the face and nose. This can occur with either internal carotid artery occlusion or brain death.

Faint visualization of the venous sagittal or transverse sinus in the absence of intracranial perfusion may be seen in 10% to 20% of patients. Although most interpret these findings as equivocal and recommend a repeat follow-up study (in hours to days), others believe it represents part of the spectrum of decreasing cerebral perfusion and brain death can be diagnosed, *if* there is unequivocal lack of arterial flow. These patients almost invariably progress to death within days.

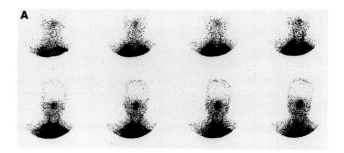

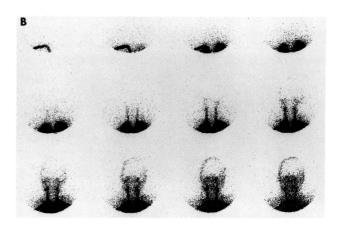

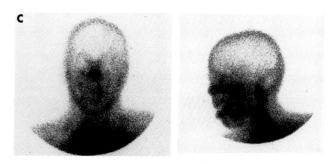

Fig. 11-13   Brain death. **A,** Tc-99m DTPA blood flow study shows activity transiting the internal carotids, but no blood flow within the brain. Note the "hot nose" due to shunting of flow from the internal to the external carotid system which supplies the face and scalp. **B,** Scintangiogram with Tc-99m HMPAO in another patient with suspected brain death shows no cerebral perfusion. **C,** Planar images obtained 15 minutes after injection of Tc-99m HMPAO show no cortical uptake. Because of the lack of cerebral blood flow, the Tc-99m HMPAO images look similar to the distribution of Tc-99m GH or DTPA. This study is diagnostic of brain death.

Accuracy

Although CT and MRI are superior overall to brain scintigraphy, the accuracy of brain scintigraphy is good (Table 11-1)

SPECT   SPECT can improve the detection of small, deep (e.g., basilar), and multiple lesions. It improves lesion characterization, better delineates the distribution

Table 11-1	Sensitivity of Conventional Brain Scintigraphy	
Entity	**Sensitivity (%)**	
Subdural hematomas		
Less than 10 days' duration	50	
Chronic	90	
Brain abscess	90	
Encephalitis	90	
Brain tumors	85	
AV malformations	95	

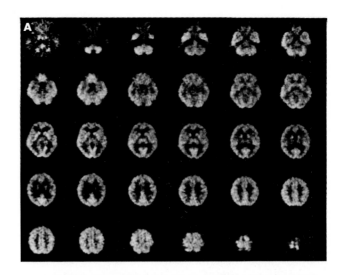

of lesions, and separates skull from intracranial abnormalities (Figure 11-10).

POSITRON EMISSION TOMOGRAPHY

A new era in nuclear medicine brain imaging emerged with the development of PET. PET is a unique tool in brain research allowing in vivo imaging of brain biochemistry and physiology. The potential of PET is that virtually any compound of biological interest (protein, sugar, fat, receptors, enzymes, etc.) can theoretically be labeled with radioactive oxygen, nitrogen, or carbon and used as a radiotracer.

Advances in cyclotrons and PET instrumentation have made this imaging modality not only a unique research instrument, but also a formidable clinical tool. Modern PET cameras have excellent resolution and, unlike SPECT instrumentation, no collimator is needed and attenuation correction can be easily and accurately performed. Cyclotrons are gradually becoming smaller. Only the cost of PET has hindered its widespread use. Most efforts in the clinical arena to date have focused on imaging and quantitating glucose metabolism with ^{18}FDG (fluorodeoxyglucose) and blood flow with $^{15}O_2$.

PET was first to demonstrate the clinical utility of functional brain imaging in the diagnosis of stroke, Alzheimer's disease, Huntington's chorea, epilepsy, and tumors (Figure 11-14A-E). Much of this work has now been replicated by SPECT cerebral perfusion imaging.

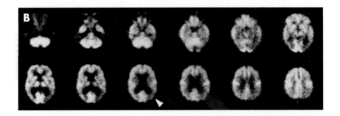

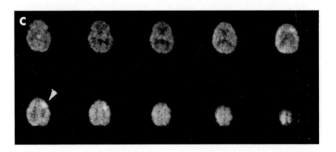

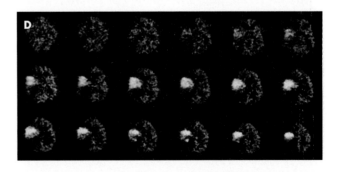

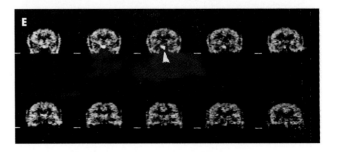

Fig. 11-14 PET images. **A**, Normal F-18 FDG scan with high-resolution cross-sectional sections. **B**, Alzheimer's disease. Note the bilateral parietal temporal hypoperfusion (*arrowheads*), although it is asymmetric, with more decrease on the left than the right. **C**, Seizure disorder. Note the focally increased uptake in the left frontal parietal region (*arrowhead*) during a seizure (ictal). **D**, Astrocytoma. Very increased focal uptake within a high-grade astrocytoma. **E**, Pituitary adenoma. Increased uptake in the region of the pituitary (*arrowhead*) on these coronal sections.

Research efforts are now concentrated in the areas of receptor imaging, tumor metabolism, and drug pharmacokinetic research. PET is likely to continue to lead nuclear medicine into new arenas, although its present clinical role in neuronuclear medicine is limited.

CEREBRAL PERFUSION IMAGING

Cerebral perfusion imaging with SPECT has revived brain imaging in clinical nuclear medicine. Although PET led the way and has the advantage that it is able to demonstrate metabolism as well as perfusion, SPECT performed with new single photon perfusion agents has been able to reproduce most of the clinical diagnostic findings initially described with PET. This has been made possible by advances in dedicated SPECT instrumentation and the development of a variety of new radiopharmaceuticals. The present clinical indications for SPECT cerebral perfusion studies are listed in Box 11-3 and described in the following sections. With cerebral perfusion imaging, SPECT is not just advantageous but mandatory.

Radiopharmaceuticals

Cerebral perfusion radiopharmaceuticals have a number of common characteristics that make them useful for regional cerebral blood flow (rCBF) scintigraphy. All are lipophilic, permitting rapid diffusion across the blood-brain barrier; they are small in molecular size, have a neutral charge, have high brain extraction proportional to blood flow, become relatively fixed in brain cells with little or no redistribution, and have progressive blood clearance at a rate that provides a good brain-to-blood ratio within 1 to 2 hours after injection.

Iodine I-123 isopropyl iodoamphetamine (I-123 IMP; Spectamine, IMP Inc., Houston), introduced in 1980, was the first brain perfusion radiotracer to be synthesized and approved for clinical use. After injection it distributes in the brain according to blood flow, with a 3-4:1 ratio of gray to white matter uptake.

Peak brain activity is reached within 20 minutes. Being lipophilic, I-123 IMP rapidly crosses the blood-brain barrier, diffuses through the interstitial space, and binds to amphetamine receptors on the brain cells. It has a high first-pass extraction fraction of greater than 95%. From 6% to 9% of the intravenously (IV) injected dose rapidly localizes in the brain (Table 11-2).

I-123 IMP is taken up by other organs, importantly the lungs, but also the liver and kidneys. There is some delayed cerebral uptake from its slow pulmonary release. Some intracranial washout occurs, as well as "redistribution." That is, metabolites of I-123 IMP are re-taken up by the cortex, but not in the same distribution as blood flow. Therefore, imaging must be done promptly, since, after an hour, delayed images show a loss of definition between cortex and white matter.

There is good correlation between initial IMP distribution and rCBF as determined by labeled microspheres and Xenon-133 washout studies. Preliminary data with another I-123-labeled perfusion agent, *I-123 HIPDM*, show many similar characteristics and clinical utility; however, the latter agent is not available for clinical use.

The I-123 radiolabel of IMP is not ideal. Images are suboptimal due to emission of other high-energy photons, the administered dose is limited to 3 to 6 mCi based on dosimetic considerations, and because it is not generator produced, there are problems of production and distribution. Therefore, Tc-99m-labeled cerebral perfusion agents were sought and investigated.

A new family of Tc-99m-based CBF radiopharmaceuticals was introduced in 1984. The most successful of this group was *hexamethylpropyleneamine oxime* (HMPAO; Ceretec; Medi-physics, Inc., Paramus, NJ). It has 80% first-pass extraction, brain uptake peaks 1 to 2 minutes after injection, and 3.5% to 7% of the injected dose remains within the brain (Table 11-2). Over the next 10 to 15 minutes there is a rapid 15% washout of brain activity. The rest remains fixed in the brain following conversion by glutathione to a hydrophilic compound that can no longer diffuse back out of the brain.

The distribution of Tc-99m HMPAO is also proportional to rCBF. However, the ratio of gray to white matter is only 2.5:1. When flow and metabolism are uncoupled, as they are in the luxury perfusion of acute stroke, Tc-99m HMPAO uptake may be normal or even increased, in contrast to I-123 IMP uptake, which always shows the metabolic defect of decreased uptake. Tc-99m HMPAO is chemically unstable in vitro and must be injected promptly after preparation.

Tc-99m ethyl cysteinate dimer (Tc-99m ECD; Neuro-

Box 11-3   Clinical Indications for Cerebral Perfusion SPECT

Stroke
Dementia
  Alzheimer's disease
  Multi-infarct dementia
  AIDS
Epilepsy
Trauma
Extrapyramidal disorders
  Parkinson's disease
  Huntington's chorea
Psychiatric disorders
Brain death

Table 11-2   Pharmacokinetics of Brain Blood Flow Radiopharmaceuticals

	Peak Brain Activity (min)	Blood T$_{1/2}$	First-Pass Extraction (%)	Brain Uptake (%)	Brain Washout
IMP	20	Slow	> 90	6.5-8.3	Redistribution
HMPAO	2	Slow	70-80	3.5-7	15% over 15 min
ECD	2	Rapid	> 70	5-7	6% per hr

lite; E.I. Dupont de Nemours Co., Billerica, Mass.), is a new cerebral perfusion agent showing considerable promise. Like Tc-99m HMPAO, it has moderate cerebral extraction and underestimates rCBF. Peak activity occurs within 1 to 2 minutes after injection, and 6% to 7% of the injected dose is retained within the brain (Table 11-2). Brain uptake is rapid and clearance from the brain is very slow. Blood clearance is rapid, resulting in a higher brain-to-background activity ratio than that of Tc-99m HMPAO. Unlike Tc-99m HMPAO, it is stable in vitro.

Methodology

Functional brain imaging requires strict adherence to a routine protocol. The radiopharmaceutical should always be injected under the same circumstances (e.g., room lighting, background noise, patient position). Otherwise different functional images will result. As an example, occipital parasagittal visual center activation depends on whether the eyes are open or closed.

SPECT is mandatory for diagnostic cerebral perfusion imaging. Although single-headed cameras can produce diagnostic images, dedicated brain SPECT and multi-headed cameras are preferable because of their superior image resolution. State-of-the-art SPECT systems can now give 6 to 9-mm resolution with imaging times of 10 to 20 minutes. The protocol in Box 11-4 specifies a three-headed rotating camera.

Quantitation of Blood Flow

Mean CBF in the normal person is 50.5 ± 6.2 mL/min/100 g. Children 3 to 10 years old have greater mean CBF, about 100 mL/min/100 g. There are substantial differences in normal regional perfusion. Mean gray matter blood flow is about 80 mL/min/100 g compared to a mean white matter blood flow of 20 mL/min/100 g.

Blood flow increases in regions of increased function and metabolic demand. For example, with unilateral hand exercise, blood flow increases markedly in the contralateral motor area of the precentral gyrus. Similarly, blood flow is increased by 30% in the occipital lobes when the eyes are opened compared to closed. Hypoxia and hypercapnia at the tissue level increase flow by local vasodila-

Box 11-4   Cerebral Perfusion Imaging With Tc-99m HMPAO or I-123 Iodoamphetamine SPECT: Protocol Summary

PATIENT PREPARATION

3 drops SSKI one-half hr prior to I-123 IMP imaging.

RADIOPHARMACEUTICAL

Tc-99m HMPAO (Ceretec), 20 mCi.
I-123 IMP (Spectamine), 6 mCi.

INSTRUMENTATION

Camera: Triple-headed SPECT camera.
Collimators: Ultra-high-resolution (or fan-beam) collimators.
Computer setup: SPECT acquisition parameters:
    Matrix size: 64 × 64.
    Zoom: 2.
    Rotation: Step and shoot.
    Orbit: Circular.
    Stops: 40 per head.
    Angle step size: 3°.
    Time per stop: 40 sec.

IMAGING PROCEDURE

Prepare dose according to package insert. Tc-99m HMPAO must be injected within 30 min (preferably 10-15 min) of preparation
Position patient so that brain is entirely within field of view of all detectors. Position collimators as close as possible to patient's head.
Begin scanning 15 min or later after injection of Tc-99m HMPAO and promptly after I-123 IMP.

PROCESSING

Filter: Hamming, 1.2 high-frequency cutoff.
Axial kernal size: 5.
Axial kernel: 1 3 5 3 1.
Attenuation correction: 0.11.

tion. The increased metabolism associated with a seizure results in similarly increased flow. Decreased blood flow may be seen diffusely (senile dementia) or regionally (occlusive cerebrovascular disease, severe brain injury).

Quantitation of CBF in mL/g/min is clinically desirable and possible but is not generally possible. The standard test for quantitation of blood flow experimentally is the microsphere method. Microsphere injection directly into the carotid artery is invasive and not practical clinically. PET, using oxygen-labeled water ($H_2^{15}O$) or carbon dioxide ($C^{15}O_2$), computer modeling, and arterial blood sampling, allows accurate quantitation of CBF, but it is not widely available.

Blood flow can also been measured by quantitating the clearance of xenon-133 from the brain. Xenon-133 is an inert gas administered by inhalation or IV injection. The lipid-soluble gas diffuses rapidly into tissues; washout is directly proportional to blood flow and can be calculated in mL/g/min. Because of its rapid clearance, multiple studies can be performed on the same day.

Xenon-133 multiprobe detectors have been widely used for quantitating cortical blood flow. Two-dimensional planar imaging is posssible but gives only limited regional information. More recently, dynamic SPECT has been utilized. Very rapid acqusition capability is required owing to xenon's fast clearance from the brain, demanding special instrumentation and software that is not generally available. Development of this methodology is ongoing. Stable xenon can by imaged by CT and used for the measurement of CBF; however, technical difficulties and low count rates have limited its clinical utility.

Quantitation of CBF with Tc-99m HMPAO and I-123 iodoamphetamine has been done; however, it requires arterial sampling and careful modeling to account for incomplete extraction, back flux from the brain, and other deviations from the theoretical model. For clinical purposes, absolute quantitation is not practical. However, relative quantitation, as exemplified by the right-to-left parietal cortex uptake ratio, often proves useful.

Dosimetry

Animal studies suggested that I-123 IMP had considerable eye uptake. However, this has not proved to be the case in humans. Sodium or potassium perchlorate must be given to prevent thyroid uptake of free iodide. The target organ is the lung (Table 11-3). The whole body uptake of Tc-99m HMPAO is very low (0.3 rads/20 mCi), and the target organs are the gallbladder and lacrimal glands (Table 11-4).

Image Interpretation

Anatomy   The cerebral cortex is composed of gray matter and anatomically divided into lobes (Figure 11-15

Table 11-3	I-123 Iodoamphetamine Dosimetry
Organ	**rads/6 mCi (cGy/222 MBq)**
Brain	0.35
Lens and retina	0.29
Lung	0.84
Liver	0.78
Bladder	1.38
Thyroid (blocked)	0.24
Testes	0.18
Ovaries	0.26
Red marrow	0.32
Total body	0.26

Modified from IMP Inc., Houston, TX, package insert.

Table 11-4	Tc-99m HMPAO Dosimetry	
Organ	**rads/mCi**	**rads/20 mCi (cGy/740 MBq)**
Lacrimal glands	0.26	5.2
Gallbladder wall	0.19	3.8
Kidney	0.13	2.6
Thyroid	0.10	2.0
Large bowel	0.08	1.6
Liver	0.05	1.1
Bladder	0.05	0.9
Brain	0.03	0.5
Ovaries	0.02	0.5
Eyes	0.03	0.5
Testes	0.01	0.1
Whole body	0.01	0.3

Modified from E.I. Dupont, Billerica, MA, package insert.

A, B). The *frontal* lobe extends fron the anterior portion of the brain to the central sulcus (fissure of Rolando). Extending along the central gyrus anteriorly is the precentral gyrus, which is the motor center of the cortex. The postcentral gyrus, the sensory center of the cortex, runs along the posterior margin of the central sulcus. The *parietal* lobe lies behind the central (rolandic) fissure. The most posterior segment of the cortex is the *occipital* lobe with the right and left visual cortex on either side of the fissure.

A large, deep fissure, the lateral sulcus or Sylvian fissure, divides the frontal and parietal lobes from the *temporal* lobe. If the temporal lobe is removed, its most medial margin is seen to lie adjacent to another series of gyri, the *insula* or central lobe, which lies hidden in the depths of the lateral sulcus. Each cerebral hemisphere is concerned with sensory and motor function for the opposite side of the body. Discrete associate areas are (1) *Broca's area,* situated in the lateral portion of the frontal

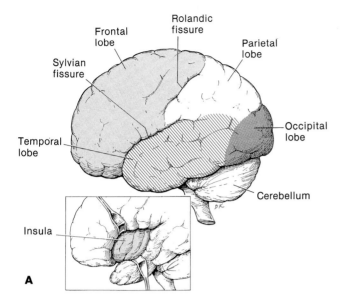

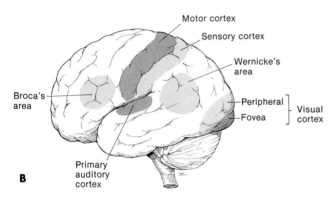

Fig. 11-15   Brain anatomy (**A**) and regional function and associative areas (**B**). See text for discussion.

lobe and controlling coordination of mouth movements into coherent speech, and (2) *Wernicke's area*, located in the temporal lobe and controlling the sensory component of speech and word selection.

Underneath the gray matter of the cerebral cortex lies the white matter, composed of myelinated fibers connecting the cortex with other parts of the brain and spinal cord. The basal ganglion (caudate nucleus, putamen, and globus pallidus) is the central gray matter of the cerebrum and lies between the insula and the thalamus, separated by the the internal capsule of the cortical white matter. The components of the basal ganglion are important in the initiation of movement. The cerebellum occupies the posterior cranial fossa and lies between the brain stem and the occipital lobes of the cerebrum. It is involved in the regulation of muscle tone and the initiation and coordination of voluntary movements.

Normal uptake and distribution of SPECT perfusion agents   SPECT cerebral perfusion agents distrib-

ute throughout the gray matter of the brain, and uptake reflects the distribution of rCBF (Figure 11-16). Uptake appears somewhat heterogeneous as a result of the normal irregular convolutions of the gyri and sulci and the limits of resolution of SPECT instrumentation. Uptake is highest in the cerebellum, followed by the temporal, parietal, and frontal lobes and the basal ganglia, which have slightly lower cortical uptake (75%-85% of the cerebellar uptake). Uptake in white matter is considerably less because of the relatively lower blood flow. Uptake in white matter is not seen well on SPECT imaging; it fades into background. The central cold area seen on cross-sectional SPECT images represents not only the ventricles, but white matter as well.

Clinical Applications

Cerebrovascular disease   Acute cerebral infarction (stroke) was the first application of SPECT perfusion imaging. Decreased rCBF is seen with SPECT immediately after the acute cerebrovascular event (Figure 11-17A,B). In contrast, CT is usually normal during the first hours to days after the ictus. During the first 8 hours after infarction, only 20% of CT scans are positive, while 90% of SPECT scans will be abnormal. MRI can usually demonstrate infarcts within 6 hours of the event.

Defects seen on SPECT are often larger than those seen on CT, suggesting an area of ischemic brain tissue surrounding the infarction that is potentially at risk for infarction (penumbra). Factors limiting SPECT's sensitivity are its lower detection rate for lacunar infarcts and the effect of luxury perfusion. Because of the latter, imaging during the subacute phase of a stroke should be approached cautiously. Decreased cerebellar perfusion contralateral to the cortical infarct (crossed cerebellar diaschisis) is often noted during the acute and subacute phases; it is thought to result from metabolic inhibition from direct neuroconnections.

Although its clinical role in acute stroke is uncertain at present, SPECT has shown the potential for detecting low flow states and for evaluating cerebrovascular reserve, which could have prognostic and therapeutic applications. Although some patients with transient ischemic attacks (TIAs) and carotid stenosis may have cortical perfusion defects, most do not. Specially performed SPECT studies and drug interventions may be able to select out those patients who could benefit from carotid endarterectomy or temporal artery to middle cerebral artery bypass operations. Several different methods have been described, and preliminary data are available.

As brain flow decreases, the normal compensatory tissue response to increase oxygen extraction is local vasodilation. This increases the blood volume-flow ratio in that region. This ratio can be quantitated with SPECT from combined brain perfusion (e.g., I-123 IMP) and

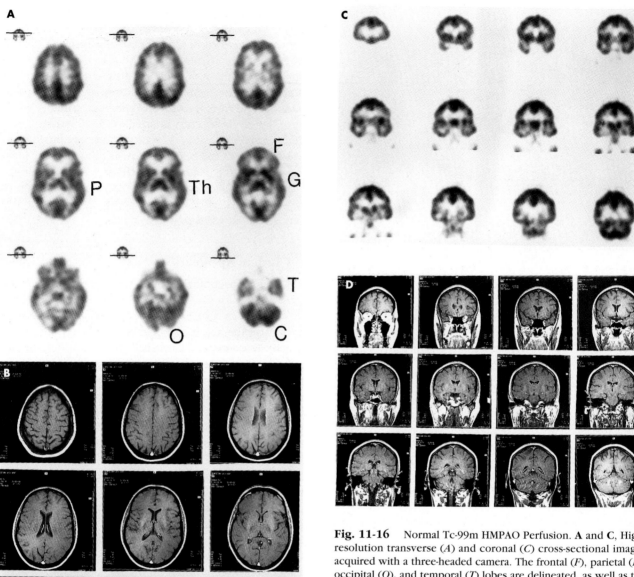

Fig. 11-16   Normal Tc-99m HMPAO Perfusion. **A** and **C**, High-resolution transverse (*A*) and coronal (*C*) cross-sectional images acquired with a three-headed camera. The frontal (*F*), parietal (*P*), occipital (*O*), and temporal (*T*) lobes are delineated, as well as the thalamus (*Tb*) and basal ganglion (caudate, putamen) (*G*). **B** and **D**, Comparable transverse (*B*) and coronal (*D*) CT sections in the same patient made for anatomic correlation. Note that the photopenic areas in the SPECT study represent not only ventricles but also white matter.

blood volume studies (Tc-99m RBC). An increased blood volume to perfusion ratio suggests ischemia and tissue at risk for infarction.

Another approach for determining the adequacy of cerebrovascular reserve is the use of acetazolamide (Diamox), a carbonic anhydrase inhibitor and cerebrovascular vasodilator. It is used in much the same way that carbon dioxide inhalation was used in the past. Normally, CBF increases fourfold with Diamox; however, regions with a perfusion reserve deficit cannot increase flow normally because vasodilation is already

maximal. This results in a Diamox-induced regional perfusion deficit. This method shows considerable promise.

I-123 IMP, because of its property of "redistribution," may be able to demonstrate viable brain in resting low perfusion states. Early studies suggest that delayed (4-hour) uptake in regions of early hypoperfusion is an indication of viable and potentially reversible ischemia (Figure 11-18). The mechanism is uncertain, but I-123 metabolites are thought to be taken up by viable brain cells. Although the mechanism differs, one could think of it as similar to Tl-201 redistribution in the brain.

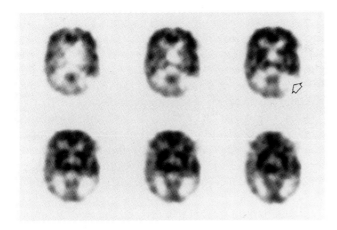

Fig. 11-17   Cerebral infarct seen with Tc-99m HMPAO. Left posterior parietal perfusion defect (*arrowhead*) seen on sequential transverse cross-sectional SPECT images in a patient with an acute right-sided stroke.

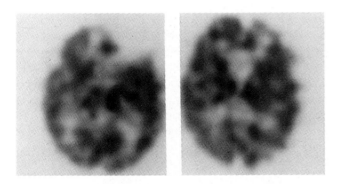

Fig. 11-18   I-123 IMP redistribution. *Left,* Immediate postinjection I-123 iodoamphetamine SPECT study shows cerebral perfusion defect noted in the left frontal cortex. *Right,* Repeat SPECT at 4 hours after tracer injection shows much improved perfusion in a comparable section, consistent with at least partially reversible ischemia.

Dementia   Dementia implies loss of mental faculties sufficient to interfere with social and occupational functioning. Deficits include memory, language, and visual-spatial perception. Psychiatric symptoms are not uncommon. The differential diagnosis is long (Table 11-5), and the entities are not always clinically distinguishable. SPECT cerebral perfusion imaging has shown clinical utility in the differential diagnosis.

Alzheimer's disease   Alzheimer's disease is now recognized as a very common cause of dementia (Table 11-5). In the past it was associated with dementia in a relatively young age group (presenile dementia). It is now appreciated that many patients previously classified as having multi-infact dementia actually had Alzheimer's and approximately 25% of patients diagnosed with Alz-

Table 11-5   Dementias

Disease	Incidence (%)
Alzheimer's disease	50-60
Multi-infarct dementia	5
Parkinsonism	15
Drugs and alchohol	10
Pick's disease	<1
Creutfeldt-Jakob discase	<1
Progressive supranuclear palsy	<1
Huntington's disease	<1
Multiple sclerosis	<1
Vitamin B$_{12}$ deficiency	<1
Endocrine (hypothyroid)	<1
Chronic infection (TB, syphilis)	<1

heimer's disease are found to have other diseases at autopsy. Clinical neurologic criteria can often differentiate these diseases, but much overlap exists. Brain biopsy is the only definitive method of diagnosis but is rarely used.

The diagnostic scintigraphic pattern on SPECT perfusion imaging is that of bilateral posterior temporal and parietal hypoperfusion (Figure 11-19). This pattern corresponds to the pathologic finding of abnormal tangles of nerve fibers and degenerative neuritic plaques, which occur in the same distribution. The patient's degree of dysfunction is related to the number of these abnormal cortical structures.

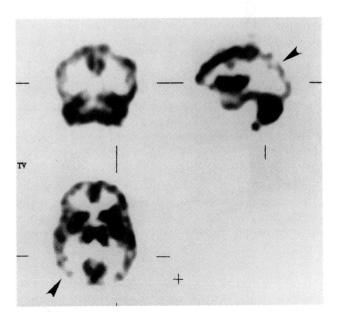

Fig. 11-19   Alzheimer's disease. The patient presented with dementia; Alzheimer's was suspected. The three-view display of selected cortonal, sagittal, and transverse Tc-99m HMPAO sections shows a classic pattern of Alzheimer's disease with bilateral temporal-parietal hypoperfusion (*arrowheads*). This is best seen in the sagittal view.

This scintigraphic pattern has a predictive value of over 80%; however, it can sometimes be seen in other diseases, including Parkinson's disease. Less frequent and less specific patterns seen with Alzheimer's disease include unilateral temporal-parietal and anterior perfusion defects. The occipital lobes, sensory motor cortex, and cerebellum are generally spared.

Frontal hypoperfusion is seen with *Pick's disease*. The scintigraphic pattern of *multi-infarct dementia* is that of multiple asymmetric perfusion defects, often involving the primary cortex and deep structures. Depression and metabolic disturbances usually have normal perfusion images.

Huntington's disease   Huntington's disease is an inherited disorder that affects middle-aged adults. Symptoms develop insidiously and usually appear between the ages of 35 to 50 years, inevitably progressing to uncontrollable choreiform movements and dementia. Pathologically, there is atrophy of basal ganglia, especially the caudate nuclei. The caudate and putamen are deficient in the inhibitory neurotransmitter γ-aminobutyric acid (GABA) and glutamic acid decarboxylase. Although it can begin asymmetrically, symmetric involvement eventually develops. Although initially described with PET, SPECT images have also shown decreased uptake in the caudate in patients with moderate to severe Huntington's disease.

AIDS dementia or HIV encephalopathy   The early clinical signs of AIDS demential complex (ADC) or HIV encephalopathy are frequently subtle and can be hard to distinguish from depression, psychosis, or focal neurologic disease. Because treatment (e.g., with AZT) can improve cognitive function, early detection is helpful. Findings on CT and MRI are not specific for ADC. Cerebral perfusion SPECT is highly sensitive for ADC and shows a typical scintigraphic pattern of multifocal or patchy cortical and subcortical regions of hypoperfusion, most frequently in the frontal, temporal and parietal lobes. Basal ganglia involvement is common. Many patients also have focal areas of increased activity. The perfusion pattern can improve with therapy. A similar brain perfusion pattern has been described in chronic cocaine and polydrug users.

Seizure disorders   Many patients with partial complex seizures unresponsive to anticonvulsant therapy may be helped by temporal lobectomy. The most common pathologic finding is mesial temporal sclerosis, thought to be due to a gliotic scar after resolution of some prior process. Excision of well-localized foci can lead to elimination of seizures or significantly improved pharmacologic control in 80% of surgical patients. However, only a few undergo surgery because of the difficulty of adequate seizure focus localization.

Surface EEG has poor spatial resolution, is dependent on cortical surface effects, and is limited by the area of brain sampled. As a result, EEG may not always be diagnostic and can sometimes be misleading. CT and MRI have low sensitivity for seizure foci detection, 17% and 34%, respectively. Surgically placed depth EEG electrodes can confirm a suspected site of seizure focus, but only limited regions can be sampled, and the technique is invasive and has some associated surgical risk.

SPECT and PET have both proved able to localize *epileptic foci*. Seizure foci are seen as areas of *hypo*perfusion interictally (Figure 11-20) and *hyper*perfusion ictally, similar to the hypo- and hypermetabolism seen with F-18 FDG PET (Figure 11-14C). The concurrence of the clinical picture, surface EEG pattern, and SPECT interictal hypoperfusion can obviate the need for more invasive diagnostic procedures. PET and SPECT studies have a similar sensitivity for detection of interictal seizure foci (65%-75%). Extratemporal seizure foci, for example in the frontal lobe, can also be identified; however, surgical results have been less successful.

I-123 IMP *ictal* studies in combination with interictal studies have been more sucessful in identifying seizure foci than interictal studies alone, although secondary generalized activation may sometimes obscure the original focus. However, true ictal studies with Tc-99m HMPAO are extremely difficult to obtain because the compound cannot be prepared in advance, owing to its chemical instability in vitro, which leads to delays between seizure onset and injection. Some preliminary data suggest that early postictal studies (within 5 minutes) may be as effective as true ictal injections. The good stability of Tc-99m ECD may make true ictal studies possible.

Wada Test   The goal of temporal lobectomy is to eliminate seizures unresponsive to medical therapy while limiting the volume of temporal lobe resected so as to minimize postoperative neurologic deficits. However, the risk of seizure recurrence is greater if the hippocampus is left intact.

The intracarotid administration of amobarbital sodium, or Wada test, has been used to predict postoperative speech and memory function in patients being considered for this surgery. Unfortunately, some patients have postoperative memory impairment despite Wada testing predictive that the contralateral hippocampus would be able to sustain memory. The patient may falsely fail the Wada test because of unintentional anesthesia of the contralateral hemisphere by flow through the circle of Willis, or because other cortical areas involved in memory processing have been anesthetized. If amobarbital does not perfuse the medial temporal lobe structures, a false negative memory test may result.

Therefore, to correctly interpret the neuropsychological results, it is important to know which areas of the brain have been anesthetized. In the past, this was determined by clinical neurologic testing, EEG, or angiography performed prior to the Wada test. On angiography, visualization of the posterior cerebral artery is taken as confir-

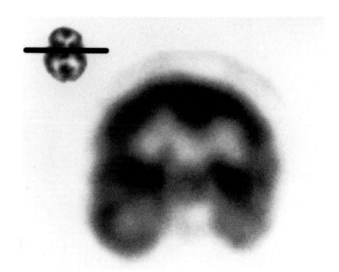

Fig. 11-20 Seizure disorder. The patient had partial complex seizures poorly responsive to conventional anticonvulsant therapy and was being considered for temporal lobectomy. The EEG and clinical history favored a left temporal focus. If the Tc-99m HMPAO study could confirm this, subdurally placed depth electrodes could be avoided. The interictal study shows hypoperfusion of the left temporal lobe (*arrows*) consistent with a left temporal lobe focus.

mation of hippocampal anesthesia. However, it is known that the laminar flow effects of rapidly injected contrast agent for angiography may result in a distribution dissimilar from the true perfusion pattern at the capillary level.

Mixing Tc-99m HMPAO with the amobarbital and injecting them simultaneously (Figure 11-21) has demonstrated discrepancies with angiography. One recent study reported that Tc-99m HMPAO activity was seen in the medial temporal lobe in less than 30% of patients injected with the amobarbital. This would explain the suboptimal results with Wada testing. The use of perfusion imaging at the time of testing could improve its predictive value.

Trauma Tc-99m HMPAO SPECT can be more sensitive than CT in detecting abnormalities in patients with a history of *traumatic brain injury,* and it can detect the changes earlier, particularly in patients with minor head injuries.

Psychiatric applications The role of PET and SPECT brain perfusion imaging in psychiatric diseases is uncertain at present. Diagnostic or prognostic functional abnormalities have not been identified in psychiatric diseases. Although frontal lobe hypometabolism and hypoperfusion have been described in schizophrenia, the findings are nonspecific. Studies in patients with depression have yielded conflicting results. However, because of the suspicion that much psychiatric disease is due to disordered metabolism, further investigation is indicated. At present, it may be of most value in identify-

ing patients with psychiatric symptoms who are suspected of having underlying organic disease.

Brain tumor imaging Most brain tumors have increased blood flow compared to surrounding normal brain tissue. This was often seen in the past on dynamic blood flow studies performed with Tc-99m pertechnetate or Tc-99m GH. PET with F-18 FDG has demonstrated increased glucose metabolism in glioblastomas, with the greatest uptake noted in the higher grade malignancies.

However, SPECT with the cerebral perfusion agents, I-123 iodoamphetamine and Tc-99m HMPAO, usually shows decreased uptake in most primary and metastatic tumors. Only a rare tumor has shown increased uptake

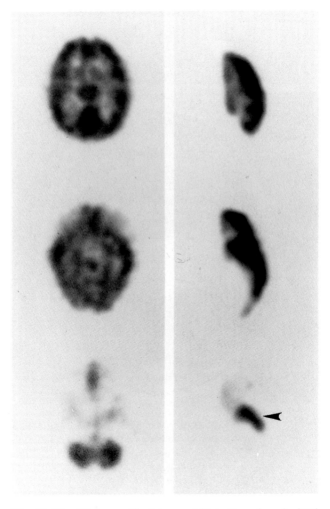

Fig. 11-21 Wada test. The intracarotid injection of amobarbital (Wada test) is used to predict speech and memory function in patients being considered for temporal lobectomy. *Left,* three cross-sectional selected sections of a routine baseline Tc-99m HMPAO study after intravenous tracer injection. *Right,* Tc-99m HMPAO was mixed with amobarbital and injected into the left carotid at the time of angiography. Transverse sections at comparable levels showed perfusion only of the left hemisphere, including left temporal lobe perfusion confirming that the clinical results of the amobarbital study truly reflected left temporal lobe function.

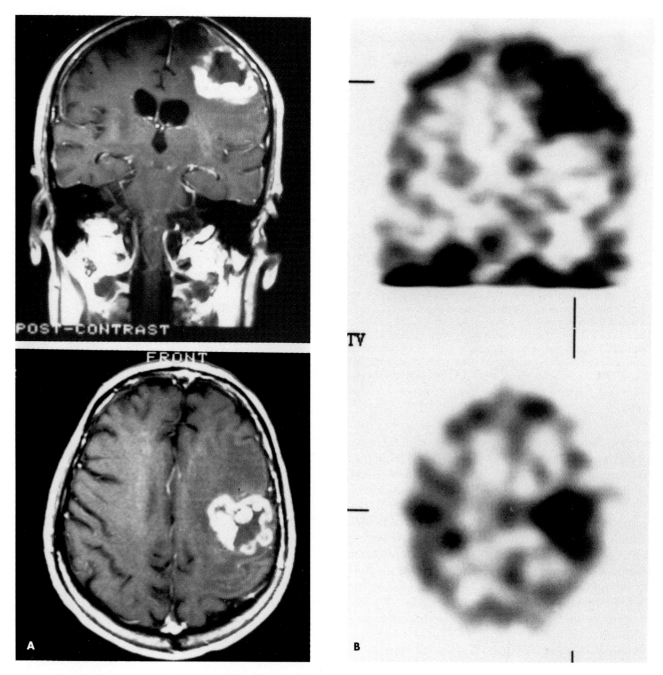

Fig. 11-22 Brain tumor imaged with Tl-201. **A,** MRI shows an astrocytoma in the left parietal region of the brain on the selected coronal and transverse sections. **B,** Corresponding sections of a Tl-201 SPECT study in the same patient. The intense uptake is consistent with a high grade malignant tumor. This test can be used to differentiate viable residual tumor from post-radiation therapy fibrosis and necrosis, often not distinguishable on CT or MRI.

on SPECT with Tc-99m HMPAO, never with I-123 IMP. The reason for the latter is thought to be due to the lack of normal receptor mechanisms on the tumor cells. However, if early dynamic SPECT acquisition is performed, increased flow to the tumor can usually be demonstrated, confirming that these tumors have increased blood flow but the tumor cannot retain the tracer.

Thallium-201, used primarily for myocardial perfusion imaging, is also taken up by a variety of human tumors. As a result, SPECT Tl-201 imaging has been successfully used to image brain tumors. As with PET, the degree of uptake in glioblastomas is proportional to the malignant grade of the tumor. Tumors with the highest grade have the most uptake, and this has prognostic implications. However, the most important clinical use of Tl-201 has been in determining tumor viability after radiation therapy. It can be very difficult to differentiate on CT or MRI residual or recurrent viable tumor from tumor necrosis and fibrosis. Both PET with F-18 FDG and Tl-201 SPECT can reliably distinguish the two (Figures 11-14D, 11-22).

Tl-201 SPECT has also been used in patients with AIDS presenting with intracerebral mass lesions. In this patient group, the diffential diagnosis is lymphoma (30% incidence) versus toxoplasmosis (60% incidence) and other atypical infectious agents. Lymphoma in AIDS patients is usually an aggressive tumor and requires prompt therapy. Usually a clinical trial of antitoxoplasmosis therapy is undertaken; however, a period of 2 to 3 weeks or longer is necessary to determine the effectiveness of therapy, often delaying appropriate therapy in patients with other causes of an intracerebral mass lesion. Intracerebral lymphoma in AIDs patients avidly takes up Tl-201; infection does not. Tc-99m sestamibi is also taken up by a variety of tumors, but its uptake in the choroid plexus may not be ideal for imaging some brain tumors.

Future applications Because a number of neurologic and psychiatric diseases may be due to abnormalities of neurotransmission, there has been considerable interest in the development of radiotracers for imaging and quantitation of neurotransmitter receptors in the hope that this approach might be useful in the diagnosis or treatment of a variety of diseases. A receptor is defined as a macromolecule that specifically binds to a ligand. Well-studied neurotransmitters include acetylcholine, endorphins, catecholamines, and serotonin. Each neuroreceptor has an effector component that initiates a biological response.

Radiolabeling neuroreceptors that could serve as imaging agents has been a challenge for the radiochemists, for these receptors represent only a very small proportion of the overall brain tissue, and very high-affinity and high-specific-activity agonists or antagonists are required to provide sufficient target-to-background ratios to permit external imaging.

Much of the early work has been done with PET; however, some single photon neuroreceptors have been developed. Changes in dopamine receptor density have been described in schizophrenia, tardive dyskinesia, Parkinson's disease, and Huntington's chorea.

I-123 QNB, a muscarinic acetylcholine receptor-binding agent, has been studied for many years in the hope that it might be useful in the diagnosis of diseases with associated receptor abnormalities, such as Alzheimer's disease. To date, this radiopharmaceutical has not found clinical utility, probably because of the nonspecificity of the ligand and the inability to differentiate presynaptic from postsynaptic binding.

I-123-IBZM is a D$_2$ receptor antagonist that locates primarily in the basal ganglion (Figure 11-23). The dopa-

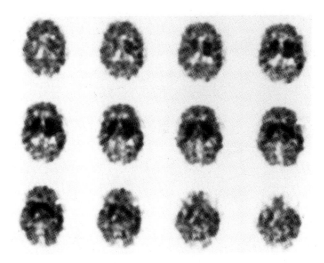

Fig. 11-23 Dopamine receptor imaging. Sequential cross-sectional transverse sections with I-123 IBZM show intense uptake in the basal ganglion bilaterally (*white arrowhead*), with much less activity in the cerebral cortex and no uptake in the cerebellum.

minergic system plays an important role in coordination. Because dopaminergic receptors serve as a site for neuroleptic drugs in the treatment of schizophrenia and Parkinson's disease, a potential use might be for determining the effective dose of antipsychotic therapy, that is, when all the receptor sites have been bound.

High concentrations of benzodiazepine receptors occur in the medial temporal cortex and are altered in partial complex epilepsy. *I-123 iomazenil* is a specific ligand for this receptor and appears to be abnormal even when perfusion studies are normal. Neuroreceptor imaging is an area of considerable promise, but at present has no defined clinical role.

CISTERNOGRAPHY

The study of cerebrospinal fluid (CSF) dynamics using radiotracers has been utilized for many years to diagnose the site of CSF leakage, to evaluate shunt patency, and for the diagnosis and management of hydrocephalus. Although CT and MRI are now commonly used for much of this evaluation, radionuclide cisternography can still play an important role because of the unique physiologic information it provides.

Radiopharmaceuticals

Various radiotracers have been used over the years, including I-131 serum albumin, Tc-99m HSA, and yterbium-169. Now that *In-111 DTPA* is widely available, it is preferred because of its better imaging characteristics, shorter half-life, and lower dosimetry.

Table 11-6	Dosimetry of In-111 DTPA for Cisternography

Organ	rads/500 μCi (cGy/18.5 MBq)
Total body	0.04
Kidneys	0.22
Spinal cord	
Surface	5.0
Average	1.5
Brain	
Surface	4.1
Average	0.5
Bladder	
2-hr void	0.2
4-hr	0.5
Testes	
2-hr void	0.04
4-hr void	0.05
Ovaries	
2-hr void	0.06
4-hr void	0.06

Modififed from package insert, Medi-physics, Inc., Arlington Heights, IL.

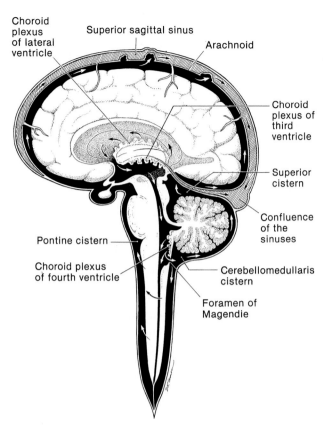

Fig. 11-24 Normal cerebrospinal fluid flow. Originating in the choroid plexus of the lateral ventricle, CSF flows through the third and fourth ventricles into the basal cisterns and then moves over the cerebral convexities, finally being reabsorbed in the superior sagittal sinus.

Dosimetry

The radiation absorbed dose will depend to some extent on the clearance dynamics in a particular patient. The spinal cord receives the highest dose, followed by the kidney and bladder next, since the radiopharmaceutical undergoes renal excretion (Table 11-6).

Mechanism of Radiopharmaceutical Uptake

CSF anatomy and physiology CSF that fills the ventricles and subarachnoid space surrounding the brain and spinal cord is secreted in the choroid plexus of the ventricles and, to a lesser extent, in extraventricular sites. The CSF normally drains from the lateral ventricles through the interventricular foramen of Monro into the third ventricle (Figure 11-24). With the additional CSF produced by the choroid plexus of the third ventricle, it passes through the cerebral aqueduct of Sylvius into the fourth ventricle and then leaves the ventricular system through the median foramen of Magendie and the two lateral foramina of Luschka. Here the CSF enters the subarachnoid space surrounding the brain and spinal cord. Along the base of the brain, the subarachnoid space expands into a number of lakes called cisterns. The subarachnoid space extends over the surface of the brain. The CSF bathes the brain and is absorbed through the pacchionian granulations of the pia arachnoid villa into the superior sagittal sinus.

Pharmacokinetics Radiopharmaceuticals injected intrathecally into the lumbar subarachnoid space are small molecules that follow the flow of the CSF without affecting the dynamics. The radiotracer normally reaches the basal cisterns by 1 hour, the frontal poles and Sylvian fissure area by 2 to 6 hour, the cerebral convexities by 12 hours, and the arachnoid villi in the sagittal sinus by 24 hours. Flow to the parasagittal region occurs through both central and superficial routes . The radiotacer does not normally enter the ventricular system because physiologic flow is in the opposite direction.

Clinical Applications

Hydrocephalus Hydrocephalus refers to a pathologic increase in CSF volume associated with enlargement of the ventricles. Table 11-7 presents a useful clinical classification of hydrocephalus. *Obstructive noncommunicating hydrocephalus* is an intraventricular obstruction occurring somewhere between the lateral ventricles and the basal cistern and may be caused by such conditions as a colloid cyst, aqueductal stenosis, Arnold-Chiari malformation, or neoplasm. It is usually diagnosed with CT

Table 11-7   Classification of Hydrocephalus

Classification	Site of Obstruction	Scintigraphy Type
Obstructive		
Noncommunicating	Intraventricular, between lateral ventricles and basal cisterns	I, II
Communicating	Extraventricular, affecting basal cisterns, cerebral convexities, and arachnoid villi	III A, III B, IV
Nonobstructive		
Generalized	Cerebral atrophy	II
Localized	Porencephaly	

or MRI. Lumbar cisternography demonstrates a normal flow pattern.

Obstructive communicating hydrocephalus refers to an extraventricular obstruction in the basal cisterns, cerebral convexities, or arachnoid villi. Common causes of the latter include a previous subarachnoid hemorrhage, chronic subdural hematoma, leptomeningitis, or meningeal carcinomatosis, and *normal pressure hydrocephalus.* CT shows a ventricular system dilated out of proportion to the cortical sulci, and prominent basal cisterns. Radionuclide cisternography shows reflux of radiotracer into the ventricles and delayed or absent movement over the convexities. A spectrum of scintigraphic findings have been described (Table 11-8). *Generalized nonobstructive hydrocephalus* refers to patients with cerebral atrophy. CT shows ventricular dilation and wide

cortical sulci. Porencephaly is a *localized nonobstructive hydrocephalus.*

Normal pressure hydrocephalus (NPH) manifests clinically with dementia, ataxia, and incontinence. The etiology and cisternographic findings do not differ from those of communicating hydrocephalus with elevated pressure; the reason for the difference is uncertain. The usual clinical problem presented to nuclear medicine is to differentiate NPH from hydrocephalus ex-vacuo (generalized brain atrophy).

CT can often make this differential based on the size of the ventricles, cisterns, and convexity sulci, but the findings overlap, and functional flow information from the radionuclide study is often helpful. Atrophy alone will cause delayed tracer movement through the enlarged subarachoid space, sometimes with transient ven-

Table 11-8   Cerebrospinal Fluid Flow Patterns in Hydrocephalus

Type	Pattern	Etiologies
I	Basal cistern, 2-4 hr Sylvian fissure, 6 hr Other convexities, 24 hr Decreased activity, 48 hr	Normal Intraventricular obstructive hydrocephalus
II	No ventricular activity Delayed migration	Cerebral atrophy Increased intracerebral pressure Advanced age Noncommunicating hydrocephalus

III A	Transient ventricular activity
	Clearance by usual
	  migration (often)
		Cerebral atrophy
		Evolving or resolving communicating
		  hydrocephalus

III B	Transient ventricular activity,
	  clearance without
	  usual migration
		Communicating hydrocephalus with alternative
		  pathway of resorption
		  (transependymal)

IV	Persistent ventricular
	  activity, inadeqate
	  clearance
		Communicating hydrocephalus

tricular reflux, but there is normal clearance over the hemispheres by 24 hours. Although the pattern with NPH is variable (Figures 11-25, 11-26), ventricular reflux does not clear, and there is delayed clearance over the cerebral hemispheres.

NPH is a progressive disease. Surgical shunting of CSF can potentially cure this cause of dementia; however, not all patients improve with surgery. Predicting which patients will be helped is problematic. Radionuclide cisternography and metrizamide CT, when used in conjunction with clinical findings such as clinical response (mental clearing) to CSF fluid reduction, can be helpful. Patients with the type IV cisternographic pattern are most likely to benefit from shunting (Figure 11-25, Table 11-8).

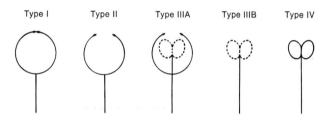

Fig. 11-25 CSF flow, abnormal patterns. See Table 11-12 for description of patterns I-IV with their respective etiologies.

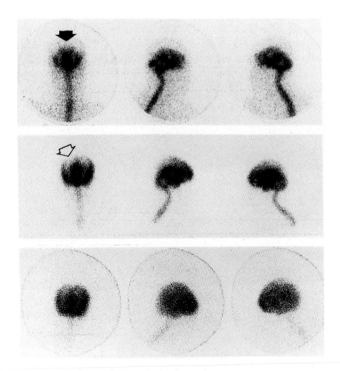

Fig. 11-26 Normal pressure hydrocephalus. Tc-99m DTPA cisternogram images acquired at 24 hours (*top*), 48 hours (*middle*), and 72 hours (*bottom*) in the anterior (*left*), right lateral (*middle*), and left lateral (*right*) views. Ventricular reflux (closed arrowhead) is present, as is very delayed flow (*open arrowhead*) over the cerebral convexities. The intracerebral activity at 72 hours was due to transependymal uptake.

Surgical shunt patency Diversionary CSF shunts (ventriculoperitoneal, ventriculoatrial shunt, or lumbo-peritoneal) are used in treating obstructive forms of hydrocephalus. There are various types of shunts and numerous variations. Complications which are not rare, may include catheter blockage, infection, thromboembolism, subdural or epidural hematomas, disconnection of catheters, and bowel perforation.

The diagnosis of shunt patency and adequacy of CSF flow can usually be made by examination of the patient and inspection of the subcutaneous CSF reservoir. When this assessment is uncertain, radionuclide studies with either In-111 DTPA or Tc-99m DTPA are useful for confirming the diagnosis (Figure 11-27). Familiarity with the specific type and configuration of shunt is important when performing a CSF shunt study. To prevent damage to the shunt, many neurosurgeons prefer and expect to inject these shunts themselves.

CSF leak Trauma and surgery (transsphenoidal and nasal) are the most common causes for CSF rhinorrhea. Nontraumatic causes include hydrocephalus and congenital defects. CSF rhinorrhea may occur anywhere from the frontal sinuses to the temporal bone (Figure 11-28). The cribriform plate is most susceptible to fracture and rhinorrhea. Otorrhea is much less common.

Accurate localization of CSF leaks is sometimes difficult. Although glucose oxidase test strips are used to confirm CSF leak, both lacrimal and nasal secretions contain glucose. The false positive rate may be as high as 50%. Radionuclide studies have proved to be a sensitive and accurate method of detection. The site is most likely to be identified during heavy leakage. Imaging in the appropriate projections is important for identifying the site of leak—lateral and anterior imaging is used for rhinorrhea and posterior imaging for otorrhea.

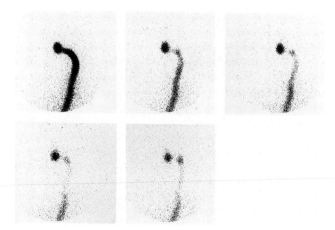

Fig. 11-27 CSF shunt patency. After injection of In-111 DTPA into the shunt reservoir, there is rapid clearance over a 30-minute observation period. An abdominal view can confirm clearance through the ventriculoperitoneal shunt into the abdominal cavity.

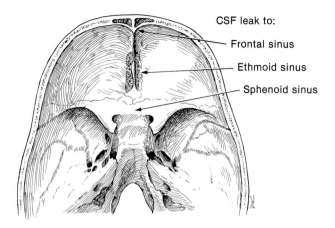

Fig. 11-28   Common sites of CSF leakage.

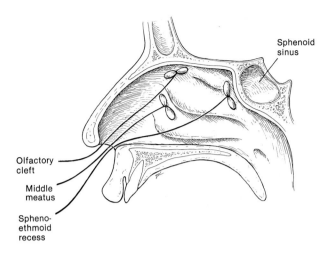

Fig. 11-29   Placement of pledgets for CSF leak study. The cotton labeled pledgets have been placed by ENT at various locations within the anterior and posterior nares to detect leakage from the frontal, ethmoidal, and sphenoidal sinuses.

To maximize the sensitivity of the test, nasal pledgets are placed in the anterior and posterior portion of each nasal region and then removed and counted 4 hours later. A ratio of nasal-to-plasma radioactivity greater than 3:1 is considered positive. It is often useful to ask the patient what position is associated with greatest leakage. This position should be reproduced during imaging.

Methodology

The cisternography protocol is described in Box 11-5. Proper lumbar puncture technique is critical. It should be performed by someone experienced in the technique to ensure subarachnoid injection.

Shunt injection should also be performed by someone very familiar with the type of shunt in place, usually the neurosurgeon. The protocol for shunt patency is described in Box 11-6.

Nose packing for CSF leak studies should be performed by an otolaryngologist (Figure 11-29). A protocol is described in Box 11-7.

Image Interpretation

Normal pressure hydrocephalus   Figure 11-25 illustrates the spectrum of findings seen with NPH, and Figure 11-26 illustrates the typical findings.

CSF shunt patency   There should be prompt flow of

Box 11-5   Cisternography: Protocol Summary

RADIOPHARMACEUTICAL

In-111 DTPA, 250 μCi.

INSTRUMENTATION

Camera: Large field of view gamma camera.
Collimator: Medium energy.

IMAGING PROCEDURE

Inject slowly into lumbar subarachoid space via a 22-gauge needle with the bevel positioned vertically.
Patient should remain recumbent for at least 1 hr after injection.
All images should be obtained for 50k counts.
Imaging times:
   1 hr: thoracic-lumbar spine for evaluation of injection adequacy.
   3 hr: base of the skull to visualize basilar cisterns.
   24, 48 hr: evaluation of ventricular reflux and arachnoid villi resorption.
Obtain anterior, posterior, and both lateral views of the head at 3, 24, and 48 hr.

Box 11-6 Shunt Patency: Protocol Summary

RADIOPHARMACEUTICAL

Tc-99m DTPA, 0.5 - 1.0 mCi, or In-111 DTPA, 250 µCi.

INSTRUMENTATION

Camera: Wide field of view with general all-purpose collimator.
Computer and camera setup: 1-min images x 30.

IMAGING PROCEDURE

Using aseptic technique. Clean the shaved scalp with Betadine.
Penetrate the shunt reservoir with a 25-35-gauge needle.
Once the needle is in place, position the patient's head under the camera with the reservoir in the middle of the field of view.
Inject the radiopharmaceutical.
Take serial images for 30 min.
If no flow is seen, place the patient in an upright position and continue imaging for 10 min.
If no flow is still seen, obtain static images of 50k after 1 and 2 hr.
If flow is demonstrated at any point, obtain 50k images of the shunt and tubing every 15 min until flow to the distal tip of the shunt tubing is identified or for 2 hr, whichever is first.
To determine proximal patency of the reservoir, the distal catheter can be manually occluded during the procedure so that the radiotracer will reflux into the ventricular system.

Box 11-7 Protocol for CSF Leak

PATIENT PREPARATION

Pledgets should be placed in the nose by ENT or other qualified physician and labeled as to location.
Maintain the patient supine (Trendelenburg) until the time of imaging to pool the radiotracer in the basal regions. Put the patient into a position that contributes to CSF leak.

RADIOPHARMACEUTICAL

In-111 DTPA, 250 µCi.

INSTRUMENTATION

Camera: Large field of view gamma camera.
Collimator: Medium energy.

IMAGING PROCEDURE

Begin imaging when activity reaches the basal cisterns (1-4 hr).
Position patient to maximize leak.
   Rhinorrhea: Lean patient's head forward and against camera face with the camera positioned in the left and right lateral positions.
   Otorrrhea: Obtain posterior images instead of lateral views.

Acquisition

Acquire 5 min/frame images for 1 hr in the selected view, then acquire the other three views (anterior, left lateral, right lateral, posterior). Then obtain 50k images every 10 min x 1 hr in the orginal view.
Remove the pledgets and draw a 5-mL blood sample.
Count the pledgets and count a 0.5-mL aliquot of plasma.
Repeat views may be indicated at 6 and 24 hr.

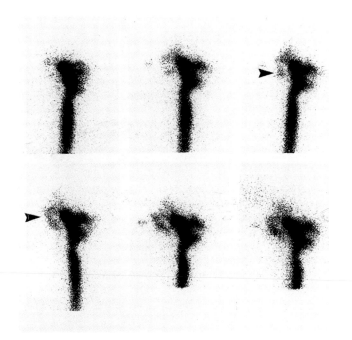

Fig. 11-30 Radionuclide CSF leak study, left lateral view. A positive In-111 DTPA study with activity increasing over time originating from the nares and seen leaking into the nose and mouth (*arrowheads*).

CSF into the distal shunt catheter (Figure 11-27). The shunt tubing will occasionally be seen. Peritoneally draining catheters will reveal increasing accumulation of radiotracer free within the abdominal cavity.

CSF leaks Localized increasing accumulation of activity is seen at the site of the leak. The pledgets can be used to determine the origin (anterior vs. posterior) of the leak (Figure 11-30).

SUGGESTED READINGS

Holman BL, editor: *Radionuclide imaging of the brain,* 1985, Churchill Livingstone.

Holman BL and Devous MD, Sr: Functional brain SPECT: The emergence of a powerful clinical method, *J Nucl Med* 33:1888-1904, 1992.

Lequin MH, Blok D, and Pauwels EKJ: Radiopharmaceuticals for functional brain imaging with SPECT. In Freeman LM, editor: *Nuclear Medicine Annual 1991*, New York, 1991, Raven Press.

Mazziotta JC and Gilman S, editors: *Clinical brain imaging: principles and applications,* Philadelphia, 1992, FA Davis & Co.

Nagel JS, Garada BM, and Holman BL: Functional brain imaging in dementia. In *Nuclear Medicine Annual 1993*, New York, 1993, Raven Press.

CHAPTER 12

Genitourinary System

Radionuclide evaluation of renal function dates back to the early 1950s (Table 12-1). A variety of radiopharmaceuticals and methodologies have been used over the years. Early studies with radiotracers and external probe detector systems produced no images but rather time-activity histograms showing uptake and excretion of the renal radiopharmaceutical. These early studies did not permit visualization of renal blood flow, parenchymal anatomy, or collecting system integrity.

Probe studies have given way to gamma camera-based evaluations that employ computer-acquired and -processed dynamic imaging studies. These contemporary studies offer the ability to do very sophisticated combined examinations of renal function, anatomy, and collecting system integrity. Reflecting these various categories of diagnostic interest, different radiopharmaceuticals have been developed.

In the lower urinary tract, radionuclide cystography has proved useful for evaluating ureteral reflux, especially

Table 12-1	Radionuclides Used for Renal Function Evaluation	
Year	**Radiopharmaceutical**	**Method**
1952	I-131 Iopax	Urine counting
1956	I-131 Diodrast	Renogram
1960	I-131 hippuran	Renogram
1968	I-131 hippuran	Lasix renography
1968	Hg-203 Cl$_2$	Individual renal function
1969	Tc-99m gluconate	Renal scan
1970	Tc-99m DTPA	Renal scan, GFR
1971	I-131 hippuran	Single sample GFR
1974	Tc-99m DMSA	Renal scan
1984	I-131 hippuran	Captopril renography
1986	Tc-9m MAG3	Renal scan

in children. Scrotal scintigraphy has played an important role in the differential diagnosis of the acute scrotum.

RENAL ANATOMY AND PHYSIOLOGY

The kidneys are paired, bean-shaped organs that measure 9 to 11 cm in length, equal to two to three vertebral bodies, and weigh about 150 grams each. The right kidney is often lower than the left. The outer cortex contains the glomeruli and proximal convoluted tubules. The renal pyramids, consisting of collecting tubules and the loops of Henle, make up the medulla. At the apex of the pyramids are papillae, which drain into the renal calyces. Cortical tissue that lies between the pyramids is known as the columns of Bertin (Figure 12-1).

The kidney is a complex organ with several functions. In addition to regulating water and electrolyte balance, it excretes products of metabolism and foreign chemicals, secretes hormones (renin, erythropoietin), and activates vitamin D.

Approximately 25% of cardiac output is delivered to the kidney via the renal artery and its tributaries (see Figure 12-1). End arterioles lead to tufts of capillaries forming glomeruli which lie within the renal cortex. Bowman's capsule surrounds the glomerulus. It is the closed end of a long, tortuous renal tubule making up the nephron, the basic functional unit of the kidney. Each kidney has over a million nephrons.

Urine formation begins with filtration of blood. The average renal plasma flow is about 600 mL/min. Twenty percent of this is filtered through the glomerulus (120 mL/min). The relatively high renal plasma flow and resistance provided by the efferent arteriole combine to maintain a presssure gradient that provides the driving force for filtration (Figure 12-2A). The resulting ultrafiltrate, consisting of water and crystaloids but no colloids or cells, enters into the renal tubule. Inulin is a drug that is

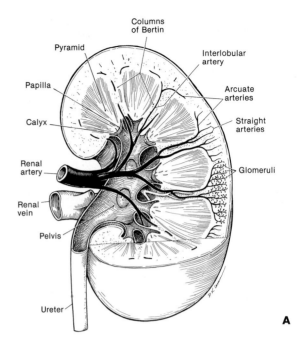

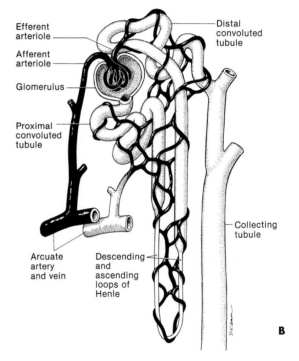

Fig. 12-1 **A**, Gross anatomy of the kidney. Cortex and medulla: The outer layer, or *cortex*, is made up of glomeruli and proximal collecting tubules; the inner layer, or *medulla*, contains the pyramids, which contain the distal tubules and loops of Henle. The tubules converge at the papillae, which empty into the calyces. The columns of Bertin, between the pyramids, are also cortical tissue. Renal vasculature: The renal artery and vein enter and leave at the hilus. The interlobular branches of the renal artery divide and become the arcuate arteries, which give rise to straight arteries, from which arise the afferent arterioles that feed the glomerular tuft. **B**, Nephron. The nephron consists of the vascular afferent and efferent blood vessels leading to a tuft of capillaries, the glomerulus, as well as to Bowman's capsule, the proximal and distal renal tubules, and the loops of Henle. Each kidney has over 1 million functioning nephrons.

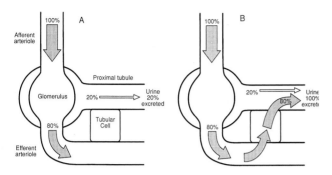

Fig. 12-2 **A,** Glomerular filtration. Twenty percent of renal blood flow to the kidney is filtered through the glomerulus. **B,** Tubular secretion. The remaining 80% of renal plasma flow is secreted into the proximal tubules from the peritubular fluid space.

entirely filtered through the glomerulus and, therefore, has been used as a standard measure of the glomerular filtration rate (GFR).

The remaining 80% of plasma not filtered enters the peritubular fluid and is actively secreted by the tubular epithelial cells into the renal tubules (Figure 12-2B). Para-aminohippurate (PAH) is the classic example of a drug that, after being partially filtered at the glomerulus (20%), is secreted into the renal tubules (80%). Therefore, PAH serves as the standard for quantitation of renal plasma flow.

Clearance from the plasma of a substance that is maintained in the blood in a steady state, such as infused inulin, PAH, or endogenous creatinine, can be used to quantify specific aspects of renal function. The formula, clearance (mL/min) = UV/P, where U = urine concentration (mg/mL), P = plasma concentration (mg/mL), and V = urine volume (mL), measures the volume of plasma completely cleared of the substance under examination each minute.

As urine passes along the tubule, the filtrate is concentrated and essential substances are conserved. The tubular epithelium actively reabsorbs water and selected substances—glucose, sodium, amino acids—into the blood. This is an energy-dependent process. Water is passively reabsorbed by the osmotic gradient set up by solutes, chiefly sodium. Sixty-five percent of sodium and water filtered at the glomerulus is reabsorbed in the proximal convoluted tubule.

The renal tubules empty formed urine into the calyces through the papillae of the medullary pyramids. From there the urine passes to the renal pelvis, ureter, and bladder.

TERMINOLOGY

The terms used to describe nuclear medicine renal studies—renal scans, renograms, renography, scintigrams, differential function, quantitative renal function, and so forth—will be used repeatedly in this chapter.

Box 12-1   Terminology for Radionuclide Renal Studies

RENOGRAM (OR RENOGRAPHY)

Time-activity curves derived historically from renal probe (nonimaging) studies or in current practice from computer-processed dynamic renal imaging studies after drawing renal ROIs.

RENAL SCAN (OR SCINTIGRAM)

Renal images are acquired using radiopharmaceuticals that fix to the cortex, or timed sequential images are acquired of radiotracer uptake and clearance in a dynamic renal study.

DIFFERENTIAL OR INDIVIDUAL RENAL FUNCTION

Percent right or left renal cortical uptake or retention as a percent of total renal uptake, derived from renal scintigraphy.

QUANTITATIVE GFR OR ERPF

Clearance (mL/min) calculation derived from either (1) blood sampling after radiotracer injection to determine blood clearance of the radiotracer or (2) computer-derived quantitative estimates of renal cortical uptake from scintigraphy. Both methods, when the appropriate radiopharmaceutical is used, can be used to derive GFR or ERPF estimates.

However, the terms are sometimes used interchangeably in different books, which can be confusing. These terms developed historically, often with the use of instrumentation that is not used today, such as renal probes (renogram) and rectilinear scanners (scan). To minimize confusion, definitions are provided in Box 12-1.

RADIOPHARMACEUTICALS

A number of radiopharmaceuticals have been used clinically over the years to evaluate renal function (Table 12-1). Those now commonly used are discussed here.

Mechanisms of Uptake

Various renal radiopharmaceuticals have different mechanisms of uptake. A functional classification of the major agents is shown in Table 12-2 and Figure 12-3.

A *glomerular agent* is a radiopharmaceutical that is cleared primarily by glomerular filtration. It is neither reabsorbed nor secreted by the renal tubules. To be freely filtered, there must be minimal or, preferably, no protein binding.

Although a number of different glomerular agents have been used for investigative and quantitative purposes (Box 12-2), the most clinically important agent is

Table 12-2   Mechanisms of Uptake of Renal Scintigraphic Agents

Mechanism of Uptake	Agent
Glomerular filtration	Tc-99m DTPA
Tubular	Tc-99m MAG3
Tubular (80%) and glomerular (20%) (ERPF)	I-131 and I-123 OIH
Cortical binding (50%)	Tc-99m DMSA
Glomerular filtration (80%) and cortical binding (20%)	Tc-99m GH

Box 12-2   Glomerular Agents Used to Quantify GFR

C-14 or H-3 inulin	Cr-51 EDTA
I-125 diatrizoate	In-111 DTPA
I-125 iothalamate	Yb-169 DTPA
Co-57 vitamin B_{12}	**Tc-99m DTPA**

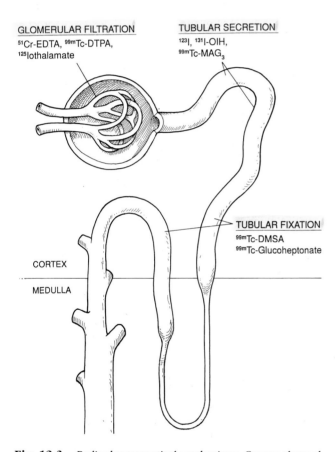

GLOMERULAR FILTRATION
^{51}Cr-EDTA, ^{99m}Tc-DTPA, ^{125}Iothalamate

TUBULAR SECRETION
^{123}I, ^{131}I-OIH, ^{99m}Tc-MAG$_3$

TUBULAR FIXATION
^{99m}Tc-DMSA
^{99m}Tc-Glucoheptonate

CORTEX

MEDULLA

Fig. 12-3   Radiopharmaceutical mechanisms. Commonly used renal radiotracers have different mechanisms of renal uptake and excretion, including one or more of the following, as shown: glomerular filtration, tubular secretion, and cortical tubular fixation.

technetium-99m diethylenetriamine pentaacetic acid (Tc-99m DTPA), also known as Tc-99m pentetate. Most criteria for a glomerular agent are met by this agent. Although there is a small amount of protein binding in some commercial preparations, this becomes important only if one wants to accurately quantify the GFR. It is of little consequence for routine scintigraphy.

Tc-99m DTPA is a versatile renal imaging agent. Prerenal blood flow, renal parenchymal function, and post-renal collecting system integrity can all be evaluated (Figure 12-4). The relatively large administered dose (20 mCi) results in good blood flow images. During the tissue (nephrogram) phase, scintigraphy demonstrates parenchmal uptake and renal anatomy. After excretion, good images of the collecting system allow assessment of its patency and can be used for evaluation of obstructive uropathy.

The next important class of renal radiopharmaceuticals consists of the *tubular* agents (see Box 12-3). To meet criteria for this category, the mechanism of renal uptake should be predominantly that of tubular secretion. The classic tubular agent is nonradioactive PAH, which is used mainly on an investigative basis to calculate renal plasma flow. I-131 ortho-iodohippurate (I-131 OIH), or hippuran, is chemically and pharmocokinetically similar to PAH and is the classic tubular agent used in nuclear medicine for many years (Figure 12-5). Like PAH, I-131 OIH is cleared partially by glomerular filtration (20%) and the remainder by tubular secretion (80%).

I-131 OIH has been used to quantify effective renal plasma flow (ERPF). The term *effective* refers to the fact that the urinary clearance of OIH is slightly lower than that of PAH. The lower clearance has been attributed to the presence of free I-131 in the preparation, plasma protein binding, and differences in tubular transport. This has only a small effect on the calculation.

More recently, Tc-99m mercaptylacetyltriglycine (Tc-99m MAG3) has been approved for clinical use. Its mechanism of renal clearance is solely tubular secretion. Its overall clearance is less than that of OIH.

For most clinical imaging purposes, glomerular and tubular radiopharmaceuticals can be used interchangeably, particularly in the setting of normal function. The major difference scintigraphically depends on the radiolabel—I-131 versus Tc-99m, for example. However, with increasing renal insufficiency, the tubular agents are superior because of their higher extraction efficiency.

Several radiopharmaceuticals demonstrate prolonged retention in the kidney. Tc-99m glucoheptonate (Tc-99m GH), or gluceptate, and Tc-99m dimercaptosuccinic acid (Tc-99m DMSA), or succimer, bind to proximal tubular cells in the renal cortex. This makes possible static imaging of the renal parenchymal cortex (Figures 12-6, 12-7). Because uptake and binding require functioning renal cel-

Flow study, planar + tomographic images of spine
                    (SPECT)
in 30 young pts c̄ back pain

Can use Free Tc-pertechnetate (NOT Tc-labelled
　　　　　　　or Iodine　　　　　　　　　　Iodine)

c̄ Renovascular disease after captopr.

Renal scan → hippuran → GFR 20%　　　　　↑ & sustained hippuran tracer
　　　　　　　　　　　+++ secretion 80%

　　us DTPA → +++ GFR (pure GFR)　　　　↓ uptake of tracer
　　　　　　　　　　100%?

Tc-glucoheptonate → Blood flow study for kidneys
　　　　　　　　　(image/4 sec × 15 ≈ 60 sec
　　　　　　　　　　of 2 min, equilibrium phase
　　　　　　　　　& can obtain both image
　　　　　　　　　of kidneys b/c 15% localizes to cortex
　　　　　　　　　　(AP + 2 Obliques)

Hippuran → 30 min. study, ≈ 15 images

Papillary CA → local invasion, neck nodes +/- chest
Follicular CA → hematogenous ⓐ bone mets, distant mets.

R/O coronary artery disease → sestamibi
⬤ Assess myocardial viability → ~~Gallium~~ Tl is better
　　　　　　　　　　　　　　　to show viable tissue
　　　　　　　　　　　　　　　(sestamibi may _ show if
　　　　　　　　　　　　　　　　isn't viable)

Gastric emptying → use any Tc-labelled compound
　　　　　　　　　(except pertechnetate which sticks mucosel lining)
　　　　　　　　　　　　of mouth   esoph.
　　→ measure counts(ROI) in stomach at t = 0
　　　then every 30 sec × total 30 min
　　　measure ROI at 30 min   see % emptying al 30 min
　　　then calculate T½ by

Sestamibi & picked up
by PT adenom / thyroid adn. (Can also code Tl
(both are perfusion)
tracers

Persantine (for stress-test)
↳ blocks adenosine breakdown
∴ vasodilates

☺

No caffeine prior to test
Contraind

Ga → Think of it as
Iron → binds to transferrin
lactoferrin (released at sites
of infection)

90
190 } → these ones are
290 }   imaged.
390 }

-capillary leak
-lactoferrin release
-tumors, why?

-excreted in GI mucosa
-taken up by lacrimals + saliv. glands
liver (iron stores)
colon

Sickle cell bone scan Tc-MDP
→

Mets → spine
sternum
prox. long bones
SI area
ribs

Martai's neuvrond

Blood Flow study prior to Tc-MDP
1) Arterial phase } image/4sec x15 = 60sec
2) capillary "
3) venous phase
4) Equilibrium phase ≈ 2min = blood pool on
" volume image
(∴ ↑ for hyperemia
which implies acute/
aggressive process

↳ ectopic
PT adenoma

(Tl) → Mercury
vs. Tc-sestamibi for 1ˢᵗ pass
            + EF

~~Need~~ Can only use ↓ dose of Tl 2m Cu
b/c of: 1) ↑ ½ life (3 days vs. 6 hrs for Tc)
        2) ↓ photopeak (∴ ↑ absorption by pt
                        keV ≈ 80
                        vs 144 for Tc 99)

For well perfusion,
        Cardiolite (Tc-sestamibi)
            ↳ gets into all cells which are active,
                eg. pecs, heart
        & later into liver, GB & excreted via biliary tree

                        taken up by
Tin-colloid   →   RES   eg. kupffer cells in liver
(vs. sulfer-colloid   WBCs in spleen
  b/c don't need   shouldn't {   up in marrow } the 1ᵉʳ this
    to heat it up   normally {   intensity is, the
    & don't need   see this. [+ up in lungs   } sharper the
    gelatin   liver isn't only
         ☺ easy to prepare   ☺ ↑ up activity
Ti   (shake & bake)   "colloid"   elsewhere
             ∴ Tin-colloid → get shift" into spleen
                        b/c longer particles in Tin
             whereas c Sulf. colloid → if there is
                    a shift (ratio ≈ spleen) ∴ ↓ T
                        = hepatic dysfunction

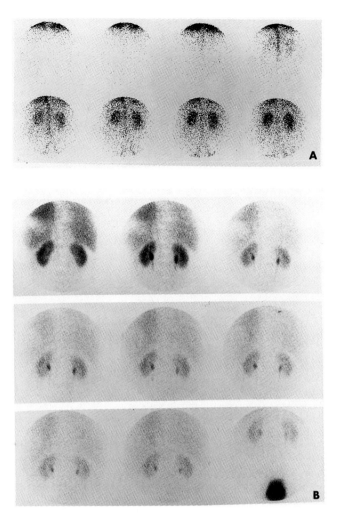

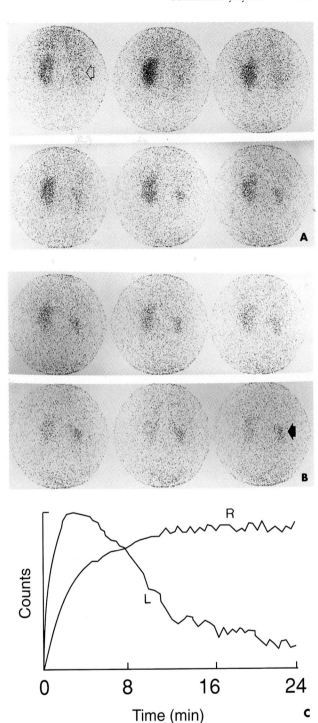

Fig. 12-4   Tc-99m DTPA normal study. **A,** The blood flow phase shows prompt perfusion to both kidneys bilaterally. **B,** Dynamic sequential images aquired for 30 minutes. The first image was acquired for 500,000 counts and taken immediately after the 60-second flow study. The second image was taken at 3 minutes, and each subsequent image was aquired every 5 minutes thereafter for equal time. The immediate blood pool image shows radiotracer in the liver, spleen, heart, and lungs, as well as in the kidneys. By the second image, cortical uptake is maximum and Tc-99m DTPA is already seen in the pelvis and ureters. Renal and background clearance are rapid, consistent with very good function. The distal ureters are never well visualized, not uncommon. In the last image, the field of view has been moved up to include the bladder.

Fig. 12-5   **A** and **B,** I-131 hippuran study in a hypertensive patient with proven renal artery stenosis of the right kidney. The image quality is inferior to that achieved with Tc-99m DTPA (see Figure 12-4). However, the kidney-to-background ratio is high. No renal flow study is possible because of the low administered dose (250 μCi). Note the initially decreased uptake in the right kidney (*open arrowhead*). With sequential images acquired every 2 minutes, the normally functioning left kidney has completely cleared by the end of the 24 minute study (*closed arrowhead*), while the poorly functioning right kidney is better seen (flip-flop) owing to delayed uptake of tracer. **C,** Time–activity curves confirm the visual impression. The left kidney exhibits normal uptake and clearance, while the right kidney has very delayed uptake.

Box 12-3	**Renal Tubular Radiopharma-**
	ceuticals for ERPF Quantitation

H-2 or C-14 PAH

I-125, I-131 iodopyracet

I-125, **I-123,** or **I-131 OIH**

Tc-99m MAG3

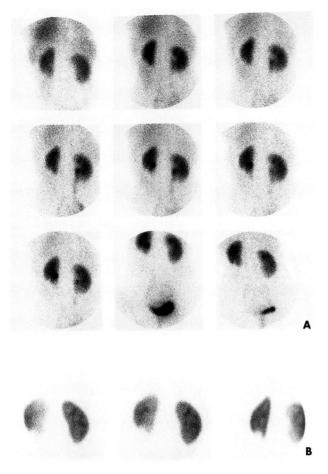

Fig. 12-6   Tc-99m glucoheptonate in a patient with known vesicoureteral reflux. Tc-99m GH permits a flow and dynamic phase study (**A**), as well as delayed cortical imaging (**B**). Both phases show a cortical defect in the lower pole of the left kidney. The delayed images were acquired using a pinhole collimator (*left to right:* RPO, posterior, and LPO views), which resulted in improved resolution.

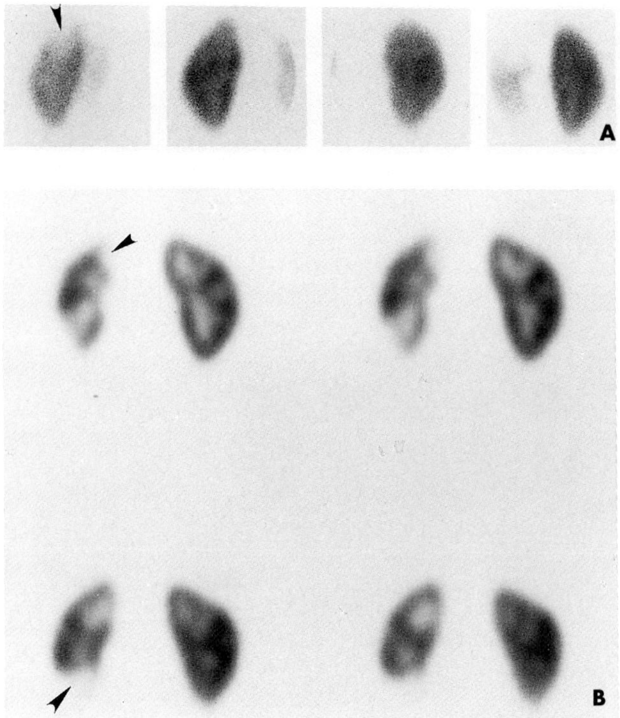

Fig. 12-7   Tc-99m DMSA planar and high-resolution SPECT images in two different patients with cortical scars secondary to reflux. **A,** Planar images acquired using a pinhole collimator. *Left to right:* LPO, posterior (left kidney), posterior, and RPO (right kidney) views. A cortical defect in the superior pole on the left (*arrowhead*) is best seen in the LPO view. **B,** High-resolution SPECT sequential 3.5-mm coronal sections showing a cortical defect in the upper pole and a larger defect in the right lower pole. Note the distinct separation of cortex from medulla and collecting system with SPECT imaging.

lular elements, the radiopharmaceutical is not taken up in cysts, tumors, scars, and so forth, which appear scintigraphically as photon-deficient areas. Due to a cortical dysfunction resulting from *acute pyelonephritis*, binding is impaired and parenchymal defects are seen. This finding is reversible with appropriate antibiotic therapy.

Glomerular and Tubular Imaging Agents

Technetium-99m DTPA

Chemistry and radiolabeling   Radiolabeling of Tc-99m DTPA is accomplished in commercial preparations by using stannous ion as a reducing agent. The DTPA molecule is a powerful chelating agent that binds Tc-99m avidly in reduced form, although the exact charge of the Tc complex is uncertain. As with all Tc-99m radiolabeled agents there is a potential for radiopharmaceutical contaminants due to oxidation of Tc-99m and/or unlabeled reduction products. In vitro, these contaminants are readily detected by radiochromatography.

In vivo, free Tc-99m pertechnetate is recognized by uptake in the thyroid, salivary glands, and stomach and by its longer persistence in the blood pool than Tc-99m DTPA. Colloidal impurities may be recognized by increased uptake and prolonged retention of activity in the liver and other reticuloendothelial system components.

Pharmacokinetics   The pharmacokinetics of Tc-99m DTPA are very similar to those of radiographic contrast media (e.g., diatrizoate and iodothalamate) because they are also "glomerular" agents. I-125-radiolabeled iothalamate is commercially available in the United States and can be used for nonimaging quantitative measurements of glomerular filtration.

After intravenous (IV) injection, Tc-99m DTPA is rapidly distributed by the arterial circulation throughout the body. This vascular phase permits an assessment of renal perfusion. It then diffuses rapidly into the extracellular fluid space of the body but does not enter cells. Peak glomerular filtration occurs 3 to 4 minutes after tracer administration. Tc-99m DTPA has a first-pass extraction fraction (arterial – venous difference) of about 20% with normal renal function, less with poor function.

Clearance is a function of the GFR, normally 120 mL/min. The biological half-life is just under 2.5 hours, with approximately 95% of the administered dose cleared from the body of normal subjects in 24 hours. During the parenchymal uptake phase the renal cortical outlines are well visualized. By 5 minutes, tracer appears in the renal collecting system, with visualization of the calyces and then the pelvis. The ureters are not always visualized in normal subjects with normal urine flow rates. Bladder activity is usually seen by 10 to 15 minutes (see Figure 12-4). The half-time of renal clearance is 15 to 20 minutes.

Ortho-iodohippuric acid

Chemistry and radiolabeling   OIH is commercially available as both an I-131- and an I-123-labeled radiopharmaceutical. It is radiolabeled by an exchange reaction. The agent has a tendency to degrade with time and should be stored at 4°C or less and be protected from light. Stabilizing and buffering agents are added for pH adjustment.

Pharmacokinetics   Because radioiodinated OIH is cleared by both tubular and glomerular mechanisms, the biological half-life is less than that of Tc-99m DTPA. In subjects with normal renal function, it is 1 hour or less. The vast majority (98%) of the administered agent is cleared within 24 hours, with a small amount excreted heterotopically in bile. The normal renal clearance half-time is about 10 to 15 minutes.

After IV administration of OIH, the kidneys are rapidly visualized, with a peak cortical concentration achieved in 3 to 5 minutes. Blood flow is not directly evaluated with I-131 or I-123 OIH because of the low administered doses (300 μCi and 1 mCi). The sequence of pelvicocalyceal and bladder visualization is similar but slightly faster than Tc-99m DTPA (see Figure 12-5). The first-pass extraction fraction of OIH is approximately 85% in subjects with normal renal function, less in those with renal insufficiency.

Patients should receive Lugol's solution or saturated solution of potassium iodide (SSKI) before administration of the radioiodinated agent to prevent any unlabeled radioiodine from being taken up by the thyroid. Free iodine should be minimized and can be assessed by radiochromatography. *United States Pharmacopeia* standards for OIH call for less than 3% free iodide. Because radioiodine crosses the placenta and is excreted in breast milk, additional precautions should be taken in women who are pregnant or breast-feeding. Conservatively, breast-feeding should be discontinued for at least 5 days.

OIH labeled with I-123 has advantages over OIH labeled with I-131. The image quality is superior and the radiation dose is less. However, the short half-life (15 hours) of I-123 and the long half-lives of its radionuclide impurities—I-124 or I-125, depending on its method of production—necessitate use on the day of calibration. I-131 has a long shelf life due to its 8 day half-life. Although initially expected to replace I-131 OIH, problems of ready availability, short shelf life, and cost have limited the widespread use of I-123 OIH.

Technetium-99m MAG3

Radiolabeling   Tc-99m MAG3 is available in kit form. The labeling procedure entails the addition of sodium pertechnetate to a reaction vial. A unique feature of the labeling process is that a small amount of air is added to the reaction vial to consume excess stannous ion for increased stability. Radiolabeling efficiency is 95% or greater.

Pharmacokinetics   Tc-99m MAG3 is an important new renal tubular agent that has been touted as a replacement for OIH because of its Tc-99m label. It is not truly an OIH analogue. Tc-99m MAG3 is a pure tubular agent, with higher protein binding, slower plasma clearance, and a smaller volume of distribution than OIH. Because of these pharmacokinetic differences, Tc-99m MAG3 cannot be used to directly calculate ERPF, although a "correction factor" has been used to translate MAG3 clearance into estimated ERPF values. Tc-99m MAG3's important alternative route of excretion is hepatobiliary.

The advantages of Tc-99m MAG3 compared to OIH include better image quality resulting from the Tc-99m versus radioiodine label and a lower radiation absorbed dose, especially in patients with diminished renal function. And, importantly, flow images can be performed. Tc-99m MAG3 is particularly useful in patients with renal insufficiency, for it produces images and time-activity curves similar but superior to those achieved with OIH. For scintigraphic purposes, Tc-99m MAG3 combines the qualities of Tc-99m DTPA and OIH and can be effectively used as an alternative (Figure 12-8). Cost is the major factor preventing its universal use.

Cortical imaging agents   The original agents for imaging the renal cortex were based on radiolabeling of the diuretic chlormerodrin with mercury-203 and then mercury-197. These agents have been abandoned in favor of the technetium-labeled radiopharmaceuticals, Tc-99m DMSA and Tc-99m GH. Both agents are supplied in kit form and employ stannous ion for reducing Tc-99m pertechnetate.

Tc-99m glucoheptonate   About 80% of Tc-99m GH is filtered through the glomerulus, the remaining 20% becoming fixed to the proximal renal tubular cells by tight sulfhydryl-group binding. Cortical images are obtained 1.5 to 2 hours after injection to allow maximal cortical uptake and renal clearance from background soft tissue and the renal collecting structures. A dynamic imag-

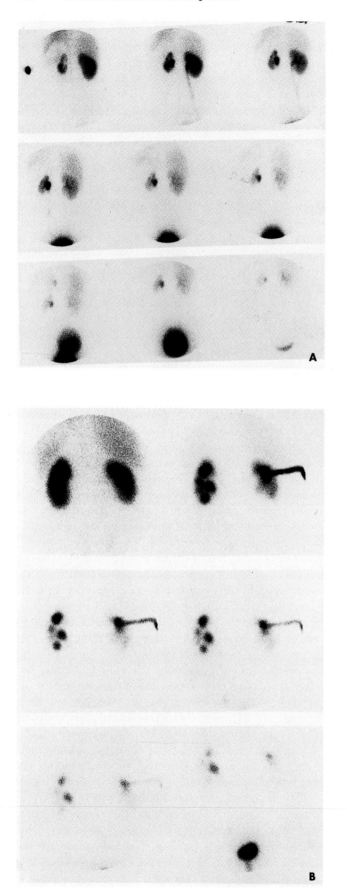

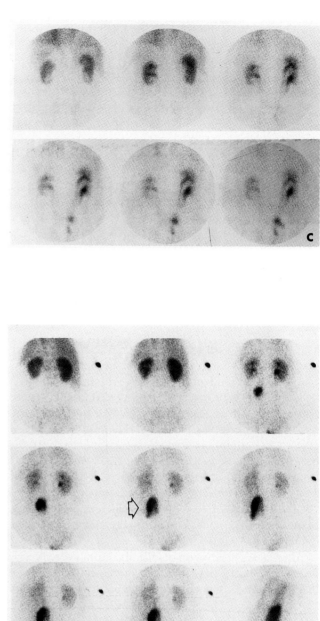

Fig. 12-8   Tc-99m MAG3 studies. **A,** Small scarred left kidney secondary to vesicoureteral reflux. Differential function was calculated to be 85% on the right and 15% on the left. Good cortical definition can be seen in both kidneys. The normal right ureter is seen. There is mildly increasing hepatic uptake over time, which is normal. Although transient residual activity is seen in the left renal pelvis, cortical clearance is bilaterally symmetric. Patient movement is noted in the lower left image. **B,** Obstruction of the right kidney secondary to cervical carcinoma. A nephrostomy tube has been placed and is draining well. Renal function appears good bilaterally. Prominent calyces on the left and the pelvis clear by the end of the study. **C,** A duplicated collecting system is seen on the left. This congenital abnormality often is associated with reflux and infection of the lower pole and obstruction of the upper pole. **D,** Post-operative patient with cervical carcinoma. Rapid ureteral leak detected early in the imaging sequence (*arrowhead*).

Table 12-3 Radiation Dosimetry for Renal Radiopharmaceuticals

Organ	I-123 OIH (rads/1 mCi)	I-131 OIH (rads/300 μCi)	Tc-DTPA (rads/20 mCi)	Tc-MAG3 (rads/8 mCi)	Tc-DMSA (rads/5 mCi)	Tc-GH (rads/20 mCi)
Bladder	0.95	1.55	5.40	4.80	0.42	2.4
Kidneys	0.05	0.05	1.80	0.14	3.78	4.8
Ovaries	0.05	0.03	0.31	0.26	0.04	0.2
Testes	0.03	0.02	0.21	0.16	0.04	0.2
Whole body	0.02	0.01	0.12	0.07	0.09	0.2

Modified from product information brochures, Medi-Physics Inc, Paramus, NJ, and Mallinckrodt Medical, Inc, St Louis, Mo.

ing sequence similar to that used with Tc-99m DTPA and Tc-99m MAG3 can be used for Tc-99m GH during the first 30 minutes after injection, giving additional information about blood flow, dynamic function, and collecting system patency (see Figure 12-6). The liver serves as the alternative route of excretion, and gallbladder uptake is occasionally seen.

Tc-99m DMSA   Maximal renal cortical uptake of Tc-99m DMSA is reached within 3 to 6 hours of radiotracer administration. Compared to Tc-99m GH, a significantly higher fraction of the dose of Tc-99 DMSA is bound to the cortex, on the order of 40% to 50%, and a smaller fraction is excreted into the urine. Because of the different administered doses (5 mCi DMSA, 15-20 mCi Tc-99m GH), the absolute amount that binds to the kidneys is comparable.

The principal advantage of the renal cortical agents is their relatively prolonged and stable retention in the kidney after background and urinary clearance. This allows high-resolution imaging with pinhole collimators or single photon emission computed temography (SPECT) (see Figure 12-7). The rapid, dynamic transit of Tc-99m DTPA, OIH, and Tc-99m MAG3 is not suited for the longer imaging times required for these high-resolution techniques.

Radiation Dosimetry

The radiation absorbed dose to the patient from renal radiopharmaceuticals (Table 12-3), even I-131 OIH, is quite low in subjects with normal renal function. In renal failure, the absorbed dose is still limited by the 6-hour half-life of Tc-99m-labeled tracers; however, with I-131-labeled agents, the absorbed dose can rise significantly (Table 12-4).

IMAGING TECHNIQUES

Renal imaging and function study protocols are modified or tailored for specific clinical applications. This section presents a basic approach to imaging with each of the three major classes of renal radiopharmaceuticals. Modifications and interventions are discussed under their respective clinical applications.

Dynamic Renal Scintigraphy for Tc-99m Agents

A similar protocol can be used for Tc-99m DTPA, Tc-99m MAG3, and Tc-99m GH (Box 12-4). Good patient hydration is important. Dehydration can result in delayed uptake and excretion, simulating poor function. The patient should be positioned supine, for ptotic kidneys move inferiorly and anteriorly when upright. Renal transplant patients are imaged anteriorly because the allograft is usually located in the extraperitoneal iliac fossa.

Table 12-4 Renal Dosimetry for I-131 OIH in Disease States

Condition	rads/mCi	rads/300 μCi
Normal	0.1	0.03
Tubular necrosis	6.0	1.80
Glomerulonephritis	67.5	20.25
Outflow obstruction (50% uptake)	400.0	120.00

Modified from Elliot AT and Britton KE: *J Appl Radiat Isot* 29:571-573, 1978.

Box 12-4   Dynamic Renal Scintigraphy With Tc-99m DTPA, Tc-99m MAG3, or Tc-99m GH: Protocol Summary

PATIENT PREPARATION

Hydration: Adults drink 300-500 mL water.
Children: IV hydration with D5W, 15 mL/kg over 30 min.
Have patient void prior to beginning study.

INSTRUMENTATION

Gamma camera: large field of view gamma camera.
Collimator: low-energy all-purpose parallel-hole collimator.
Photopeak: 15%-20% window centered over 140 keV (Tc-99m) or 159 keV (I-123) window.

PATIENT POSITION

Supine. Image posteriorly, except in renal transplant patients, who are imaged anteriorly.

RADIOPHARMACEUTICAL

Tc-99m DTPA:
Adult: 15 mCi.
Pediatric dose: 200 μCi/kg, 2 mCi minimum, 10 mCi maximum.

Tc-99m GH:
Adult: 20 mCi.
Pediatric dose: same as for Tc-99m DTPA.

Tc-99m MAG3:
Adult: 8 mCi.
Pediatric dose: 100 μCi/kg, 1 mCi minimum, 5 mCi maximum.

COMPUTER ACQUISITION

1-sec frames × 60, then 30-sec frames × 25 min.

STATIC OR ANALOG IMAGE FORMAT

2-sec flow images.
Dynamic images: immediate image for 500 k count, then acquire images every 5 min for equal time for study duration.
Obtain a postvoiding image.

PROCESSING

Draw ROIs on computer around kidneys and background. Generate time-activity curves for 60-sec flow phase and 25-min study.

Commonly used adult doses are 15 mCi for Tc-99m DTPA, 20 mCi for Tc-99m GH, and 8 mCi for Tc-99m MAG3. Doses in children are lower. Various methods for estimating pediatric doses have been used, including methods based on age (Webster's rule: [age + 1] / [age + 7] × adult dose) or nomograms based on weight or body surface area.

The study is usually performed in two phases: a "flow" or perfusion phase (radionuclide angiography) followed by a dynamic functional phase demonstrating uptake and clearance of the radiotracer.

In contemporary practice computer acquisition and analysis is mandatory. With older but still commonly used analog cameras, data are acquired simultaneously on film directly from the gamma camera and separately on computer after analog-to-digital conversion. Analog film parameters must be preset on the camera formatter (e.g., 2-second flow images × 30, then a 500 k count immediate image, followed by images acquired for an equal time every 5 minutes × 5). With the newer digital cameras, hard copy formatting is done directly from the computer after acquisition in whatever format is desired: images can be summed according to a routine protocol or determined on an individual basis. Computer acquisition permits improved qualitative and quantitative analysis.

Dynamic Renal Scintigraphy for Radioiodinated OIH

Patient preparation and positioning are the same for studies with OIH as for studies with Tc-99m DTPA. The usual adult dose of I-131 OIH is 300 μCi and for I-123 OIH it is 1.0 mCi. The protocol for OIH is similar to the Tc-99m studies, except that flow studies are not performed (Box 12-5). I-131 OIH requires a high energy collimator.

Renal Cortical Imaging

With Tc-99m DMSA, dynamic imaging is not useful because background clearance is slow and only a relatively small percentage of radiotracer (25%) is cleared by the kidney. Only delayed cortical planar or SPECT imaging is required. Planar imaging is performed in multiple views, such as the posterior and left and right posterior oblique views, using a high-resolution pinhole collimator (Figure 12-7). Box 12-6 describes a typical protocol. High-resolution SPECT affords excellent cortical imaging, even in small children; however, a multi-headed camera is required (Figure 12-9). Single-headed SPECT resolution is insufficient for quality imaging. Sedation may be needed for small children. Tc-99m GH can be imaged similarly.

COMPUTER PROCESSING OF RENAL STUDIES

Computer processing of renal studies can be a valuable aid in evaluating renal blood flow, function, and collecting system patency. Mentally integrating all the information in the acquired images, however, can be difficult, even for the experienced observer. Computer-processed time-activity curves give a two-dimensional representa-

---

Box 12-5   Imaging with I-131 and I-123 OIH: Protocol Summary

PATIENT PREPARATION

Hydration: oral or IV. See Box 12-4.
Patient should void prior to initiation of study.

INSTRUMENTATION

Gamma camera: large field of view gamma camera in adults.

Collimator:	high-energy parallel-hole for I-131, LEAP for I-123.
Photopeak:	20% window over 364 keV I-131 or 159 keV I-123 photopeak.

PATIENT POSITION

Supine. Image posteriorly, except in renal transplant patients who are imaged anteriorly.

RADIOPHARMACEUTICAL

Inject IV.

I-131 OIH:	Adult—300 µCi; Children—3 µCi/kg.
I-123 OIH:	1 mCi.

ANALOG FILM ACQUISITION

I-131 OIH:	2-min images immediately after injection and every 5 min for 20 min.
I-123 OIH:	500 k count images immediately, then acquire images every 5 min for equal time.

Acquire a postvoiding image.

COMPUTER ACQUISITION

60-sec frames × 20, then 1-min frames × 19

PROCESSING

ROIs placed around kidneys and background. Generate time-activity curves.

Box 12-6   Protocol for Renal Cortical Imaging With Tc-99m DMSA or Tc-99m GH

RADIOPHARMACEUTICAL

Tc-99m DMSA:	Adult: 5 mCi.
	Pediatric dose:50 µg/kg (minimum dose, of 600 µCi).
Tc-99m GH:	Adult: 15-20 µCi. Child: 200 µCi/kg.

INSTRUMENTATION

Planar Imaging

1. Pinhole collimator for cortical imaging. A converging collimator can be used for adults and large children.
2. Wide field of view camera with low-energy all-purpose collimator for anterior and posterior images for quantitation of relative renal function.
3. SPECT: Dual- or triple-headed SPECT camera.

PROCEDURE

1. Inject radiopharmaceutical IV.
2. Have patient void prior to imaging.
3. Begin imaging 2 hr post injection.
4. Acquire pinhole images for 100 k counts per view. Position patient to image each kidney separately in the posterior, RPO, and LPO views.
5. Acquire anterior and posterior views for 500 k counts using a parallel-hole collimator to include both kidneys for quantitation of differential function. Acquired on computer.
6. Quantitate differential function by drawing ROIs on anterior and posterior views for both kidneys. Calculate the geometric mean (square root of the product) counts for each kidney and differential function.

SPECT

Camera:	triple-headed with low-energy, ultra-high-resolution collimator.
Matrix:	128 × 128.
Zoom:	adjusted so that outside distance between kidneys on the posterior view is between 50 and 64 pixels.
Orbit:	noncircular body contour, rotate 180°, step and shoot 40 views/head, 3° per stop, 40 sec per acquisition.
Reconstruction:	64 × 64.
	Hamming filter with high cutoff 2.0. Smoothing kernel 1 3 5 3 1. Attenuation correction: 4 pt ellipse, attenuation coefficient = 0.11.

---

tion of the temporal changes in flow and function that can aid in assimilating this data.

The time-activity curves and quantitative indices derived should never be interpeted alone, but rather in conjunction with image review. The reasons for discrepancies must be understood and explained. Time-activity curves can be affected by a number of variables, especially the specific renal and background regions of interest (ROIs) selected.

Radionuclide Renography

The renogram or time-activity curve shows the renal uptake and transit of the radiopharmaceutical and is classically divided into three phases (see Figure 12-9): the *tracer appearance* phase (blood flow), characterized by a sharp rise in the curve due to radioactivity in the blood pool; the *uptake* phase, in which the time-activity curve rises owing to parenchymal accumulation of tracer, either filtered by the glomerulus, secreted by the tubules, or both, depending on the radiopharmaceutical; and the *excretory* phase, in which the time-

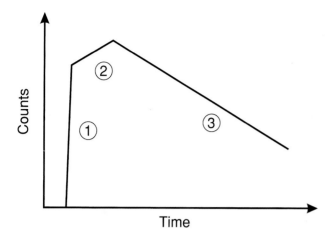

Fig. 12-9 Schematic diagram showing the three phases of a renogram: *1*, the initial blood flow phase (30–60 seconds), *2*, the cortical uptake phase (normally between 1 and 3 minutes) and *3*, the clearance phase representing cortical excretion and collecting system clearance.

activity curve falls as tracer leaves the cortex and urinary collecting system.

Renal flow   Time-activity curves can be generated for the 60-second flow study (Figure 12-10). ROIs are drawn for the kidney and the adjacent artery, which is the aorta for subjects with two kidneys and the aorta or iliac artery for renal tranplant patients. Background ROIs are not usually necessary because there is not significant background during the arterial flow phase. The computer-generated time-activity curves can be quite helpful in deciding the importance of flow differences noted on the 2- to 3-second images. They can help the observer determine, for instance, whether there is a true flow abnormality or simply a poor bolus injection (see Figure 12-10C). Time-activity curves are particularly useful for comparing serial studies done over time, as in renal transplant recipients.

Absolute flow measured in milliliters per kilogram per minute, cannot be determined using the radiotracers discussed; however, relative flow parameters can be helpful. Semiquantitative indices can be derived from time-activity curves. One common method is to calculate a ratio of the upslope of the early portion of the time-activity curves for the kidneys compared to the arterial supply, such as the aorta (K/A ratio). The slopes should be similar. Another method uses a ratio of the total counts integrated under the two curves. Both methods are subject to technical errors, and attention to detail is needed to use these numbers appropriately.

These indices are most valuable for following the course of an individual subject undergoing serial studies. Similar ROIs must be used for all studies. Quantitation is not mandatory. The relative upslopes of the time-activity curves can be judged subjectively quite easily and used clinically without specific quantitation.

Renal function   Time-activity curves should be routine for evaluation of dynamic renal function with Tc-99m DTPA, Tc-99m MAG3, Tc-99m GH, I-123 OIH, and I-131 OIH. The curves should be generated for the entire 25 minute study. Considerable information can be derived from these curves. Uptake and clearance of the radiotracer can be quickly appreciated (Figures 12-5C, 12-11).

Care should be taken in proper kidney ROI selection. The correct ROI depends to some extent on the information needed. Whole kidney ROIs can be used for cortical function curves if collecting system activity clears without delay. However, with calyceal retention of tracer, a 2-pixel ROI along the cortical edge would likely be more accurate. However, differential function requires ROIs that include the entire kidney, because excluding the pelvis and calyces will likely exclude the cortex, making quantitation erroneous. Differential renal uptake will be accurate because it is determined before the tracer appears in the collecting system (1-3 minutes). In contrast, diuretic renography demands ROIs that include all the collecting system, as discussed later.

Various parameters of function have been derived from these time-activity curves, among them time to peak activity, slope of uptake, rate of clearance, percentage clearance at 20 minutes, and so forth. No general standard exists, and personal preference and experience determine the use of these and other derived parameters. Again, qualitative analysis of the curves without quantitation can be very valuable. Quantitation must always be used in conjunction with image analysis.

Individual renal function   Individual or differential renal function studies should be routinely performed in all patients with two kidneys. This is information that cannot easily be obtained from any nonradionuclide method. Individual renal function represents the percentage of radiotracer taken up by each kidney and, in essence, the percent functional mass of each kidney. Whole kidney ROIs are chosen and background corrected.

Differential function is calculated using the uptake counts following the flow phase but before the radioactive tracer arrives in the collecting system (extraction phase), usually the time period between 1 and 3 minutes after tracer administration. Differential function is calculated by dividing the background subtracted counts of one kidney by the total background-corrected counts of the two kidneys.

With Tc-99m DMSA and Tc-99m GH cortical imaging, background correction is also usually performed but is less critical because of the relatively high uptake in the cortex compared to background during the 2-hour imaging period. Background becomes more critical in subjects with renal insufficiency.

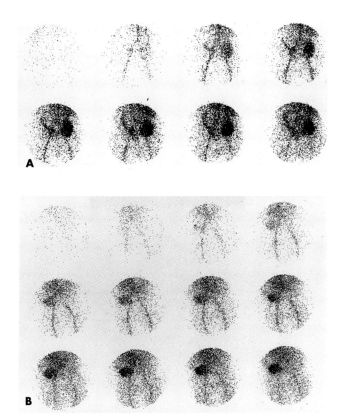

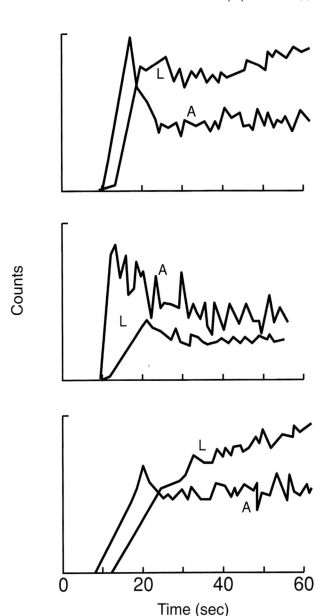

Fig. 12-10 **A,** Radionuclide angiogram in a diabetic patient with a recently tranplanted kidney and pancreas. Imaged anteriorly, the 2-second frames show the bolus rapidly transiting the aorta and the iliac vessels with good perfusion of the pancreas (*right*) and kidney (*left*). **B,** Poor blood flow or poor bolus? Two-second-per-frame images in a different patient show slow transit and fragmentation of the bolus as it passes through the aorta and iliac vessels. This might be misinterpreted as delayed renal flow. A time-activity curve can be quite helpful in differentiating the two. **C,** Flow time-activity curves derived from ROIs flagged for the arterial vessel (*A*) and the kidney (*L*) in three different renal transplant patients. With good flow (top), the initial slopes of the arterial and renal curves are steep and similar. With very poor flow (*middle*), the upslope is much less steep and delayed compared to the arterial curve. With a poor bolus (*bottom*), neither the arterial nor the renal upstrokes are steep, and both equally delayed.

The appropriate choice of background ROIs is also important. Unfortunately, true background cannot be determined. There is some difference of opinion as to the ideal background ROI. Commonly, 2-pixel semilunar ROIs adjacent and inferolateral to the kidneys are chosen (Figure 12-12). Others encircle the whole kidney; yet others have used a single region located between the two kidneys. Caution is necessary when the liver and spleen overlap the kidneys, especially in the setting of renal insufficiency. This is a special problem with Tc-99m MAG3 because of its alternative hepatobiliary route of excretion.

The accuracy of background subtraction decreases

with poor renal function. In such patients, methods that result in the least background may be more accurate, such as the use of Tc-99m DMSA or Tc-99m OIH as tracer. With Tc-99m DMSA or Tc-99m GH, imaging can be delayed for up to 24 hours to maximize background clearance. Normal values for differential function vary between 45% and 55%.

Quantitative renal function Clinical assessment of renal function is relatively crude. Patients may have a significant reduction in renal function before the serum blood urea nitrogen (BUN) or creatinine levels rise. The 24-hour urinary creatinine clearance rate is more accurate but requires urine collection with its associated diffi-

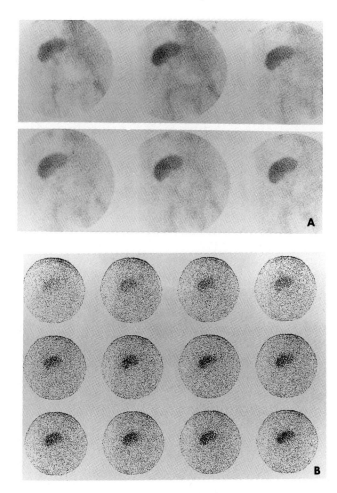

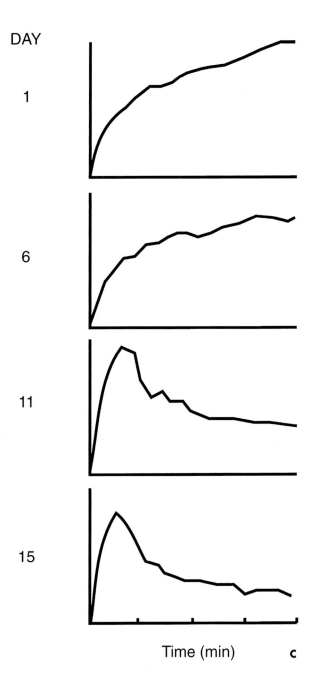

Fig. 12-11   Acute tubular necrosis following renal transplantation. Blood flow to the kidney was normal (not shown). **A**, The Tc-99m DTPA study shows poor renal uptake and no excretion, resulting in a high persistent level of background activity over the 30 minute study. **B**, I-131 hippuran study in the same patient performed immediately after shows a similar pattern of delayed uptake and no clearance. Unlike Tc-99m DTPA, no vascular structures are seen. **C**, Time-activity curves for I-131 OIH on day 1 (this study) and follow-up studies on days 6, 11, and 15. ATN resolved over a 2-week period. Note that as function improves, the curves change from having a gradual upslope without a plateau to having a clear-cut early peak and definite clearance.

culties. Accurate quantitation of GFR or ERPF with non-radioactive inulin or PAH, respectively, requires a constant infusion technique, multiple blood and urine samples, and chemical analysis—none of these tests that are routinely performed on a clinical basis.

A number of quantitative radionuclide methods for measuring renal function have been developed. They can be divided into blood sampling techniques and camera-based methods. Tc-99m DTPA is most commonly used in the United States to calculate GFR because of its low cost and widespread availability. However, I-125 iodothalamate is commercially available for use in the

United States, and Cr-51 EDTA is available in Europe. I-123 or I-131 OIH is used to calculated ERPF.

Accurate renal function can be quantified from the plasma disappearance curve derived from multiple blood samples. The more samples, the more accurate is the analysis. However, simplified methods using two or even one blood sample have been validated. A popular one-sample technique for determining the GFR that uses Tc-99m DTPA as the tracer requires a single sample drawn at 3 hours. For I-131 OIH tracer determination of the ERPF, 44 minutes appears to be the optimal time.

Camera-based methods have been validated for use

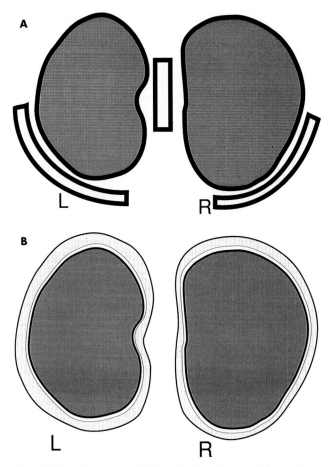

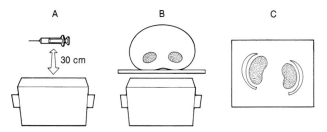

Fig. 12-13 Gamma camera technique for quantitative GFR calculation. **A,** A 1-minute image is acquired of the Tc-99m DTPA syringe before and after injection 30 cm from the center of the collimator. After injection, 15-seconds-per-frame images are acquired for a total of 6 minutes. Kidney and background ROIs are selected. The background-corrected net renal cortical uptake as a percentage of the injected dose for each kidney is determined. Attenuation correction is performed using the patient's height and weight. To estimate GFR, these data are inserted into a regression analysis formula derived from studying in an identical manner a group of patients who also had GFRs calculated by a standardized method.

Fig. 12-12 Background ROI selection. Three different background ROIs are selected. Each has been recommended and used in different laboratories. **A,** The curvilinear ROI around the inferior lateral aspect of both kidneys is most commonly used with dynamic renal scintigraphy. The single interrenal ROI is less commonly used. **B,** The 1- to 2-pixel ROI surrounding the entire kidney is often utilized with cortical imaging.

with modern gamma cameras. These methods require no blood sampling and no more than 15 minutes of imaging time (Figure 12-13). The basis for this technique is that early radiotracer uptake by each kidney is directly proportional to its clearance. Once the mathematical relationship between uptake and some measurement of renal function—GFR, creatinine clearance rate, or ERPF—has been established over a range of renal function, it can be applied clinically. The software to make these determinations is now available for most nuclear medicine computer systems.

It should be emphasized that the simplified radionuclide methods for quantifying renal function are estimates of function, with clinically acceptable levels of error. The error of the estimate typically increases in the setting of very poor renal function, but so does the error associated with presently used biochemical tests, such as the creatinine clearance rate.

To be useful clinically, a method need not be highly accurate; it is more important that it be reproducible. For example, the creatinine clearance rate is commonly used clinically basis to estimate GFR. However, this endogenous substance is reabsorbed and secreted by the renal tubules, as well as being filtered through the glomerulus. Thus, the GFR so determined is not an "accurate" measurement but a clinical estimate. Normal GFR is 100 mL/min, while the normal creatinine clearance rate is 120 mL/min. Therefore, the method is not very accurate but it is reproducible and has been found useful for following patients over time.

One problem limiting the more general acceptance of radionuclide methods is cost, which is often greater than that of the biochemical tests generally used. Radionuclide methods are most useful clinically in patients in whom urine collection is difficult, among them poorly cooperative patients, children, and in those with renal insufficiency. Camera-based methods offer another advantage: quantitation of *individual* renal function.

CLINICAL APPLICATIONS OF RADIONUCLIDE STUDIES

Scintigraphic Pattern in Normal Subjects

Once the peak of the arterial bolus has reached the level of the abdominal aorta, the outlines of the normal kidneys are completely visualized within 4 to 6 seconds. Any significant asymmetry in tracer distribution suggests decreased renal perfusion to that side. Delayed visualization of both kidneys is due either to a poor bolus, which can be assessed visually and confirmed with an aortic time-activity curve, or is the result of a bilateral renal flow abnormality.

The spleen is seen simultaneously with flow to the kidneys. The liver is visualized during the venous phase because of its predominant portal blood flow. In normal subjects there is no confusion in differentiating the kidneys, spleen, and liver. However, in patients with diminished renal function or lacking a left kidney, the spleen may be mistaken for the left kidney.

During the parenchymal tissue phase (1-3 minutes) of studies using either glomerular or tubular agents, the kidneys progressively accumulate radiotracer (see Figures 12-4, 12-5, 12-8). The renal cortex appears homogeneous without focal areas of decreased accumulation. With good-resolution images, the calyces and pelvis are seen as photopenic areas.

In the clearance phase, calyceal structures fill in, and over the following 10 to 15 minutes net activity in the kidney and the collecting structures decreases. In some healthy subjects, pooling of activity in the calyces results in focal hot spots, because imaging with the patient supine makes some calyces dependent with respect to the level of the ureteropelvic junction. Persistent pooling or visualization of pyelocalyceal structures overlapping the cortex or projecting well outside the renal outlines suggests hydronephrosis.

The normal ureter may or may not be visualized, depending on the urinary flow rate. Prolonged and especially unchanging visualization suggests ureteral dilation. The bladder is well seen in normal subjects. In small children and infants, the bladder can appear quite large and may project close to the kidneys, even occasionally overlapping the lower poles.

Radionuclide Evaluation of Urinary Tract Obstruction

The diagnosis and management of urinary tract obstruction is an important problem in both pediatric and adult urology. The clinician is often confronted with a dilated collecting system and must determine if it is obstructed or whether the dilation is a consequence of muscular atony or a structural abnormality. The distinction between significant mechanical obstruction and dilation not associated with obstruction is fundamental and critical to patient management. Uncorrected obstruction can lead to recurrent infection and ultimately to loss of renal function and parenchymal atrophy.

The sequence of pathophysiologic events leading to renal atrophy is complex and not completely understood. The process appears to be cyclical. Obstruction leads to increased pressure within the collecting structures. This pressure is transmitted through the luminal structures to the renal parenchyma, resulting in a reduction in parenchymal blood flow. A subsequent reduction in urine formation temporarily relieves the increased pressure while leaving the kidney with a lower func-

tional capacity. The pressure then gradually increases again and the cycle is repeated, with progressive loss of function and nephron dropout.

The changes due to obstruction can be arrested and to a certain extent reversed after surgical intervention. On the other hand, surgical intervention is not indicated in cases of dilation not associated with obstruction, such as vesicoureteral reflux.

Contrast intravenous urography (IVU), ultrasonography (US), and conventional radionuclide renography are unreliable for differentiating obstructive from nonobstructive causes of hydroureteronephrosis, owing to the overlap in findings between the conditions. Dilation, delayed opacification, and delayed washout are the hallmarks of obstruction on contrast-enhanced urography but may also be seen secondary to virtually any cause of collecting system dilation. US is a sensitive technique for detecting hydroureteronephrosis but does not depict urodynamics.

The *Whitaker test*, first described in the early 1970s, is used to measure pressure-flow relationships in the renal pelvis. The technique entails fluoroscopically guided insertion of a trocar, or in more recent practice, a 22-gauge spinal needle into the renal pelvis and bladder catheterization (Figure 12-14). Pressure in the renal pelvis and bladder is measured under basal conditions and after perfusion of a dilute solution of contrast medium at the rate of 10 mL/min. In a dilated, nonobstructed collecting system, the differential pressure between kidney and bladder remains low (<10-12 cm H_2O). In obstructed systems, the equilibrium perfusion pressure exceeds 15 cm H_2O, and is frequently much higher.

The percutaneous perfusion technique is contraindicated in patients with acute pyelonephritis. Pyelotubular backflow may occur with pelvic pressures greater than 30 cm H_2O and result in systemic infection. The technique is also contraindicated in patients with bleeding diatheses. It is associated with a significant radiation dose when done fluoroscopically. Owing to the need for a cannula in the renal pelvis, the technique does not lend itself to frequent follow-up studies. Variable results may be obtained, dependent on technical factors such as needle size, volume of the hydronephrotic collecting system, and flow rates.

Diuresis renography   For the study of urinary tract obstruction, conventional radionuclide renography has been modified to include an interventional maneuver, the administration of a potent diuretic. The fundamental hypothesis underlying the diuretic renography is that the prolonged retention of radioactivity seen in nonobstructed, dilated systems is due to a reservoir effect. Increased urine flow, as produced by a diuretic, will produce a prompt washout of activity in a dilated, nonobstructed system. In cases of mechanical obstruction with a narrowed and fixed luminal cross-sectional area at the ureteropelvic or ureterovesical junction, the capacity to augment washout is much

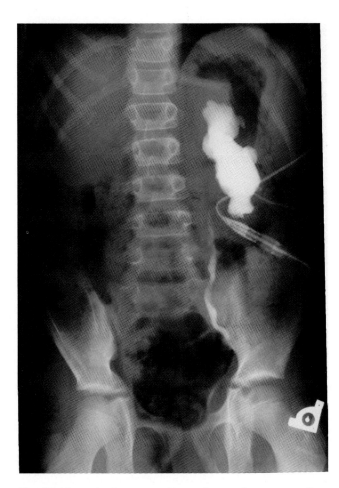

Fig. 12-14   Whitaker test. A dilute solution of contrast medium is infused into a dilated renal pelvis at the rate of 10 mL/min. Pressure measurements are obtained to evaluate for suspected obstruction.

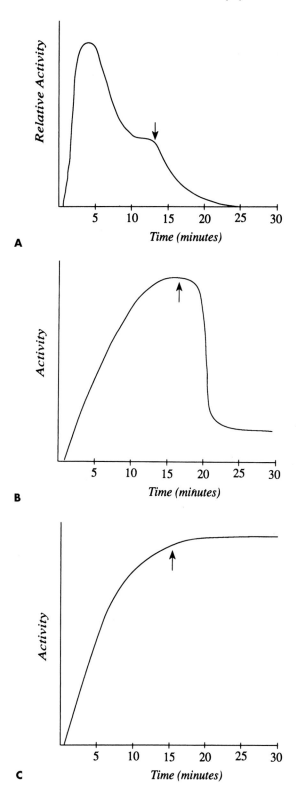

Fig. 12-15   Diuresis renography time-activity curves. In these examples, the diuretic is given at the time of peak collecting system filling. **A,** Normal kidney response to diuretic. The short plateau before further emptying represents diuretic-induced flow just prior to rapid clearance. **B,** Dilated nonobstructed kidney. The slowly rising curve represents progressive pelvicocalyceal filling. With diuretic administration (*arrow*), rapid clearance occurs. **C,** Obstructed kidney. The diuretic has no effect on the abnormal time-activity curve.

less, resulting in prolonged retention of tracer proximal to the obstruction (Figure 12-15).

For this method to be successful, renal function must be sufficient to promote a significant diuresis. Response patterns will depend on the timing of diuretic injection, the amount and type of diuretic, the route of administration, and the state of hydration of the patient.

Methodology   A typical imaging protocol for diuresis renography is detailed in Box 12-7. There are a number of variations of this technique. An attempt has been made to standarize the methodology for pediatric patients. Using the same technique is quite important when comparing data between institutions or in the same patient when studies are done serially over time.

Radiopharmaceuticals   The original agent used for diuresis renography was I-131 OIH. However, Tc-99m DTPA is more suited to studies with the gamma camera and has been used extensively. Tc-99m MAG3 is being increasingly utilized because of its better renal uptake in patients with renal insufficiency.

Box 12-7   Diuresis Renography: Protocol Summary

INDICATION

Evidence of pelvico-calyceal retention of radiotracer at end of routine renal scintigraphy using Tc-99m DPTA or Tc-99m MAG3.

PATIENT PREPARATION

Hydration described in protocol for dynamic renal scintigraphy. Place Foley catheters in children; optional for adults. If catheter is not used, complete bladder emptying is necessary prior to diuretic injection.

FUROSEMIDE DOSE

Approximate adult furosemide dose based on patient's creatinine:

Serum Creatinine	Creatinine Clearance	Furosemide Dose
1.0 mg/dL	100 cc/mL	20 mg
1.5	75	40
2.0	50	60
3.0	30	80

Furosemide dosage for children with normal renal function: 1 mg/kg.

INSTRUMENTATION

Camera: same as for dynamic renal scintigraphy.
Computer setup: 30-sec frames × 20 min.

PROCEDURE

Start computer and run for at least 60 sec prior to diuretic injection.
Inject Lasix slowly IV over 60 sec.
Obtain postvoiding image in patients without catheters.

PROCESSING

On computer, draw ROI around entire kidney, including pelvis. A ureteral ROI may be useful when dilated.
Generate time-activity curves.
Calculate a half-emptying time or fitted $T_{1/2}$.

Diuretic administration   Furosemide is the diuretic routinely used. It acts through inhibition of sodium and chloride reabsorption in the proximal and distal tubules and the ascending loop of Henle. IV administration of furosemide is required, because the peak effect following oral ingestion may not occur for an hour or longer. The injection is given slowly over 1 to 2 minutes. Onset of action occurs within 30 to 60 seconds. Side effects are unusual. A small number of patients experience nausea; syncope occurs rarely.

In the past, and still at some institutions, the diuretic is given as soon as pelvic filling is seen on the oscillo-scope or computer monitor, typically at 15 to 20 minutes (see Figure 12-15). For reasons of standardization, many institutions have adopted a two-phase study, particularly for children. First, routine dynamic renal scintigraphy is performed, as previously described. The second phase, diuretic renography, requires a second computer setup for an additional 20 minutes. Digital acquisition of data by computer is required to generate time-activity curves and calculate a half-emptying time.

Patients must be well hydrated so that fluid is available for mobilization in response to diuresis and to prevent dehydration. Other medical conditions must always be considered in managing fluid intake. If a catheter is not placed in the urinary tract, increased pressure from bladder filling can be transmitted, blunting the diuretic effect. Children and infants must be catheterized for the study, as must older subjects who are unable to void voluntarily. If no catheter is used (e.g., in an adult), the subject must void prior to the study.

Image analysis   Total ureteral obstruction of more than 24 hours' duration may result in a nonfunctioning kidney. With high-grade but lesser obstruction, scintigraphy will show poor blood flow, decreased function, and no evidence of radiotracer entering the collecting system (Figure 12-16). With lower-grade obstruction, the kidney will retain good blood flow and function and the radiotracer will empty into a hydronephrotic collecting system. However, during the 30-minute duration of the study, no pelvic or calyceal clearance will occur. During this period, the observer often cannot differentiate nonobstructed from obstructed hydronephrosis (Figures 12-17 to 12-19). Delayed imaging at about 4 hours can be helpful; for an obstructed kidney will show little change and a nonobstructed kidney will have been cleared of tracer. But this observation is variable, delays diagnosis, and is not quantitative. Images made during diuretic renography may show prompt clearance in a nonobstructed kidney and no clearance in an obstructed kidney. However, it is often not an all-or-none phenomenon, and time-activity curves can be quite valuable for interpretation of diuretic renography (see Figures 12-17 to 12-19).

Data analysis   Each kidney and ureter is analyzed separately with the aid of a computer. The entire study is first inspected frame by frame to assess renal cortical and collecting system morphology and to select appropriate frames for use in assigning ROIs. This step is also useful to make sure the patient has not moved during the study, which can invalidate time-activity curve data.

In practice it is useful to add early and late frames together to ensure that ROIs include the entire desired structures and do not overlap unwanted structures. For example, ureteral ROIs are flagged to avoid overlap with the renal pelvis and the bladder. Separate regions are flagged for each kidney and ureter. Additional ROIs are drawn for background correction.

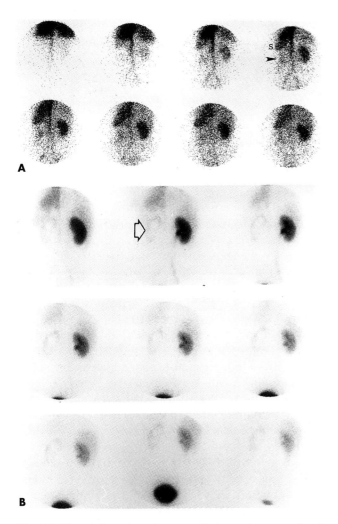

A

B

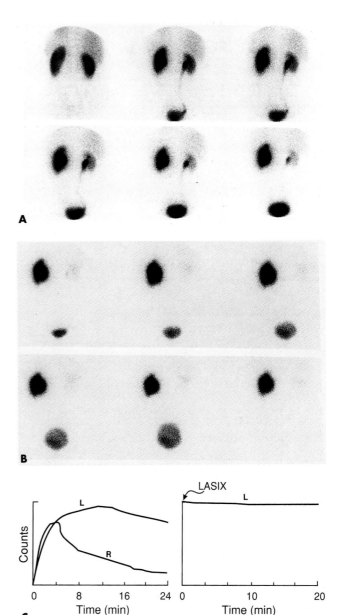

A

B

Fig. 12-16 High-grade vesicoureteral obstruction secondary to tumor. **A**, Flow study shows very decreased perfusion of the left kidney (*arrowhead*). Do not confuse the spleen (*S*) with the kidney. **B**, Dynamic sequential images acquired every 5 minutes show only a thin rim of cortex with poor uptake (*open arrowhead*) and a very large central photopenic collecting system consistent with hydronephrosis. Diuresis renography would not be indicated or useful, since no tracer fills the collecting system. This is a very high-grade obstruction.

Fig. 12-17 Obstructed hydronephrosis, TC-99m MAG3 study. **A**, Hydronephrosis on the left. There is continued filling of an enlarged collecting system on the left, while the right kidney clears. **B**, Diuresis renography shows no significant clearing of the hydronephrotic left kidney after furosemide administration. This is a high-grade partial obstruction and requires intervention. **C**, Time-activity curbes before (*left*) and after (*right*) Furosemide administration confirm the imaging findings, showing an extremely poor response to the diuretic.

Interpretation The significance of time-activity response patterns is based on empirical correlations with both surgical results and long-term clinical follow-up. The literature is replete with attempts to refine and quantify response patterns. Conservatively, the diuresis renogram should be taken as only one indicator of renal function. It has limitations (discussed later) and sometimes must be interpreted as indeterminate or nondiagnostic. Serial studies can be done to determine whether there is change over time.

NORMAL PATTERN In normal pelvicalyceal systems, the conventional radionuclide time-activity curve shows increasing activity that reaches a sharp peak within sev-

eral minutes after radiotracer injection. This is followed by a spontaneous, rapid decline in activity. Furosemide diuresis accelerates the rate of tracer washout (see Figure 12-15A).

In the normal ureter, the time-activity histogram is usually flat, indicating a small, constant amount of activ-

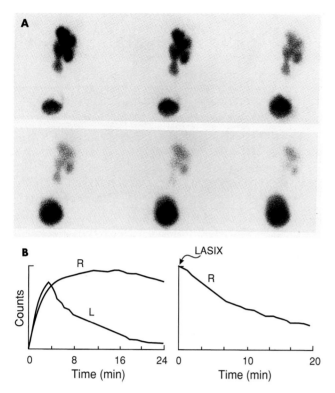

Fig. 12-18 Nonobstructed hydronephrosis. **A**, Diuresis renography in a patient with a history of surgically treated vesicoureteral obstruction of the right kidney who was being followed postoperatively. After the first 30-minute study (not shown), the post-furosemide images show that the very prominent hydroureteronephrosis responds rapidly to the diuretic, with almost complete clearance. **B**, Patient's time-activity curves for the pre- (*left*) and postdiuretic (*right*) phases. Before diuretic administration, the curve of the hydronephrotic kidney plateaus. After furosemide administration, the curve promptly declines, signifying no significant obstruction.

ity. There is frequently a transient spike of activity after diuretic injection, indicating passage of a bolus of accumulated activity from the renal pelvis.

DILATED NONOBSTRUCTED PATTERN In dilated but nonobstructed kidneys with good function, the initial portion of the time-activity curve may be quite similar to that seen in normal kidneys, but accumulation is progressive, without a sharp, narrow peak in the time-activity curve. The curve frequently reaches a plateau at 20 to 30 minutes after tracer injection. After furosemide diuresis, the level of activity decreases rapidly, indicating diuresis-induced washout (see Figure 12-15B). The rate and degree of decrease reached by 20 to 30 minutes after diuretic injection are quite variable. A half-time of washout of less than 10 minutes is generally taken as an indication that significant mechanical obstruction is not present. A half-time of washout greater than 20 minutes is consistent with obstruction. A half-time between 10 and 20 minutes is considered an indeterminate response: obstruction cannot be ruled out.

The larger the collecting system, the less "crisp" is the response. The relationship between volume and flow is given by the equation:

$$\bar{t} = \frac{V}{F},$$

where $\bar{t}$ is the time of a tracer through a system, V is the volume of the system, and F is the flow through it. According to this formula, the larger the volume, the more prolonged will be the transit time at a given flow rate, and for any given volume the transit time will be longer at lower rates of flow. Thus, extremely large, hydronephrotic systems may appear to exhibit delayed washout regardless of whether they are obstructed or not. Likewise, renal units with impaired function and diminished response to the diuretic will exhibit prolonged washout, whether they are obstructed or not. These are two situations in which indeterminate or nondiagnostic patterns may occur and represent a limitation of the test.

Time-activity curves for dilated, nonobstructed ureters are similar to those for kidneys. After diuretic injection there is a lag in response, owing to the serial nature of the washout phenomenon from renal pelvis to ureter.

OBSTRUCTED PATTERN The initial slope of the time-activity curve in obstructed kidneys is frequently somewhat less steep than in normal kidneys, and either there is progressive accumulation of activity or a plateau is reached within 20 to 30 minutes. After furosemide diuresis, the time-activity histogram of the obstructed kidney most frequently shows a flat response without significant washout (see Figures 12-15C, 12-17, 12-19). In some cases, progressive accumulation actually continues, and in a few cases, there is a transient decrease in activity followed by reaccumulation. In patients with reasonably good function, a time-activity histogram showing equal or greater activity at 10 minutes after diuretic administration compared with the preinjection level indicates significant mechanical obstruction.

The pattern for obstructed ureters is similar qualitatively. There is a failure of activity to decrease following diuresis.

Clinical applications Clinical conditions studied by diuresis renography are summarized in Box 12-8. The most common clinical problem encountered is suspected ureteropelvic junction obstruction (see Figures 12-17 to 12-19). When dilated collecting systems referred for evaluation are demonstrated not to be obstructed, this eliminates the need for more invasive procedures or a prolonged series of contrast-enhanced urograms for follow-up. The sensitivity of the study for mechanical obstruction has been variably reported as between 60% and 90%.

Although diuresis renography is often performed to differentiate obstructive from nonobstructive hydronephrosis, it is also used in patients to determine the clinical significance of a known partial obstruction, as in

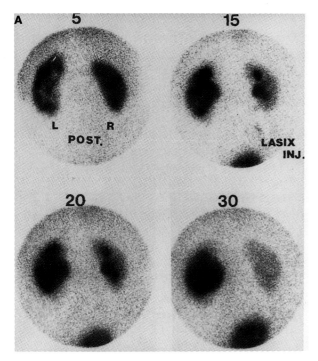

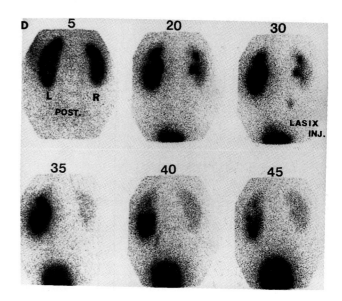

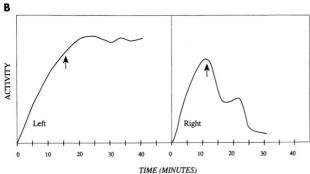

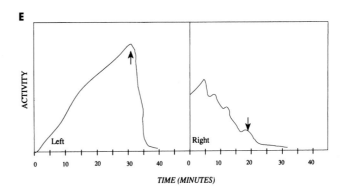

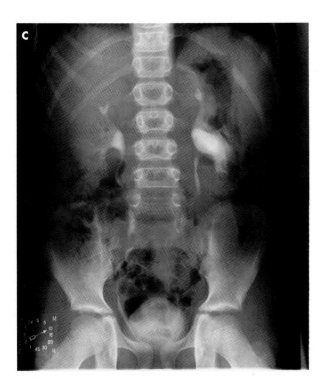

Fig. 12-19 Pre- and postoperative diuresis renography: utility of follow-up. **A**, In an 8-year-old boy with a history of abdominal pain, images obtained with Tc-99m DPTA (15 minutes) before Lasix administration reveal minor dilation of the collecting structures on the right and marked left-sided hydronephrosis. After Lasix injection, there is prompt washout from the right kidney but progressive accumulation on the left (30 minutes). **B**, Time-activity curves confirm the imaging findings. No response to Lasix injection (*arrows*) is seen on the left, confirming the diagnosis of obstruction. **C**, The patient underwent a left pyeloplasty and returned 2 months later for follow-up IVU. The postoperative IVU shows dilation on the left with contrast material accumulating in the pelvis and calyces, especially inferiorly. The adequacy of surgery is uncertain. **D**, Diuresis renography again demonstrates hydronephrosis on the left prior to Lasix administration. After injection of the diuretic, there is prompt washout of activity, except for minimal residual tracer in the left inferior pole. **E**, Time-activity curves confirmed prompt bilateral clearance.

patients with cervical carcinoma. A high-grade obstruction will result in renal damage and dysfunction, while a lower-grade obstruction may be compensated for and cause only dilation, without an adverse affect on renal function. Diuresis renography can determine whether aggressive intervention is indicated (e.g., stenting or surgery).

A kidney from which tracer does not wash out with furosemide is signficantly obstructed; that is, it can be predicted that renal function will deteriorate if there is no intervention. In contrast, a collecting system from which tracer is washed out with furosemide will usually retain good function in the immediate future. Serial studies, perhaps done every few months, can be used to follow the course of the partial obstruction.

A number of other less frequently encountered conditions also lend themselves to evaluation by diuresis renography (see Box 12-8). For example, some degree of hydronephrosis and hydroureter is extremely common in patients with long-standing ileal loop diversions. The degree of hydronephrosis can be quite alarming and may also be associated with reflux. Other conditions such as prune-belly syndrome are associated with structural dysmorphism and flaccidity of the collecting structures.

Pitfalls and limitations   The problem of the equivocal or indeterminate diuresis renogram is discussed in the section on time-activity curve patterns. Limited renal function undermines the rationale for the procedure. A flat response or failure of response to occur after diuretic injection in a patient with significantly impaired renal function is moot, for the renal function may be inadequate for effective diuresis.

Good criteria are not available in the literature to definitively determine when renal function is adequate to meet the rationale of the test. However, if the uptake in the kidney is poor or the collecting structures are not clearly visualized, caution should be used in interpretation. The serum creatinine level may be normal in the setting of unilateral renal impairment and is not a reliable indicator in the face of unilateral disease.

In infants and children younger than 5 years, radioactivity in the bladder may overlap and obscure the lower ureters and in some cases reach the level of the kidneys. Importantly, increased pressure in the abdomen and collecting system due to a filled bladder may alter the washout response pattern. Therefore, whenever bladder activity and associated increased pressure are likely to confuse the results, the bladder should be catheterized before the study is initiated. This should probably be routine for younger subjects. A special problem arises with low-lying or pelvic kidneys, in which case overlap is invariable and catheterization is required.

Determining the cause of neonatal hydronephrosis can be problematic. Neonates have functionally immature kidneys. Even without hydronephrosis, uptake and clearance of radiotracer may be delayed in this age group, especially in premature infants. Even in those with hydronephrosis without obstruction, diuresis renography may suggest obstruction. Those patients without clear-cut obstruction should be followed with serial diuresis renograms. Surgeons prefer to operate when the infant and the genitourinary system are larger and more mature.

In some patients with hydroureteronephrosis, dialation is associated with reflux rather than obstruction. Reintroduction of tracer in the upper tracts as a result of reflux is a theoretical problem that can cause an upward deflection on the time-activity histogram. In practice, this is generally recognized by reviewing the sequential images and by assessing the bladder time-activity curve, which shows a reciprocal downward deflection as significant reflux occurs.

Several technical errors can invalidate the results of diuresis renography. One obvious potential error is infiltration of the diuretic dose. Because it is somewhat painful, infiltration is generally recognized in adult subjects but may not be as easily recognized in infants and small children. From a practical standpoint, an IV "keep open" line should be used in children and checked for free flow just before the diuretic is injected. This also reduces the chance for patient motion during the venipuncture.

Motion artifacts are another potential problem in diuresis renography. During the procedure, subjects must remain still for a minimum of 30 minutes and possibly as long as 60 minutes, which is difficult for most patients, especially children. Motion artifacts can be minimized by ensuring that the patient's position is comfortable before starting the examination. Motion is easily recognized by rapid sequential viewing of the images on the computer screen and should be suspected if the renal time-activity curves are irregular.

Radionuclide Evaluation of Renal Transplants

Radionuclide methods have been applied extensively in the evaluation of renal allografts after transplantation. Radiotracer techniques are noninvasive and are easily repeated to clarify the evolving clinical findings.

Kidneys for transplantation come from either living donors related to the patient or cadaveric donors. Potential donors typically undergo extensive anatomic and functional evaluation as well as immunologic matching. Cadaveric kidneys are carefully preserved and stored in regional organ banks, then distributed to transplantation centers when needed. The surgical technique is well established (Figure 12-20). The superficial placement of the graft in the anterior iliac fossa allows palpation for assessment of change in size as well as easy access for biopsy and surgical repair.

Although renal allografts from living-related donors are considerably more successful than cadaveric grafts, only about 35% of transplanted kidneys come from living-related donors. Most come from unrelated people who have died of head injuries. One-year graft survival rates are 86% for HLA-identical siblings, 82% for living-related donors, but only 56% for cadaver transplants.

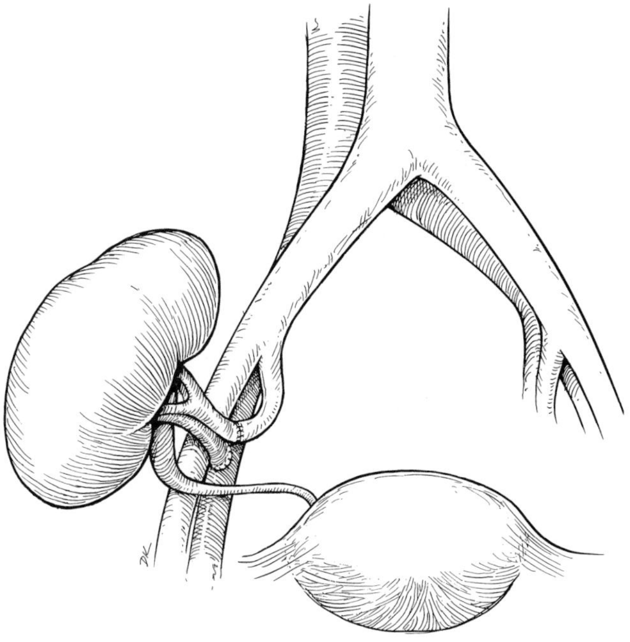

The time after transplantation is a key factor in determining what nuclear medicine procedure to apply and in interpreting the significance of the findings. Table 12-5 summarizes the major complications based on their time of occurrence.

Medical complications Early complications include ischemic damage to the donor kidney that results in *acute tubular necrosis* (ATN). ATN invariably occurs with cadaveric allografts but much less commonly with living-related donor grafts. A prolonged time between the donor's death and transplantation increases the severity of ATN.

ATN is characterized scintigraphically by well-preserved perfusion but poor renal function and decreased urine excretion. In severe cases, no urine is produced at all. These findings are usually seen on a baseline scan performed within 24 hours of surgery. The ischemic damage resolves over 1 to 3 weeks, and renal function and urine excretion return (see Figure 12-11). In laboratories using quantitative measurements of renal function, ERPF is decreased. The severity of ATN varies considerably and the condition may be superimposed on other complications.

Hyperacute rejection refers to an immediate reaction of preformed antibodies in the recipient's circulation with the graft. The surgeon often recognizes this event as soon

Fig. 12-20 Renal transplant surgery. For technical reasons, the initial allograft is placed in the right iliac fossa. The donor renal artery is anastomosed end-to-end to the hypogastric artery and the renal vein end-to-side to the external iliac vein. The ureter is attached to the recipient's ureter or, more often, implanted directly into the bladder. Second grafts are commonly placed in the left iliac fossa. When a pancreas is transplanted simultaneously with the kidney in a diabetic patient, the transabdominal approach is used.

Table 12-5	Complications After Renal Transplantation	
Complication	**Usual Time of Occurrence**	**Comments**
Acute tubular necrosis	Minutes to hours postoperatively	Cadaveric transplant
Rejection		
Hyperacute	Within minutes to hours	Preformed antibodies; irreversible
Accelerated	1-5 days	Occurs after previous transplant or transfusions
Acute	After 5 days; Most common during first 3 months	Cell-mediated; responsive to treatment
Chronic	Months to years	Humoral; irreversible
Cyclosporin toxicity	Months	Reversible with drug withdrawal
Surgical		
Urine leak	Few days or weeks	
Hematoma	First few days	
Wound infection	First few days	
Obstruction	Days, months, years	Clots, scar, calculi
Lymphocele	2nd to 4th month	
Renal artery stenosis	After 1st month	

as the vascular clamp is released following anastomosis. The kidney turns blue. There is thrombosis of the renal vasculature and irreversible destruction of the donor kidney. This complication is infrequent in contemporary practice with the ability to comprehensively screen the donor and recipient immunologically. Prior transplantation and a history of blood transfusions are risk factors.

Although rarely seen, the scintigraphic appearance of hyperacute rejection is that of absent perfusion to the transplanted kidney and no evidence of function. The kidney appears as a photon-deficient area with high background activity due to tracer retained in the extracellular fluid space. This pattern is identical to that seen in *acute arterial or venous thrombosis* (Figure 12-21). The clinical significance of renal vein thrombosis is much greater in the newly transplanted kidney than in native kidneys because the allograft has no venous collaterals. From a practical standpoint, venous thrombosis has the same significance as arterial obstruction in the immediate transplant period.

Acute rejection may occur as early as 5 to 7 days after transplantation and is most commonly seen in the first 3 months, although it can occur years later. It is a cell-mediated immunologic process. Clinically, acute rejection manifests with symptoms of fever, transplant tenderness, and enlargement. Laboratory values, such as the sedimentation rate and serum β_2-microglobulins, may rise. Untreated, acute rejection results in allograft death due to vascular and tubular damage; however, it often responds to appropriate immunosuppressive therapy. *Accelerated acute rejection* occurs in a sensitized patient as a result of previous transplantation and blood transfusions. It can be seen during the first week of transplantation.

The scintigraphic hallmark of acute rejection is a decrease in transplant perfusion. With a good bolus injection and a framing rate of 2 to 3 seconds per frame, the kidney should normally become the "hottest" structure in

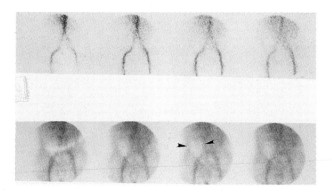

Fig. 12-21   Renal artery thrombosis. *Top,* radionuclide angiogram demonstrates no perfusion to the renal transplant. *Bottom,* dynamic images acquired immediately after the flow study and sequentially every 5 minutes show a photopenic defect (*arrowheads*) due to a nonviable allograft causing attenuation but having no radiopharmaceutical uptake.

the field of view within one or two frames of appearance of the tracer bolus at the level of the iliac artery. Failure of the kidney to show uptake in the setting of adequate bolus injection is indicative of reduced perfusion (Figure 12-22). A baseline study prior to the fifth post-transplant day is useful for comparison purposes.

With acute rejection, renal uptake and excretion are reduced. The baseline scintigrams and renogram curve should be used for comparison to assess the contribution of preexisting ATN (see Figure 12-22). When comparing sequential renogram curves, it should be remembered that ATN is most severe initially and should resolve with time, usually over 1 to 2 weeks. Thus, interval changes in the curve indicating slower uptake, more prolonged retention, and less excretion typically indicate acute rejection in the appropriate time interval after transplantion.

Quantitative measurements of GFR or ERPF are both diminished in acute rejection. Their significance is greatest when baseline and sequential values are available to differentiate changes of acute rejection from preexisting damage due to ATN.

In addition to conventional renography with either tubular or glomerular agents, other radiotracer methods have been proposed for evaluation of acute transplant rejection. Gallium-67 citrate (Ga-67) accumulates to some degree in acute rejection. However, it is excreted through the kidney in the first 24 hours after injection, and only delayed uptake is a reliable indicator. This is not clinically useful, for treatment decisions must be made promptly.

Tc-99m sulfur colloid (Tc-99m SC) has been used to diagnose acute rejection (Figure 12-23). In rejecting kidneys, the colloidal particles become trapped in fibrin thrombi that develop in the vessels of rejecting transplants. Although this method has some utility in detecting the first episode of acute rejection, delayed return to normal makes the use of Tc-99m SC problematic thereafter.

Mixed populations of In-111-labeled leukocytes and of In-111-labeled lymphocytes have both been tried. Both tracers accumulate avidly in rejecting grafts. However, the specificity is poor, with frequent false positive results (e.g., due to infection or hematoma). There is limited but promising experience with In-111-labeled platelets. Avid uptake is seen in acute rejection, although false positive studies have been reported in patients receiving cyclosporin therapy. It is likely that any cause of inflammation will result in localization of leukocytes, lymphocytes, and platelets.

Chronic rejection is a delayed phenomenon that occurs months to years after transplantation. The course is insidious, and gradual deterioration of transplant function results. It is a humorally mediated process. Renal perfusion, GFR, and ERPF are diminished. These changes are all reflected scintigraphically as decreased perfusion,

A

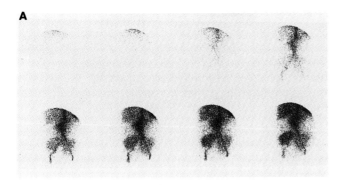

B

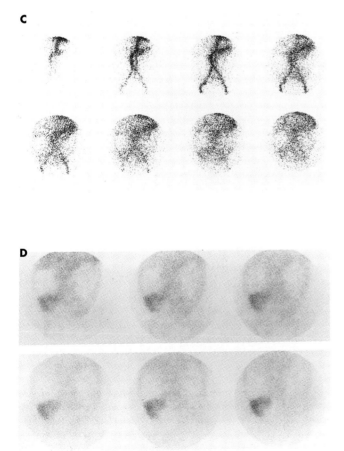

E

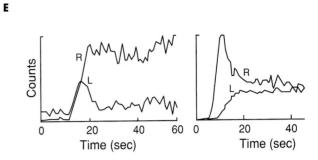

Fig. 12-22 **A** through **E**, Acute transplant rejection. **A** and **B**, Tc-99m MAG3 study at the end of the first week following transplantation. Good blood flow (A) and function (B) of the allograft in the right iliac fossa are seen. **C** and **D**, Two days later the patient had low-grade fever, transplant tenderness, and rising serum creatinine levels. The follow-up flow study (**C**) shows very poor blood flow and function (**D**). **E**, Flow time-activity curves show good blood flow before rejection (*left*) but delayed flow of the transplant during rejection. *R*, arterial curve and *L*, transplant.

C

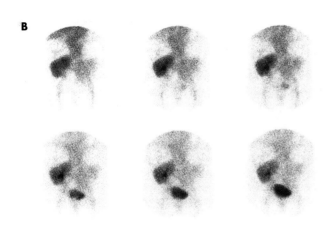

D

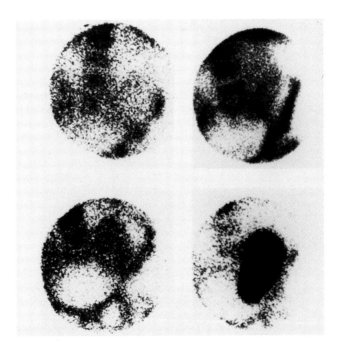

Fig. 12-23 Images in four different patients obtained 20 minutes after injection of Tc-99m SC showing varying degrees of radiocolloid uptake within the renal transplant in the left iliac fossa, from none (*upper left*), to mild (*upper right*), moderate (*lower left*), and marked (*lower right*). Uptake is characteristic but not specific for rejection.

reduced and slow accumulation of tracer, and reduced urine formation (Figure 12-24).

Surgical complications A variety of surgical complications can also be detected scintigraphically. A *urinary leak* secondary to necrosis of the ureteral anastomosis may occur in the immediate postoperative period. When rapid, this may be easily recognized from tracer accumulation in the area of leak (Figure 12-25). Only a photopenic defect adjacent to the kidney may be seen with slower leaks, due to the nonlabeled urinoma. Delayed imaging can sometimes detect active but slow leakage.

Hematomas are also seen in the transplant bed and are recognized as fixed photon-deficient areas (Figure 12-26). Another cause of photon-deficient areas around the kidney is a *lymphocele*. Lymphoceles most commonly occur 2 to 3 months postoperatively. Because the transplanted kidney does not have lymphatic connections, disruption of lymph channels in the transplant bed can result in lymphocele formation. This may occur in as many as 10% of transplants, but it is clinically important only if it displaces the kidney or impinges on the ureter or renal vascular pedicle.

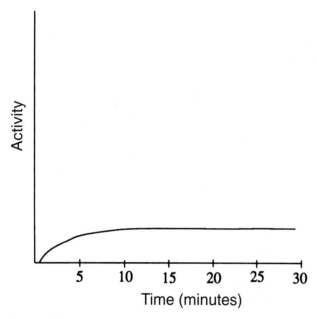

Fig. 12-24 Chronic allograft rejection. The creatinine clearance rose slowly over the preceding 3 years. The transplant was placed 6 years earlier. The time-activity curve shows poor uptake and clearance, consistent with chronic rejection.

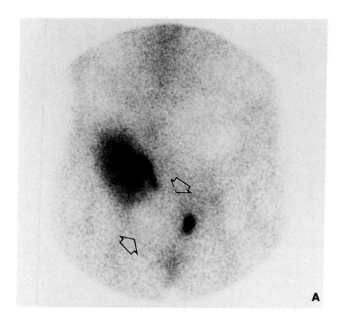

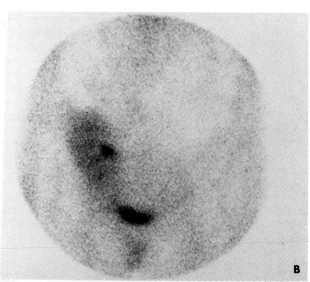

Fig. 12-26 Partial ureteral obstruction of a renal transplant. **A,** Postoperative study showing dilated calyces and renal pelvis with an abrupt cutoff of the ureter. Note the adjacent relatively photopenic area just inferiorly (*arrowheads*) because of a hematoma. **B,** Repeat study performed 3 weeks postoperatively shows complete self-resolution of the obstruction.

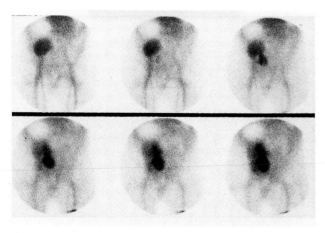

Fig. 12-25 Postoperative transplant study showing a rapid urine leak caused by a disrupted surgical anastomosis. Note accumulation of radiotracer just inferior to the transplant but superior and lateral to the bladder. No bladder filling is seen.

Ureteral obstruction can be caused by kinking, compression by an extrinsic mass such as a hematoma or lymphocele, intraluminal obstruction by a blood clot, or calculous and periureteral fibrosis (see Figure 12-26). Some degree of collecting system dilation is often seen after transplantation without significant mechanical obstruction.

Arterial stenosis of the allograft should be suspected in patients who develop hypertension after tranplantation. Captopril renography may prove useful in selected cases.

RADIONUCLIDE EVALUATION OF RENOVASCULAR HYPERTENSION

Hypertension is a common clinical problem afflicting over 50 million people in the United States. In more than 90% of patients, there is no identifiable cause of "essential hypertension" and no prospect for cure. It usually requires lifelong medical management with drug therapy. However, in a small percentage of patients, hypertension is due to a potentially curable cause such as coarctation, an endocrine-related defect, and renovascular hypertension.

Renovascular hypertension refers to hypertension caused by renal arterial hypoperfusion secondary to a stenotic vessel. Renovascular disease may or may not cause sufficient hypoperfusion to set off the process that leads to hypertension. For example, almost half of normotensive patients over age 60 have atherosclerotic lesions in their renal vessels. In a nonselected hypertensive population, the prevalence of renovascular hypertension is less than 1%. Among patients ultimately referred for renal diagnostic studies, 2% to 4% have renovascular hypertension.

Pathogenesis of Renovascular Hypertension

There has been much research and controversy regarding the etiology of renovascular hypertension since 1934, when Goldblatt first induced hypertension in dogs by partially occluding one renal artery. It is now generally agreed that increased renin secretion is responsible for the hypertension caused by renal hypoperfusion, whereas renal sodium retention is the primary mechanism for hypertension resulting from loss of renal parenchyma.

Although there are two main causes of renovascular hypertension, atherosclerosis and fibromuscular dysplasia, with somewhat different clinical pictures, repair of any form of *functional* renovascular disease is indicated. The earlier an arterial stenosis causing hypertension is corrected, the greater is the chance for cure. Otherwise, widespread arteriolar damage and glomerulosclerosis in the contralateral kidney can result from prolonged exposure to hypertension and high levels of angiotensin II.

Diagnostic Tests

The patient's history and physical examination findings can help in selecting patients with an increased likelihood of renovascular hypertension. These factors include a rapid and recent onset of hypertension, hypertension refractory to therapy, generalized systemic vascular disease, abdominal bruits, young patients with significant hypertension, and patients who experience renal failure during treatment with angiotensin-converting enzyme (ACE) inhibitors.

However, these selection criteria are far from specific, and the false positive rate would be extremely high if all were subjected to angiography, an invasive procedure.

Considerable effort has been expended to find a non-invasive screening test that could predict which patients might benefit from surgery. In the recent past, peripheral blood renin levels and IVU were advocated as screening tests for renovascular hypertension. However, serum renin is not specific, and the "hypertensive IVU" suffers from an unacceptably high percentage of false positive and false negative results, on the order of 25% each. Subsequently it was recommended that fewer patients be screened and that those with suggestive clinical features should undergo selective renal arteriography.

The use of conventional radionuclide renography to diagnose renovascular hypertension was abandoned because of a similarly poor specificity. This was the situation until the development of an interventional maneuver, the *captopril-stimulated* study, which has led to a renaissance in the use of radionuclide renography to make the diagnosis of a renin-dependent renovascular hypertension. Captopril-stimulated plasma renin levels have also been advocated, but specificity is poor. Lateralization of renal vein renin values can confirm the diagnosis, if needed after angiography.

Radionuclide evaluation of renal artery stenosis The close link between the rate of radiopharmaceutical accumulation and renal blood flow forms the basis of the nuclear medicine approach. Although the radionuclide angiogram may show decreased blood flow on the stenotic side, sensitivity is not high. The primary focus for making a diagnosis of renal vascular hypertension has been the second phase of the renogram (see Figure 12-5). In patients with renovascular hypertension, the second phase of the classic renogram is often flattened, with a less steep upslope. The peak of the curve may be blunted and the third phase prolonged without a crisp, concave appearance. However, this pattern is not specific. The accuracy of this finding is only slightly better than that of "hypertensive" IVU.

Captopril renography It was observed clinically that some patients receiving captopril, an ACE inhibitor, for the treatment of hypertension developed renal failure, which was usually reversible. These patients were found to have bilateral renal artery stenosis. This observation led to the clever idea that ACE inhibitors could be used to make the diagnosis of renovascular hypertension.

Mechanism   Glomerular filtration is driven by pressure at the renal glomerulus. When perfusion pressure drops, renal filtration, as measured by the GFR, also decreases. In the normal compensatory response, renin is then released by the juxtaglomerular apparatus. Renin converts angiotensinogen made in the liver to angiotensin I, which is converted to angiotensin II in the lungs by ACE. Angiogensin II is a powerful vasoconstrictor that, in addition to peripheral vasoconstriction, produces constriction of the efferent arterioles of the glomerulus (Figure 12-27). This raises the filtration pressure, thus maintaining GFR. However, this normal compensatory mechanism has its limits. If renal blood flow continues to decrease, GFR will deteriorate. With time, the kidney will become scarred and contracted.

ACE inhibitors work by blocking the conversion of angiotensin I to angiotensin II (Figure 12-28), preventing this normal compensatory mechanism. Postglomerular resistance decreases, and therewith the transcapillary driving force that maintains filtration is decreased in kidneys with renin-dependent, hemodynamically significant renal artery stenosis. GFR will fall in the involved kidney.

Oral captopril has been most commonly used as the ACE interventional agent in combination with Tc-99m DTPA, I-131 OIH, and more recently Tc-99m MAG3. Conventionally, two radionuclide studies are performed, one with and one without captopril stimulation. In normal subjects and patients with hypertension unrelated to renal artery stenosis, the renogram curve remains unchanged compared to baseline after administration of the ACE inhibitor. In patients with hemodynamically significant renal artery stenosis, a reduction in renal function of the affected kidney will occur. The reduced GFR is seen scintigraphically as delayed uptake and cortical retention (Figures 12-29, 12-30).

In patients with unilateral disease and renal asymmetry on the baseline renogram, the administration of captopril may result in greater asymmetry. A severely diseased and shrunken kidney may not respond to captopril, being no longer renin dependent. It should be emphasized that ACE inhibitor has no effect on the flow phase of the study.

In a commonly used protocol (outlined in Box 12-9) the captopril-stimulated study is performed first. If it is completely normal, no baseline study is required. However, if any abnormality is noted, a baseline study without captopril is performed similarly on another day. Furosemide is often given simultaneously with the radionuclide to clear collecting system activity, which can affect visual and renographic interpretation. IV enalapril, another ACE inhibitor, is being investigated as an alternative to oral captopril.

Accuracy   Investigators have reported the test to be approximately 90% sensitive and more than 95% specific. False positive results are extremely rare. The accu-

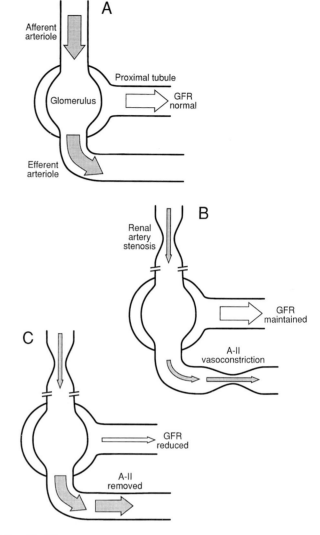

Fig. 12-27   Pathophysiology of renin-dependent renovascular disease and the pharmacologic effect of captopril. **A,** Normal glomerular perfusion. **B,** Renal artery stenosis. Because of reduced renal plasma flow, filtration pressure and GFR fall. Increased renin and resulting angiotensin II (see Figure 12-28) produces vasoconstriction of the efferent glomerular arterioles, raising glomerular pressure and maintaining GFR. **C,** Captopril blocks the normal compensatory mechanism described in **B,** and GFR falls.

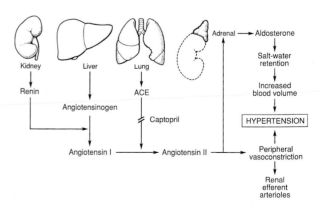

Fig. 12-28   Renin-angiotensin-aldosterone physiology and site of ACE inhibitor (captopril) blockage. See text for details.

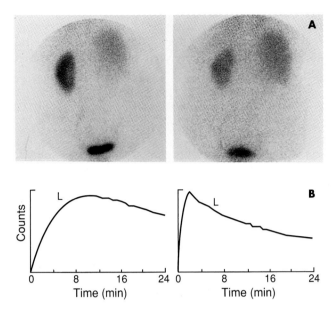

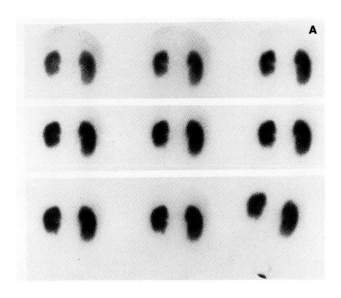

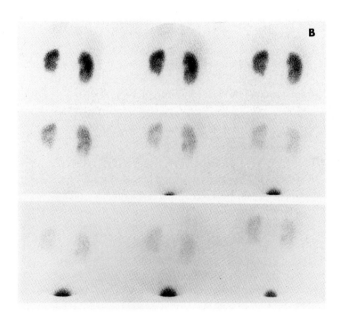

Fig. 12-29 Positive captopril-stimulated study in a patient with only one functioning kidney (left). **A,** Only the last sequential Tc-99m MAG3 image at 30 minutes is shown for comparison of the baseline and captopril-stimulated study. *Left,* captopril study shows prominent cortical retention. *Right,* baseline study without captopril does not show cortical retention. Also compare the renal-to-liver uptake ratio between the two studies. **B,** Baseline (*left*) and postcaptopril study (*right*) time-activity curves confirm the imaging findings and are diagnostic of renin-dependent renal artery stenosis. The capopril study shows delayed uptake and clearance, whereas the baseline time-activity curve is normal.

racy of Tc-99m MAG3 seems equally high. The sensitivity falls in the setting of renal insufficiency, and the test is not useful in evaluating small, poorly functioning kidneys. In those cases, captopril renography can still be used to evaluate the contralateral kidney. Captopril renography should be limited to patients with symptoms or signs suggestive of renovascular hypertension.

RENAL CORTICAL SCINTIGRAPHY

Distinguishing upper from lower urinary tract infection on a clinical basis can be difficult. Symptoms and signs are often indistinguishable. The long-term complications of and therapeutic implications for parenchymal infection are very different from those of lower urinary tract disease. Cortical scarring can lead to renal failure and hypertension. Tc-99m DMSA and Tc-99m GH can make this distinction.

In the past, the standard method for detecting pyelonephritis and renal scarring was IVU, and most of the epidemiologic data on the incidence of acute pyelonephritis and its sequelae—scarring, hypertension and renal failure—were based on this technique. Since the mid-1980s, studies have demonstrated the superiority of radionuclide renal cortical imaging for detecting both

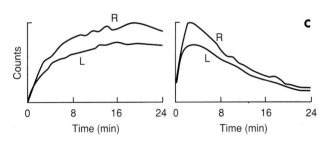

Fig. 12-30 Bilateral renal artery stenosis studied with Tc-99m MAG3. **A,** Captopril-stimulated study: bilateral cortical retention and minimal urinary bladder clearance over 30 minutes. **B,** Baseline study without captopril shows normal cortical function and good clearance into the bladder. This is diagnostic of bilateral renal artery stenosis. **C,** Time-activity curves confirm the diagnosis (*left,* captopril-stimulated study; *right,* baseline study).

Box 12-9 Captopril Renography: Protocol Summary

PATIENT PREPARATION

NPO after midnight.

RADIONUCLIDE

Tc-99m MAG3, 8 mCi.

POSITIONING

Supine.

PROCEDURE

IV hydration: normal saline, 10 mL/kg over 1 hr to a maximum of 500 mL, prior to radionuclide. KVO during entire study.

Captopril, 25 mg orally 1 hr prior to starting the radionuclide study. Children: 0.5 mg/kg (maximum, 25 mg).

Monitor blood pressure and record every 15 min before and during study. A large drop in pressure may require saline infusion.

Give IV furosemide at the time of radionuclide injection. Dosage is similar to that used for Lasix renography.

Inject radiopharmaceutical IV.

Imaging is similar to that described for dynamic renal scintigraphy.

INTERPRETATION

If the images and time-activity curve are normal, a renin-dependent renovascular hypertension is excluded.

Evidence of cortical retention on scintigrams and an abnormal time-activity curve (delayed peak and clearance) require a repeat study without captopril for comparison.

---

acute pyelonephritis and renal scarring when compared to IVU and US.

Pathophysiology of Acute Pyelonephritis

Pyelonephritis results from vesicoureteral reflux of infected urine. Although only a portion of the cortex drained by a refluxing papilla may be involved in any one infection, the remaining cortex often becomes infected on repeated occasions until all functioning renal tissue drained by that papilla is destroyed. Repetitive infection may also occur during a single clinical episode if it is not promptly and appropriately treated. In addition, infection with certain strains of *E. coli* has been shown to paralyze the ureter and cause a functional obstruction. For this reason, pyelonephritis may be seen in the cortex of even a normally nonrefluxing papilla.

Renal infection induces rapid activation of serum complement and granulocyte aggregation at the site of infection; vascular occlusion and renal ischemia result.

In areas of acute inflammation, the renal microcirculation becomes impaired due to interstitial edema, with compression of glomeruli, small peritubular capillaries, and the vasae rectae.

Imaging of Pyelonephritis and Cortical Scarring

Cortical scintigraphy demonstrates approximately twice as many defects as US and four times as many defects as IVU. Color Doppler imaging has improved the sensitivity of US, but it remains inferior to that of scintigraphy. Studies suggest that computed tomography (CT) may also be an accurate method, although no direct comparison studies have been performed. However, CT is more expensive, has the associated risk of contrast agent reaction, and results in a higher radiation absorbed dose to the patient.

Ga-67 and In-111 leukocyte imaging can demonstrate infection; however, delayed imaging is required (24 hours for In-111 WBCs and 48 hours for Ga-67) and both studies are associated with a relatively high radiation dose. Therefore neither is widely used in children.

Scintigraphic Pattern in Acute Pyelonephritis and Scarring

Pyelonephritis may be seen as a solitary defect involving only a portion of one kidney, as multiple focal defects involving one or both kidneys, or as diffuse involvement of an entire kidney. A follow-up study should be performed 3 to 6 months after the acute infection to determine if the infection has resolved or if there has been renal scarring (Figure 12-31).

Scarring is seen as volume loss, whether focal or global (see Figure 12-6). Volume loss may even occur in the absence of focal defects and present only as atrophy. More commonly it is seen as small, large, single or multiple focal cortical defects and/or cortical thinning.

Mechanism of Decreased Tc-99m DMSA Uptake in Pyelonephritis

There is good agreement between an abnormal cortical scintigram and the histopathology of pyelonephritis in animal studies. Two mechanisms have been proposed. One is that the decreased uptake is due to the decreased blood flow and ischemia associated with pyelonephritis. The other is that toxic byproducts of granulocyte lysis paralyze the active tubular transport mechanism responsible for DMSA tubular localization.

Other Clinical Applications

Renal cortical scintigraphy has been used for evaluating renal tumors and trauma. Tumors and cysts would not be expected to accumulate renal radiopharmaceuticals and appear as "cold" or photon-deficient areas. However, other imaging modalities, such as CT and US, are better for this purpose. The one exception is the ability of scintigraphy to confirm functioning renal tissue, for example in differentiating a renal tumor from a *pseudotumor*, as seen with a hypertrophied column of Bertin.

RADIONUCLIDE CYSTOGRAPHY

Radionuclide cystography was introduced in the late 1950s to diagnose vesicoureteral reflux and is increasingly being accepted as the technique of choice for the evaluation and follow-up of children with urinary tract infections and reflux. The radionuclide method is more sensitive than contrast-enhanced cystography for detecting reflux and results in considerably less radiation exposure to the patient. In many centers, contrast voiding urethrocystography is reserved for the initial workup of male patients to exclude an anatomic cause for reflux, such as posterior urethral valves.

Pathogenesis of Vesicoureteral Reflux

Untreated reflux and infection are associated with subsequent renal damage, scarring, hypertension, and chronic renal failure. Vesicoureteral reflux is caused by a failure of the ureterovesical valve. The normal ureter passes obliquely through the bladder wall and submucosa to its opening at the trigone. As urine fills the bladder, the valve passively closes, preventing reflux. If the intramural ureteral length is too short in comparison with its diameter or if the course too direct, the valve will not close completely and reflux results. As a child grows, the ureter usually grows in length more than diameter, resulting in

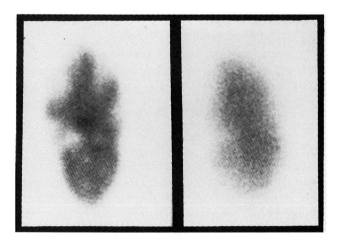

Fig. 12-31 Acute pyelonephritis in an 11-year-old child studied with Tc-99m DMSA and imaged with a pinhole collimator. *Left*, note multiple cortical defects, particularly in the upper pole. *Right*, a follow-up scan obtained 6 months later, after appropriate antibiotic therapy, shows resolution of most cortical defects.

decreased reflux and eventual resolution in 80% of patients.

Patients with severe vesicoureteral reflux are more likely to have renal damage than those with mild or moderate grades of reflux. Reflux by itself is not pathologic—that is, sterile low-pressure reflux does not cause renal injury. The intrarenal reflux of infected urine is required for damage to develop. The goal of therapy is to prevent infection of the kidney until reflux resolves spontaneously.

Methodology

Two forms of radionuclide cystography have been used, direct and indirect. *Indirect* radionuclide cystography is performed as part of routine dynamic renal scintigraphy with Tc-99m DTPA or Tc-99m MAG3. The child is asked not to void until the bladder is maximally filled. When the bladder is as full as can be tolerated, a prevoiding image is obtained. Dynamic images are then recorded continuously during voiding. After voiding is complete, a postvoiding image is obtained.

The indirect method is no longer commonly used. Although the advantage of this method is that bladder catheterization is unnecessary, upper tract stasis often poses a problem for interpretation, good renal function is necessary, and the method cannot be used to identify patients who experience reflux only during the filling phase (20%).

Direct radionuclide cystography is the technique most commonly performed. It is usually performed as a three-phase procedure, with continuous monitoring during filling of the bladder, micturition, and after voiding. The procedure can determine the presence or absence of reflux and measure the postvoiding residue in the bladder.

A standard protocol is described in Box 12-10. The study is performed dynamically and acquired on computer. Tc-99m SC is the radiotracer of choice, since Tc-99m pertechnetate may be absorbed through the bladder systemically, particularly if the bladder is inflamed (a similar concern exists with the use of Tc-99m DTPA). A solution of 1.0 mCi/500 mL provides sufficient concentration.

Urinary tract catheterization of the child is an important step in the procedure, and personnel involved should be taught appropriate sterile technique. The catheter selected should be large enough to permit filling of the bladder within 10 minutes. The patient's cooperation is extremely valuable to avoid premature voiding around the catheter and resultant contamination of the imaging field. As capacity is reached, voiding may occur spontaneously, especially in young children and infants.

Radiation Dosimetry

The radiation absorbed dose is quite low. There is 50 to 200 times less radiation to the gonads with the radionuclide method than with contrast cystography (Table 12-6).

Box 12-10   Radionuclide Retrograde Cystography: Protocol Summary

RADIOPHARMACEUTICAL
1 mCi Tc-99m SC.

CAMERA
Large field of view.

COMPUTER SETUP
64 × 64 word mode.

FILLING
10-sec frames × 60.

PREVOID
30-sec image.

VOIDING
2-sec frames × 120.

POSTVOID
30-sec image.

COLLIMATOR
Converging for newborn to 1 yr; LEAP for > 1 yr of age.

PATIENT PREPARATION
Insert and secure a urinary catheter.

PATIENT POSITION
Supine with the bladder, ureters, and kidneys in the field of view (symphysis pubis to xiphoid). Image posteriorly with camera under table.

PROCEDURE
Hang 500 mL normal saline 25 cm above the table.
Inject radiotracer into the catheter.

Filling phase
Fill bladder to maximum capacity with IV drip open. Bladder capacity can be estimated by the formula: (age [yr] + 2) × 30 = mL.
Filling should be continued until the drip slows, or there is backup of flow into tubing or voiding around catheter. Observe the oscilloscope for reflux.

Voiding phase
In patients able to void on request:
1. Place camera perpendicular to table.
2. Position patient sitting on bedpan with back to camera.
3. Have patient void.
4. Measure volume.
In patients too young to void on request:
1. Change diaper and put on a preweighed dry diaper.
2. Deflate Foley.
3. Record volume of saline infused at initiation of reflux and the voided volume. Weigh diaper.
Total bladder volume, residual postvoid volume, and bladder volume at initiation of reflux can be determined.

Residual bladder volume (mL) =

$$\frac{\text{Voided volume (mL)} \times \text{residual counts/min}}{\text{Initial counts/min} - \text{Residual counts/min}}$$

Table 12-6   Radiation Dosimetry for Tc-99m Retrograde Cystography

Organ	mrads/mCi
Bladder	18-27
Ovaries	1-2
Testicle	< 1-2
Kidneys	0.02-0.04 mrads/mL of reflux/min of residence in collecting system

Modified from Willi UV and Treves ST: Radionuclide voiding cystography. In Treves ST, editor: *Pediatric nuclear medicine*, New York, 1985, Springer Verlag.

Image Interpretation

In a normal study, no tracer is seen in the region of the ureters or kidneys. Any reflux is abnormal and readily detected from the presence of activity above the bladder. Reflux can be graded using criteria devised for contrast cystography (Figure 12-32); however, anatomic resolution and the detail available with scintigraphy are significantly less than with conventional x-ray cystography. Because scintigraphy does not have adequate resolution to permit visualization of calyceal morphology, the following criteria are used instead to grade of reflux: level reached, degree of dilation of the renal pelvis, and degree of dilation and tortuosity of the ureter. Generally, reflux is considered minimal when confined to the ureter, mild to moderate when it reaches the pelvicocalyceal system, and severe when a distended collecting system and/or a redundant ureter are noted (Figure 12-33).

The volume of the bladder and the residual volume after voiding can be calculated by measuring the change in count rate before and after voiding and relating it to the urine volume (see Box 12-10).

Accuracy

Radionuclide cystography is more sensitive than the radiographic contrast technique. The radionuclide technique permits detection of reflux volumes on the order of 1.0 mL. In one comparison study, 17% of reflux events were seen only on the radionuclide study when compared to the radiographic contrast method. Repeating the filling and micturation phases of the radionuclide study can improve the sensitivity for detecting reflux, although this is not routinely done.

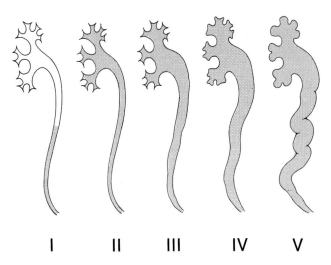

Fig. 12-32 Contrast cystography grading system for vescio-ureteral reflux as put forth by the International Reflux Study Committee:

Grade I   Ureteral reflux only.

Grade II   Reflux into ureter, pelvis, and calyces. No dilation; normal calyceal fornices.

Grade III Mild to moderate dilation and/or tortuosity of ureter and mild to moderate calyceal dilation, but no blunting of fornices.

Grade IV   Moderate dilation and tortuosity of ureter and moderate dilation of renal pelvis. Angles of fornices are obliterated, but papillary impressions are maintained.

Grade V   Gross dilation and tortuosity of the ureter and gross dilation of renal pelvis and calyces. Papillary impressions are no longer visible in most calyces.

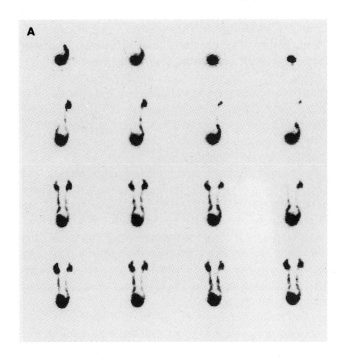

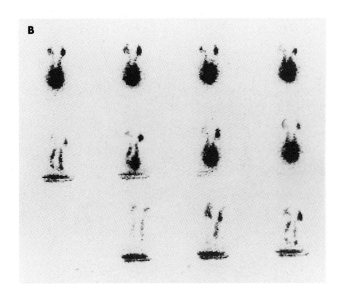

Fig. 12-33 Scintigraphic appearance of vesicoureteral reflux. **A,** During the filling phase, reflux is first seen on the right, then bilaterally. **B,** On voiding, the left side clears better than the right. Postvoiding images (*bottom*) show bilateral pelvic reflux recurring (*bottom*).

SCROTAL SCINTIGRAPHY

Scintigraphy has been used to diagnose the cause of *acute* scrotal pain since the early 1970s. Its utility lies in the ability to differentiate acute testicular torsion from inflammation, most commonly epididymitis.

Testicular viability after torsion of the spermatic cord depends on the length of time between onset of pain and surgical reduction. Atrophy may occur after as little as 4 hours of ischemia and is inevitable by 10 hours after torsion. Therefore, testicular torsion is a surgical emergency. Scintigraphy can promptly confirm the clinically suspected diagnosis of torsion and direct that patient to surgery. It can also minimize unnecessary exploration in patients with an inflammatory cause of their pain.

Color flow Doppler imaging is now being used to evaluate acute scrotal pain; however, there are no comparison studies. For *chronic* or painless disorders of the scrotum, US is the method of choice, and scintigraphy does not play an important role.

Pathogenesis of Testicular Torsion

Developmental abnormalities of testicular descent and attachment predispose to spermatic cord torsion. The testicle is a retroperitoneal structure. During fetal growth, the testis and its aortic blood supply descend from the midabdomen through the inguinal canal into the scrotum. The tunica vaginalis, formed as an outpouching of the retroperitoneal lining, covers the developing testis and muscular and fascial layers of the abdominal peritoneum, and descends into the developing scrotal pouch. Normally the tunica vaginalis covers the testes anteriorly only. The testis is anchored inferiorly and posteriorly through attachments to the posterior scrotal wall (Figure 12-34A).

The most common developmental abnormality leading to torsion of the spermatic cord is the "bell clapper" testis (Figure 12-34B). This abnormality results in complete encirclement of the testis, epididymis, and spermatic cord by the tunica vaginalis, preventing normal posterior and inferior anchoring of the testis. The testis and vascular bundle are suspended freely like the clapper of a bell between the layers of the tunica. The abnormality is usually bilateral.

The incidence of torsion is tenfold higher in undescended testes than in those that have descended normally; however, the former circumstance is rare. Torsion of an incompletely descended testis above the inguinal ring is difficult to detect scintigraphically owing to the large amount of background activity.

Blood Supply to Testes and Scrotum

The testes and scrotum have separate blood supplies. The spermatic cord vessels supplying the *testes* include the testicular artery, which arises from the abdominal aorta just below the orgin of the renal arteries, and the cremasteric and deferential arteries (Figure 12-35). The *scrotum* receives blood supply ultimately from the femoral and internal iliac arteries via the superficial, deep external, and internal pudendal arteries. These separate blood supplies can sometimes be distinguished scintigraphically. The spermatic cord has a steeper and more vertical axis than the scrotal vessels, which enter more horizontally.

Radiopharmaceutic and Physiologic Mechanism

Tc-99m pertechnetate is used for testicular scanning. It serves as a blood flow and blood pool (extracellular fluid space) radiomarker. Evidence of asymmetric blood

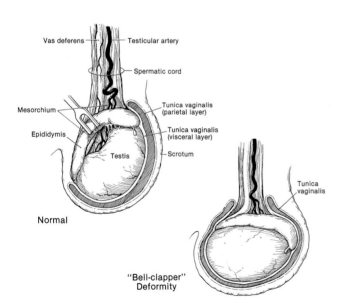

Fig. 12-34 A, Normal scrotal anatomy, right lateral view. The normal testis is a retroperitoneal organ with both layers of the tunica vaginalis anterior to it. The epididymis is attached to the posterolateral margin of the testis. These structures are normally anchored to the posterior scrotal wall by the testicular mesorchium. **B,** "Bell-clapper" deformity. In this congenital abnormality, which usually occurs bilaterally, the tunica vaginalis completely invests the testes. The normal posterior mesorchial anchor is absent, allowing the testis to twist on its vascular pedicle. The posterior midtesticular insertion of the testicular artery results in a horizontal lie of the testis, which is diagnostic of bell-clapper deformity.

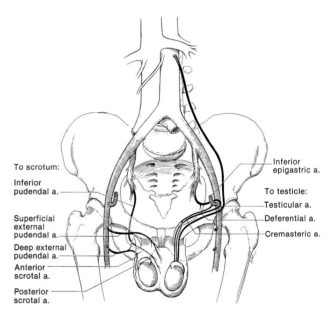

Fig. 12-35 Blood supply to the testes and scrotum. The testes and scrotum have separate blood supplies. The spermatic cord vessels enter the scrotum more superiorly and vertically than the scrotal vessels, which enter more horizontally and laterally. The *spermatic cord vessels* include the testicular artery, which arises from the abdominal aorta just below the orgin of the renal arteries; the cremasteric artery, which arises from the inferior epigastric artery; and the deferential artery, which originates from either the internal iliac or vesical artery. The *scrotal vessels* include the superfical external pudendal artery, arising from the femoral artery; the anterior scrotal artery, arising from the deep external pudendal artery, which orginates from the femoral artery below the superficial external pudendal artery; and the posterior scrotal artery, which arises from branches of the internal pudendal artery, which originates from the internal iliac artery.

flow or tissue blood pool distribution is diagnostic. Inflammation and infection produce hyperemia and increased flow and tissue phase distribution on the involved side, while ischemia results in decreased delivery of radiotracer.

Methodology

Correct positioning is extremely important to compare right and left sides. A marker should be placed on the right thigh to ensure correct right/left orientation. The testicles may be supported with a scrotal sling so that the camera can be positioned as close as possible. In some patients with marked enlargement of one hemiscrotum, it may be necessary to tape the scrotum to prevent the enlarged side from rotating and overlapping the noninvolved side.

Physician involvement is critical for the proper performance and interpretation of this study. The patient should be examined and testicular findings noted. Rubberized lead should be cut to size and placed immediately behind the testes to shield background thigh activity. Gentle retraction over the shield may be necessary if testis redux (involuntary contraction of the cremasteric muscle) occurs. On a late tissue phase image, a "hot" marker should be placed on the abnormal testicle to ensure correct interpretation. A lead median raphe marker placed between the two testicles can also sometimes aid in interpretation. The entire examination should take only 15 to 20 minutes. A typical protocol is described in Box 12-11.

Shielding

Correct placement of an appropriate size lead shield is critical for acquiring an interpretable study. It must be large enough to shield thigh activity behind the scrotum but not so large as to obscure iliac and femoral vessel flow. One approach has been to use no shield during the flow phase and place it before acquiring tissue phase images. A logistically easier method is to cut and fit the shield correctly before starting the study so that no time is lost during imaging.

The study should be performed with a gamma camera interfaced to a nuclear medicine computer system so that image intensity can be optimized retrospectively and, if necessary, selected images from the flow phase can be added together to increase count density.

In young children, a converging collimator can be used for magnification and improved image resolution. A pinhole collimator has been advocated for use in very small children. However, a flow study must be done with another camera, and positioning becomes critical, for slight misalignment of the collimator orientation with the field of view can distort scrotal anatomy.

Box 12-11   Testicular Scintigraphy: Protocol Summary

PATIENT PREPARATION

Oral potassium or sodium perchlorate, 8 mg/kg to a maximum of 500 mg, administered 15–30 min prior to imaging.

RADIOPHARMACEUTICAL

Tc-99m pertechnetate, 10 mCi IV. Children: 250, uCi/kg (minimum, 2 mCi).

CAMERA

Large field of view gamma camera.
Collimator
    Adults: low-energy, all-purpose collimator.
    Children: converging low-energy collimator.

COMPUTER SETUP

Magnification to limit field of view from umbilicus to junction of upper and middle thirds of the femur.
Flow: 2 sec frames for 60 sec.
Tissue phase: 5 sequential static images for 500k counts with a 10-sec delay between images to add or remove markers.

PROCEDURE

1. Position patient supine with towel roll between knees. Tape legs together at knees to prevent movement. Support scrotal contents with tape sling to allow close placement of camera.
2. Place individually fitted rubber lead shield behind scrotum to block background. Do not obscure femoral or iliac vessels.
3. Tape penis up to the lower abdomen so that it does not overlap scrotal contents.
4. Place marker on right thigh.
5. Start computer.
6. Inject radiopharmaceutical.
7. Acquire 60-sec flow study as described above.
8. Then obtain 5 sequential images: 1-3, 500k static images; 4, hot marker on symptomatic testicle; 5, lead marker along median raphe between testicles.

Radiation Dosimetry

The target organ is the stomach, followed by the unblocked thyroid (Table 12-7). However, the thyroid should be blocked with oral perchlorate if time permits.

Image Interpretation

A practical way of analyzing the scrotal scintigram is to divide the images into three phases: spermatic cord flow in the early dynamic flow phase, hemiscrotal flow

Table 12-7	Radiation Dosimetry With Tc-99m Pertechnetate Testicular Scintigraphy
Organ	**rads/mCi**
Stomach	2.50
Colon	0.60
Thyroid	1.30 unblocked
Ovaries	0.20
Testicles	0.09

Modified from MIRD Dose Estimate Report No. 8, *J Nucl Med* 17:74, 1976.

in the late flow phase, and hemiscrotal static activity from the sequential tissue phase images. In each phase the activity on the symptomatic side is compared with that on the opposite side.

Spermatic cord flow can be seen in the frames following tracer appearance in the iliac artery. Hemiscrotal flow appears later in the dynamic flow phase, in the region of the testicle itself. Blood flow is graded as increased, decreased, or equal with respect to blood flow on the asymptomatic side. Hemiscrotal tissue phase activity is assessed on immediate and sequential high count images by comparing the symptomatic and asymptomatic sides.

Normal findings   On flow images, the iliac arteries should be seen simultaneously and should appear symmetric in the amount of radioactivity and the time course of its passage. Because of the relatively low blood flow to the normal scrotal contents, only low-grade, diffuse, symmetric flow is seen bilaterally. On static tissue phase images, scrotal uptake is also low grade and symmetric, usually somewhat less than in the thighs.

Bladder accumulation of radiotracer is increasingly seen on sequential tissue phase images. Activity at the base of the penis may be seen in the midline and should not be misinterpreted. Diffusion of activity into the scrotal contents on later images may decrease the contrast between structures, making image interpretation more difficult. Therefore, the later images are best used for marker placement.

Acute testicular torsion   The scintigraphic findings in acute testicular torsion depend on the time that has elapsed since the acute event. In early torsion, with a few hours of onset, flow images may show no significant asymmetry during either the spermatic cord or later hemiscrotal phase. Occasionally a small projection of activity medial to the iliac artery on the affected side due to activity in the proximal portion of the obstructed spermatic vessels ("nubbin" sign) can be seen. On the static tissue phase images, decreased activity may be seen in the region of the involved testicle (Figure 12-36).

It cannot be emphasized enough that the diagnosis of early testicular torsion is not based on the demonstration of decreased flow. Moreover, in the face of unequivocal clinical findings of an acute hemiscrotum, an apparently "negative" scrotal scintigram must be taken as evidence of acute torsion. The reasoning behind this observation comes from two factors. First, it is not usually possible to distinguish "normal" from "decreased" flow by radionuclide scrotal scintigraphy. Second, compensatory changes may obscure the decreased testicular uptake that should theoretically be seen on high count images in acute torsion. Lead shielding

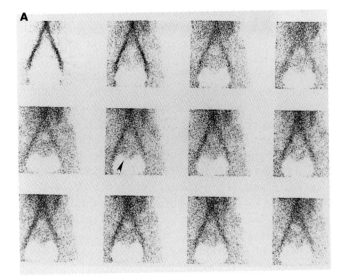

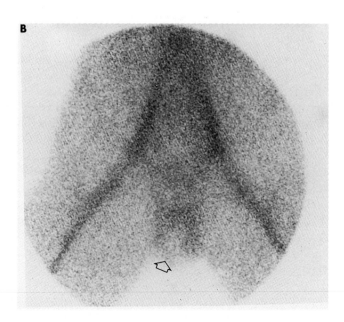

Fig. 12-36   Acute torsion. **A,** The flow phase shows minimal asymmetry, with slightly decreased flow seen on the right (*arrowhead*). **B,** This static high-count blood pool image shows decreased activity on the right (*open arrowhead*) consistent with right testicular torsion. This was confirmed at surgery.

to reduce scatter and shine-through background activity is particularly valuable in early subtle cases.

Later in the course of torsion, the image findings change significantly. Increased perfusion is actually demonstrated on the affected side as a result of scrotal flow from the pudendal arteries. The delayed dynamic flow phase images show increased scrotal activity. The ischemic testicle is seen as an area of relatively decreased activity on static tissue phase images. A distinct surrounding halo (Figure 12-37) of increased activity develops and is due to hyperemia of the dartos, the superficial smooth muscle in the scrotum.

As the time that has elapsed since the acute torsion event increases, the findings of hemiscrotal hyperemia, the nubbin sign, and the dartos halo all become increasingly prominent. The term *missed torsion* is sometimes used to describe the late findings of torsion; however, *delayed torsion* is preferable and more accurate. Although the involved testis may not be salvageable, it is important to recognize a late torsion, for it identifies patients who should undergo prophylactic contralateral orchiopexy, for the predisposing developmental abnormality is usually bilateral.

Acute epididymitis Bacterial epididymitis and epididymo-orchitis usually occur coincident with the onset of sexual activity; the peak incidence is in the late teens and early adult years. Inflammatory disease in prepubertal children is more commonly caused by a virus.

The scintigraphic findings in acute epididymitis are dramatically different from those of acute or delayed torsion. The early dynamic phase images demonstrate markedly increased activity in the spermatic cord vessels (Figure 12-38). The hemiscrotal phase dynamic images also demonstrate asymmetry with intensely increased localization on the affected side. Classically in this phase there is a crescent configuration of increased activity laterally in the epididymis. On static images, diffusely increased uptake is seen in the region of the epididymis,

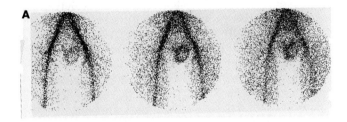
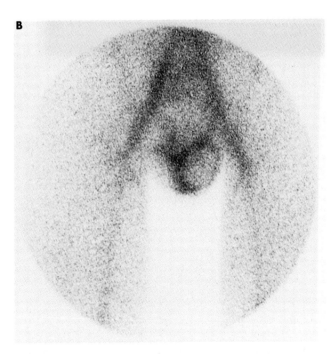

Fig. 12-37 Delayed torsion. Pain in the left testicle began 24 hours earlier. **A,** Two-second frames show increased flow to the left hemiscrotum. **B,** High-count blood pool images shows a "halo" pattern on the left, consistent with delayed torsion. At surgery, this testicle was not viable and was removed. Orchiopexy was subsequently performed on the right.

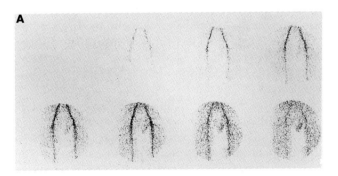
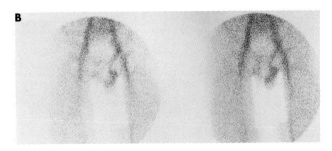

Fig. 12-38 Acute epididymitis. The patient complained of recent onset of pain in the left testicle. **A,** There is increased flow to the left lateral scrotum. **B,** High-count blood pool images show a similar pattern of uptake, most consistent with acute epididymitis. The symptoms resolved over a week while the patient took antibiotics.

but activity is normal within the testicle. With testicular involvement (epididymo-orchitis) the entire hemiscrotum shows asymmetrically increased activity.

Torsion of a testicular appendage Torsion of one of the testicular appendages, although painful, is not serious and always resolves spontaneously. Management is conservative and nonoperative. This condition commonly occurs in boys 7 to 14 years old and has a frequency similar to that of spermatic cord torsion. On physical examination there may be a palpable nodule at the upper pole of the involved testis, and a "blue dot" may be seen deep in the soft tissues with transillumination of the scrotum.

Radionuclide scrotal scintigraphy may be normal or may show low-grade inflammation. Mildly increased flow can be seen, mainly in the venous phase, as a result of inflammation of overlying dartos. In the tissue phase, there may be a focal area of increased activity at the upper pole.

Other testicular diseases Scrotal scintigraphy is not the primary imaging modality of choice in most other conditions affecting the scrotal contents or testis. *Testicular abscesses* exhibit very increased flow on the dynamic phase images. Hyperemia surrounding the abscess produces an appearance not unlike the halo seen in delayed or missed torsion. *Hydroceles* and *hematomas* appear as photon-deficient areas. Uncomplicated hydroceles are not associated with increased flow.

The appearance of *testicular tumors* is quite variable. They can be hyperemic with increased flow on the dynamic images and increased tracer localization corresponding to the tumor. With necrotic tumors, photon deficient areas are seen within the lesion. The appearance can be deceptively similar to that of missed torsion, although the clinical history is usually of a longer standing process.

Varicoceles can be quite dramatic by radionuclide imaging. The later venous portions of the dynamic flow sequence demonstrate increased tracer localization in the pampiniform venous plexus. Because the key to the diagnosis of varicocele is late accumulation of activity in the venous structures, Tc-99m-labeled RBCs can be used to make this diagnosis. Varicoceles are associated with an increased incidence of sterility.

Accuracy

Testicular scintigraphy is an accurate technique for differentiating acute testicular torsion from epididymoorchitis if the examination is performed within 24 hours of the onset of symptoms. In the appropriate clinical seeting, the sensitivity and specificity approach 95%. The study is not as reliable if pain and swelling have been present for a longer time. The halo sign of peripheral hyperemia is nonspecific and can be seen in other conditions.

SUGGESTED READINGS

Blaufox MD, editor: *Evaluation of renal function and disease with radionuclides*, ed 2, 1989, S Karger.

Chen DCP, Holder LE, and Melloul M: Radionuclide scrotal imaging: further experience with 210 patients. Part I and Part II, *J Nucl Med* 24:735-742, 841-853, 1983.

Eggli DF and Garcia JE: Radionuclide imaging of the acutely painful scrotum. In Van Nostrand D and Baum S, editors: *Atlas of nuclear medicine*, Philadelphia, 1988, JB Lippincott.

Eggli DF and Tulchinsky M: Scintigraphic evaluation of pediatric urinary tract infection, *Semin Nucl Med* 23: 199-218, 1993.

Eshima D, Fritzberg AR, and Taylor A Jr: Tc-99m renal tubular function agents: current status, *Semin Nucl Med* 20:28-40, 1990.

Fommei E, Ghione SS, Hilson AJW et al: Captopril radionuclide test in renovascular hypertension: a European multicentre study. *Eur J Nucl Med* 20:617-623, 1993.

O'Reilly PH: Diuresis renography 8 years later: an update, *Urol* 136:993-999, 1986.

Tauxe WN and Dubovsky EV, editors: *Nuclear medicine in clinical urology and nephrology*, Norwalk, Conn, 1985, Appleton-Century-Crofts.

Thrall JH, Koff SA, and Keyes JW Jr: Diuretic radionuclide renography and scintigraphy in the differential diagnosis of hydroureteronephrosis, *Semin Nucl Med* XI: 89-103, 1981.

CHAPTER 13

Endocrine System

Studies of the endocrine system are among the original procedures in nuclear medicine. Iodine-131 was made available to the medical community in the United States after World War II by the Atomic Energy Commission. It was quickly recognized by thyroidologists that the percentage uptake of radioiodine at a fixed point in time after administration was a measure of thyroid function. This early measurement was further enhanced by suppression and stimulation interventions aimed at determining thyroid autonomy and thyroid functional reserve, respectively. By the early 1950s, gamma ray scintillation detectors had been coupled to mechanical devices to permit systematic rectilinear scanning to form functional image maps (scans) of the thyroid gland. These studies of the thyroid gland were a stimulus to the early development of the entire field of nuclear medicine.

In the ensuing decades further advances occurred in the instrumentation and pharmaceuticals used for thyroid imaging, and scintigraphic techniques were applied to imaging other endocrine organs, with variable success. The singular strength of the radiotracer approach in the endocrine system is the ability to use a wide variety of endocrine hormone precursors and analogues to create radiopharmaceuticals that become incorporated into endocrine metabolic pathways.

THYROID IMAGING AND FUNCTION STUDIES

Thyroid scintigraphy and radiotracer uptake studies remain an important part of the practice of nuclear medicine, although they are not used as frequently today as they were two and three decades ago. For example, ultrasonography (US) and fine needle aspiration biopsy have partially supplanted thyroid scintigraphy in the evaluation of patients with clinically palpable thyroid nodules.

Thyroid scintigraphy remains uniquely suited to the determination of the functional status of thyroid nodules, the detection of extrathyroidal metastases from differentiated thyroid carcinoma, and in establishing the thyroid as the tissue of origin of mediastinal masses. The thyroid scintigram has the advantage over cross-sectional techniques of depicting the entire gland in a single image and allows physical findings to be correlated with specific abnormalities in the image.

Radiopharmaceuticals

The principal radiopharmaceuticals employed for thyroid imaging include iodine-131, iodine-123, and technetium-99m. Thallium-201 has also been used selectively in studies of thyroid cancer.

Rationale   Iodine is a precursor in thyroid hormone synthesis. The thyroid gland traps iodine and can concentrate it with a ratio of over 100:1, compared to plasma. The iodine in the gland is incorporated into thyroid hormone (organification) and subsequently bound to thyroglobulin. The pertechnetate ion (TcO_4^-) is trapped and concentrated by the thyroid gland but does not undergo organification or incorporation into thyroid hormone. The normally high concentration of these radiotracers in the thyroid gland affords excellent visualization of the thyroid unless thyroid uptake and function are impaired.

Physics and dosimetry   I-131 undergoes beta minus decay with a principal gamma photon energy of 364 keV. The energy of the principal beta particle is 0.606 MeV and the half-life is 8.06 days (Box 13-1). I-131 is formulated as a sodium salt for clinical use.

The presence of beta particle emissions, the relatively high energy of the principal gamma ray emissions, and the long half-life of I-131 are disadvantages to the use of this tracer. The particulate emissions and long half-life result in a higher than optimal radiation dose to the thyroid gland (see Box 13-1). This in turn restricts the size of the administered dose. The principal photon energy is higher than ideal for use with gamma scintillation cameras. Negative factors related to high energy include image degradation through septal penetration of the collimator and poor detection sensitivity in the relatively thin sodium iodide crystals of gamma cameras.

For these reasons, I-131 is not considered the agent of choice for routine diagnostic thyroid scintigraphy. However, its long half-life is well suited to delayed studies at 24, 48, and even 72 hours after injection. Delayed imaging improves tracer clearance from nontarget tissues, which is a distinct advantage in detecting thyroid cancer metastases and evaluating mediastinal masses.

In many respects I-123 is a better agent than I-131 for thyroid imaging. The principal gamma energy is 159 keV, which is ideally suited for gamma scintillation cameras (Box 13-2). The half-life of 13.3 hours is also well suited to the time frame for most thyroid imaging and uptake studies. The mode of decay is electron capture, and there are no primary particulate emissions.

A number of drawbacks have kept I-123 from becoming universally employed for thyroid scintigraphy. First, most methods of preparing I-123 result in longer-lived radionuclidic impurities (I-124 and I-125) that result in higher radiation doses to the thyroid than would be calculated from I-123 alone. Second, commercial availabil-

---

Box 13-1   Iodine-131: Summary of Physical Characteristics and Dosimetry

PHYSICAL CHARACTERISTICS

Mode of decay:	Beta minus.
Physical half-life ($T_{1/2}$):	8.1 days.
Photon energy:	364 keV.
Abundance:	81%.

DOSIMETRY*: SODIUM IODIDE 131 ADMINISTERED ORALLY

Organ	rads/100 μCi
Thyroid (15% uptake)	78
Bladder	0.27
Stomach wall	0.15
Small intestine	0.11
Liver	0.028
Testes	0.018
Ovaries	0.012
Red marrow	0.021
Total body	0.047

*Modified from product information comparative data, Mallinckrodt Medical Inc., St. Louis, Mo.
Note: All values assume 15% thyroid uptake.

Box 13-2   Iodine-123: Summary of Physical Characteristics and Dosimetry

PHYSICAL CHARACTERISTICS

Mode of decay:	Electron capture.
Physical half-life ($T_{1/2}$):	13.2 hr.
Photon energy:	159 keV.
Abundance:	83.4%.

DOSIMETRY*: SODIUM IODIDE CAPSULES ADMINISTERED ORALLY

Organ	rads/400 μCi
Thyroid (15% uptake)	7.7
Bladder	0.16
Stomach wall	0.089
Small intestine	0.065
Liver	0.010
Testes	0.007
Ovaries	0.017
Red marrow	0.012
Total body	0.014

*Modified from product information for sodium iodide-123 capsules, Mallinckrodt Medical Inc., St. Louis, Mo.
Note: All values assume thyroid uptake of 15% at time of calibration.

ity has been limited, resulting in higher cost for this agent. The short physical half-life also makes it more difficult to keep I-123 reliably available on a routine basis.

Technetium-99m pertechnetate is a frequently used alternative to radioiodine for thyroid scintigraphy. As noted previously, the physical characteristics of Tc-99m are ideal for use with gamma scintillation cameras (Box 13-3). Sodium pertechnetate is readily and reliably available in nuclear medicine clinics from Mo-99/Tc-99m generator systems, so that supply is not a problem, as it is with I-123. The lack of particulate emissions and the short half-life of Tc-99m result in the lowest radiation dose per unit of administered activity of any of the thyroid imaging agents (see Box 13-3).

Pharmacokinetics Radioiodine is rapidly absorbed from the gastrointestinal tract after oral administration. Radioactivity is detectable in the gland within minutes and, in euthyroid subjects, reaches the thyroid follicular lumen within 20 to 30 minutes. Thus, the uptake and organification of iodine are quite rapid. The several-hour delay selected for imaging studies using I-123 and the 1-day delay typically chosen for studies with I-131 are dictated by the desire for background clearance and not by slow uptake in the gland. The normal range for percent uptake is 10% to 30% of the administered dose.

The pharmacokinetics for Tc-99m pertechnetate are also rapid. The tracer is typically administered intravenously (IV) for thyroid imaging studies and the trapping process begins essentially immediately. Optimal uptake is achieved by 20 to 30 minutes, which is also selected as the time to begin imaging. At this time, approximately 0.5% to 3.75% of the radiopertechnetate is in the gland of euthyroid subjects.

The pertechnetate ion is avidly trapped but not organified by the thyroid. In the vast majority of circumstances there is concordant localization and identical scintigraphic visualization with pertechnetate and radioiodine. In a small percentage of thyroid nodules there is a discordance between the scintigraphic pattern of radioiodine and radiopertechnetate owing to loss of the organification function in the nodular tissue. This will be discussed further in the section on clinical applications.

Precautions Radioiodine is excreted in human breast milk, and nursing should be stopped following diagnostic or therapeutic studies with radioiodine. With I-123, nursing can be resumed after several days if the amount used does not exceed 30 μCi. However, the usual imaging dosage is 100 to 400 μCi, and a longer interval is necessary. For I-131, nursing must be terminated for many weeks after even small doses before safe levels are achieved. With Tc-99m pertechnetate, nursing can be resumed in 24 hours.

Pregnancy is also a special precaution for studies with radioiodine. The fetal thyroid concentrates radioiodine after the 12th week of gestation. Radioiodine crosses the

---

Box 13-3 Technetium 99m: Summary of Physical Characteristics and Dosimetry

PHYSICAL CHARACTERISTICS

Mode of decay:	Isomeric transition.
Physical half-life ($T_{1/2}$):	6 hr.
Photon energy:	140 keV.
Abundance:	89%.

DOSIMETRY*: SODIUM PERTECHNETATE ADMINISTERED INTRAVENOUSLY

Organ	rads/mCi
Thyroid	0.130
Bladder wall	0.085
Stomach	0.05
Large intestine	0.11
Red marrow	0.02
Testis	0.01
Ovary	0.03
Total body	0.01

*Modified from product information brochure for sodium pertechnetate, Dupont Company, Billerica, Mass.

---

placenta, and significant exposure of the fetal thyroid can occur and may even result in cretinism following therapeutic doses to the mother.

A more practical and common problem with thyroid studies is the interference of stable iodine contained in foods and medications. Table 13-1 summarizes some of the more commonly encountered ones as well as several non-iodine-containing drugs that affect thyroidal radioiodine uptake. The suppression of uptake may be sufficient to preclude successful imaging but is even more important in assessing the results of radioiodine percent uptake studies of thyroid function. As little as 1 mg of stable iodine can cause significant reduction of the 24-hour radioiodine uptake, and as little as 10 mg can effectively block the gland, with a 98% reduction in uptake. Radiographic contrast media are a common source of iodine in hospitalized patients that may interfere with thyroid imaging and uptake studies. A food and drug history should be obtained from all patients undergoing thyroid imaging and function studies.

Technique

The gamma scintillation camera with pinhole collimator is the usual instrument of choice for thyroid imaging. This combination has replaced the rectilinear scanner. The combination of gamma camera and pinhole collimator offers the flexibility of obtaining multiple views of the thyroid. The magnification made possible by the pinhole

Table 13-1 Nonthyroidal Causes of Increased and Decreased Thyroidal Uptake of Radioiodine

Cause	Duration of Effect (wks)
DECREASED UPTAKE	
Thyroid hormones	
Thyroxine (T$_4$)	4-6
Triiodothyronine (T$_3$)	2-3
Excess iodine (expanded iodine pool)	
Lugol's solution	2-4
SSKI	2-4
Some mineral supplements, cough medicines, and vitamin preparations	2-4
Iodine food supplements	
Iodinated drugs	2-4
Iodinated skin ointments	2-4
Radiographic contrast media	
Water-soluble intravascular media	2-4
Oral cholecystographic agents	4 to indefinite
Fat-soluble media (lymphography)	Months to years
Non-iodine-containing drugs	Variable
ACTH, adrenal steroids	
Monovalent anions (perchlorate)	
Penicillin	
Goitrogenic foods (cabbage, turnips)	
INCREASED UPTAKE	
Iodine deficiency	
Pregnancy	
Rebound after therapy (thyroid hormones, antithyroid drugs)	
Recovery from subacute thyroiditis	
Choriocarcinoma, hydatidiform mole	
Renal failure	

Box 13-4 Tc-99 Pertechnetate Thyroid Imaging: Protocol Summary

PATIENT PREPARATION

Discontinue any medications that interfere with thyroid uptake of Tc-99m pertechnetate (Table 13-1).

DOSAGE AND ROUTE OF ADMINISTRATION

1-10 mCi (37-370 MBq) Tc-99m pertechnetate administered IV.

TIME OF IMAGING

20 min after radiopharmaceutical administration.

PROCEDURE

Use a gamma camera with a 3-6-mm-aperture pinhole collimator and a 20% energy window centered at 140 keV.

Position the patient supine with the chin up and neck extended.

Position the collimator so that the thyroid fills about two thirds of the diameter of the field of view.

Obtain anterior and 45° left anterior and right anterior oblique views (move the collimator, if possible, rather than the patient).

Obtain 200,000 - 250,000 counts per view.

Mark the chin and suprasternal notch.

Note the position and mark palpable nodules and surgical scars.

Marker sources may be placed lateral to the thyroid to calibrate size.

---

collimator allows resolution of nodules smaller than possible with parallel-hole collimators. Nodules as small as 3 to 5 mm in diameter can be detected in ideal situations.

Radiopertechnetate imaging For studies with Tc-99m pertechnetate, 1 to 10 mCi is administered IV with imaging begun 20 minutes post injection (Box 13-4). A standard field of view gamma camera equipped with a pinhole collimator and 3- to 6-mm insert is used with a 20% window centered at 140 keV. The patient is positioned supine with the neck extended so that the plane of the thyroid gland is parallel to the crystal face of the camera. The collimator is positioned so that the thyroid gland fills approximately two thirds to three quarters of the field of view. In patients with normal thyroids, this is achieved with a 6- to 8-cm distance from the collimator to the surface of the neck. It is useful to put a radioactive marker on the sternal notch and chin, and most laboratories use a 4- to 5-cm line marker or two point sources 4 to 5 cm apart on the neck just lateral to the thyroid lobes

and parallel to their long axis (Figure 13-1). The marker permits size estimates of observed structures, including nodules, by allowing correction for the pinhole magnification effect.

Images are obtained in the anterior and both the 45° right anterior oblique and 45° left anterior oblique views (Figure 13-2). Each image is obtained for 200,000 to 250,000 counts. Marker source images may be obtained for fewer counts. It is preferable to keep the patient in one position and move the camera and collimator. This is more reproducible than moving the patient and does not distort the thyroid.

Before the patient is placed in position for imaging, a physical examination of the thyroid gland is performed to identify the location of nodules. Locations are verified in the imaging position, and during a separate acquisition a Tc-99m marker source is used to locate palpable nodules for functional correlation. If all images are obtained with a computer system, the distance calibration

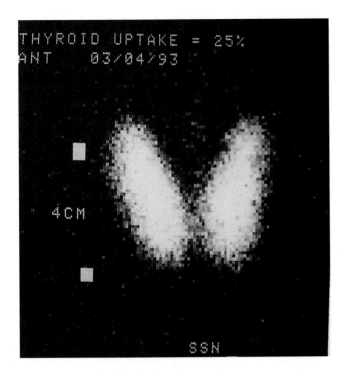

Fig. 13-1 Normal thyroid scintigram obtained with I-123. The sternal notch is indicated, and there are electronic markers providing a 4-cm scale adjacent to the right thyroid lobe. Radioiodine uptake is 25%.

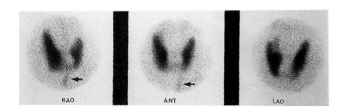

Fig. 13-2 Anterior and both anterior oblique views obtained with Tc-99m pertechnetate. Note the esophageal activity below the thyroid to the left of midline (*arrows*).

images as well as images obtained for nodule localization purposes with marker sources can be readily superimposed on each other for analysis.

Radioiodine-123 Studies with I-123 are also obtained with a standard field of view gamma camera equipped with a pinhole collimator and a 3- to 6-mm insert (Box 13-5). The tracer is administered orally in capsule form as sodium iodide. Imaging may be accomplished at 6 and 24 hours, depending on laboratory preference. A 20% window is used and centered at 159 keV. The imaging sequence is the same as with radiopertechnetate. For each image, 200,000 to 250,000 counts are obtained. The chin and suprasternal notch are marked on the scan. All palpable nodules, masses, and scars are also noted

---

Box 13-5   Thyroid Imaging With I-123 (Sodium Iodide): Protocol Summary

PATIENT PREPARATION

Discontinue any medications that interfere with thyroid uptake of radioiodine.

DOSAGE AND ROUTE OF ADMINISTRATION

100-400 μCi administered orally in capsule form.

TIME OF IMAGING

Image at 6 and/or 24 hr.

PROCEDURE

Use a gamma camera with a 3-6-mm-aperture pinhole collimator and a 20% energy window centered at 159 keV.

Position the patient supine with the chin up and the neck extended.

Position the collimator so that the thyroid fills about two thirds of the diameter of the field of view.

Obtain anterior and 45° left anterior and right anterior oblique views (move the collimator, if possible, rather than the patient).

Obtain 200,000-250,000 counts per view.

Mark the chin and suprasternal notch.

Note the position and mark palpable nodules and surgical scars.

Marker sources may be placed lateral to the thyroid to calibrate size.

---

both on the physical examination and, when appropriate, by radioactive marker sources on the scan.

Thallium-201   Thallium-201 chloride has been used for tumor imaging, including thyroid carcinoma. The uptake is nonspecific and is seen in benign as well as malignant conditions. Tl-201 has not found widespread application in the initial diagnosis of thyroid cancer. Some proponents have championed the use of Tl-201 for thyroid cancer follow-up imaging, where differentiating uptake in normal tissue and benign lesions from tumor is not an issue. One advantage is that patients apparently need not be taken off thyroid hormone replacement therapy for imaging to be performed. However, this approach has not found wide acceptance and should be used with caution. It may be useful for locating metastases in patients with increased thyroglobulin levels and negative radioiodine whole body scintigrams.

Iodine-131: Postoperative and follow-up imaging for thyroid carcinoma   Radioiodine-131 is administered orally in a dose of 2 to 10 mCi (Box 13-6). A large field of view gamma camera equipped with a high-energy

---

Box 13-6   I-131 Whole Body Imaging in Thyroid Cancer: Protocol Summary

PATIENT PREPARATION

Discontinue thyroid hormone for a sufficient period (T_4 for 6 wk, T_3 for 2-3 wk) to ensure an endogenous TSH response.

DOSAGE AND ROUTE OF ADMINISTRATION

2-5 mCi (74-185 MBq) administered orally.

IMAGING TIME

Image at 24 hr Repeat at 48 and 72 hr for equivocal findings.

PROCEDURE

Use a wide field of view gamma camera with computerized data acquisition.

Use a high-energy parallel-hole collimator and a 20% window centered at 364 keV.

Obtain 20-min spot views of the head, neck, and chest and other clinically indicated areas.

Box 13-7   Clinical Indications for Thyroid Scintigraphy

Further evaluation of physical examination findings.
Detection of metastases in patients with thyroid carcinoma.
Follow-up after radioiodine therapy for differentiated thyroid cancer.
Determination of functional status of thyroid nodule.
Differential diagnosis of mediastinal masses.
Detection of extrathyroidal tissue (lingual thyroid).
Screening after head and neck irradiation.

---

parallel-hole collimator is used with a 20% window centered at 364 keV. The single most important view is the anterior view of the head, neck, and chest. However, it is more complete to obtain views from head to pelvis. Computer acquisition is helpful to accommodate a wide range of possible count densities in the image. Many laboratories image for a fixed period of time, typically 10 to 20 minutes per view. The pinhole collimator may also be used to obtain higher resolution spot views of positive areas. Marker sources are used to indicate the location of the chin, suprasternal notch, and xiphoid.

Imaging is often first accomplished at 24 hours. If initial images are equivocal or negative in the setting of high clinical suspicion, further delayed imaging at 48 and 72 hours is done, and even further delays may be necessary. Some laboratories acquire initial images at 48 to 72 hours.

Clinical Applications

The major clinical applications of thyroid scintigraphy are summarized in Box 13-7. In current practice, perhaps the most common indications are the further evaluation of equivocal or confusing findings on physical examination and the follow-up of patients with thyroid cancers.

Appearance of the normal thyroid scintigram   In the euthyroid adult the thyroid gland weighs approximately 15 to 20 grams. It has a butterfly shape with lateral lobes extending along either side of the thyroid car-

tilage of the larynx (see Figures 13-1, 13-2). The lateral lobes are connected by an isthmus that crosses the trachea anteriorly below the level of the cricoid cartilage. The detailed appearance of the gland is highly variable from patient to patient. The right lobe is often slightly larger than the left. The lateral lobes typically measure 4 to 5 cm from superior to inferior poles and have a variable breadth of 1.5 to 2 cm. The pyramidal lobe is a paramedian structure that arises from the isthmus (Figure 13-3). It may arise either to the right or left of the midline and represents functioning thyroid tissue in the thyroglossal duct tract.

In the normal euthyroid subject, there is homogeneous and uniform distribution of radiotracer throughout the gland. Some variation in intensity may be seen in the middle or medial aspects of the lateral lobes due to the thickness of the gland in this location. The amount of activity in the isthmus is highly variable between patients. In some subjects little or no activity is seen, while in others it may be quite prominent. Likewise, in the majority of normal adults, little or no activity is seen in the pyramidal lobe. It is often seen in patients with Graves' disease due to hyperplasia of the tissues in the duct.

In studies obtained with Tc-99m pertechnetate, the salivary glands are routinely visualized (see Figure 13-3) and should not be mistaken for the thyroid or thyroid cancer metastases. Because of the later imaging time for studies with I-123, the salivary glands are not usually seen; the tracer has already been cleared. It is also very common to see some activity in the esophagus (see Figures 13-2, 13-3). The activity is frequently not in the midline, because the esophagus is displaced by the trachea and cervical spine when the neck is hyperextended in the imaging position. The esophageal activity is more commonly seen just to the left of midline and can be confirmed by having the patient swallow a drink of water to cleanse the esophagus, followed by repeat imaging.

Interpretation of the Abnormal Thyroid Scan   A systematic and complete interpretation of the thyroid scintigram requires assessments of thyroid size and con-

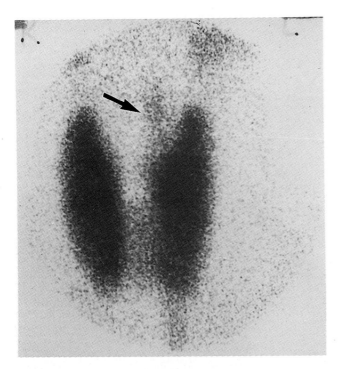

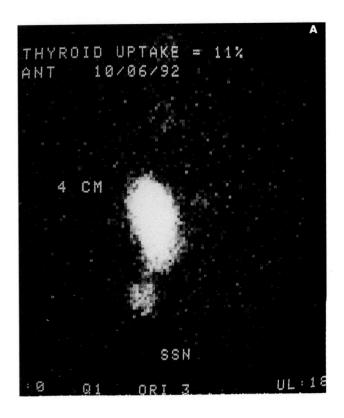

Fig. 13-3 A small pyramidal lobe is seen arising from the medial aspect of the upper pole of the left lobe of the thyroid (*arrow*). A small amount of activity is present below the left lobe in the esophagus. The study was obtained with Tc-99m pertechnetate, and some activity is seen in the region of the salivary glands.

figuration and the identification and description of focal abnormalities, including hot and cold nodules and extrathyroidal activity in the neck or mediastinum. A complete scintigraphic evaluation also entails a close correlation of palpable abnormalities and surgical scars with scintigraphic findings (Figures 13-4 through 13-6). This is frequently critical in assigning significance to a palpable abnormality.

Goiter The term *goiter* simply refers to an enlargement of the thyroid gland. The term itself has no further implication or meaning but is often qualified to indicate the cause of the enlargement. Prior to the addition of iodine supplements to salt and the use of periodates in food, goiter was endemic in the northern United States and in scattered locations in Europe, including southern Germany, and other locations throughout the rest of the world. These endemic goiters typically were composed of colloid nodules, and the vast majority were benign. These goiters are also referred to as *colloid nodular goiters* or *nontoxic goiters*.

The pathogenesis of nodule formation appears to be iodine deficiency-induced hyperplasia followed by the formation of functioning nodules that undergo hemorrhage and are replaced by lakes of colloid. Over time,

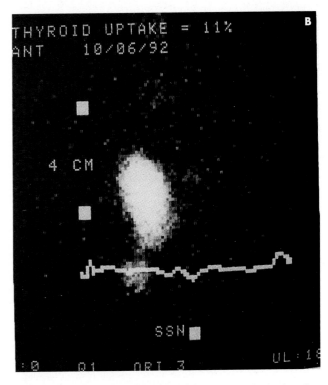

Fig. 13-4 **A,** Thyroid scintigram in a patient who had undergone thyroidectomy for thyroid carcinoma. **B,** Repeat image indicating location of surgical scar on the neck.

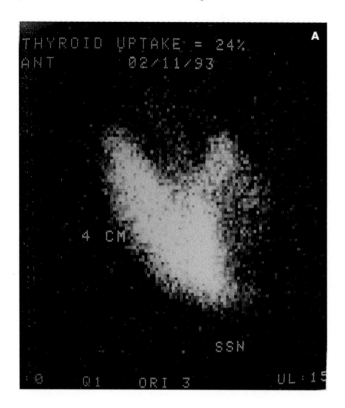

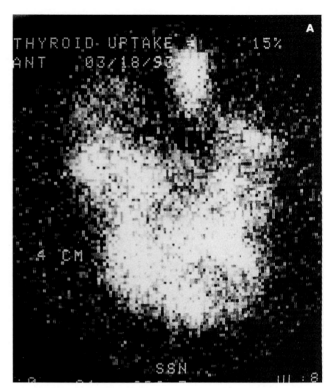

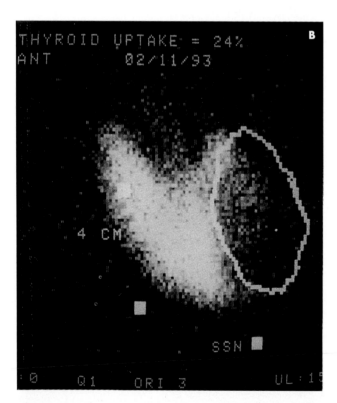

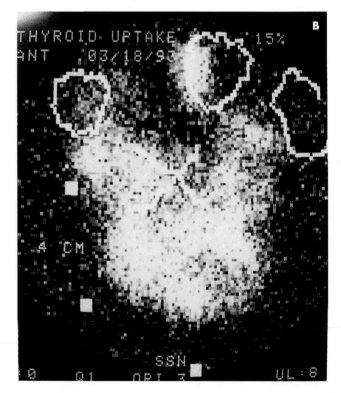

Fig. 13-5 **A**, Thyroid scintigram in a patient presenting with a large solitary nodule in the region of the left lobe. **B**, Repeat scintigram with outline of the clinically palpated nodule superimposed. The nodule is cold and measures approximately 5 × 2.5 centimeters.

Fig. 13-6 **A**, Thyroid scintigram in a patient with a large goiter. Distribution of tracer is inhomogeneous, with numerous cold areas scattered throughout the gland. **B**, Repeat scintigram with the location of three discretely palpable nodules marked on the image.

a repetition of this process leads to overall glandular enlargement, with nonfunctioning colloid nodules the dominant histopathologic feature.

The typical scintigraphic appearance of these benign multinodular colloid goiters is inhomogeneous uptake of tracer with cold areas of various size (Figures 13-6, 13-7A). The incidence of thyroid carcinoma in endemic goiter is low (1%-5%). However, if a patient has a dominant cold nodule, out of proportion in size to other cold areas or enlarging suddenly, it should be regarded with suspicion.

Another important cause of goiter is Graves' disease (toxic goiter) (Figure 13-7B). In this condition the gland is diffusely hyperplastic. The scintigraphic appearance of Graves' disease is uniform and intensely increased uptake. The pyramidal lobe is frequently seen due to hyperplasia of the thyroid tissues in it. In current practice, Graves' disease is not generally considered an indication for obtaining a thyroid scintigram, but imaging has been used in some institutions for help in estimating the size of the thyroid gland to calculate the dosage for I-131 therapy.

Thyroid enlargement can also be due to thyroid carcinoma or involvement of the thyroid by other neoplasm such as lymphoma (Box 13-8). The thyroid may also be enlarged in active phases of thyroiditis.

Thyroid nodules Thyroid nodules are extremely common and the incidence increases with age. Nodules are more common in women than men. The presence of multiple nodules (see Figures 13-6, 13-7), indicating multinodular goiter, significantly reduces the likelihood of malignancy compared to the likelihood of cancer in patients with a solitary "cold" nodule (<5% vs. 15%-40%). The thyroid scintigram may be used to confirm the presence of a clinically palpable nodule, to determine whether other nodules are present, and to assess the functional status of the detected nodule (see Box 13-7). As noted earlier, cold nodules as small as 3 mm in diameter may be detected using the pinhole collimator. Box 13-8 provides a differential diagnosis for thyroid nodules.

Thyroid nodules are classified scintigraphically as being "cold" (nonfunctioning), "hot" (functioning), or indeterminate. The latter category may be assigned when a nodule demonstrates function equal to that of the surrounding normal thyroid. It may also be assigned when a cold or nonfunctioning nodule arises from the anterior or posterior surface of the gland, with normal glandular activity superimposed over the area of the nodule on the scintigram. Although the problem is not common, the possibility of an indeterminate nodule should be borne in mind and highlights the need for close correlation between physical findings and scintigraphic findings. Oblique views with a pinhole collimator can be helpful in separating the nodule from adjacent thyroid tissue. For management purposes, an indeterminate nodule has the same significance as a cold nodule.

"Cold" nodules The vast majority of thyroid nodules

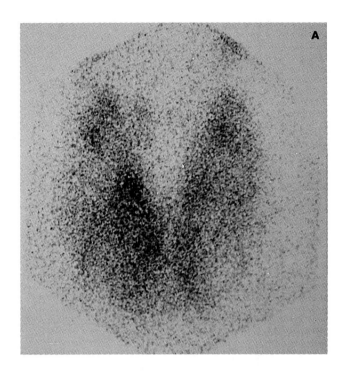

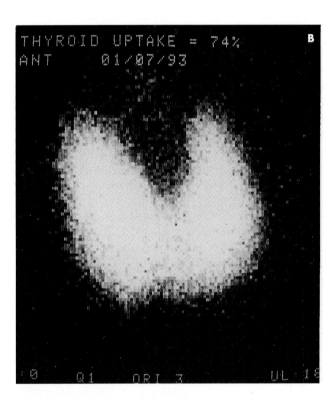

Fig. 13-7 **A,** Typical colloid nodular goiter with enlargement of the thyroid, inhomogeneous tracer distribution and focal cold areas corresponding to nodules. **B,** Thyroid scintigraphy in a patient with Graves' disease. The gland is uniformly enlarged, with homogeneous tracer uptake and distribution. The radioiodine percent uptake is markedly increased at 74%.

Box 13-8   Differential Diagnosis of Thyroid Nodules

BENIGN

Colloid nodule
Simple cyst
Hemorrhagic cyst
Adenoma
Thyroiditis (focal)
Abscess
Parathyroid cyst or adenoma

MALIGNANT

Thyroid cancer
  Papillary
  Follicular
  Anaplastic
  Medullary
Lymphoma
Metastatic carcinoma
  Lung
  Breast
  Melanoma
  Gastrointestinal
  Renal

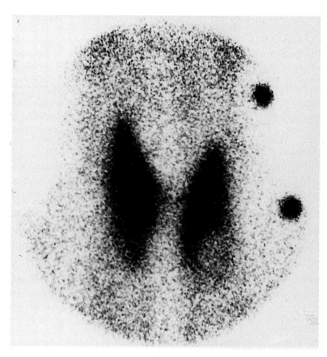

Fig. 13-8   Solitary "cold" nodule in the lower pole of the left lobe.

---

are cold or nonfunctioning (Figures 13-5, 13-8). In reported surgical series, the incidence of thyroid carcinoma in solitary cold nodules ranges from 5% to 40%. An important factor associated with a higher likelihood of cancer is a prior history of radiation to the head and neck or mediastinum. Several decades ago, it was common to use external radiation therapy to shrink the thymus gland and to treat enlarged tonsils and adenoids. Radiation up to 1,500 rads has been conclusively shown to result in an increased incidence of thyroid cancer, and there is increased concern when a cold nodule is detected in a patient with a history of such radiation exposure. Above 1,500 rads, the risk actually appears to decrease, presumably due to destruction of tissue in the gland. Thyroid scintigraphy is more sensitive in detecting nodules than physical examination and has proved useful in screening populations of irradiated patients.

Age and sex are also important factors influencing the likelihood that a solitary cold nodule represents cancer. Because the incidence of benign nodules increases with age there is much more concern over the presence of a nodule in a young individual than in an older subject. Incidental nodules are also more common in women than men. Thus, solitary cold nodules in young men are of particular concern. The other end of the probability spectrum is represented by a multinodular goiter in an older woman.

The thyroid scintigram cannot be used to rule out or

rule in malignancy in cases of solitary cold nodules, and each physician or clinic should have a systematic approach to the workup of such cases. Some physicians advocate US as the next step in the workup. Purely cystic lesions are rarely due to cancer. However, cancers can demonstrate cystic degeneration, and the results of US can be misleading. There are proponents of going directly to fine needle aspiration biopsy without performing scintigraphy as a more direct means of establishing the histology of solitary nodules. This approach is subject to negative sampling errors and requires an experienced cytopathologist.

"Hot" nodules   Hyperfunctioning or "hot" nodules may be either autonomous or under hormonal feedback control (Figure 13-9). Radiotracer uptake in autonomous nodules is not suppressed with administration of thyroid hormone (discussed under Thyroid Function Studies, later in this chapter). Autonomous nodules larger than 3 to 4 cm in diameter typically produce enough thyroid hormone to suppress the pituitary feedback loop. In this case the extranodular thyroid tissues are not visualized scintigraphically (Figure 13-10). In cases with smaller hot nodules producing less hormone, significant uptake may still be visualized in the extranodular structures (Figure 13-11). Hot nodules may undergo spontaneous involution and may have areas of cystic degeneration within them (Figure 13-12).

The importance of demonstrating radioiodine uptake

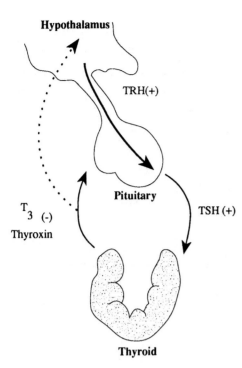

Fig. 13-9 Schematic of the thyroid-pituitary feedback loop. The normal thyroid is under the control of thyroid-stimulating hormone (TSH). The hypothalamic production of thyroid-releasing hormone (TRH) and the pituitary release of TSH are decreased or suppressed as circulating levels of thyroid hormone increase.

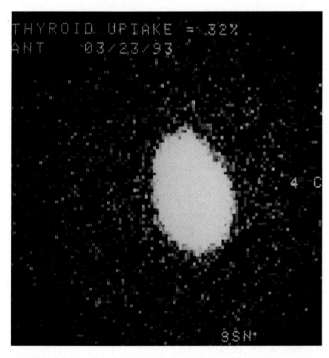

Fig. 13-10 Thyroid scintigram demonstrating a large functioning nodule. No extranodular tissues are seen, indicating suppression of the pituitary feedback loop. Radioiodine uptake is increased, and the patient is clinically hyperthyroid ("toxic" nodule).

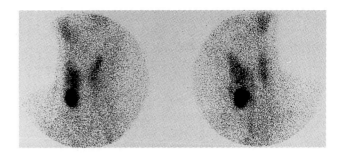

Fig. 13-11 Thyroid scintigram demonstrating a small "hot" nodule arising from the lower pole of the right lobe. The extranodular thyroid tissues are clearly visualized.

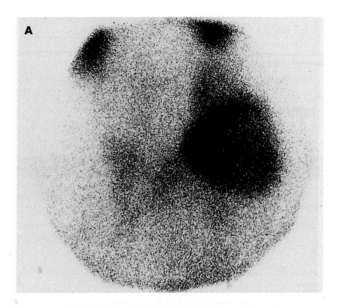

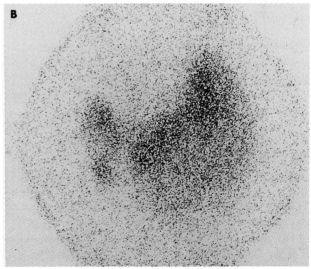

Fig. 13-12 **A,** Thyroid scintiscan showing a large "hot" nodule in the left lobe of the thyroid. The center of the nodule appears to have less intense tracer activity than the periphery, suggesting central degeneration. **B,** Follow-up scintigraphy 1 year later reveals complete involution of the previously seen hot nodule, with residual distortion of the gland.

in a nodule is in the reduced likelihood of cancer compared to solitary cold nodules. Less than 1% of hot nodules harbor malignancy, and a critical review of the literature suggests the likelihood is even lower if incidental cancers adjacent to hot nodules are excluded.

Functioning nodules may be associated with hyperthyroidism (see Figure 13-10). This usually requires a large nodule, 3 to 4 cm or more in diameter, or the presence of multiple functioning nodules. Thyrotoxicosis associated with autonomous (autonomous toxic nodule) functioning nodules is referred to as Plummer's disease.

The clinical management of patients with hyperfunctioning nodules is influenced by the presence of local symptoms in the neck and by whether the patient is euthyroid or thyrotoxic. Locally asymptomatic hot nodules in euthyroid subjects can often be followed clinically. In some cases the nodules continue to grow in size with the development of thyrotoxicosis. In other cases the nodules stabilize or even regress or undergo involution.

In thyrotoxic subjects, surgical removal, typically by lobectomy, is often recommended. An alternative approach is treatment with radioiodine. Proponents of this approach note that there is selective delivery of radiation to the hyperfunctioning tissue with sparing of the extranodular tissues. This treatment should not be used if there is any suspicion of thyroid cancer.

"Discordant" nodules An important aspect of thyroid scintigraphy is the possibility of "discordance" between radioiodine and radiopertechnetate scintigrams. Because Tc-99m pertechnetate is trapped but not organified, a nodule may appear hot on pertechnetate imaging and cold on radioiodine imaging (Figure 13-13). This occurs in approximately 2% to 3% of radiopertechnetate hot nodules. Conservatively, a single hot nodule identified on radiopertechnetate imaging should not be considered a functioning nodule until confirmed by radioiodine studies. Case reports in the literature describe thyroid cancers maintaining the trapping but not the organification function. The problem of the discordant nodule is a drawback to the use of Tc-99m pertechnetate for routine thyroid scintigraphy.

Substernal thyroid Thyroid scintigraphy is used occasionally in the differential diagnosis of mediastinal masses. Substernal thyroid tissue may be the result of goitrous enlargement with downward extension or may be due to abnormal migration during development (Figure 13-14).

The ability to perform delayed imaging after tissue and blood pool clearance of background activity is a major advantage of I-131 for this application. Tc-99m pertechnetate is not a good choice, owing to the high mediastinal blood pool activity at the 20- to 30-minute imaging time typically used with this tracer (Figure 13-15). Function and tracer uptake in substernal goiters are frequently poor, and the highest target-to-background ratio possible is desirable. Delayed imaging at 48 and 72 hours may be required.

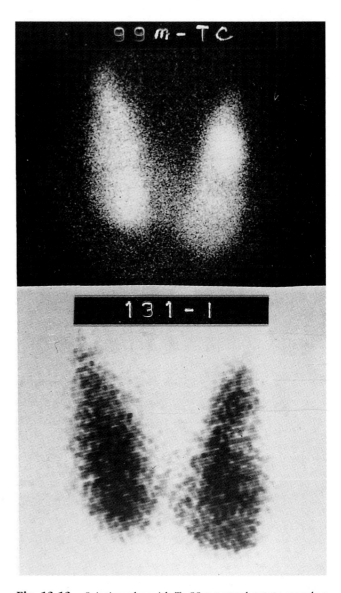

Fig. 13-13 Scintigraphy with Tc-99m pertechnetate reveals a functioning nodule in the left upper pole. In the corresponding I-131 radioiodine scintigram, the nodule is cold. This is referred to as "discordance" between radioiodine and radiopertechnetate. (Courtesy Steven M. Pinsky, M.D., University of Illinois, Chicago.) (From Keyes JW Jr, Thrall JH, and Carey JE: Technical considerations in In Vivo Thyroid studies. *Semin Nucl Med*, VIII, 43, 1978.)

The usual cervical location of the thyroid gland should always be imaged when searching for substernal goiter because the vast majority of cases demonstrate continuity with the cervical portion of the gland. In some cases, there is only a fibrous band connecting the substernal and cervical thyroid tissues, but in almost all cases there is some abnormality of the main gland.

Other ectopic thyroid tissue The thyroglossal duct runs from the foramen cecum at the base of the tongue to the thyroid. Rarely, the thyroid fails to migrate from its anlage. Complete failure to migrate results in a *lin-*

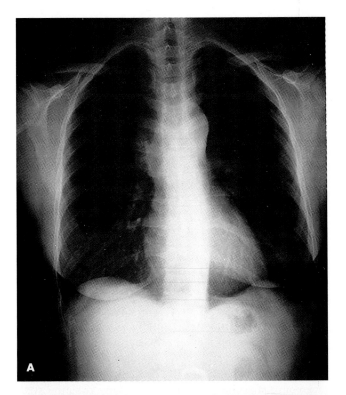

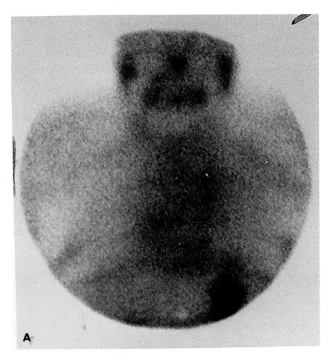

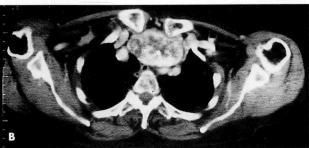

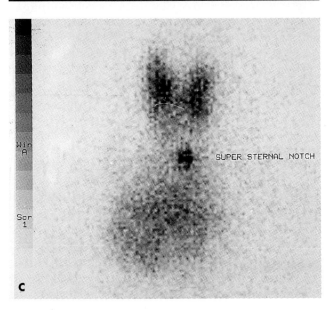

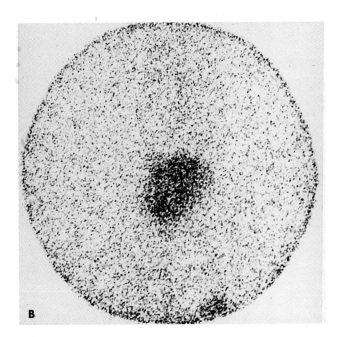

Fig. 13-14   **A**, Chest radiograph reveals a superior mediastinal mass. **B**, CT confirms the presence of the mass, which demonstrates inhomogeneous density. **C**, Subsequent radioiodine scintigraphy reveals a large substernal goiter.

Fig. 13-15   **A**, Tc-99m pertechnetate study in a patient with suspected substernal goiter. High background activity and activity in the large vascular structures of the mediastinum obscure visualization of thyroid tissue in the mediastinum. **B**, Subsequent I-131 scintigraphy demonstrates uptake with good target-to-background ratio.

gual thyroid. This can be demonstrated scintigraphically. The typical appearance is absence of tracer uptake in the expected cervical location with a focal or nodular accumulation at the base of the tongue. Thyroid tissue may also be found anywhere along the tract of the thyroglossal duct.

Thyroiditis   Subacute thyroiditis (deQuervain's disease) is a nonsuppurative granulomatous inflammatory process that may affect all or part of the thyroid. The etiology is unproved but speculated to be viral. During the active phase the thyroid scintigram demonstrates decreased or absent uptake in the affected part of the gland (Figure 13-16). Adjunctive scintigraphic methods such as

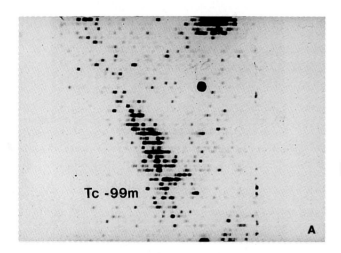

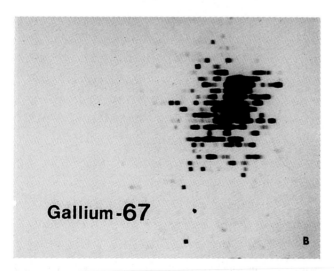

Fig. 13-16   **A**, Tc-99m pertechnetate scintigraphy in a patient with subacute thyroiditis affecting the left lobe. There is virtually complete lack of tracer uptake in the left lobe and decreased accumulation in the right lobe. **B**, Corresponding Ga-67 citrate scintigram obtained while the patient was still symptomatic reveals marked focal accumulation in the area of the left lobe, indicating the inflammatory nature of the process.

gallium-67 imaging have been used to demonstrate the inflammatory nature of the process.

The clinical picture can be confusing if there are minimal local symptoms. Often there is a history of recent upper respiratory tract infection and neck tenderness. Plasma levels of thyroid hormone are increased in the initial phase due to an outpouring of stored hormone occasioned by the inflammatory process in the gland. Patients may appear thyrotoxic clinically and may be mistaken for having Graves' disease. However, the percent uptake of I-131 is typically decreased in subacute thyroiditis. The possibility of subacute thyroiditis should always be borne in mind before a patient is treated with radioiodine for thyrotoxicosis.

Chronic thyroiditis or Hashimoto's thyroiditis is characterized by a lymphocyctic infiltration of the gland. It occurs most frequently in women and may manifest with goiter or hypothyroidism. Rarely, a patient presents with hyperthyroidism and the slang term "Hashitoxicosis" is used. Scintigraphic findings are highly variable and depend on the stage in the natural history during which imaging is performed. The scintigram may be normal early in the course of the process. Later, diffuse enlargement may be demonstrated. Many patients with Hashimoto's thyroiditis eventually become hypothyroid. The scintigram often appears inhomogeneous with hot and cold areas.

Acute thyroiditis due to suppurative bacterial infection is rare. The thyroid is typically enlarged and tender. Associated focal abscess may appear as a cold nodule scintigraphically. Reidel's thyroiditis or struma is also uncommon. The gland is replaced by fibrous tissue.

Scintigraphic detection of thyroid cancer metastases   Extended field of view and/or whole body imaging is useful in detecting metastatic deposits from differentiated thyroid cancer. Follicular thyroid carcinoma has the capacity to concentrate radioiodine and can be demonstrated scintigraphically. Mixed papillary-follicular carcinomas can also be demonstrated, but medullary carcinomas do not concentrate radioiodine and are not detected with thyroid scintigraphy. However, in the case of a histologic diagnosis of papillary carcinoma, it is still often worthwhile to image with radioiodine because thyroid cancer can be multifocal and can have different histologic types.

The most common sites of metastasis are locally in the lymph nodes of the neck, the lung, and the skeleton (Figures 13-17, 13-18). Nodal activity is typically focal and, if sufficiently intense, may result in a starburst pattern on parallel-hole collimators (see Figure 13-17). The intensity of uptake in residual normal tissue in the thyroid bed after thyroidectomy may preclude visualizing more subtle areas of uptake outside the thyroid. The intense activity in the thyroid bed may require shielding. Imaging is now typically performed 48 to 72 hours after

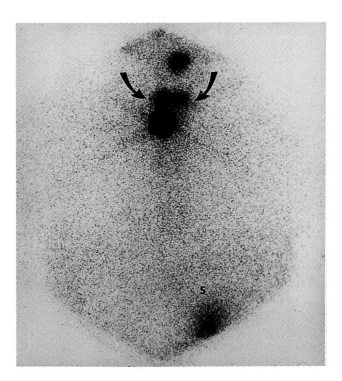

Fig. 13-17 Radioiodine imaging in a patient following thyroidectomy for thyroid cancer. There is residual activity in the thyroid bed (*arrows*). There is also activity in lymph nodes above and below the thyroid. Note the starburst artifact associated with the intense uptake in the lymph node below the thyroid bed. Uptake in the lower left-hand portion of the image is radioiodine in the stomach (S).

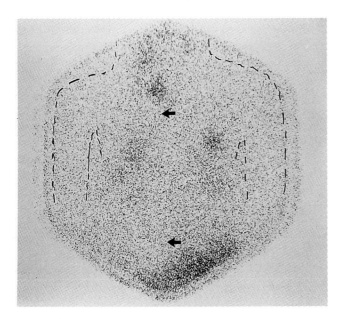

Fig. 13-18 Neck and chest images acquired after thyroidectomy for thyroid cancer reveal some residual activity in the thyroid bed and significant uptake in both lungs (*upper arrow* indicates suprasternal notch, *lower arrow* indicates the xiphoid).

radioiodine administration. More lesions are demonstrated in this time frame than at 24 hours.

The preparation of patients for follow-up imaging and the details of dose selection are somewhat controversial. In one school of thought, thyroid hormone replacement therapy is withdrawn for 4 to 6 weeks so that patients may achieve a maximal endogenous thyroid-stimulating hormone (TSH) response. Another approach is to switch patients to a triiodothyronine (T_3) preparation for a period of time and then discontinue the T_3 for 2 weeks. This protocol reduces the problem of symptomatic hypothyroidism but its efficacy is not as well established as 6 weeks of abstinence from thyroid hormone. Last, some centers have used bovine TSH before imaging. This is not considered as satisfactory for increasing I-131 uptake, and there is a significant incidence of allergic reactions to the bovine preparation. Whichever approach is used, it is important to achieve adequate uptake of tracer. Inadequate preparation can result in false negative scintigrams.

Selection of the scanning dose is also subject to debate between medical centers. The literature suggests that higher doses of I-131 reveal greater numbers of metastases. It is not clear that there is a consensus dose at the current time, but the literature supports the use of 2 to 10 mCi of I-131.

Thyroid function studies

Thyroid percent uptake The radioactive iodine uptake test was among the earliest applications of radiotracers in medicine. The degree of radioiodine uptake parallels the functional activity of the thyroid gland in producing thyroid hormone. The test is used clinically to differentiate Graves' disease from most other causes of hyperthyroidism and to guide selection of the therapeutic dosage of I-131.

The greatest experience with thyroid uptake studies has been with radioiodine-131. The test is performed using a nonimaging probe detector with a 2 × 2-inch or larger sodium iodide crystal. Six to 10 μCi of I-131 is given orally. The sodium iodide may be in either liquid form or in solid, capsule form. From a health physics standpoint, capsules are preferable because they reduce airborne exposure of workers to radioiodine and are more convenient for handling. An early problem with commercial capsules was incomplete dissolution in the gut, resulting in falsely low 24-hour uptake values. This is no longer a problem.

The uptake measurement is accomplished by counting the patient's neck and a standard dose of equal activity to that given to the patient in an appropriate neck phantom. The probe is typically positioned 10 inches from the anterior surface of the neck. A single-hole collimator designed to encompass the entire thyroid gland is used on the probe. Background correction may be accomplished either by using a lead thyroid shield and obtaining measurements with and without the shield or by counting the patient's thigh activity at the same 10-inch distance. The formula for computing the percent uptake is given in Box 13-9.

In the United States, the normal range for percent uptake of radioiodine in a thyroid is 10% to 30%. Before the widespread use of periodate in bread and the iodination of table salt, the normal range was substantially higher, and each laboratory should keep an actual running correlation to ensure the appropriate values for normal. Table 13-1 summarizes some of the common nonthyroidal causes of increased and decreased radioiodine percent uptake. As noted, a history of drug use should be obtained in conjunction with the radioiodine percent uptake test.

The availability of sensitive and accurate thyroid function tests, including tests for determining serum T_4 and T_3 values, has diminished the role of the radioactive iodine uptake test in determining the functional status of the thyroid. However, the test is uniquely suited to the differential diagnosis of hyperthyroidism. It is classically elevated in Graves' disease and Plummers' disease and decreased in hyperthyroidism due to subacute thyroiditis and thyrotoxicosis factitia.

There are a number of variations on the standard percent uptake. If hyperthyroidism is suspected, earlier measurements at 2, 4, or 6 hours should be considered. In some patients with florid hyperthyroidism, the uptake actually peaks before 24 hours and the measurement at 24 hours is misleadingly low.

Suppression test In the thyroid suppression test, a baseline 24-hour uptake is determined. The patient then receives 25 μg of T_3 four times a day for 8 days. The 24-hour uptake is repeated beginning on day 7. Some residual activity may be in the thyroid, and the neck is counted prior to administration of the repeat uptake dose. A normal response to thyroid suppression is a fall in the percent uptake to less than 50% of the baseline value and less than 10% overall. The thyroid suppression test is not often used in current practice. Its utility was in diagnosing patients with borderline Graves' disease and autonomous functioning glands. The thyrotropin-releasing hormone (TRH) infusion test is now used. After TRH administration, TSH is sampled for 30 minutes. In patients with Graves' disease, TSH is suppressed and does not rise with TRH.

Stimulation test The thyroid stimulation test also is infrequently used today. It was indicated to distinguish primary from secondary (pituitary) hypothyroidism. Failure to respond to exogenous TSH is indicative of primary hypothyroidism. Patients with secondary hypothyroidism have increased radioiodine uptake after TSH stimulation.

The stimulation test is performed by determining a baseline 24-hour radioiodine percent uptake. The patient then receives 10 units of TSH intramuscularly. The radioiodine uptake is repeated beginning the next day. In healthy subjects and patients with secondary hypothyroidism (hypopituitarism), the uptake should double, whereas there is no response in primary hypothyroidism.

In some centers TSH stimulation is used to prepare patients for follow-up scintigraphy after surgery or radioiodine studies for thyroid cancer. It should be borne in mind that TSH is a bovine protein and there is a significant incidence of adverse reactions, especially with repeated exposures.

Perchlorate discharge test A third interventional modification of the percent uptake test is the perchlorate discharge test. This procedure demonstrates disassociation of the trapping and organification functions in the thyroid. Dissociation occurs in certain rare congenital enzyme deficiencies, certain types of chronic thyroiditis, and during therapy with propylthiouracil. The patient receives a tracer dose of radioiodine. The percent uptake is measured at 1 to 2 hours, and 1 gram of potassium perchlorate is given orally. The percent uptake is measured hourly. In normal subjects or patients with hyperthyroidism on inadequate antithyroid drug therapy, less than a 10% discharge of radioiodine is demonstrated. A greater than 10% workout suggests the presence of an organification defect.

Box 13-9 Calculation of Thyroid Percent Uptake of Radioiodine

INPUT DATA

Phantom count with radioiodine standard sample.
Neck count.
Background count.

CALCULATION

$$\text{Thyroid percent uptake} = \frac{\text{Neck count} - \text{Background count}}{\text{Phantom count}}.$$

$$\begin{array}{c}\text{Microcuries of radioiodine}\\ \text{taken up in thyroid}\end{array} = \begin{array}{c}\text{\% uptake} \times \text{microcuries}\\ \text{in patient dosage.}\end{array}$$

RADIOIODINE TREATMENT OF HYPERTHYROIDISM AND THYROID CANCER

Radioiodine has been used for the treatment of hyperthyroidism for more than five decades. Box 13-10 presents a classification of hyperthyroidism and indicates causes potentially treatable with radioactive iodine. The vast majority of patients with primary hyperthyroidism

---

Box 13-10 **Classification of Hyper-thyroidism: Indications for I-131 Therapy**

I-131 POTENTIALLY INDICATED IN

- Graves' disease (diffuse toxic goiter)
- Plummer's disease (toxic nodular goiter)
- Functioning thyroid cancer

I-131 NOT GENERALLY INDICATED OR CONTRAINDICATED IN

- Thyrotoxicosis factitia
- Subacute thyroiditis
- "Silent" thyroiditis (atypical, subacute thyroiditis, lymphocytic thyroiditis, transient thyroiditis, postpartum thyroiditis)
- Struma ovarii
- Thyroid hormone resistance (biochemical and/or clinical manifestations)
- Secondary hyperthyroidism (pituitary tumor)

Box 13-11 **Calculation of I-131 Therapy Dose**

INPUT DATA

Gland weight: 60 g
24-hr % uptake: 80%
Desired dose to be retained in thyroid (selected to deliver 8,000-10,000 rads to the thyroid): 100 μCi/gm

CALCULATIONS

Required dose (μCi):

$$\frac{60 \text{ g} \times 100 \text{ μCi/g}}{0.80} = 7,500.$$

$$\text{Dose in mCi:} \quad = \frac{7,500}{1,000} = 7.5 \text{ mCi}$$

---

have Graves' disease (diffuse toxic goiter) and are candidates for I-131 therapy. A small percentage have one or more toxic nodules and, as discussed earlier, may also be candidates for therapy. As noted in Box 13-10, there are a number of causes of hyperthyroidism for which I-131 therapy is not indicated and could be potentially harmful.

The therapeutic goal in treating hyperthyroidism is to render the patient euthyroid in a reasonable length of time with a single radioiodine therapy dose. Empirically, this is achieved in Graves' disease when 80 to 100 μCi is retained in the gland per gram of tissue. Box 13-11 shows a typical calculation of an individualized treatment dose based on estimated thyroid gland weight and measurement of the 24-hour radioiodine percent uptake. Alternatively, some centers have abandoned the attempt to individualize therapy and give a standard dose in the 5 to 10 mCi range to all patients with diffuse toxic goiter.

More than 90% of patients who undergo radioiodine therapy are cured with a single dose. However, the therapeutic effects are not instantaneous because stored hormone must be released and used up. Also, the majority of patients eventually become hypothyroid and need replacement hormone therapy. Treatment with radioactive iodine obligates the patient to lifelong follow-up.

Patients with hyperthyroidism due to toxic nodules (Plummer's disease) are generally thought to be more difficult to treat with radioiodine than patients with diffuse goiter. The tissue is relatively radioresistant, possibly due to its inhomogeneity. The radioiodine dose is frequently increased into the range of 15 to 29 mCi. The extranodular tissue is spared, since uptake in it is suppressed, and

after successful therapy may resume function.

Radioactive iodine is also used in the treatment of differentiated thyroid cancer. It is not useful for treating anaplastic and medullary tumors. It is fair to say that there is a vast divergence of opinion on how and when to employ radioactive iodine.

Metastatic disease is most common locally in the neck. Distant metastases are most common in the lung and skeleton. An initial dose of 150 to 200 mCi is administered after appropriate patient preparation. Repeated doses up to a total of 1 Ci may be required. Skeletal metastases are more difficult to eradicate than lung metastases.

Patients are prepared for therapy by being taken off thyroid replacement and suppressive therapy. A diagnostic scan is typically done to establish the presence of metastatic lesions. Patients must be hospitalized and remain isolated until retained activity is less than 30 mCi. It is often useful to obtain a repeat whole body scintigram using the therapeutic dose. The patient is then placed back on thyroid hormone replacement or suppressive therapy. Retreatment is usually not considered for at least 6 months and preferably 12 months to avoid bone marrow suppression.

ADRENAL SCINTIGRAPHY

Separate classes of radiopharmaceuticals are available for scintigraphic imaging of the adrenal cortex and the adrenal medulla. Adrenal cortical scintigraphy enjoyed a brief vogue prior to the development of body CT. Nuclear imaging studies of the adrenal cortex are not frequently performed in current practice but retain a limited utility in assessing the functional status of adrenal cortical tissue when CT findings are indeterminate. In particular, incidental adrenal nodules demonstrated by CT can be assessed for functional status by adrenal cortical scintigraphy.

Scintigraphic studies of the adrenal medulla and related tissues have created significant interest and have found an expanding role in contemporary practice.

Adrenal Cortical Scintigraphy

Radiopharmaceuticals   The first successful radiopharmaceutical for adrenal visualization was I-131-19-iodocholesterol. The current agent of choice is I-131-6β-iodomethyl-19-norcholesterol (NP-59). This agent was identified as an impurity in the original formulation.

The mechanism of localization of I-131-6β-iodomethyl-19-norcholesterol by the adrenal cortex is related to the transport and receptor systems for serum cholesterol bound to low-density lipoprotein (LDL). Factors affecting cholesterol uptake into the adrenal also affect uptake of the radiopharmaceutical. An increase in the serum cholesterol reduces the percent uptake. Increases in plasma adrenocorticotropic hormone (ACTH) result in increased radiocholesterol uptake. The radiopharmaceutical is stored in adrenal cortical cells and is esterified but not incorporated into adrenal hormones.

The uptake of I-131-6β-iodomethyl-19-norcholesterol is progressive over several days following tracer administration. The background clearance is also relatively slow, and for routine or baseline studies, imaging is typically performed several days after tracer injection. Background tissues demonstrating significant localization include the liver, colon, and gallbladder.

Technique   Patients should be pretreated for at least 1 day with Lugol's iodine, three drops twice daily or equivalent, to block uptake of free radioiodine in the thyroid. This is continued for 7 days.

The usual dose of I-131-6β-iodomethyl-19-norcholesterol is 1.0 mCi/1.7 m² of body surface area. The dose is administered IV over a 1- to 2-minute interval.

For routine or baseline studies imaging is accomplished 4 to 5 days after radiopharmaceutical administration. A large field of view gamma scintillation camera with a high-energy parallel-hole collimator is used and a 20% window is centered at 364 keV. Ideally all images are acquired with a dedicated nuclear medicine computer system. This permits a standardized time per image with intensity optimization after data acquisition. With this approach a standard imaging time of 20 minutes per view is used. The most important view is a posterior view that includes both adrenals. Anterior views may be helpful to assess adrenal asymmetry. Lateral views with a line marker source on the middle of the back are obtained to determine adrenal gland depth for percent uptake calculations and to help differentiate gallbladder uptake from activity in the right adrenal gland.

Suppression studies   Routine or baseline adrenal cortical scintigraphy is typically employed in patients with hypercortisolism. In patients with abnormalities of the zona glomerulosa (production of aldosterone) or the zona reticularis (production of androgens), it is often desirable to suppress ACTH secretion and thereby adrenal uptake of radiocholesterol in the zona fasciculata. This is accomplished by administering dexamethasone, 2 mg every 6 hours beginning 2 to 3 days prior to radiopharmaceutical administration and continuing until imaging is completed.

Percent uptake determination   The relative percent uptake of radiocholesterol in the adrenal is a crude marker of adrenal functional activity and may be calculated in a manner similar to the thyroid radioactive iodine uptake. A standard sample is counted on the gamma camera to determine the count rate of the injected dose. The net count rate from the individual glands is determined by background-corrected regions of interest (ROIs) defined on the posterior view. Tissue attenuation is corrected by measuring the left and right adrenal gland depths from the lateral view. The percent uptake of 6β-iodomethyl-19-norcholesterol in healthy subjects is approximately 0.16% of the administered dose per gland (range, 0.073%-0.26%).

Interpretation of the normal adrenal cortical scintigram   In normal subjects, radiotracer uptake in the adrenal cortex increases over the first 2 days after injection. Background activity is still relatively high at this time, especially in the liver, and imaging may be delayed until day 4 or 5.

The two adrenals are not symmetric anatomically and most often have a different appearance scintigraphically. The right adrenal is typically applied to the superior pole of the right kidney and is slightly cephalad to the left adrenal. It appears round and in most subjects is slightly more intense than the left adrenal gland. The greater intensity is due to its more posterior location in the body and hence less soft tissue attenuation. There is also superimposed liver activity. The left adrenal is typically applied to the anteromedial border of the left kidney and may extend inferiorly to the renal hilum. Scintigraphically it appears more caudad and has an oval rather than round configuration. It frequently appears less intense owing to its more anterior location and the lack of additive background activity from the liver.

Activity in the gallbladder may be confused for right adrenal activity. The gallbladder can be emptied by administering a cholecystagogue. It is also of occasional value to administer a renal agent to localize the kidneys and establish the relationship of kidneys to the adrenals.

Clinical applications

Cushing's syndrome   A schematic presentation of scintigraphic patterns in Cushing's syndrome is provided in Figure 13-19. In patients with biochemically proven hypercortisolism, symmetric visualization of the adrenals is invariably due to adrenal hyperplasia (Figure 13-20). The most common cause is Cushing's disease or pituitary excess ACTH. Less commonly, ectopic ACTH syndromes may be the cause. The percent uptake is increased in Cushing's disease to an average of 0.50% of the injected dose per gland. The highest uptakes are seen in ectopic ACTH syndromes and adrenal macronodular hyperplasia, which result in uptakes of 1.2% ± 0.30% per gland of the injected dose. Uptakes greater than 0.26% per gland are invariably associated with Cushing's syndrome. However, even in patients with Cushing's, the serum cholesterol has an inverse effect on percent uptakes.

In a small number of patients both glands are visualized but are asymmetric. Mild to moderate asymmetry may be seen with hyperplasia. More striking asymmetry may be due to macronodular hyperplasia, the concomitant presence of adenoma on one side, or prior surgery with asymmetric adrenal remnants.

Unilateral visualization is classically seen in patients with glucocorticoid-producing adrenal adenomas (Figure 13-21). The autonomous production of cortisol in the adenoma feeds back to shut off pituitary ACTH secretion and thereby shuts off uptake in the contralateral adrenal (Figure 13-22).

Bilateral adrenal nonvisualization in patients with Cushing's syndrome is indicative of adrenal carcinoma. The tumors can be quite large and are often first manifested clinically by signs and symptoms of hormone excess. However, the function per gram of tumor tissue is typically very low, and tracer uptake is insufficient to visualize the tumor. The contralateral adrenal is typically not visualized because the cortisol production in the cancer shuts down pituitary ACTH secretion (see Figure 13-22).

Biochemical proof of hypercortisolism and CT demonstration of a large lesion in the adrenal are considered sufficient evidence and scintigraphy is not needed. However, if CT findings are negative or equivocal, adrenal cortical scintigraphy can be quite helpful. Another potential use of adrenal cortical scintigraphy in patients with Cushing's syndrome, even in the era of MRI and CT, is in

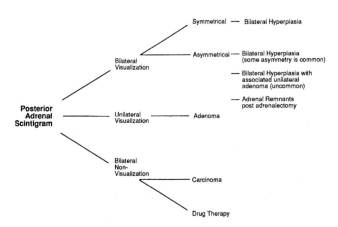

Fig. 13-19 Diagnostic patterns for adrenal cortical scintigraphy in patients with biochemically proven Cushing's syndrome.

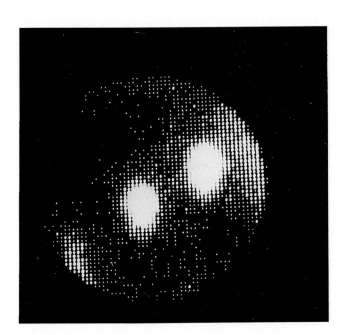

Fig. 13-20 Adrenal cortical scintigraphy in a patient with Cushing's disease. Note the bilateral and fairly symmetric uptake.

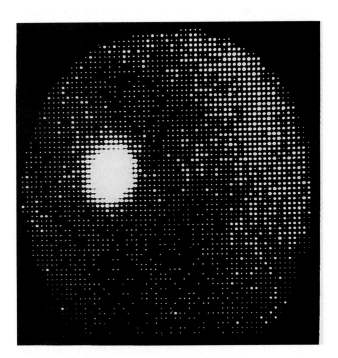

Fig. 13-21 Adrenal cortical scintigraphy reveals unilateral uptake in the left adrenal in a patient with an adrenal adenoma.

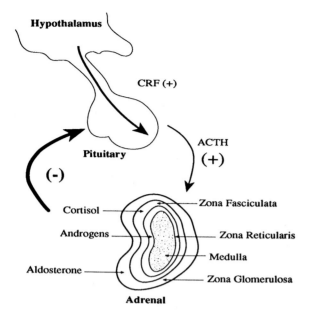

Fig. 13-22 The pituitary-adrenal feedback loop. Function in the zona fasciculata is stimulated by ACTH. Pituitary secretion of ACTH decreases as circulating levels of cortisol increase.

the detection of postsurgical adrenal remnants. These remnants may result in recurrent disease and may be difficult to localize in a surgically altered anatomy. They are readily detected by adrenal cortical scintigraphy.

Aldosteronism The principal clinical question in aldosteronism is the distinction of adenoma from hyperplasia. Aldosteronomas are typically small, and CT or MRI often is not diagnostic. Aldosterone is produced in the zona glomerulosa of the adrenal cortex. This hormone does not affect the pituitary-ACTH feedback loop, and the dexamethasone suppression scan is necessary in evaluating patients with aldosteronism. Normal uptake in the zona fasciculata can obscure asymmetry due to small nodules and adenomas in the zona glomerulosa. The suppression scan is performed sequentially over a number of days. Early (<5 days) unilateral "breakthrough" indicates aldosteronoma. Bilateral, delayed breakthrough typically indicates hyperplasia.

Androgen excess The adrenal may be a source of androgen excess. Scintigraphic patterns are similar to those found in aldosteronism. That is, patients with bilateral hyperplasia demonstrate bilateral breakthrough on dexamethasone suppression scans, and adenomas are characterized by marked scintigraphic asymmetry.

Adrenal Medullary Scintigraphy

Adrenal medullary scintigraphy has proved useful in the management of patients with functional adrenergic tumors. These include paragangliomas, neuroblastomas, ganglioneuroblastomas, and ganglioneuromas. Pheo-

chromocytomas are paragangliomas that arise in the adrenal medulla. Paragangliomas are associated with a number of important familial syndromes, including multiple endocrine neoplasia (MEN) type IIA (medullary carcinoma of the thyroid, pheochromocytoma, hyperparathyroidism) and MEN type IIB (medullary carcinoma of the thyroid, pheochromocytoma, ganglioneuromas). Other associations are von Hippel-Lindau disease and neurofibromatosis.

Radiopharmaceuticals Scintigraphic studies of the adrenergic nervous system became possible with the invention of metaiodobenzylguanidine (MIBG). This pharmaceutical is an analogue of guanethidine. Localization appears to be through the type I, energy-dependent, active amine transport mechanism. The tracer is taken up and further localized in cytoplasmic storage vesicles in presynaptic adrenergic nerves. In addition to the uptake in the adrenal medulla and other adrenergic and neuroblastic tumor tissues noted above, the tracer localizes avidly in other organs with rich adrenergic innervation, including the heart, salivary glands, and spleen. Both I-131 and I-123 have been used as radiolabels. I-123 has the advantage of a lower radiation dose to the patient, while I-131 facilitates delayed imaging.

Technique The tracer is taken up rapidly by adrenergic tissues. To achieve sufficient target-to-background ratios, imaging is typically delayed for 1 day following tracer administration and may be repeated at 2 or 3 days.

For studies with I-131 MIBG, patients are given a blocking dose of either saturated solution of potassium iodide (SSKI) or Lugol's solution. The usual adult dose of I-131 MIBG is 0.5 mCi/1.7 m². The tracer is administered IV over a 15- to 30-second interval. Higher doses have been used postoperatively to look for residual remnant tissues. When MIBG is radiolabeled with I-123, up to 10 mCi/m² can be administered with the same radiation dose to the patient as is received from 0.5 mCi/m² of I-131 MIBG.

Initial images with I-131 MIBG are usually obtained at 24 hours, with further delayed imaging at 48 and 72 hours after injection. A wide field of view gamma scintillation camera equipped with a high-energy parallel-hole collimator is used for all computerized image acquisition. Computer acquisition permits a fixed time per image to be used, typically 20 minutes. The views obtained are determined by the clinical condition under evaluation. For pheochromocytoma, the single most important view is the posterior view of the midabdomen to include the region of the adrenals. Additional images from pelvis to base of skull are indicated to detect extraadrenal pheochromocytoma (paraganglioma).

With I-123 MIBG, initial images may be obtained at 2 to 3 hours, with delayed imaging at 24 hours and 48 hours. Single photon emission tomography is feasible with I-123 MIBG.

Precautions A number of drugs interfere with MIBG

uptake, and a drug history should be obtained prior to imaging. Interfering drugs include tricyclic antidepressants, reserpine, guanethidine, certain antipsychotics and cocaine, and the alpha and beta blocker labetalol.

Interpretation of the normal MIBG scintigram
With the usual doses employed for I-131 MIBG imaging, only faint visualization of the normal adrenal medulla is achieved in 10% to 15% of patients. Visualization increases with time but the image remains faint. The normal adrenal is visualized somewhat more frequently with I-123 MIBG and with therapeutic doses of I-131 MIBG. Early images reveal activity in the spleen, heart, salivary glands, and liver. These areas clear with time. Some bladder activity may be visualized due to free radioiodine. The colon is also seen transiently in 20% to 25% of cases.

Clinical applications   The greatest clinical experience with MIBG is in the evaluation of patients with suspected intra-adrenal paraganglioma or pheochromocytoma. The characteristic appearance is unilateral, focal uptake in the tumor (Figure 13-23). The literature consensus sensitivity for detection of pheochromocytoma is in the range of 90% or better, with a specificity above 95% in reported series. In approximately 10% of cases, pheochromocytoma is bilateral. In 10% to 20% of cases the tumors are extra-adrenal, in which case they are referred to as paragangliomas. Note has already been made of the increased incidence of pheochromocytomas in conjunction with other neuroectodermal disorders including neurofibromatosis, tuberous sclerosis, Carney's syndrome, and von Hippel-Lindau disease. Paragangliomas may be found from the bladder up to the base of the skull.

Scintigraphy with MIBG is not a screening procedure for pheochromocytoma and should only be applied after biochemical tests suggest the diagnosis. Many centers first use CT to evaluate the adrenals. If an adrenal mass is demonstrated, the diagnosis is inferred and further workup prior to surgery is not considered indicated. MIBG is particularly helpful in surveying the entire body for extra-adrenal and metastatic lesions.

Patients with MEN IIA develop adrenal medullary hyperplasia. This condition is difficult to diagnose with CT or MRI. MIBG scintigraphy is uniquely suited to detect medullary hyperplasia and has been used to assist decision making for timing of surgery (Figure 13-24).

Although the greatest experience with MIBG imaging has been with pheochromocytomas, there has also been significant experience in imaging neuroblastoma. Reported sensitivity is variable between studies but is in the range of 60% to 90%, with a high degree of specificity. Other tumors demonstrating uptake of MIBG include carcinoids and medullary carcinoma of the thyroid.

The successful scintigraphic visualization of these tumors as well as pheochromocytoma has led a number of investigators to attempt therapy with I-131 MIBG. Therapeutic applications are still experimental, and the work has been restricted largely to patients in whom prior conventional therapies have failed.

PARATHYROID SCINTIGRAPHY

A number of imaging techniques have been proposed for visualizing the parathyroid glands. US with high-resolution small parts transducers (10 MHz) is the imaging technique of choice in most centers. US has the addi-

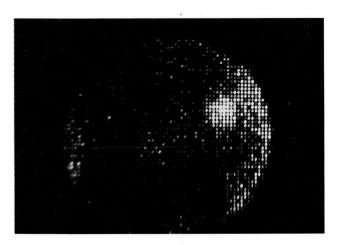

Fig. 13-23   Adrenal medullary scintigraphy reveals unilaterally increased uptake in the region of the left adrenal due to pheochromocytoma.

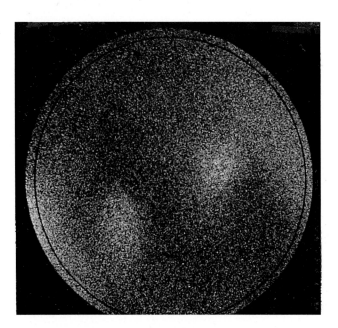

Fig. 13-24   Adrenal medullary scintigraphy in a patient with multiple endocrine neoplasia type IIA demonstrates bilateral uptake due to adrenal medullary hyperplasia.

tional advantage that it can be used to guide needle biopsies and even percutaneous ablation of parathyroid adenomas or hyperplastic glands. Scintigraphy has also proved useful in many institutions.

The first radiopharmaceutical used to any extent for parathyroid scintigraphy was Se-75-selenomethionine. The rationale for this tracer is the incorporation of selenomethionine in areas of protein synthesis as an amino acid analogue of methionine. Both the sensitivity and the specificity in the detection of parathyroid adenomas were poor, and this tracer has been largely abandoned.

The current scintigraphic technique uses combined Tc-99m pertechnetate/Tl-201 subtraction imaging. The rationale is that thallium is avidly accumulated in both parathyroid tissue and thyroid tissue, while Tc-99m pertechnetate is only accumulated in thyroid tissue. Thus, the subtraction of normalized Tc-99m pertechnetate activity from a thallium image should theoretically remove the contribution from the thyroid and leave only activity due to Tl-201 accumulation in the parathyroids (Figure 13-25). If the parathyroid adenoma is adjacent to the thyroid rather than behind it or in it, visualization is usually

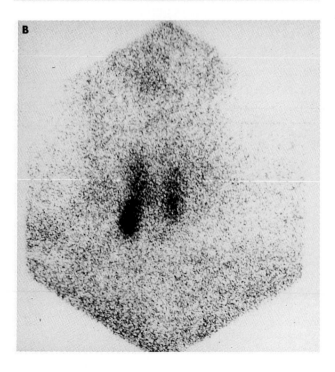

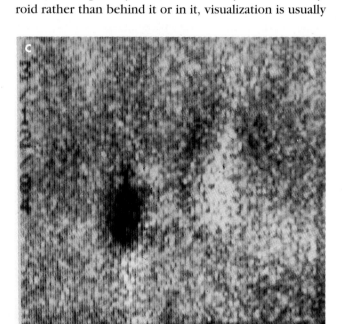

Fig. 13-25   **A**, Tc-99m pertechnetate scintigraphy in a patient with suspected parathyroid adenoma is essentially normal. **B**, Corresponding Tl-201 scintigraphy reveals an apparent area of increased uptake adjacent to the lower pole of the right lobe. **C**, Subtraction of the Tc-99m pertechnetate study from the Tl-201 study confirms the presence of a parathyroid adenoma.

obvious without the need for subtraction.

Techniques have been described for the initial injection of either Tc-99m or Tl-201, although most laboratories use Tl-201 first because of its lower energy. Either approach is probably valid. When Tl-201 is administered first, images are acquired with a nuclear medicine computer system in several projections. The view thought to be most indicative of possible abnormality is selected, and the patient is repositioned in that view. A baseline Tl-201 image is obtained. The patient is then given 1 to 2 mCi of Tc-99m pertechnetate, with image acquisition repeated 10 minutes after tracer administration. A normalization factor is computed by comparing the count rates on the respective thallium and pertechnetate images in areas of normal thyroid tissue. Care must be used in flagging the regions of interest for the normalization calculation to avoid abnormal areas.

The sensitivity of the technique depends on the size of the parathyroid adenoma being sought. For lesions over 1.0 gram in size, sensitivity is reported to be over 95%. The sensitivity falls off for smaller lesions. The smallest lesion detectable by this technique is on the order of 0.3 gram.

There are a number of pitfalls to the technique. First, the relative uptake of Tc-99m pertechnetate and Tl-201 chloride throughout the thyroid gland may not be equal and constant in the setting of thyroid pathology such as multimodular goiter or follicular adenoma. Second, other lesions, including primary metastatic cancer, that take up Tl-201 can mimic parathyroid adenomas. Third, patient motion can cause misregistration of data on the two images, with inaccurate subtraction.

Recently, Tc-99m sestamibi has been successfully used for parathyroid imaging. The slower washout of this agent from hyperfunctioning parathyroid glands compared to thyroid tissue permits diagnosis by observing differential clearance over time.

SUGGESTED READINGS

Ferlin G, Borsato N, Camerani M, Conte N, and Zotti O: New perspectives in localizing enlarged parathyroids by technetium-thallium subtraction scan, *J Nucl Med* 24:438-441, 1983.

Freitas JE, Gross MD, Ripley S, and Shapiro B: Radionuclide diagnosis and therapy of thyroid cancer: current status report, *Semin Nucl Med* 15:106-131, 1985.

Gelfand MJ: Meta-iodobenzylguanidine in children, *Semin Nucl Med* 23:231-242, 1993.

Giulette TMD, Brownless SM, Taylor WH, Shields R, and Simkin EP: Limits to parathyroid imaging with thallium-201 confirmed by tissue uptake and phantom studies, *J Nucl Med* 27:1262-1265, 1986.

Gross MD, Shapiro B, Freitas JE, Thrall JH, and Beierwaltes: The scintigraphic imaging of the endocrine organs, *Endocrine Rev* 5:221-281, 1984.

Sandler MP and Patton JA: Multimodality imaging of the thyroid and parathyroid glands, *J Nucl Med* 28:122-127, 1987.

Sandler MP, Patton JA, Gross MD, Shapiro B, and Falke THM: *Endocrine Imaging*, Norwalk, 1992, Appleton & Lange.

Sisson JC et al: Scintigraphic localization of pheochromocytomas, *N Engl J Med* 305:12-17, 1981.

CHAPTER 14

Pearls, Pitfalls, and Frequently Asked Questions

The purpose of this chapter is to have a little fun and to reinforce concepts already presented in this book. Every student of medicine gathers pearls of wisdom from his or her mentors that may not fit well into a didactic treatment of a subject but are extraordinarily valuable in day-to-day practice. Likewise, we all learn to avoid pitfalls that arise in situations that have somehow escaped our formal education. In a slightly different vein, questions that are posed for us at the viewbox or elsewhere often require assembling multiple bits of information for a correct answer. Somehow these questions are never presented in quite the same way that subject material is presented didactically!

By the nature of this chapter it is neither comprehensive nor weighted to the relative importance of the topics. It is an experiment that we hope is successful. Feedback from readers will tell us, so let's take the plunge together.

BASIC PHYSICS

Q: What is the difference between *isotopes, isobars,* and *isotones?*
A: *Isotopes* are varying forms of a given element and by definition possess the same number of protons but different numbers of neutrons. *Isobars* are atoms that have the same total number of nucleons (protons and neutrons) but are different elements and hence have different numbers of protons. *Isotones* are atoms with the same number of neutrons but are of different elements and, therefore, have different numbers of protons. Remember that *isomers* are simply different energy states of nuclei of the same isotope (same atomic number, same number of neutrons, and same mass number).

Q: What is the difference between x-rays and gamma rays?
A: Both x-rays and gamma rays are types of ionizing radiation. By definition, x-rays originate outside of the atomic nucleus and the gamma rays originate in the atomic nucleus. The respective energy spectra for x-rays and gamma rays substantially overlap each other at the high-energy end of the spectrum for all kinds of electromagnetic radiation.

Q: What is the energy equivalent of the rest mass of an electron?
A: 511 keV.

Q: What is the difference between the *rad, roentgen,* and *rem?*
A: These terms are frequently confused with each other but have important distinctions. *Rad* stands for **r**adiation **a**bsorbed **d**ose. A rad is equal to the absorption of 100 ergs per gram of absorbing material. The rad is the traditional unit of absorbed dose. The gray (Gy) is the unit of absorbed dose in the international system (SI). One gray = 100 rads.

Rem is an acronym for **r**oentgen **e**quivalent **m**an. The rem is calculated by multiplying the absorbed dose in rads by a factor to correct for the *relative biological effectiveness* (RBE) of the kind of radiation in question. The rem is the traditional unit. In the SI system the term sievert (Sv) is used. One sievert = 100 rem.

The *roentgen* (R) is a unit of radiation *exposure*. It is defined as the quantity of x-radiation or gamma radiation that produces one electrostatic unit of charge per cubic centimeter of air at standard temperature and pressure. In the international unit system, radiation exposure is expressed in terms of coulombs per kilogram (C/kg). One roentgen is equal to 2.58×10^{-4} C/kg air.

Q: Which is more penetrating in soft tissues, alpha particles or beta particles of the same kinetic energy?

A: Alpha particles have very low penetration in soft tissue owing to their rapid loss of kinetic energy through interaction of their electrical charge with electrons in the tissues. Beta particles of the same respective kinetic energy of alpha particles have higher velocity, lower mass, and a single negative charge. They demonstrate significantly greater penetration in soft tissues, although penetration still is typically measured in millimeters.

Q: Define the two systems for expressing radioactive decay.

A: The traditional unit of radioactive decay was the *curie* (Ci). One curie is equal to 3.7×10^{10} disintegrations per second (dps). This number was derived from the decay rate of 1 gram of radium. (Modern measurements indicate that the actual decay rate for 1 gram of radium is 3.6×10^{10} dps.)

In the international system, decay is expressed in becquerels (Bcq). One becquerel equals one disintegration per second.

Q: How are the "half-life" and the "decay constant" related?

A: The physical half-ife ($T_{1/2}$) of a radionuclide is defined as the time for half of the atoms in a sample to decay. The half-life is expressed in units of time, typically seconds, minutes, hours, days, or years.

The decay constant indicates the fraction of the sample decaying in a unit of time. The units of the decay constant are "per unit time" (per second, per hour).

Mathematically, the half-life ($T_{1/2}$) and the decay constant (λ) are related by the following equation:

$$T_{1/2} = \frac{\ln 2}{\lambda}.$$

Q: Which is longer, the biological half-life or the effective half-life?

A: The effective half-life is always shorter than either the biological half-life or the physical half-life because biological clearance and physical decay take place simultaneously. In calculating radiopharmaceutical dosimetry, the conservative assumption is sometimes made that biological half-life is infinite. This is probably never completely correct but simplifies calculations because the effective half-life may be taken simplistically as the physical half-life.

Q: After a photon has undergone Compton scattering, how does the energy of the scattered photon compare to the original photon energy?

A: In Compton scattering, the photon gives up energy to a recoil or Compton electron. The "scattered" photon has correspondingly lower energy. The amount of energy lost increases as the angle of scattering increases.

Q: What factors speed up or slow down radioactive decay?

A: Unlike chemical reactions, radioactive decay is a physical constant that cannot be sped up or slowed down by heating or cooling a specimen or application of other physical or chemical influences.

Q: How many observed counts are necessary to have a percent fractional standard deviation of 5%, 2%, and 1%, respectively?

A: 400, 2500, 10,000.

Q: What is the maximum number of electrons that can occupy the outermost shell of an atom?

A: 8.

Q: What special term is used to designate the electrons in the outermost shell of an atom?

A: They are called *valence* electrons and are responsible for many of the chemical characteristics of the element.

Q: What is the binding energy of an electron?

A: The concept of binding energy refers to the amount of energy required to remove that electron from the atom. Electrons in shells close to the nucleus have higher binding energy than electrons farther from the nucleus. This energy is typically expressed in terms of electron volts (eV).

Remember that the binding energy for each electon shell and subshell is characteristic for the respective element and that the higher the atomic number of the element, the greater is the binding energy for each shell and subshell.

RADIATION DETECTION AND INSTRUMENTATION

Q: What are some examples of the uses of ionization chambers in nuclear medicine?

A: Ionization chambers are commonly used in radiation survey meters and some pocket dosimeters. The radionuclide dose calibrator incorporates an ionization chamber.

Q: What is the purpose of the thallium impurity added to sodium iodide crystals?

A: The thallium is used to "activate" the sodium iodide crystal. The thallium impurity provides "easier" pathways for the return of electrons from the conduction band of the crystal to the valence bands of atoms.

Q: What is the relationship between photon energy and detection efficiency in a sodium iodide crystal?

A: For a given crystal size, detection efficiency decreases with increasing photon energy.

Q: Why do photopeaks appear as bell-shaped curves in pulse height spectra rather than as discrete spikes corresponding to the energy of the gamma ray?

A: Although gamma rays have discrete energies, the detection process is subject to statistical factors at each step of the process. The bell-shaped curve corresponding to the gamma ray photopeak reflects these statistical variations, which results in different events being measured as having slightly different energies. The better the "energy resolution" of a pulse height analyzer, the narrower is the bell-shaped curve.

Q: In using a gamma scintillation camera, what does it mean to "set" the energy window?

A: Gamma cameras are equipped with pulse height analyzers that allow the operator to select a range of observed energies for accepting photons to be used in making the scintigraphic image. The "window" is usually described by giving the photopeak energy of interest and a percentage range that defines the limits of acceptance above and below the photopeak energy. A typical window for the 140 keV photon of technetium-99m is 20%, or ±14 keV.

Pitfall: Some nuclear medicine clinics use radioactivity in the patient to confirm the window setting. This can be a pitfall because scattered photons are included in the observed spectrum and can actually shift the apparent location of the photopeak. Ideally, a sample of the radionuclide to be imaged should be used for "peaking" in the gamma camera energy window.

Q: What effects do Compton-scattered photons have on scintigraphic image quality?

A: Compton scattered photons are the enemy! Scattered photons that fall within the acceptance limits of the energy window are included in the image. They represent false data because they are recorded in a different spatial location than the origin of the primary photon. Thus, Compton scattering reduces image contrast and spatial resolution. Also, Compton-scattered photons falling outside the energy window still must be processed by the gamma camera pulse height analyzer circuitry. These rejected events contribute to dead time and reduce the count rate capability of gamma cameras.

Q: What photons are desired in the scintigraphic image?

A: Primary (unscattered) photons that arise in the organ of interest in the body and travel parallel to the axis of the gamma camera collimator field of view are the photons desired in the image. Intuitively, one may think of these as "good" photons. All other photons are "bad" photons! These include primary (unscattered) photons that arise in the object or organ of interest but travel "off axis," primary photons that arise in front of or behind the organ of interest (background photons), and all scattered photons.

Q: What is the purpose of the collimator?

A: The collimator defines the geometric field of view of the gamma camera crystal. Off-axis photons, whether they are primary photons or scattered pho-

tons, are absorbed in the septa of the collimator.

Pearl: Pinhole collimators allow resolution of objects below the spatial resolution of the gamma camera through geometric magnification.

Q: What is the theoretical advantage of an asymmetric window?

A: Asymmetric windows that encompass the gamma ray photopeak but offset to the high side contain a higher ratio of primary photons to scattered photons than symmetric windows. Asymmetric windows are feasible with modern high-performance gamma cameras. In older cameras, the photomultiplier tube energy response was too variable between the multiple tubes for effective use of asymmetric windows.

Q: How does poor energy resolution degrade spatial resolution?

A: In gamma cameras with poor energy resolution there is a reduced ability to reject scattered photons on the basis of pulse height analysis. There is also a reduced ability for accurate determination of x and y coordinates for spatial localization of events.

Q: What special importance does the biological half-life of a radiotracer have in SPECT imaging?

A: In SPECT imaging data are acquired sequentially from different sampling angles. If significant biological redistribution of a radiopharmaceutical takes place between the start of data acquisition and completion, the reconstruction of tomographic images can be significantly distorted.

NUCLEAR PHARMACY

Q: What relationship between the half-lives of a parent radionuclide and a daughter radionuclide is necessary for a generator system?

A: The parent radionuclide must have a long enough half-life to permit formulation and distribution of the generator. The daughter half-life must be reasonable for clinical application. A longer-lived parent decays to a shorter-lived daughter in all generator systems in use.

Q: How are parent and daughter radionuclides separated in generator systems?

A: Because the parent and daughter are different elements, they can be chemically separated.

Q: What is the major drawback of molybdenum-99 prepared by neutron activation?

A: When molybdenum-99 is prepared from molybdenum-98 by neutron activation it is not possible to separate the two isotopes, and there is significant molybdenum-98 carrier in the preparation. This ultimately results in low specific concentration eluates of Tc-99m from the generator system.

Q: What is the difference between "transient" equilibrium generators and "secular" equilibrium generators?

A: In "secular" equilibrium generators the half-life of the parent is far longer than the half-life of the daughter. If the generator system is left alone, the activity of the daughter becomes equal to the parent. In generator systems where the parent half-life is on the order of 10 to 100 times that of the daughter, a condition of transient equilibrium occurs if the generator is not eluted. The point of transient equilibrium is defined as the time at which the ratio of the daughter and parent activities becomes a constant. Because the parent half-life is longer, the daughter appears to decay with the same half-life. The Mo-99/Tc-99m generator system is an example of transient equilibrium.

Q: What is the practical problem with having carrier Tc-99 in the generator eluate?

A: Tc-99 and Tc-99m behave identically from a chemical standpoint. Therefore, if there is excessive Tc-99 in the eluate, labeling efficiency can be impaired. For example, in a kit preparation using stannous chloride as a reducing agent, there may be unreduced Tc-99 and Tc-99m left in the preparation, with the consequent presence of radiochemical impurities in the final preparation.

Q: When is the buildup of Tc-99 at its highest?

A: Because Tc-99 has a far longer half-life than Tc-99m, the longer the interval between generator elutions, the greater the buildup of Tc-99. The first elution after commercial shipment or following a long weekend will have the highest content of Tc-99.

Q: What is the legal limit for Mo-99 in Tc-99m-containing radiopharmaceuticals?

A: The Nuclear Regulatory Commission limit is 0.15 µCi of Mo-99 activity per 1.0 mCi of Tc-99m activity in the administered dose.

Q: How does the ratio of Mo-99 to Tc-99m change with time?

A: In any preparation where the radionuclidic contaminants have longer half-lives than the desired radionuclide label, the relative activity of the contaminant increases with time. This is an issue for I-123 preparations that have longer-lived radioiodine contaminants as well as for the Mo-99 contamination in Tc-99m preparations.

Q: What is the purpose of stannous ion in Tc-99m labeling procedures?

A: Stannous ion is a reducing agent used to reduce Tc from a +7 valence state in pertechnetate to lower valence states necessary for labeling a wide range of agents. The development of this approach was one of the true breakthroughs in nuclear pharmacy.

Q: What constitutes a misadministration of a radiopharmaceutical?

A: There are four basic categories of misadministration. An agent can be given to the wrong patient, or a patient may receive the wrong radiopharmaceutical. The wrong route of administration may be used, or the administered dose may differ from the prescribed dose by greater than an allowable standard. The standard varies depending on the kind of preparation in question, as described in Chapter 3.

Q: Describe the general response to the spill of radioactive material.

A: In general, the person who recognizes that a spill has occurred should notify all persons in the vicinity and the area should be restricted. If it is possible to identify the spill it should be covered. For minor spills, cleanup using appropriate disposable and protective clothing can be accomplished until background or near-background radiation levels are observed. For major spills, the source of the radioactivity should be shielded. For both major and minor spills, all personnel potentially exposed in the area should be surveyed, with appropriate removal of contaminated clothing and decontamination of skin. The radiation safety officer should be notified of all spills and has the primary responsibility for supervising cleanup for major spills and determining what reports must be made to regulatory agencies.

CARDIOVASCULAR SYSTEM

Pearl: Think of the myocardial perfusion scintigram, whether acquired with single photon or PET agents, as a "map" of relative blood flow to viable myocardium. That is, in order for activity to be recorded in the image it must be delivered (blood flow) and taken up by a myocardial cell (viable myocardium).

Q: How does the extraction of thallium-201 passing through the myocardial capillary bed compare with the extraction of Tc-99m sestamibi and Tc-99m teboroxime?

A: Tl-201 has a myocardial extraction fraction of approximately 0.85 in normal subjects at normal flow rates. Tl-201 is in the middle. The myocardial extraction of Tc-99m teboroxime is greater and the myocardial extraction of Tc-99m sestamibi is lower.

Pitfall: If imaging is begun too soon following exercise in myocardial perfusion SPECT studies, the position of the heart may change during the study as the patient's respiratory rate returns to baseline. The term *cardiac creep* has been used to describe this phenomenon. Replaying the multiple projections from the SPECT data acquisition readily identifies the phenomenon. Imaging can be started in most patients by 10 to 15 minutes after exercise. *to avoid "cardiac creep" phenomenon.*

Pearl: The left anterior oblique (LAO) view is the single planar view in which the most lesions are seen by Tl-201 scintigraphy. Some departments obtain an LAO planar image prior to beginning a SPECT study. This also permits assessment of lung activity.

Q: What is the rationale for a second injection of Tl-201 versus simple delayed imaging to distinguish fixed from reversible defects?

A: Relying solely on delayed imaging overestimates the number of fixed myocardial defects. Internal redistribution may take longer than the usual 3- to 4-hour delay and may not even be complete by 24 hours.

Pitfall: Incomplete normalization does not equate with a fixed defect. Insisting on complete normalization before accepting an abnormality as not "fixed" results in underdetection of ischemic areas versus scarred areas.

Q: What is the relationship between the time after myocardial infarction and the sensitivity of perfusion imaging?

A: The sensitivity of perfusion imaging for detecting defects due to acute MI is greatest right after the infarct and diminishes with time. This is different from "hot spot" imaging with Tc-99m pyrophosphate, in which the greatest sensitivity does not occur for a day or two after infarction.

Pitfall: Although myocardial perfusion scintigrams are positive immediately after infarction, it is not possible to determine whether a given defect is new or old. A given cold area may be due to myocardial scar or acute infarction.

Pitfall: In most laboratories the greatest single cause of false negative Tl-201 exercise studies in the diagnosis of coronary artery disease is failure to achieve adequate exercise.

Pearl: After exercise, significant Tl-201 localization in the liver usually indicates a poor exercise level. At peak exercise, blood flow is diverted from the splanchnic circulation.

Q: What is the mechanism of action of dipyridamole?

A: Dipyridamole inhibits the action of adenosine deaminase. By augmenting the effects of endogenous adenosine, dipyridamole is a powerful vasodilator.

Q: What effect can a cup of coffee have on a dipyridamole stress test?

A: Caffeine in coffee, tea, soft drinks, or foods such as chocolate can block the effect of dipyridamole and should be avoided prior to dipyridamole pharmacologic stress.

Q: What is the significance of lung uptake on Tl-201 exercise studies?

A: Patients with left ventricular failure during exercise have higher lung-to-heart ratios than normal subjects. Signifcantly increased lung uptake during exercise is a secondary sign of heart disease.

Q: What percentage stenosis at rest is necessary in the coronary arteries for resting blood flow to be affected?

A: Coronary artery stenosis greater than 85% to 90% is required before flow is diminished at rest. Remember that not all stenoses are created equal. Long irregular stenotic segments have more effect than discrete short-segment stenoses.

Q: What percentage of Tl-201 localizes in the heart?

A: On the order of 4% to 5% of the administered dose localizes in the heart in normal subjects.

Q: What factors can increase the Tl-201 washout rate from the myocardium after excercise?

A: Eating and the administration of glucose and insulin both can increase the washout rate.

Q: What is the relative biological half-time of Tl-201 in the myocardium compared to Tc-99m sestamibi and Tc-99m teboroxime?

A: The biological half-time for Tc-99m teboroxime is the lowest (fastest washout). Technetium-99m sestamibi has the longest half-time in the myocardium, with thallium having an intermediate half-time.

Q: What is the route of excretion of Tc-99m teboroxime?

A: Technetium-99m teboroxime is cleared through the hepatobiliary system. Liver uptake can obscure the inferior wall of the heart.

Q: Why is imaging delayed for 30 to 90 minutes after administration of Tc-99m sestamibi?

A: Although myocardial uptake is rapid with Tc-99m sestamibi, lung and liver uptake are also significant. These organs clear more rapidly, so that the target-to-background ratio improves with time.

Q: To what part of the red cell does the Tc-99m label bind?

A: Tc-99m binds to the beta chain of hemoglobin when the stannous pyrophosphate technique is used.

Pitfall: Injection of labeling materials through a heparinized intravenous line can significantly decrease the yield with in vivo RBC labeling.

Pearl: For multiple first-pass studies, choose an agent that is rapidly cleared from the blood, such as Tc-99m sulfur colloid or Tc-99m DTPA.

Q: What are the considerations for selecting the number of frames in a gated blood pool study?

A: Selecting the number of frames to divide the cardiac cycle is a balance between having enough frames to capture the peaks and valleys of the ventricular time-activity curve versus the need to acquire a statistically valid number of counts in each frame. In most applications, 16 to 24 frames achieves this compromise. Too few frames will "average out" the peaks and valleys. Too many frames increases the imaging time required for a given number of counts per frame.

Pitfall: In calculating the left ventricular ejection fraction, too high an estimate of the background counts per pixel will result in a falsely high ejection fraction. This can happen if the background area includes activity from the spleen.

Pearl: Variations in the length of the cardiac cycle can be recognized on gated blood pool studies if the time-activity curve trails off or fails to approximate the height of the initial part of the curve. Significant asymmetry (greater than 10%) of the height of the curve at the beginning and the end may indicate significant arrhythmia.

Q: What do amplitude and phase images portray?
A: Amplitude and phase images are parametric or derived images. The amplitude image portrays the maximum count difference at each pixel location during the cardiac cycle. High ejection fraction areas have high amplitude, background areas have low amplitude. The phase image portrays the timing of cyclic activity with respect to a reference standard, usually the R wave.
Q: What is the hallmark of a ventricular apical aneurysm by phase analysis?
A: Aneurysms demonstrate paradoxical motion. Activity in the area of the aneurysm is typically 180° out of phase with the rest of the ventricle.
Q: What factors help to distinguish true from false aneurysms?
A: True aneurysms have all of the layers of the heart. They typically have a wider mouth than false aneurysms and are most commonly located anteriorly or anteroapically. False aneurysms are due to actual rupture of the myocardium, covered only by epicardium. False aneurysms classically have narrow necks and are most commonly located posterolaterally. Both kinds of aneurysms distort the ventricular contour and exhibit paradoxical wall motion.

SKELETAL SYSTEM

Q: What is the difference between phosphate and phosphonate compounds?
A: Skeletal-seeking radiopharmaceuticals are based on both classes of compounds. The phosphate compounds are inorganic and have a basic P-O-P structure. Phosphonate compounds are organic and have a basic P-C-P structure. Both classes of compound demonstrate avid skeletal localization.
Q: What are the potential impurities in technetium-labeled pyrophosphate and diphosphonate compounds, based on their biodistribution?

A: Activity in the orophyarynx, thyroid gland, and stomach suggests free pertechnetate. Activity in the liver suggests that a colloidal impurity is present. Occasionally activity is seen in the gut due to excretion of activity through the biliary system. The mechanism is not well understood. Other increased soft tissue or renal activity is usually due to a disease process rather than to tracer impurity.
Q: What percentage of the Tc-99m-labeled compounds is retained in the skeleton at the usual time of imaging?
A: In normal adult subjects, on the order of 40% to 60% of the injected dose is in the skeleton 2 to 3 hours after tracer administration.
Q: What is the distribution of metastatic deposits from epithelial primary malignancies in the skeleton?
A: A rough rule of thumb is that 80% of metastases are found in the axial skeleton (spine, pelvis, ribs, and sternum). The remaining are distributed equally between the skull (10%) and the long bones (10%).

Pearl: The majority of epithelial tumor metastases localize first in the red marrow. The skeletal tracers do not localize in the tumor tissue per se but in the reactive bone around the metastatic deposits.

Pitfall: A small amount of activity is frequently seen at the injection site; this should not be confused with a metastatic lesion. Likewise, variable degrees of urinary contamination on the skin may be superimposed on skeletal structures and be confused with activity due to metastatic disease.

Q: How can the radiation dose to the bladder, ovaries, and testes be reduced?
A: The radiation dose to these structures is largely due to radioactivity in the bladder. Frequent voiding reduces the radiation dose.

Pearl: When using a multiple spot view technique for whole body skeletal imaging, consider obtaining pelvic views first immediately after the patient has emptied his or her bladder to begin the examination. When performing SPECT of the pelvic area, the same consideration of emptying the bladder applies.

Q: What factors distinguish a superscan due to metastatic disease versus a superscan due to metabolic disease?
A: In the usual superscan due to metastatic disease the increased uptake is restricted to the axial skeleton and the proximal parts of the femurs and humeri, the red marrow-bearing areas. In metabolic bone disease the entire skeleton is typically affected, with increased uptake seen in the extremities as well as in the axial skeleton. In some cases due to secondary hyperparathyroidism,

increased activity will also be seen in the lung and stomach.

Pearl: Faint or absent visualization of the kidneys is one of the findings on superscans that should alert the observer. This has been misinterpreted by many people as indicating lack of excretion of tracer through the kidneys. In cases of superscan due to metastatic disease, there are two different reasons for faint visualization of the kidneys. First, the skeleton does accumulate more tracer than usual, leaving less available for renal excretion. Also, because of the increased skeletal tracer uptake, the renal activity may actually fall below the density threshold of the recording medium. For images obtained using digital computers, the presence of renal activity is readily established by adjusting the window and center on the cathode ray tube.

Pitfall: The greatest pitfall in interpreting skeletal scintigrams is failure to understand the inherent non-specificity of skeletal imaging. In our zeal to "not miss the cancer," many incidental areas of abnormally increased tracer accumulation are incorrectly attributed to metastatic disease. The most common pitfalls are diagnosing areas of arthritis or prior trauma as metastases.

Q: Which factors favor osteoarthritis versus metastatic disease as the cause of increased activity?
A: Osteoarthritis has characteristic locations in the extremities. Because metastatic lesions are relatively rare below the proximal femurs or beyond the proximal humeri, osteoarthritis should be considered first in the elbows, wrists, hands, knees, and feet of older subjects. Involvement of both sides of a joint is common in arthritis but unusual in metastatic disease. The lower lumbar spine is the most problematic area because both arthritis and metastases are common there.
Q: What is the mechanism of the "flare" phenomenon?
A: In some patients treated with chemotherapy for metastatic disease, regression of the tumor burden is associated with increased osteoblastic activity, presumably due to skeletal healing. This can appear on skeletal scintigrams as a paradoxical increase or apparent "worsening" of the abnormal tracer uptake.
Q: Describe the postmastectomy appearance of the thorax.
A: With radical mastectomy, the majority of the soft tissue is removed from the corresponding anterior thorax. The ribs appear "hotter" than on the contralateral side. This is probably due to a combination of less attenuation of rib activity in soft tissue and possibly some uptake associated with postsurgical healing. (Note, however, that if the patient is imaged with a prosthesis in place, the rib activity may be attenuated.)
Q: What factors contribute to prolonged fracture positivity on scintigrams?
A: Displaced and comminuted fractures and fractures involving joints tend to have prolonged positivity scintigraphically.
Q: What factors favor shin splints versus stress fracture scintigraphically in the tibia?
A: Stress fractures are classically focal or fusiform. The uptake can involve the entire width of the bone. Shin splints are classically located along the posterior tibial cortex and involve a third or more of the length of the bone. In pure shin splints a focal component should not be present.

Pitfall: False negative scintigrams may be seen in neonates with osteomyelitis. False negatives may also be seen in very old or debilitated patients and in patients who have received a course of antibiotic therapy before scintigraphy is performed.

PULMONARY SYSTEM

Q: What is the most commonly used agent for ventilation imaging?
A: Xenon-133.
Q: What are the half-lives of Xe-133 and Xe-127?
A: The half-life of Xe-133 is 5.3 days and the half-life of Xe-127 is 36.4 days.
Q: What are the principal photon energies of Xe-133 and Xe-127?
A: The principal photon energy of Xe-133 used for imaging is 81 keV. The principal photon energies of Xe-127 are 172 and 203 keV.
Q: What is the minimum number of particles recommended for pulmonary perfusion imaging?
A: Pulmonary perfusion scanning assumes a statistically even distribution of particles throughout the lung. This requires at least 60,000 particles in normal adults, and many authorities recommend a minimum of 100,000 particles.
Q: How should the dose of Tc-99m MAA be adjusted in pediatric patients?
A: Radiopharmaceutical doses are always adjusted with respect to radioactivity in the pediatric population. With Tc-99m MAA it is also necessary to adjust the number of particles.
Q: What is the size range of macroaggregated albumin particles?
A: In commercial preparations the majority of particles are in the range of 20 to 40 microns.

Pitfall: If blood is withdrawn into the syringe along with Tc-99m MAA particles it is possible to create a small radioactive embolus that shows up as a "hot spot" on subsequent images.

Pitfall: Failure to resuspend the Tc-99m MAA particles prior to administration may result in clumping of particles together and the presence of "hot spots" on subsequent imaging.

Q: What is the biological fate of MAA particles?
A: MAA particles are physically broken down in the lung. Delayed imaging performed several hours after pharmaceutical administration demonstrates activity in the reticuloendothelial system due to phagocytosis of the breakdown particles.

Pearl: One way to determine whether radioactivity outside of the lungs is due to free Tc-99m or shunted Tc-99m MAA is to image the brain. Free pertechnetate should not localize in the brain, whereas Tc-99m MAA particles that gain access to the systemic circulation will lodge in the first capillary bed that they encounter, including the capillary bed in the brain.

choroid plexus?

Q: What is the preferred patient position during administration of Tc-99m MAA?
A: Administering Tc-99m MAA with the patient supine results in a more homogeneous distribution of particles in the lung than when the patient is sitting or standing. Gravitational effects result in more basilar distribution when injection is accomplished with the patient upright.
Q: What is the major drawback to the use of Xe-133 for ventilation imaging?
A: The principal photon energy of Xe-133 is 81 keV, which is below the energy of Tc-99m. Thus, imaging with Xe-133 is problematic after the perfusion portion of a V/Q study. Ideally, one would like to do the perfusion study first and then position the patient in the view that would best evaluate demonstrated perfusion defects. *Xe-133 must be done prior to perfusion study (NOT OPTIMAL)*

Pitfall: In lateral views of the lung obtained for a fixed number of counts, "shine through" from the contralateral lung can give the false impression of activity arising from the side being imaged. This is most dramatically demonstrated in patients following pneumonectomy in whom no activity is demonstrated on anterior or posterior views but a near-normal appearance can be seen due to the shine-through phenomenon.

Pitfall: In analyzing perfusion scintigrams, failure to recognize the significance of *decreased* versus *absent* activity is a potential pitfall. Not every clot is 100% occlusive of the circulation. Significantly diminished activity needs to be recognized as one of the patterns caused by pulmonary emboli.

Pitfall: In some patients with fatty liver, retained activity in the liver on Xe-133 scans can be confused with retained activity or delayed washout at the right base.

Remember that xenon is fat soluble and will show significant accumulation in patients with fatty liver. *→ can look like RLL delayed washout.*

Pitfall: The pulmonary hili are photon-deficient structures due to the displacement of lung parenchyma by large vascular and bronchial structures. Failure to remember this can result in false positive interpretations, especially for defects seen on posterior oblique images.

Pitfall: If the patient is placed supine for V/Q imaging but the chest radiograph was obtained with the patient upright, it can be difficult to correlate findings on the examinations. For example, free fluid may collect in a subpulmonic location or obscure the lung base in the upright position. With the patient supine, the fluid may layer out posteriorly or collect in the fissures. Also, the apparent height of the lungs may be different, as may the heart size. Ideally, imaging studies should be performed with the patient in the same position for all examinations. On the other hand, if there is significant pleural fluid, it may be desirable to image the patient in more than one position to prove that a defect is due to mobile fluid.

Q: What is the stripe sign?
A: The stripe sign refers to a stripe or zone of activity seen between a perfusion defect and the closest pleural surface. Because pulmonary emboli are typically pleural based, the stripe sign suggests another diagnosis, often emphysema. Rarely, in the resolution of pulmonary emboli a stripe sign develops as circulation is restored. *"melting sign" on CXR*
Q: What is the physiologic basis for perfusion defects in areas of poor ventilation?
A: The classic response to hypoxia at the alveolar level is vasoconstriction. Shunting of blood away from the hypoxic lung zone maintains oxygen saturation.
Q: What is the shrunken lung sign?
A: The lungs may appear smaller than usual in patients sustaining multiple small emboli, such as fat emboli, that distribute uniformly around the lung periphery.
Q: What is the classic appearance of multiple pulmonary emboli on lung perfusion scintigraphy?
A: Multiple pleural based, wedge-shaped areas of significantly diminished or absent perfusion. The size of the defects may vary from subsegmental to segmental or even involve an entire lobe or lung.
Q: What are the most commonly observed clinical signs and symptoms in patients with confirmed pulmonary embolism?
A: In the PIOPED study the three most common presenting symptoms (and approximate percentage frequency) were dyspnea—80%, pleuritic chest pain—60%, and cough—40%. Hemoptysis (15%) and leg pain (25% to 30%) were less common. On physical examination, lung crackles (60%) were encountered much more often than leg swelling (30%) or pleural friction rub (5%). Both the heart rate and the respiratory rate were elevated on average in

the PIOPED study in patients with pulmonary embolism.

Q: What is the sensitivity of the high-probability scan category for detecting pulmonary embolism?

A: In the PIOPED study, 41% of patients with pulmonary embolism had a high-probability scintigraphic pattern.

INFECTION AND INFLAMMATION

Q: The mechanism of Ga-67 uptake in patients with infection includes which of the following factors?

a. increased vascular permeability
b. binding to lactoferrin
c. binding to bacteria (siderophores)
d. binding to white blood cells
e. all of the above

A: *e.* Increased vascular permeability and binding to lactoferrin released from degranulated white blood cells at the site of infection are probably the predominant mechanisms.

Q: Which organs normally have the greatest uptake of Ga-67 and In-111 oxine-labeled WBCs?

A: The highest normal Ga-67 uptake is seen in the liver, followed by the skeletal system. In-111 oxine-labeled WBCs have highest uptake in the spleen, followed by the bone marrow.

Pearl: Ga-67 is taken up by bone and the bone marrow. In-111 oxine–labeled WBCs are taken up by the bone marrow only.

Q: What are the four photopeaks of Ga-67 and their percent abundance?

A: 91 keV (41% abundance), 185 keV (23%), 300 keV (18%), and 394 keV (4%). Only the lower three photopeaks are used for imaging.

Q: Which organ receives the highest radiation absorbed dose from Ga-67 and In-111 oxine-labeled leukocytes?

A: For Ga-67 imaging, the large intestine has the greatest exposure, 4.5 rads. For In-111 imaging the spleen receives 20 rads.

Q: Which collimator should used for In-111 and Ga-67 imaging?

A: The medium-energy collimator. A high-energy collimator can be used, although its efficiency is less and image acquisition time is longer.

Q: Ga-67 uptake is seen in all of the following diseases with lung involvement except: → Re: ≤140 → low energyc.
140-400 → medium " "
>400 → high " "

a. tuberculosis
b. histoplasmosis
c. sarcoidosis
d. *Pneumocystis carinii* infection
e. Kaposi's sarcoma
f. cytomegalovirus
g. lung cancer
h. pneumoconioses

A: *e.* Kaposi's sarcoma *is* not Ga-67 avid.

Pearl: However, Kaposi's sarcoma *is* Tl-201 avid. This can help in the differential diagnosis of AIDS-related pulmonary disease.

Q: True or false? The most sensitive test for the diagnosis of active pulmonary sarcoidosis is Ga-67 scintigraphy.

A:. True. Increased lung uptake is diagnostic of an active pulmonary alveolitis. Ga-67 uptake may be markedly increased in the setting of a normal chest radiograph in early disease; it may be negative in setting of an abnormal chest radiograph consistent with sarcoidosis. In the latter situation, the chest radiograph shows the chronic changes of sarcoidosis but the the negative Ga-67 study indicates the disease is inactive.

Pearl: Certain scintigraphic findings are characteristic of sarcoidosis: (1) the "lambda" sign, representing uptake in the paratracheal and hilar lymph node groups, and (2) the "panda" sign, or prominently increased uptake seen in the nasopharyngeal region, parotids, and salivary glands.

Q: Ga-67 resolution is not as good as that achieved with Tc-99 agents for which of the following reasons?

a. poor collimator efficiency
b. decreased crystal sensitivity for high-energy photons
c. scatter and septal penetration from high-energy photons
d. multiple photopeaks
e. low administered dose
f. high background activity

A: All except *d.*

Q: Drug toxicity is one cause of increased pulmonary Ga-67 uptake. Which drug is most commonly associated with this finding?

A: Bleomycin. Pulmonary uptake is also seen with cytoxin, nitrofurantoin, and amiodarone.

Q: To which blood cells does In-111 oxine bind to?

a. granulocytes
b. lymphocytes
c. monocytes
d. platelets
e. erythrocytes
f. all of the above

A: *f.* Although In-111 oxine binds to all of these cellular elements, platelets are low in number and erythrocytes are removed by sedimentation and centrifigation. → if not, you get blood pool activity.

Q: Which of the following statements are true?

a. In-111 oxine–labeled leukocytes are useful for evaluating inflammatory lung diseases.
b. Ga-67 is the radiopharmaceutical of choice for imaging abdominal infection. F
c. In-111 oxine-labeled leukocytes have a high sensitivity for detecting osteomyelitis of the lumbar spine.

Ga-67
vs.
In-111wbc

d. Ga-67 should only be used when the peripheral leukocyte count is greater than 3,000/mm³.

A: None of the statements is true. Ga-67 should be used for evaluating inflammatory lung disease. Clearance of Ga-67 through the bowel limits its applicability in the abdomen. False positive In-111 oxine-labeled leukocyte studies for the diagnosis of osteomyelitis in the lumbar spine are not infrequent. Ga-67 does not depend on labeling leukocytes for is distribution and uptake. Therefore it may be useful in severely leukopenic patients who cannot tolerate In-111 oxine.

Q: In-111 leukocyte uptake is commonly seen in which of the following diseases?
   a. bacterial endocarditis
   b. active inflammatory bowel disease
   c. acute myocardial infarction
   d. nonrejecting transplants
   e. parasitic infections
   f. tuberculosis
   g. fungal infections

A: *b, c, and d.* Bacterial endocarditis is usually negative on radionuclide imaging. Any uptake in the small vegetations is not usually seen, even with SPECT. Labeled WBCs can be very useful for localization of active inflammatory bowel disease. Uptake in acute myocardial infarction has been reported but is not used clinically. In-111-labeled leukocyte uptake is common in transplants, whether rejecting or not. Parasitic and fungal infections are more likely to be detected with Ga-67.

Pearl: Tc-99m HMPAO preferentially labels granulocytes, while the usual In-111 oxine–labeled preparation is a mixed population of leukocytes.

Q: Tc-99m HMPAO leukocytes should not be used to diagnose which of the following?
   a. inflammatory bowel disease
   b. osteomyelitis of the feet
   c. lung infection
   d. sinus infection
   e. acute cholecystitis

A: Tc-99m HMPAO is excreted in the bowel, complicating interpretation of *a* and *e*. *abdominal processes*

Q: Regarding osteomyelitis, which of these statements is false?
   a. The three-phase bone scan is a sensitive test for the diagnosis.
   b. The bone scan is a specific test for the diagnosis.
   c. A negative flow phase study almost always rules it out.
   d. In patients with prostheses, a bone marrow study can be useful to rule out a false positive In-111 WBC scan.
   e. Increased uptake in areas of reactive bone will be seen on Ga-67 scans, complicating their interpretation.

A: *b.* The bone scan is the most sensitive test for osteomyelitis; however, it is not specific. For example, a three-phase bone scan can be seen with fracture, a Charcot joint, tumor, and so forth. Although false negative bone scans are rare, ischemia due to arteriosclerotic vascular disease can result in a false negative Tc-99m MDP bone scan for osteomyelitis. A bone marrow study in conjunction with a labeled leukocyte study is the most accurate method for diagnosing an infected prosthesis. Ga-67 is likely to be hot even without infection due to reactive bone 2.

TUMORS

Q: What is the mechanism of Ga-67 uptake in tumor imaging?

A: Ga-67 binds to serum transferrin and is transported to the tumor, where it enters the extracellular fluid space via the tumor's leaky capillary endothelium. It is bound to the tumor cell surface by tranferrin receptors and then transported into the cell, where it binds to iron-binding proteins such as ferritin and lactoferrin, which are in increased concentration in tumors.

Q: Ga-67 uptake is normally seen in which of the following organs?
   a. salivary glands
   b. lacrimal glands
   c. thymus
   d. spleen
   e. breast
   f. heart

A: *a-e.* Salivary gland and lacrimal gland uptake is variable. Thymus uptake may be seen in children, especially after they have received chemotherapy. The spleen has uptake, but it is low in intensity. Breast uptake is variable and is most prominent post partum. Heart visualization may be seen with acute and chronic myocarditis, pericarditis, and the like, but not normally.

Pitfall: Surgical wounds normally have increased uptake for 1 to 2 weeks postoperatively and there may be faint activity for 3 to 4 weeks. Focal bone uptake may be seen after bone marrow biopsy. Lymphangiography can produce prominent pulmonary uptake.

Q: On a scale of 1 to 3 (1 being highest), grade the likelihood of good uptake by the following tumors:
   a. Hodgkin's disease
   b. non-Hodgkin's lymphoma
   c. hepatoma
   d. soft tissue tumors
   e. melanoma
   f. lung cancer
   g. head and neck tumors 2
   h. abdominal and pelvic tumors 3

A: *a—*1, *b—*1, *c—*1, *d—*1 (although Tl-201 may be superior), *e—*1, *f—*2, *g—*2, *h—*3.

Q: Which of the following statements is associated with Hodgkin's disease and which with non-Hodgkin's lymphoma?

    a. Orderly contiguous spread of lymph node involvement in young patients. H

    b. Multicentric disease with a highly variable clinical course and a high incidence of extranodal tumor involvement. NHL

    c. Mediastinal masses are common. H

    d. Abdominal involvement of mesenteric and retroperitoneal nodes is common. NHL

    e. High cure rate. H

    f. Variable clinical course that can be indolent or rapidly lethal. NHL

A: Hodgkin's disease: *a, c, e*; non-Hodgkin's lymphoma: *b, d, f.*

Pearl: Ga-67 can be used to determine tumor viability after a course of chemotherapy or radiation therapy. It is particularly useful in determining whether post-therapy masses represent residual tumor or fibrosis, necrosis, or scarring.

Pitfall: A pre-therapy study is required to ensure initial Ga-67 uptake at sites involved with disease before the study can be used to evaluate the effectiveness of therapy.

Q: Factors affecting Tl-201 uptake in tumors cells include which of the following?:

    a. blood flow

    b. viability

    c. binding to intracellular proteins

    d. tumor type

    e. increased cell membrane permeability

    f. sodium-potassium-ATPase system

A: All but *c.*

Q: Tl-201 tumor imaging has been found useful in which of the following tumors?

    a. brain tumors

    b. primary tumors of bone

    c. lung cancer

    d. breast tumors

    e. thyroid cancer

    f. islet cell tumors of the pancreas

A: *a-e.* Radiolabeled ocreotide, a somatostatin receptor, is taken up by neuroendocrine tumors, such as islet cell tumors of the pancreas, carcinoid, gastrinoma, medullary carcinoma of the thyroid, pituitary tumors, paragangliomas, and so on.

Q: What are two clear-cut indications for OncoScint CR/OV monoclonal antibody imaging in patients with cancer of the colon?

A: (1) In patients with a rising CEA level but no clinical or imaging evidence of a site of recurrence, and (2) in patients with a single known site of recurrence who are potential surgical candidates, to confirm preoperatively that this is, indeed, the only recurrence site.

Pearl: CT is superior to OncoScint scintigraphy in the liver, whereas OncoScint scintigraphy is superior to CT in the extrahepatic abdomen.

Q: Besides colon cancer, what other cancer has OncoScint been approved for?

A: Ovarian cancer.

Q: Human antimouse antibodies (HAMA) develop in 40% of patients injected for imaging. What is the clinical significance?

A: The development of antibodies would suggest that either a repeat study at a later time or therapy with the same antibody might result in an allergic reaction, although further investigation is required to determine if this is indeed true. At present, only single administrations have been approved, although a few patients have received repeat injections without problems. In 50% of cases, assays positive for HAMA become negative over time. To date, no correlation has been found between the development of antibodies and adverse reactions. However, HAMA can intefere with murine-based immunoasays of CEA and Ca-125, producing falsely high values. Alternative assay methods are available.

Q: How can lymphoscintigraphy give useful clinical information in patients with melanoma?

A: It can demonstrate the drainage pattern and potential sites of nodal spread in patients with a midtrunk lesion and in this way help the surgeon identify nodes at risk that should be resected. Performing the study preoperatively has been shown to improve prognosis in patients with Stage 1 disease.

HEPATOBILIARY SYSTEM

Q: Name four different types of radionuclide liver studies using different radiopharmaceuticals and the mechanism of uptake for each.

A:

Tc-99m sulfur colloid:	Kupffer cell extraction
Tc-99m IDA:	hepatocyte extraction
Intra-arterial Tc-99m MAA:	blood flow distribution
Tc-99m-labeled RBCs:	blood pool distribution

Pearl: Tc-99m IDA is extracted pharmacologically similar to bilirubin but it is not conjugated. Tc-99m SC is extracted by the reticuloendothelial system, including the spleen and bone marrow. → Liver, SP, BM

Q: What are the two FDA-approved Tc-99m IDA radiopharmaceuticals in use, and how are they different?

A: Tc-99m DISIDA and Tc-99m mebrofenin. The latter has better hepatic extraction, 98% versus 88%, and less renal excretion, 1% versus 9%. Mebrofenin is preferable in the setting of hepatic insufficiency.

Q: What is the most important question to ask a patient before starting cholescintigraphy for suspected acute cholecystitis, and why?

A: "When did you last eat?" If the patient has eaten in the last 4 hours, the gallbladder may be contracted secondary to endogenous stimulation of cholecystokinin, and therefore radiotracer cannot gain entry into the gallbladder. If the patient has not eaten in over 24 hours, the gallbladder may not have had the stimulus to contract and will be full of thick, concentrated bile, which may prevent tracer entry.

Q: How frequently are cystic duct stones seen with US in acute cholecystitis?

A: In less than 10% of patients. Gallstones are commonly seen, but they are not diagnostic of acute cholecysitis but rather are associated with chronic disease.

Q: In what clinical settings are false positive HIDA studies likely to occur when performed to rule out acute cholecystitis?

A: In patients who have fasted less than 4 hours or more than 24 hours, and in the settings of hyperalimentation, chronic cholecystitis, hepatic insufficiency, intercurrent serious illness, and alcoholism and pancreatitis.

Pitfall: False positive HIDA studies are most likely to occur in sick, hospitalized patients. They are much less common in outpatients. In patients who have been fasting or are on hyperalimentation, CCK is administered in an attempt to empty the gallbladder prior to Tc-IDA administration.

Q: What is the "rim sign" seen in cholescintigraphy, and what is its significance?

A: The rim sign consists of increased uptake and delayed clearance of activity in the liver adjacent to the gallbladder fossa. It has been associated with perforation and gangrene and is seen in more severe cases of acute cholecystitis.

Pearl: The rim sign is a very specific sign of acute cholecystitis and therefore can be a useful finding in patients who are at risk of having a false positive study.

Q: At what time after HIDA injection is nonfilling of the gallbladder diagnostic of acute cholecystitis?

A: If CCK has been given prior to the study, 1 hour. If no CCK has been given, 1 hour is abnormal, but repeat images at 2 to 4 hours are needed to determine if there is delayed gallbladder visualization. Delayed visualization is most commonly seen in chronic cholecystitis. It is also seen with hepatic insufficiency.

Q: What is the most common cholescintigraphic finding in chronic cholecystitis?

A: A normal study. Less than 5% of patients with chronic

cholecystitis have delayed filling. Other associated findings include delayed biliary-to-bowel transit time and, rarely, nonvisualization of the gallbladder or intraluminal filling defects.

Q: What is acute acalculous cholecystitis?

A: Acute acalculous cholecystitis is cholecystitis without a stone occluding the cystic duct. The obstruction may be due to debris or inflammatory changes, or the cholecystitis may be limited to the gallbladder wall due to infection, ischemia, or secondary to toxins. It occurs in hospitalized patients who have sustained serious trauma, burns, sepsis, or other serious illness and who frequently have an underlying chronic illness. It presents atypically and is associated with a high morbidity and mortality.

Pearl: The sensitivity of cholescintigraphy is about 90% for acute acalculous cholecystitis, perhaps slightly lower than for calculous cholecystitis. False positive studies occur in increased incidence for the same reasons as in acute calculous cholecystitis: in sick patients with intercurrent illnesses, in NPO patients, and in patients on hyperalimentation.

Pearl: Because cholescintigraphy has a false negative rate of 10% and a false positive rate of 20% to 30%, the diagnosis of acute acalculous cholecystitis may require confirmation by other means, such as the diagnostic findings of acute cholecystitis on US. In-111 oxine-labeled leukocyte imaging can confirm or rule out the diagnosis if it is still in question.

Q: The diagnosis of common duct obstruction is usually made by seeing a dilated common duct on US. In what clinical situations would cholescintigraphy be helpful?

A: In early acute obstruction (<24 hours), before the duct has had time to dilate, and in patients with previous obstruction or ductal instrumentation. Once the common duct dilates, it usually does not return to normal size. In both these situations, a Tc-IDA study can be diagnostic.

Q: What are the cholescintigraphic findings of complete (high-grade) common duct obstruction? Partial common duct obstruction?

A: Complete common duct obstruction usually demonstrates good hepatic uptake, but the biliary duct is not visualized. In partial common duct obstruction there is visualization of the biliary ducts and one or more of the following: delayed biliary-to-bowel transit time, segmental narrowing, prominence of the duct above the narrowing, or intraluminal filling defect.

Pearl: Delayed biliary-to-bowel transit time may be a normal variant; it is seen in 20% of healthy subjects. It is also seen in patients pretreated with CCK. In this situation, (re)administration of CCK will result in prompt clearance in healthy subjects, but not in those with partial common duct obstruction.

Q: What is the difference in clinical presentation and clinical course of patients with focal nodular hyperplasia (FNH) and hepatic adenoma?

A: FNH is asymptomatic and found incidentally, while adenomas often present with hemorrhage and are life-threatening. Adenomas are closely associated with the use of birth control pills, which must be discontinued.

Q: What are the Tc-99m SC scintigraphic findings in FNH and hepatic adenoma?

A: Hepatic adenomas do not show Tc-99m SC uptake, because they usually do not have Kupffer cells. FNH is associated with increased blood flow. Uptake may be increased, normal, or none. Two thirds of cases of FNH show some SC uptake.

Q: What are the cholescintigraphic findings in FNH and hepatoma?

A: FNH shows increased flow, normal uptake, and delayed clearance time. Hepatomas are cold on early images but often fill in on delayed images (2 hour). The hepatoma is functional, but hypofunctional compared to normal liver.

Q: Chronic acalculous cholescystitis is usually diagnosed on which of the following:

    a. ultrasonography
    b. oral cholecystography
    c. conventional cholescintigraphy
    d. CCK cholescintigraphy

A: *d.* Studies a, b, and c are often normal. A low gallbladder ejection fraction (<35%) on CCK cholescintigraphy is diagnostic.

Q: The sensitity for detecting liver hemangiomas with Tc-99m-labeled RBCs depends on which of the following factors:

    a. lesion size
    b. instrumentation used (e.g., SPECT vs. planar)
    c. location (e.g., superficial or deep, near large vessels)
    d. the phase of the moon

A: *a, b, c.*

Q: Characterize each of the following statements as true or false in regard to the diagnosis of hemangiomas:

    a. US is neither sensitive nor specific
    b. CT is not very sensitive when strict criteria are used and not specific when liberal criteria are used
    c. MRI is sensitive, has a distinctive pattern (light-bulb sign), and is much more specific than CT or US, but other benign and malignant tumors may have a similar MRI appearance as hemangioma.
    d. The positive predictive value of RBC scintigraphy is very high, with few false positive studies reported.

A: All true.

Q: What are the characteristic planar and SPECT imaging findings in liver hemangioma?

A: On planar imaging, the flow study is usually normal, the immediate blood pool images show a cold defect, and delayed images acquired 1 to 2 hours after tracer administration show increased uptake within the lesion compared to normal liver, often equal to uptake in the spleen and heart. On SPECT, increased uptake is seen in hemangiomas compared to normal liver.

Q: Besides FNH, name other causes of increased focal uptake on Tc-99m SC imaging.

A: Superior vena cava syndrome (with arm injection), inferior vena cava syndrome (with leg injection), Budd-Chiari syndrome, and cirrhosis with a regenerating nodule.

Pearl: The last two entitles do not truly show an absolutely increased uptake but a relatively increased uptake compared to the surrounding liver. In Budd-Chiari syndrome, the caudate has relatively more uptake owing to impaired venous drainage of the remainder of the liver and subsequent decreased function. The caudate lobe retains function because of its direct venous drainage into the inferior vena cava.

Q: What is functional asplenia?

A: Nonvisualization of the spleen on a Tc-99m SC study when the spleen is anatomically present and functions other than reticuloendothelial extraction are intact. Functional asplenia is due to an acquired dysfunction of the reticuloendothelial system (e.g., sickle cell anemia) or to a disruption of the blood supply (splenic artery occlusion). Functional asplenia is reversible in the case of sickle cell disease but irreversible when due to thorotrast irradiation, chemotherapy, or amyloid. Radiotracers with different mechanisms of splenic uptake will demonstrate the spleen, among them In-111 oxine-labeled WBCs, and Tc-99m-labeled RBCs.

Q: Regarding regional intra-arterial chemotherapy, which of the following statements is/are true?

    a. Hepatic arterial chemotherapy preferentially perfuses the tumor, with relative sparing of uninvolved liver.
    b. Systemic toxicity is directly related to the amount of chemotherapeutic agent that reaches the systemic circulation.
    c. The response to therapy can be predicted from Tc-99m MAA hepatic arterial perfusion scintigraphy.
    d. Symptoms of drug toxicity can be easily differentiated clinically from the progression of liver metastases.

A: *a.* True. Tumor in the liver receives its blood supply primarily from the hepatic artery, while the normal liver receives approximately 70% of its blood supply from the portal vein.

b. True. For example, arteriovenous shunting will increase the amount of chemotherapeutic agent reaching the gastrointestinal epithelium and marrow, with resulting toxicity.

c. True. Evidence of proper catheter placement and perfusion of tumor nodules is associated with a good response to therapy.

d. False. The symptoms are identical. Only the Tc-99m MAA study can make that differentiation by determining the adequacy of perfusion and the presence or absence of extrahepatic perfusion.

Q: True or false: Colon cancer metastases are known to be relatively hypovascular and therefore may not respond to intra-arterial chemotherapy.

A: False. Although in the past, metastatic colon metastases appeared to be hypovascular in celiac angiography, when selective contrast heptic artery angiography is performed, colon cancer metastastases are, in fact, hypervascular. Large tumors may only show this hypervascularity at the periphery of the tumor where there is active tumor growth (neovascularity). With intra-arterial administration of Tc-99m MAA these tumors are almost always hyperperfused.

Q: What is the significance of the extrahepatic perfusion seen on Tc-99m MAA hepatic arterial perfusion studies in patients receiving intra-arterial chemotherapy for liver metastases?

A: Extrahepatic perfusion of abdominal viscera, most commonly the stomach, but also the bowel, pancreas, and spleen, is associated with a high incidence of adverse symptoms (nausea, vomiting, abdominal pain), in the range of 45%, compared to a 16% incidence of similar symptoms in patients treated identically but without evidence of extrahepatic perfusion on the Tc-99m MAA study.

GASTROINTESTINAL SYSTEM

Q: What is achalasia, and how can radionuclide studies help in making the diagnosis and following the patient's course?

A. Achalasia is characterized by absence of peristalsis in the distal two thirds of the esophagus, increased lower esophageal sphincter (LES) pressure, and incomplete sphincter relaxation after swallowing. It is associated with symptoms of dysphagia, weight loss, nocturnal regurgitation, cough, and aspiration. The diagnosis can be confirmed by esophageal manometry. Radionuclide esophageal transit studies have a high sensitivity for making the diagnosis and, importantly, can evaluate the effectiveness of esophageal dilatation.

Q: Characterize the following statements as true or false in regard to reflux and apiration studies:

a. The milk study is a sensitive method for diagnosing reflux

b. The milk study is a sensitive method for diagnosing aspiration

c. Frequent image acquisition improves the sensitivity of the milk study.

d. The salivagram is a sensitive method for diagnosing aspiration.

A: *a.* True.

b. False. Only rarely will aspiration be seen on delayed imaging.

c. True.

d. True.

Q: Which anatomic portions of the stomach are responsible for solid emptying and which for liquid emptying?

A: Liquid emptying is largely due to the slow contractions of the proximal fundus, while the distal stomach, or antrum, is responsible for the grinding and sieving of solid food.

Q: Which of these factors will affect the rate of gastric emptying?

a. meal content

b. time of day

c. sex

d. position (standing, sitting, lying)

e. stress

f. exercise

g. all of the above.

A: *g.*

Q: Describe the difference in emptying patterns between solids and liquids.

A: Liquids empty exponentially, whereas solid emptying is biphasic, with an initial lag phase until linear emptying begins. The lag phase represents the time required for the food to be broken down into small enough pieces that it can pass through the pylorus.

Q: Which of the following statements is or are true for gastric emptying studies?

a. Attenuation results in an underestimation of gastric emptying when performed in the anterior view.

b. A solid gastric emptying time-activity curve shows a rise in activity after ingestion in the anterior view.

c. The geometric mean method of attenuation correction is considered the reference standard.

d. The LAO method of attenuation correction is superior to the geometric mean.

A: *a.* True.

b. True.

c. True.

d. False. Attenuation is a particular problem in obese patients. The rising activity curve is due to the fact that food is moving from the relatively posterior fundus to the more anterior antrum, closer to the camera. The LAO method of attenuation correction is an accurate and simple clinical method of correcting for attenuation, but incompletely corrects for attenuation in some patients for anatomic reasons.

Q: When might the use of Tc-99m SC offer advantages over Tc-99m RBCs for the diagnosis of acute GI bleeding?
A: With very rapid bleeding and vascular instability, the radiotracer can be injected and the study completed in 15 minutes. It is likely to be positive with a rapid hemorrhage when transfusions cannot keep up with the bleeding rate. The patient can then go directly to angiography; the radionuclide study will save the angiographer and patient time and contrast.

Q: List in increasing order the labeling efficiency of methods to label Tc-99m RBCs: in vivo, in vitro, and in vivtro.
A: In vivo,75%; in vivtro or modified in vivo, 85%; and in vitro, 98%. A kit method for labeling Tc-RBCs is now available and is the method of choice, particularly for GI bleeding studies.

Q: Why is the Tc-99m RBC method for detecting GI bleeding more sensitive than the Tc-99m SC method?
A: Delayed imaging can be performed for up to 24 hours with RBC labeling.

Q: What are the criteria needed to confidentally diagnose the site of bleeding on a radionuclide study?
A: (1) A radiotracer "hot spot" appears where there was none and conforms to bowel activity, (2) the activity increases over time, and (3) the activity moves antegrade or retrograde.

Pitfalls: A poor label can result in bladder activity that might be misinterpreted as rectal bleeding, or in gastric activity that might be construed as upper GI bleeding.

Pearl: Look for thyroid and salivary gland uptake when in doubt.

Pearl: A lateral view of the pelvis should be routine to confirm rectosigmoid bleeding in order to differentiate bladder, rectal, and penile activity. The latter can be a particularly embarrassing error which your colleagues will not soon forget, not to mention the error that could result in inappropriate diagnostic and therapeutic attempts.

Pitfalls: Focal activity that does not move may be anatomic (e.g., kidney, accessory spleen, hemangioma, varices, aneurysm).

Pearl: Contrast angiography can detect bleeding rates of about 1 mL/min, compared to 0.1 mL/min for the radionuclide study.

Q: Ectopic gastric mucosa is most commonly seen clinically in Meckel's diverticulum. What other gastric abnormalities may contain gastric mucosa?
A: Duplication of the GI tract, Barrett's esophaus, and a retained gastric antrum after gastrectomy. In addition, ectopic gastri mucosa may occcur in gastrogenic cystis, and has been found in the pancreas, duodenum, and colon.

Pearl: Studies have shown that the mucin cells in the stomach are responsible for gastric uptake of Tc-99m pertechnetate, not the parietal cells, as might be supposed.

Q: What is the origin of Meckel's diverticulum?
A: It is the most common congentital anomaly of the GI tract and results from failure of closure of the omphalomesenteric duct of the embryo, which connects the yolk sac to the primitive foregut via the umbilical cord.

Pearl: This true diverticulum arises on the antemesenteric side of the bowel, usually 80 to 90 cm proximal to the ileocecal valve, although it can occur elsewhere.

Pearl: Gastric mucosa is present in 10% to 30% of all Meckel's diverticula, in 60% of symptomatic patients, and in 98% of those with bleeding.

Pitfalls: A number of false positive studies have been reported over the years in scans for Meckel's diverticula, including those of urinary tract origin (e.g, horseshoe kidney, ectopic kidney), those due to inflammation (e.g, inflammatory bowel disease, neoplasms), bowel obstruction (seen most commonly with intussusception and volvulus), and other areas of ectopic gastric mucosa.

CENTRAL NERVOUS SYSTEM

Q: Which radiopharmaceuticals have been used for conventional brain scanning?
A: Tc-99m pertechnetate, Tc-99m DTPA, and Tc-99m glucoheptonate. Only the latter two are now used clinically because of their faster background clearance, lack of choroid plexus uptake, and lower radiation dose.

Q: What is the "flip flop" phenomenon seen with conventional scintigraphy, and what is its significance?
A: On the flow phase, parenchymal uptake and clearance are delayed on the abnormal side compared to the contralateral normal side. So, as the normal cortex clears, uptake in the abnormal side peaks. This may be seen with a high-grade carotid artery stenosis with or without cerebral infarction. Delayed carotid flow is seen concomitantly.

Pearl: A "hot nose" may be seen on the flow phase images and delayed images due to shunting of blood from the internal to the external carotid system that supplies the face and nose in patients with severe carotid stenosis, brain death, psychoactive drug use, and use of other drugs that cause nasal congestion.

Q: What is luxury perfusion?

A: Increased perfusion may be seen in the region of an infarct after a recent stroke (at approximately 5 days), representing an uncoupling of blood flow from metabolism and oxygen demand.

Q: How is brain death diagnosed?

A: The diagnosis is primarily clinical. The patient must be in deep coma with total absence of brain stem reflexes and spontaneous respiration. Reversible causes (drugs, hypothermia, etc.) must be excluded, the cause of the dysfunction must be diagnosed (trauma, stroke, etc.), and the clinical findings of brain death must be present for a defined period of observation (6-24 hours). Confirmatory tests such as electroencephalography and radionuclide imaging may be used to increase diagnostic certainty, but the diagnosis is clinical.

Q: Which radiopharmaceuticals are used to evaluate brain death, and what are the advantages of each?

A: Tc-99m flow agents, such as Tc-99m DTPA or Tc-99m pertechnetate, are inexpensive; all that is required is a 60-second flow study, and it can be interpreted at the bedside. Because Tc-99m HMPAO fixes in the cortex, delayed static images can be obtained and interpreted for diagnosis. The clinician is not dependent on a flow study, which demands a good bolus and good timing with proper computer acquisition. However, it is more expensive.

Q: The first radiopharmaceutical approved for cerebral perfusion imaging was I-123 iodoamphetamine. What are some of its unique characteristics?

A: In addition to distributing in the brain according to blood flow, it is also taken up in the lungs, from which it is slowly released and is the dominant source of radiotracer that "redistributes to the brain"; this is manifested by a decreasing target-to-background ratio over time, but can be used diagnostically to detect reversible cerebral ischemia on delayed imaging in patients with carotid stenosis, analogous to the way in which Tl-201 is used to evaluate cardiac ischemia.

Q: What distinguishes Tc-99m HMPAO from I-123 iodoamphetamine besides its Tc-99m label?

A: The ratio of gray to white matter is slightly less with Tc-99m HMPAO than with I-123 IMP (2.5:1 compared to 3-4:1). With uncoupling of flow and metabolism (e.g., in stroke), I-123 will show decreased uptake, while Tc-99m HMPAO may show the increased uptake of luxury perfusion. Tc-99m HMPAO is chemically unstable in vitro and must be injected promptly after preparation.

Q: Name two other cerebral perfusion agents and discuss their advantages and disadvantages.

A: Tc-99m ECD has a higher brain-to-background ratio than Tc-99m HMPAO and is stable in vitro. Xenon-133 can be used to quantify blood flow in (mL/g/min), but requires a special high-sensitivity camera, since the tracer is washed out very rapidly.

Q: How can SPECT brain perfusion or PET FDG imaging be useful in the differential diagnosis of dementia?

A: Multi-infarct dementia is characterized by multiple areas of old infarcts, recognized as areas of decreased uptake that correspond to the vascular distributions. Alzheimer's disease exhibits a characteristic pattern of bitemporal and parietal hypoperfusion and hypometabolism. Pick's disease is associated with decreased frontal lobe uptake. AIDS dementia is associated with a pattern of multifocal or patchy cortical regions of decreased uptake, seen particularly in the frontal, temporal, and parietal lobes and the basal ganglion.

Pearl: Although Alzheimer's disease has a characteristic bitemporal parietal-pattern on perfusion imaging, it is often *not* symmetric. Decreased frontal lobe uptake may also be seen. This pattern cannot be differentiated from the imaging pattern of Parkinson's disease, although they typically have very different clinical presentations.

Q: How can cerebral perfusion imaging help in patients with seizures? What is the expected PET or SPECT pattern?

A: PET F-18 FDG or SPECT cerebral perfusion studies can often localize the seizure focus in patients requiring surgery (typically temporal lobectomy) for seizure control. Interictally, a seizure focus will have decreased metabolism (FDG) on PET and decreased perfusion on SPECT; increased activity will be seen during a seizure (ictally). Normally perfusion follows metabolism. In many surgical seizure centers, depth electrodes are not required preoperatively if the clinical picture, EEG, and SPECT study are all consistent as to the location of the seizure focus.

Q: Which radiopharmaceuticals have been found useful in imaging brain tumors, and what is their clinical utility?

A: F-18 FDG PET imaging demonstrates increased uptake in tumors due to increased glycolysis. Uptake of FDG has been shown to be proportional to the malignant grade of glioblastomas. PET has been used clinically to determine tumor viability after radiation therapy. SPECT with Tl-201 and Tc-99m sestamibi can be used in a similar manner. Both Tl-201 and PET FDG can differentiate lymphoma from infection, most commonly toxoplasmosis, in AIDS patients. Uptake of Tl-201 or FDG is indicative of lymphoma.

Q: Name the radiopharmaceutical used for cisternography and the most common clinical indication for this study.

A: In-111 DTPA. The most common use of this radiopharmaceutical in modern practice is to confirm the diagnosis of normal pressure hydrocephalus (NPH), an obstructive communicating form of hydrocephalus. The next most common use is to localize CSF leaks.

Pearl: The symptoms of NPH are wet, wacky, and wobbly (incontinence, dementia, and gait disturbance).

Q: What is the characteristic pattern of NPH on radionuclide cisternography?
A: Persistent ventricular filling and evidence of a convexity block.

GENITOURINARY SYSTEM

Q: What percentage of renal plasma flow is filtered through the glomerulus and what percentage is secreted by the tubules?
A: Twenty percent of renal plasma flow is cleared by glomerular filtration and 80% by tubular secretion.
Q: Which nonradioactive drugs used to calculate glomerular filtration rate (GFR) and effective renal plasma flow (ERPF) are considered to be the reference standards?
A: Inulin for GFR and para-aminohippurate (PAH) for ERPF.
Q: Which radiopharmaceuticals are most commonly used clinically for measurement of GFR and ERPF?
A: Tc-99m DTPA for GFR and I-131 OIH for ERPF.
Q: What is the mechanism of renal uptake uptake for I-131 OIH, Tc-99m MAG3, Tc-99m DTPA, Tc-99m DMSA, and Tc-99m GH?
A: Tc-99m DTPA, glomerular filtration; Tc-99m MAG3, tubular secretion; I-131 OIH, tubular secretion and glomerular filtration; Tc-99m GH, cortical binding and gomerular filtration; and Tc-99m DMSA, cortical binding.
Q: What is the percent cortical binding of Tc-99m DMSA and Tc-99m GH?
A: Tc-99m DMSA, 40% to 50%; Tc-99m GH, 10% to 20%

Pearl: The two radiopharmaceuticals bind to the proximal convoluted tubules in the cortex.

Q: The radiation dose to normal kidneys from I-131 OIH is considerably higher than that of technetium-labeled agents. True or false?
A: False. The radiation dose of I-131 is high with renal insufficiency or obstruction but not in the setting of normal function. With worsening renal function, the radiation dose becomes increasing dependent on the physical half-life of the radiopharmaceutical and less dependent on body clearance.
Q: Why can't radionuclide angiography (flow study) be done with I-131 OIH?
A: The low allowable administered dose (300 µCi) results in insufficient count statistics for a diagnostic flow study.
Q: What is Webster's rule?
A: Pediatric radiopharmaceutical doses can be estimated using the formula (age + 1)/(age +7) × adult dose.

Q: The time-to-peak activity of a renal time-activity curve represents which of the following:
    a. The end of extraction.
    b. The beginning of renal clearance.
    c. The time point where the amount of cortical uptake of the radiopharmaceutical is equal to clearance.
A: *c.* Uptake and clearance are occurring simultanously over a period of time due to several factors, including an imperfect bolus, the first-pass extraction fraction of the radiotracer and the amount of recirculating radiotracer, and the normal variability of nephron function.
Q: What is the proper renal ROI selection on the computer for:
    a. diuresis renography
    b. captopril renography
A: *a.* For diuresis renography, the ROI should include the dilated pelvis and the cortex. Because of hydronephrosis, the dilated collecting system counts predominate.
    b. For captopril renography, a whole kidney ROI is adequate if there is no pelvic retention. Lasix is often given with the radiopharmaceutical to ensure pelvicocalyceal clearance. When there is pelvicocalyceal activity, a peripheral 2-pixel cortical ROI should be selected to avoid the effect of these counts on the time-activity curve. A drop in GFR with captopril is manifested as a deterioration in the cortical time-activity curve (delayed peak and clearance). An identical ROI should be used for the baseline comparison study.
Q: Differential renal function is evaluated by drawing kidney and background ROIs. The relative uptake of the two kidneys after background correction is determined. Which time interval is used to calculate differential renal function?
    a. entire 30-minute study
    b. 15 minutes is adequate
    c. 1 - 3-minute interval
    d. 1 - 2-minute interval
A: *c.* One is interested in cortical uptake of the renal radiopharmaceutical. Therefore, the optimal time interval is after the initial flow but before the collecting system has cleared, usually between 1 and 3 minutes. With good function, activity may be seen before 3 minutes, especially in children. Radiopharmaceuticals with higher extraction will also clear faster. It has been recommended that with Tc-99m DTPA the 1- to 3-minute interval is usually optimal, while with I-131 OIH the 1- to 2-minute interval is preferable because of its faster clearance. Ideally one should review the dynamic frames to determine when calyceal clearance occurred and use the 60- to 90-second interval prior to that.
Q: What are the two general methods for calculating absolute GFR?

A: Blood sampling methods and camera-based methods.

Q: At what step in the renin-angiotensin-aldosterone cascade does captopril work? In what organ does this occur?

A: Captopril blocks the conversion of angiotensin I to angiotensin II in the lungs.

Pearl: The usual captopril dose, 25 to 50 mg, although pharmacologically effective on the renal vasculature, is usually inadequate to produce peripheral vasodilation and hypotension. Rarely, a patient will develop hypotension requiring prompt fluid administration to maintain intravascular volume and pressure.

Q: True or false? In renal artery stenosis, the effect of captopril is manifested by a reduction in blood flow to the kidney which can be seen on radionuclide angiography.

A: False. Blood flow is not affected by captopril. If it is poor to begin with, it will remain poor. If it is normal, no change is seen. The compensatory mechanism for maintaining GFR is renin dependent and results in a drop in GFR following captopril administration.

Q: Which of these factors affects the accuracy of diuresis renography?

  a. state of hydration
  b. renal function
  c. dose of diuretic
  d. radiopharmaceutical used
  e. bladder capacity

A: *All.* Adequate hydration is required for good urine flow and adequate response to the diuretic. A full bladder may cause a functional obstruction. Intravenous hydration and urinary catheterization are strongly suggested, especially in children. Tc-99m DTPA, Tc-99m MAG3, and I-131 OIH have all been successfully used. Because of its better extraction efficiency and good image resolution, Tc-99m MAG3 is the agent of choice in renal insufficiency. I-131 OIH can also be useful in renal insufficiency; however, there is poor cortical versus collecting system differentiation due to poor image resolution. Tc-99m DTPA works well in the setting of good renal function. Renal insufficiency is a definite limitation to diuresis renography. The kidney must be able to respond to the diuretic challenge. Therefore the dose of diuretic must be increased in renal insufficiency. But the exact dose required is only an educated estimate.

Q: A good diuretic response rules out a partial obstruction. True or false?

A: False. In fact, diuretic renography is often performed to determine the functional significance of a known partial obstruction, such as in patients with cervical or bladder cancer. A poor diuretic response indicates impending deterioration in renal function if intervention is not performed. If the postdiuretic clearance is good, no immediate intervention is required.

Q: What is the most sensitive technique for diagnosing scarring secondary to reflux?

A: Tc-99m DMSA cortical imaging. US and IVU have much lower sensitivity.

Q: How can radionuclide imaging differentiate upper from lower tract urinary tract infection, and why is this differentiation important?

A: Tc-99m DMSA shows regional dysfunction as manifested by decreased uptake in patients with parenchymal infection. Upper tract infection has prognostic implications, as it may lead to subsequent renal scarring, hypertension, and renal failure.

Q: Why is radionuclide cystography preferable to the contrast method in most cases? What is the exception?

A: The radionuclide test is more sensitive for detection of reflux than contrast-enhanced voiding cystourethrography and results in much less radiation exposure (50- to 200-fold less) to the patient. The only exception is in the first evaluation of a male, where the better resolution of the contrast study can permit the diagnosis of an anatomic abnormality such as posterior urethral valves.

Q: Which is the preferred method for performing radionuclide cystography, direct or indirect?

A: Direct cystography, that is, cystography requiring urinary tract catheterization and infusion of radiotracer into the bladder, is a more sensitive method for detecting vesicoureteral reflux. It can be used to detect reflux during bladder filling as well as voiding, in contrast to the indirect method, which cannot be used to detect reflux during the bladder filling stage because radiotracer is flowing through the collecting system antegrade.

Q: What is the most common developmental abnormality leading to testicular torsion?

A: The bell-clapper testis.

Pearl: It is a congenital abnormality and usually bilateral. Prophylactic surgery is performed on the asymptomatic side.

Q: What is the difference in blood supply to the testes and scrotum?

A: The testes receive blood predominantly from the testicular artery, while the scrotum receives its supply from the pudendal vessels.

ENDOCRINE SYSTEM

Pearl: Swallowed activity from salivary secretions on radiopertechnetate scans occasionally remains in the esophagus and can be confusing. The nature of the activity is readily established by having the patient take a drink of water, followed by reimaging of the thyroid gland.

Q: What has happened to the range for normal percent thyroid uptake of radioiodine in the United States over the last 50 years?

[handwritten: % uptake]

A: The normal range has dropped significantly due to iodination of salt and the use of iodine in other foods. In many laboratories the range was 20% to 45% as recently as the mid-1960s but is now in the range of 10% to 30%.

[handwritten: at 24 hrs.]

Pearl: I-131 is preferred over Tc-99m for the detection of substernal goiter. The key factor is the ability to perform delayed imaging at 24 or even 48 hours, after vascular and background activity have cleared.

Q: What is the origin of lingual and sublingual thyroid tissue?

A: The main thyroid anlage begins as a downgrowth from the foramen cecum. Thyroid tissue may be seen anywhere along the tract of the thyroglossal duct from the foramen cecum to the usual location of the gland. However, with lingual thyroid tissue, there is usually a failure of normal development and no tissue in the normal location of the thyroid.

Q: What do perchlorate and thiocyanate have in common?

A: They are both monovalent anions that block iodine trapping competitively.

Q: What is the mechanism of action of propylthiouracil (PTU) and methimazole (Tapazole)?

A: Both propylthiouracil and methimazole are antithyroid drugs that work by preventing organification of iodine.

Q: What is meant by the "organification" of iodine?

A: In thyroid metabolism iodide is oxidized to iodine and incorporated into tyrosine to form either monoiodotyrosine or diiodotyrosine. A deficiency in peroxidase, which catalyzes the reaction, is a cause of congenital hypothyroidism.

[handwritten: cyclotron keV = 159 T½ = 13 hrs]

Pearl: The recommendation is usually made to use preparations of I-123 on the day of calibration. The reason for this is the presence of longer-lived radioiodine contaminants (I-124, I-125). The longer the interval before dosage administration, the higher is the relative contribution of the contaminants.

Q: What is the rationale underlying thyroid/parathyroid subtraction imaging?

A: For subtraction imaging to work best, uptake of both tracers in the organ to be "subtracted" should be identical. In the case of thyroid/parathyroid subtraction imaging with Tl-201 and Tc-99m pertechnetate, this is not always the case. Some thyroid abnormalities demonstrate Tl-201 accumulation but not uptake of radiopertechnetate. When this happens, a false positive study can result.

Q: What medical conditions are associated with an increased incidence of paragangliomas (pheochromocytomas)?

A: Both forms of multiple endocrine neoplasia type II are associated with pheochromocytoma, as are von Hippel-Lindau disease and neurofibromatosis.

Pitfall: Autonomous nodules are not synonymous with toxic nodules. Patients with small autonomous nodules (<3 cm in diameter) are most often euthyroid.

Index